Nursing Knowledge and Practice

Foundations for Decision Making

Third Edition

Edited by

Maggie Mallik   BSc(Hons) MPhil DipNursing(Lond) PGCertEd RGN

Research Fellow, School of Nursing, Midwifery and Physiotherapy, Faculty of Medicine and Health Sciences, The University of Nottingham, Queen's Medical Centre, Nottingham, UK

Carol Hall   BSc(Hons) PhD DipNursing(Lond) PGDipAdEd PGDip(Research Methods) RGN RSCN

Associate Professor and Child Health Lead, School of Nursing, Midwifery and Physiotherapy, Faculty of Medicine and Health Sciences, The University of Nottingham, Queen's Medical Centre, Nottingham, UK

David Howard   MEd PhD CertEd DipNursing(London) RGN RMN

Associate Professor, School of Nursing, Midwifery and Physiotherapy, Faculty of Medicine and Health Sciences, The University of Nottingham, Queen's Medical Centre; Senior Fellow, Institute of Mental Health, Nottingham, UK

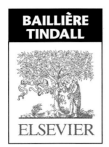

BAILLIÈRE TINDALL

ELSEVIER

EDINBURGH LONDON NEW YORK OXFORD PHILADELPHIA ST LOUIS SYDNEY TORONTO 2009

BAILLIÈRE
TINDALL
ELSEVIER

ISBN 978-0-7020-2940-0

British Library Cataloguing in Publication Data
A catalogue record for this book is available from the British Library

Library of Congress Cataloging in Publication Data
A catalog record for this book is available from the Library of Congress

Notice
Knowledge and best practice in this field are constantly changing. As new research and experience broaden our knowledge, changes in practice, treatment and drug therapy may become necessary or appropriate. Readers are advised to check the most current information provided (i) on procedures featured or (ii) by the manufacturer of each product to be administered, to verify the recommended dose or formula, the method and duration of administration, and contraindications. It is the responsibility of the practitioner, relying on their own experience and knowledge of the patient, to make diagnoses, to determine dosages and the best treatment for each individual patient, and to take all appropriate safety precautions. To the fullest extent of the law, neither the Publisher nor the Editors assume any liability for any injury and/or damage to persons or property arising out of or related to any use of the material contained in this book.

The Publisher

ELSEVIER your source for books,
journals and multimedia
in the health sciences
www.elsevierhealth.com

Working together to grow
libraries in developing countries

www.elsevier.com | www.bookaid.org | www.sabre.org

ELSEVIER   BOOK AID International   Sabre Foundation

The Publisher's policy is to use **paper manufactured from sustainable forests**

Printed in China

Contents

Contents on *Evolve* website: http://evolve.elsevier.com/Mallik/nursing/

Contributors

Janet H. Barker *BSc(Hons) PGDipAdEd PhD SRN RMN ONC*
Associate Professor, School of Nursing, Midwifery and Physiotherapy, Faculty of Medicine and Health Sciences, The University of Nottingham, Lincoln, UK

Lindsey Bellringer *RGN BSc(Hons) PGDipEd*
Skills for Practice Lead, Salisbury NHS Foundation Trust, Salisbury, UK

Brian Brown *BSc PhD*
Principal Lecturer and Reader in Health Communication, Faculty of Health and Life Sciences, De Montfort University, Leicester, UK

Roderick Cable *BSc MMedSci DipAdEd RN*
Lecturer, School of Nursing, Midwifery and Physiotherapy, Faculty of Medicine and Health Sciences, The University of Nottingham, Nottingham, UK

Anita Counsell *RGN*
Clinical Nurse Specialist Continence and Urology, Urology Out-Patients, King's Treatment Centre, Derby City General Hospital, Derby, UK

Paul Crawford *BA(Hons) PhD PGCHE DPSN RMN FRSA*
Humanities Professor of Health, School of Nursing, Midwifery and Physiotherapy, Faculty of Medicine and Health Sciences, The University of Nottingham, Nottingham; Education Centre, Derbyshire Royal Infirmary, Derby, UK

Jan Dewing *BSc PhD DipNursing DipNursEd RGN RNT MN*
Independent Consultant Nurse; Honorary Research Fellow, University of Ulster, Belfast, UK; Visiting Fellow, Northumbria University, Newcastle, UK; Professorial Fellow, University of Wollongong, NSW, Australia

Steve Eastburn *BSc(Hons) MSc NDNCert DipAdEd RGN*
Lecturer (Adult Nursing), School of Nursing, Midwifery and Physiotherapy, Faculty of Medicine and Health Sciences, The University of Nottingham, Lincoln, UK

Jeff Evans *PGCEd PGCert RN BN*
Senior Lecturer, Life Sciences, Faculty of Health, Sport and Science, University of Glamorgan, Cardiff, UK

Carol Hall *BSc(Hons) PhD DipNursing(Lond) DipAdEd PGDip(Research Methods) RGN RSCN*
Associate Professor and Child Health Lead, School of Nursing, Midwifery and Physiotherapy, Faculty of Medicine and Health Sciences, The University of Nottingham, Queen's Medical Centre, Nottingham, UK

David Howard *MEd PhD CertEd DipNursing(Lond) RMN RGN*
Associate Professor, School of Nursing, Midwifery and Physiotherapy, Faculty of Medicine and Health Sciences, The University of Nottingham, Queen's Medical Centre; Senior Fellow, Institute of Mental Health, Nottingham, UK

Karen L. Jackson *MSc PGDipAdEd RGN RSCN NDN(Cert) RNT*
Lecturer, School of Nursing, Deakin University, Geelong, VIC, Australia

Alison Kelley *BSc(Hons) DipNursing DipNursEd RGN RNT*
Lecturer, School of Nursing, Midwifery and Physiotherapy, Faculty of Medicine and Health Sciences, The University of Nottingham, Nottingham, UK

Kerry Lewis *BA MSc PGCE RGN RCNT*
Health Lecturer, School of Nursing, Midwifery and Physiotherapy, Faculty of Medicine and Health Sciences, The University of Nottingham, Nottingham, UK

Paul Linsley *BMedSci MMedSci PGDipEd ADIP CertMHS RMN RGN*
Senior Lecturer, Faculty of Health and Social Science, The University of Lincoln, Lincoln, UK

David Lomas *BSc PGCertLT PGCertErg*
Senior Lecturer in Physiotherapy, Clinical Education Co-ordination Team, Faculty of Health and Wellbeing, Sheffield Hallam University, Sheffield, UK

Maggie Mallik BSc(Hons) MPhil DipNursing(Lond) PGCertEd RGN ONC
*Research Fellow, School of Nursing, Midwifery and
Physiotherapy, Faculty of Medicine and Health Sciences,
The University of Nottingham, Queen's Medical Centre,
Nottingham, UK*

Rachel Peto BSc(Hons) RGN
*Health Lecturer, School of Nursing, Midwifery and
Physiotherapy, Faculty of Medicine and Health Sciences,
The University of Nottingham, Nottingham, UK*

Lorraine Roberts BSc(Hons) MA RGN
*Lecturer, School of Nursing, Midwifery and Physiotherapy,
Faculty of Medicine and Health Sciences, The University of
Nottingham, The Education Centre, Pilgrim Hospital,
Boston, UK*

Kevin Rowan BA(Hons) MSc
*Associate Director of Service Reliability and Safety,
Southend University Hospitals NHS Foundation Trust,
Westcliff-on-Sea, UK*

Brenda Rush BA MSc PhD CertEd RCNT RN
*Associate Professor, School of Nursing, Midwifery and
Physiotherapy, Faculty of Medicine and Health Sciences,
The University of Nottingham, County Hospital, Lincoln, UK*

Jane Seymour BA(Hons) MA PhD RGN
*Sue Ryder Care Professor of Palliative and End of Life Studies,
School of Nursing, Midwifery and Physiotherapy, Faculty of
Medicine and Health Sciences, The University of Nottingham,
Queen's Medical Centre, Nottingham, UK*

Jane Smallwood BSc(Hons) MSc RGN
*Senior Lecturer (Nursing), Faculty of Health and Well-Being,
Sheffield Hallam University, Sheffield, UK*

Helen Swain BSc(Hons) MSc DipEd RGN RSCN RNT
*Lecturer, School of Nursing, Midwifery and Physiotherapy,
Faculty of Medicine and Health Sciences, The University
of Nottingham, Nottingham, UK*

Editors' introduction

Nursing and the role of the nurse continue to evolve and change in response to people's health needs, their care expectations and the increasing complexity of information and choice available to meet those needs. The explosion in information available via the internet means that all health professionals are stimulated and challenged by well informed and questioning individuals. Alongside these changes, the organization and financing of healthcare delivery systems remain subject to political will, with change a constant experience for all healthcare workers.

For the student nurse entering a programme of study for the first time, the amount of knowledge needed, both in classroom and in practice learning, to achieve competence and proficiency for registration may seem daunting. Acceptance by the student that learning is lifelong and that foundation knowledge is just the beginning is essential to cope with the ever changing healthcare landscape. Earlier editions of this textbook emphasized the need for the integration of the knowledge base from subject areas within the nursing curriculum through a focus on the needs of service users. We continue to emphasize the integration of knowledge from theory and practice as essential to the total learning experience and for decision making that is applicable to all branches of nursing.

In the third edition of this foundation textbook we have responded to our reviewers' comments and have kept the core design, layout and organization of chapter content the same as for the previous two editions. We have retained popular features, such as the annotated readings and websites, and have added electronic ancillaries on the Evolve website as a new feature. These may be accessed via Elsevier's website

(http://evolve.elsevier.com/Mallik/nursing/) and provide supplementary information, additional suggestions for experiential learning, decision-making exercises and further annotated websites (see 'How to use this book'). All chapters have been updated with acknowledgment of the increasing shift towards interprofessional learning and consumer input to care.

The following changes have also been made in the third edition

- A new introductory chapter, 'Nursing knowledge and practice', explores the role and context of nursing, nationally and internationally, providing foundation information on core knowledge areas common to all nursing curricula.
- The 'Handling and moving' and 'Mobility' chapters have been amalgamated under a new title, 'Mobility and moving'.
- The chapter on 'Death and dying' has been completely rewritten and given the new title of 'End of life care' by its new author.
- Chapters have been reviewed by recognized experts in their respective fields (see Acknowledgements).

Maggie Mallik
Carol Hall
David Howard
Nottingham 2008

Acknowledgements

We wish to acknowledge our anonymous reviewers: we value their critical commentary on the second edition of this book as well as their suggestions for improvements to be made in this third edtion.

We thank all the contributors to our first and second editions who were willing to update and refocus their original chapters and to add new material where appropriate. We welcome and acknowledge our new contributors, who have had to shape their knowledge and expertise to suit the structured framework of this book or have had to reshape and update the material of a previous contributor.

We are grateful to all our expert external reviewers (see list below) for giving their time to read and comment on the content of selected chapters. Where appropriate, we have encouraged our authors to make changes suggested; however, responsibility for the content of all chapters belongs to the individual authors and editors of this third edition.

Acknowledgement goes to Ninette Premdas, Sheila Black, Gail Wright and the rest of the team at Elsevier for their advice and support during the whole process of completing this third edition.

This third edition could not have been completed without the love and continual support of our families: our partners Penny Howard, Rich Hall and Alan Mallik, and our children, Simon and Peter Howard, James and Rachel Hall and Catherine Mallik.

External reviewers

Nick Allcock (Chapter 11)
Associate Professor of Nursing, School of Nursing, Midwifery and Physiotherapy, Faculty of Medicine and Health Sciences, The University of Nottingham, Nottingham, UK

Peter Bentley (Chapter 7)
Senior Lecturer Applied Biological Sciences, City University, London, UK

Sally Candlin (Chapter 2)
Honorary Senior Research Fellow, Macquarie University, Sydney; Adjunct Associate Professor of Nursing, University of Sydney, Sydney, NSW, Australia

Mark Collier (Chapter 15)
Lead Nurse Consultant – Tissue Viability, United Lincolnshire Hospitals NHS Trust, Boston, UK

Alison Coutts (Chapter 8)
Lecturer, Applied Biological Sciences, City University, London, UK

David T. Evans (Chapter 16)
Educational Consultant in Sexual Health and doctoral student in Education (EdD), Freelance and University of Greenwich, London, UK

Kathryn Getliffe (Chapter 18)
Formerly Professor of Nursing and Associate Dean, Faculty Graduate School, University of Southampton, Southampton, UK

John Hurley (Chapter 12)
Lecturer, School of Nursing, University of Dundee, Dundee, UK

B. Meriel Hutton (Chapter 10)
Independent Consultant, Birmingham, UK

Rebecca Jester (Chapter 19)
Head of School (Nursing and Midwifery), Faculty of Health, Keele University, Stoke on Trent, UK

Howard Kahn (Chapter 9)
Senior Lecturer, Department of Management, Heriot-Watt University, Edinburgh, UK

Julia Love
Registered Member NBE, Moving and Handling Coordinator, LPS Training & Consultancy Ltd, Leeds, UK

Maggie Nicol (Chapter 14)
Professor of Clinical Skills, City University, London, UK

Natalie Vaughan (Chapter 5)
Senior Nurse Infection Control, Nottingham Universities Hospital NHS Trust, Queen's Medical Centre, Nottingham, UK

How to use this book

Each chapter is structured into the following four sections:

1. **Subject knowledge**, which incorporates two subdivisions:
   – Biological knowledge
   – Psychosocial knowledge
2. **Care delivery knowledge**
3. **Professional and ethical knowledge**
4. **Personal and reflective knowledge.**

In addition, each chapter is designed to contain a number of features that will guide you around the topic as well as encourage you to reflect on your learning and your experiences in practice.

At the start of each chapter

- A **Key issues** list provides a succinct menu of topics covered within the chapter for quick and easy reference.
- The **Introduction** and **Overview** provide a guide to the chapter, indicating how and why this topic is an important component of nursing practice.

Within the chapter

Each chapter contains a number of different types of information and activity that are highlighted within the text. They are designed to help you reflect on your own knowledge, consider the basis of nursing decisions and demonstrate the evidence base for practice.

Reflection and portfolio evidence

Reflection is a very important process to develop in order to aid your learning. You can learn from your practice experience and also from your reactions to the knowledge presented in texts and the classroom. The main focus of the reflective exercises in this text is on yourself and your reactions and how these interact with the particular situation observed or reflected upon. There are many models that can be used to guide and structure your reflections. You will be advised and supported in the use of any one of these models by your teacher or education facilitator. Many of the exercises will focus on dilemmas where there is no right or wrong answer but one that is negotiated to suit the specific situation. You may find these exercises particularly useful as a basis for discussion and debate in a group. Writing up your reflections in a 'reflective diary' or 'learning journal' helps to fix the knowledge gained and allows you to review your learning experiences over time.

These exercises also offer helpful suggestions and hints as to what can be included in your Portfolio of Evidence of Learning.

Decision-making exercises

Decision-making exercises are generally related to material presented in the chapter; however, they may require you to complete further work that will take you outside the scope of the text. Founded on the philosophy of problem-based learning where you are given a short scenario, critical incident or case study from practice (broadly defined), you are asked to review information already obtained from whatever source, collect further information and then make decisions as to what actions you would take, supporting this with the rationale for your actions.

Guidance may be given, as well as helpful references, but some exercises will be open-ended, as textbooks and articles go out of date quickly. It is important to do a literature search for up-to-date and local material that may be relevant to the topic being explored.

There is an assumption that you are able to use the appropriate internet and library facilities to find the relevant material. These are skills you should develop and maintain throughout your professional career.

Finally, discussion with your peers, teachers and practitioners will help you to focus your learning within the exercises.

Evidence-based practice

Brief summaries of a research study or several studies are presented in order to provide support for evidence-based practice. Although this is not explicitly stated in the book, you are encouraged to obtain a copy of the full report, read and critically appraise the study. Where you can, you should also link these studies with your practice experiences. Research evidence, where at all possible, is from studies completed from the early to mid 2000s onwards; however, you must remember that these research briefings can quickly become out of date, so they should serve as the starting point for further investigation.

Evolve ancillaries

Scattered through the chapters, you will find references to Evolve ancillaries which are PowerPoint® presentations. They can be accessed on the Evolve website (http://evolve.elsevier.com/Mallik/nursing/) managed by Elsevier, the publishers of this textbook. These ancillaries provide you with more information on a topic which could not be covered in the same depth within the chapter. They are also used to provide additional reference sources, annotated websites for information and exercises that you can complete to test your knowledge level.

Case studies

In the **Personal and reflective knowledge** section of each chapter you will find four case studies. These are designed to show how core nursing knowledge is relevant across all the four branches of nursing. Each case study provides an opportunity for you to consider nursing decisions and to appreciate how knowledge from different sources is integrated in nursing practice. They may also act as a stimulus for you to explore in greater depth issues related to your chosen branch of nursing. You may wish to read them before reading the chapter.

At the end of each chapter

A **Summary** section at the end of each chapter provides a reminder of the key content of the chapter and can be used to evaluate the learning gained through reading the chapter.

An **Annotated further reading and websites** section provides guidance on sources of relevant information if you wish to pursue particular interests further. Each suggested item has a brief commentary explaining why it has been recommended. These resources are in addition to the extensive list of **References**.

Abbreviations

ABPM	ambulatory blood pressure measurement	CHD	coronary heart disease
ACLS	advanced cardiac life support	CHI	Commission for Health Improvement
ACP	advance care planning	CINAHL®	Cumulative Index to Nursing and Allied Health Literature
ADH	antidiuretic hormone		
ADL	activities of daily living	CJ	cranberry juice
ADP	adenosine diphosphate	CJD	Creutzfeldt–Jakob disease
AED	advisory external defibrillator	CLDT	community learning disabilities nurse
AIDS	acquired immune deficiency syndrome	CNA	certified nursing assistant
ALS	advanced life support	CNST	Clinical Negligence Scheme for Trusts
AMPS	assessment of motor and process skills	CoA	coenzyme A
ATP	adenosine triphosphate	COHSE	Confederation of Health Service Employees
BAN	British Approved Name	COPD	chronic obstructive pulmonary disease
BCA	back care adviser	COSHH	Control of Substances Hazardous to Health
bd (b.d.)	twice a day, usually morning and evening	COT	College of Occupational Therapists
BLS	basic life support	CPN	community psychiatric nurse
BMI	body mass index	CPPIH	Commission for Patient and Public Involvement in Health
BMR	basal metabolic rate		
BNF	British National Formulary	CPR	cardiopulmonary resuscitation
BNF	British Nutrition Foundation	CPS	Crown Prosecution Service
BOE	brief, ordinary and effective	CSF	cerebrospinal fluid
BSA	body surface area	CSP	Chartered Society of Physiotherapists
BSE	bovine spongiform encephalitis	CST	cognitive stimulation therapy
CA	care assistant	DAFNE	dose adjustment for normal eating
CAF	Common Assessment Framework	DDA	Disability Discrimination Act
CAPE	Clifton assessment procedures for the elderly	DES	Department of Education and Science
CAPT	Child Accident Prevention Trust	DIPC	director of infection prevention and control
CASU	Controls Assurance Support Unit	DLF	Disabled Living Foundation
CBT	cognitive behavioural therapy	DH	Department of Health
CCTV	closed circuit television	DNAR	do not attempt resuscitation
CDSC	Communicable Diseases Surveillance Centre	dpm	drops per minute
CFSMS	Counter Fraud and Security Management Service	DRC	Disability Rights Commission
		DRE	digital rectal examination

EBL	enquiry based learning	LIDS	Liverpool infant distress score
EFL	enquiry focused learning	LINks	Local Involvement Networks
ECG	electrocardiograph	LOLER	Lifting Operations and Lifting Equipment Regulations
ECM	Every Child Matters		
EEG	electroencephalograph	LPA	lasting power of attorney
EFN	European Federation of Nurses	LREC	Local Ethics Research Committee
EHR	Electronic Health Records	MAG	Malnutrition Advisory Group
ENSA	European Nursing Students Association	MDMA	3,4-methylene-dioxymethamphetamine (ecstasy)
EoLC	end of life care		
EPR	Electronic Patient Records	MDRTB	multidrug resistant tuberculosis
EPUAP	European Pressure Ulcer Advisory Panel	MET	medical emergency team
ERC	European Resuscitation Council	MHOR	Manual Handling Operations Regulations
EU	European Union	MHRA	Medicines and Healthcare products Regulatory Agency
EWS	early warning system		
FBAO	foreign body airway obstruction	MMR	measles mumps rubella
FLACC	face, legs, activity, cry, consolability	MPET	multiprofessional education and training
FSA	Food Standards Agency	MQS	Medication Quantification Scale
GP	general practitioner	MRSA	meticillin-resistant *Staphylococcus aureus*
HAI	hospital acquired infection	MS	multiple sclerosis
HCAI	healthcare associated infections	NAO	National Audit Office
HDL	high density lipoprotein	NBE	National Back Exchange
HEI	higher education institution	NCEPOD	National Confidential Enquiry into Patient Outcome and Death
HIS	Hospital Infection Society		
HIV	human immunodeficiency virus	NCHSPCS	National Council for Hospice and Specialist Palliative Care Services
HSAC	Health Services Advisory Committee		
HSE	Health and Safety Executive	NDE	near death experience
IASP	International Association for the Study of Pain	NG	nasogastric
ICAS	Independent Complaints Advocacy Service	NHS	National Health Service
ICLP	infection control link practitioner	NHSLA	National Health Service Litigation Authority
ICN	International Council of Nurses	NICE	National Institute for Health and Clinical Excellence
ICNP	International Classification for Nursing Practice		
ICP	integrated care pathway	NIMHE	National Institute for Mental Health in England
ICP	intracranial pressure		
ICU	Intensive Care Unit	NIP	nurse independent prescriber
IDDM	insulin dependent diabetes mellitus	NMC	Nursing and Midwifery Council
IHD	ischaemic heart disease	NMSC	non-melanotic skin cancer
ILCOR	International Liaison Committee on Resuscitation	nocte	at night
		NPSA	National Patient Safety Agency
IV	intravenous	NRL	natural rubber latex
JANET	joint assessment nursing education tool	NRLS	National Reporting and Learning System
LGBT	lesbian, gay, bisexual and transgender	NSF	National Service Framework
		OAG	oral assessment guide
LDL	low density lipoprotein	OCD	obsessive compulsive disorder

OPSI	Office of Public Sector Information		**RP**	received pronunciation
PALS	paediatric advanced life support		**RPST**	Risk Pooling Scheme for Trusts
PALS	Patient Advice and Liaison Services		**SARS**	severe acute respiratory syndrome
PBL	problem based learning		**SBS**	sick building syndrome
PCA	patient controlled analgesia		**SHA**	Strategic Health Authority
PCT	Primary Care Trust		**SIDS**	sudden infant death syndrome
PEA	pulseless electrical activity		**SLE**	systemic lupus erythematosus
PEWS	paediatric early warning system		**SOLER**	sit squarely – open posture – lean forwards – eye contact – relax
PFMT	pelvic floor muscle training			
PHLS	Public Health Laboratory Service		**SRRS**	Social Readjustment Rating Scale
PMP	pain monitoring programme		**STI**	sexually transmitted infection
PN	parenteral nutrition		**SWOT**	strengths, weaknesses, opportunities, threats
POVA	protection of vulnerable adults		**tds (t.d.s.)**	three times a day
PPE	personal protective equipment		**TENS**	transcutaneous electric nerve stimulation
PPI	patient and public involvement		**THROAT**	the holistic and reliable oral assessment tool
PRN	*pro re nata* – when necessary		**TILER**	task – individual – load – environment – resources
PTSD	post-traumatic stress disorder			
PVS	persistent vegetative state		**TNP**	topical negative pressure
qds (q.d.s.)	four times a day		**UKCC**	United Kingdom Central Council for Nurses, Midwives and Health Visitors
RCN	Royal College of Nursing			
RDA	recommended daily allowance		**UTI**	urinary tract infection
REM	rapid eye movement		**VAC**	vacuum assisted closure
RIDDOR	Reporting of Injuries, Diseases and Dangerous Occurrences Regulations		**vCJD**	variant Creutzfeldt–Jakob Disease
			VF	ventricular fibrillation
RN	registered nurse		**VMC**	vasomotor centre
RoSPA	Royal Society for the Prevention of Accidents		**WHO**	World Health Organization

Chapter 1

Nursing knowledge and practice

Maggie Mallik, Carol Hall and David Howard

INTRODUCTION

Nursing care is provided for people with widely diverse health and sick care needs in multiple contexts worldwide. The knowledge and competence to meet such a wide variety of care needs may be daunting for the student starting a programme of study to become a registered nurse. Nursing programmes are designed to allow knowledge and practice experience to be accumulated and assimilated by the nursing student within the 3 or 4 year course period. However, learning is lifelong, and the journey of learning through a pre-registration nursing programme is only the beginning.

In the United Kingdom (UK), the knowledge and skills necessary to become registered as a nurse are primarily structured so that a student can focus on developing proficiencies to provide care for particular patient/client groups (Nursing and Midwifery Council 2004). Two of the groupings are age related, i.e. you register to deliver nursing care specifically to adults or specifically to children, usually with physical healthcare needs. The other two groupings are health condition related, i.e. nursing care is focused on people (children and adults) with mental health problems or people with learning disabilities. These 'branches' of nursing have their basis in the history of the development of nursing in the UK (Dingwall et al 1988, Nolan 1998). Following a 1-year common generic programme, students begin to accumulate knowledge and experience specific to their chosen branch of nursing.

Curricula for nursing courses worldwide are broad ranging and usually include an eclectic mix of the following areas:

- Knowledge about the individual person, i.e. physical, psychological, social, cultural and spiritual in health and in sickness
- Knowledge about the environment of care to include safety, policy and politics in the delivery of health care
- Knowledge on how to provide evidence-based nursing care to promote health and care for the sick

- Knowledge of the nursing profession to include its evolution, theoretical underpinnings, ethical and legal position, and its unique role as a profession in healthcare delivery.
- Knowledge of self as a person, as a learner, and as a future professional nurse.

Nursing, along with all the other professions involved in the delivery of health care, is a practice based profession. This means that completion of a university academic course leading to a degree or diploma is not sufficient for professional registration. All students must also learn to nurse patients/clients in the real world of health care. A substantial part of any nursing course is spent learning to nurse in a wide variety of healthcare contexts (in the UK this is currently 50% of the course programme; Nursing and Midwifery Council 2004). Knowledge gained in practice is unique for every student, as practice placement learning depends on the individual healthcare encounters experienced by each student. Making learning explicit is dependent on the interpretation of experience and events made by the learner alone and/or with their practice mentor/supervisor. Knowledge gained in this way is very personal and often depends on the reflective skills of the student and the reflective and learning facilitation skills of the practice mentor/supervisor.

In this first chapter we are presenting an overview of the generic underpinning knowledge that supports the role of the registered nurse in any branch of nursing or context of care. All other chapters of the book focus on knowledge for decision making in providing care to meet specific patient/client needs. The organization of the content of each chapter follows the same pattern as this first chapter.

OVERVIEW

Subject knowledge

This section outlines definitions of nursing and their implications for the development of the nursing profession in the UK and worldwide. An overview of theories and models of nursing, first developed in the United States of America (USA), is presented along with a brief summary of one particular model widely applied in UK nursing. There is an overview of how the image and role of the nurse is perceived by society. Knowledge of people's needs in health and illness and the policy and politics around the delivery of health care in the UK is outlined. There is an introduction to the globalization of healthcare delivery and the impact of the international movement of the nursing workforce.

Care delivery knowledge

This section focuses on the need for evidence-based health care. It outlines the processes needed to access quality evidence on which to base clinical decisions in the delivery of care. Methods of organizing nursing and other healthcare professions to deliver patient/client centred care is presented with an emphasis on the need for interprofessional learning and working. An overview of the scope of practice available in each of the four branches of nursing is presented.

Professional and ethical knowledge

Accountability and autonomy are central to any profession. This section explores the professional, legal and ethical underpinnings of nursing with an overview of virtue ethics and the impact of the Human Rights Act.

Personal and reflective knowledge

Learning to be a nurse provides an introduction to how a nursing course might be delivered, with an overview of problem based learning and an account of reflective learning. There is an introduction to keeping a Portfolio of learning. One family case study with questions will help you check and consolidate your learning from the chapter.

SUBJECT KNOWLEDGE

DEFINITIONS, THEORIES AND MODELS

The verb 'to nurse' is used in everyday language as meaning 'to care for', 'look after', 'tend', 'foster', 'nurture'; and it can be applied in many different everyday situations. Here we are looking at the definitions applied to professional nursing, that is where a person completes a recognized course of study and is assessed as competent and fit to be registered to practise. Registration is usually regulated by a national Nursing Board and is specific to individual countries of the world. Transferability of registration from one country to another is at the discretion of the host country (see Contexts of Care, below).

According to the Royal College of Nursing (RCN; 2003: 1), most countries have a legal definition of the title 'nurse' and some also have a legal definition of 'nursing'. The legal definition in the UK is policy orientated and focused around distinguishing between what care should be delivered by registered nurses as opposed to unregistered carers (Office of Public Information 2001). A professional definition is necessary to provide a framework for outlining the scope of practice of the registered nurse and to guide codes of ethics and professional conduct (Royal College of Nursing 2003).

Professional definitions are available and have changed over time. In the 20th century, the definitions most often quoted in the literature were those written by Florence Nightingale (1859) and Virginia Henderson (1960). Both focus on the activities of the nursing role:

Nature alone cures ... And what nursing has to do ... is to put the patient in the best condition for nature to act upon him. (*Nightingale 1859*)

to assist the individual, sick or well, in the performance of those activities contributing to health or its recovery (or to a peaceful death) that he would perform unaided if he had the necessary strength, will, or knowledge. (*Henderson 1960*)

The World Health Organization (WHO; 2002) and the International Council of Nurses (ICN; 1987, 2002) have provided more recent definitions. The ICN definition below attempts to include the broad scope of nursing roles within this abridged version of their 1987 definition of nursing:

Nursing encompasses autonomous and collaborative care of individuals of all ages, families, groups and communities, sick or well, and in all settings. Nursing includes the promotion of health, prevention of illness, and the care of ill, disabled and dying people. Advocacy, promotion of a safe environment, research, participation in shaping health policy and in patient and health systems management, and education are also key nursing roles. (*International Council of Nurses 2002*)

In the UK, the Royal College of Nursing's (2003: 3) document *Defining Nursing* provides a more comprehensive examination of the nursing role in the 21st century. Alongside a short definition statement it describes nursing as:

the use of clinical judgement in the provision of care to enable people to improve, maintain or recover health, to cope with health problems, and to achieve the best possible quality of life, whatever their disease or disability until death ...

It further outlines the defining characteristics of nursing as including:

1. a particular purpose for nursing
2. a particular mode for nursing interventions
3. a particular domain
4. a particular focus
5. a particular value base
6. a commitment to partnership.

These six defining characteristics of nursing provide a succinct overview of the broad scope of the nursing role in the 21st century.

Reflection and portfolio evidence

- Reflect on your perceptions of the role of the nurse prior to commencing your course. Who and what influenced your perceptions?
- Ask your friends who are not nurses what they think about the nursing profession.
- Refer to some of the definitions quoted and debate which definition helps you to define your understanding and experience of the role of a registered nurse.
- Debate your thoughts and ideas with your peer group.

Throughout the 20th century, particularly in the USA, nursing theories and models were developed (Fawcett 2004, McKenna et al 2008). Learning about these theories has been part of nursing curricula, despite the relative lack of application of many of them in the practice setting (Wimpenny 2002; see Table 1.1 for list of the main theories and their focus). The most popular nursing model, and one which did become embedded in practice settings in the UK, is that of Roper, Logan and Tierney (1980, 2000; Holland et al 2003). This model focuses on the delivery of nursing care through viewing people as having 12 activities of daily living, with care being targeted on promoting and enabling independence in these activities. In spite of its popularity, an increasing focus on collaborative multiprofessional working, with concurrent concerns about cost and quality, means that individual professional models are now being replaced by a 'care pathways' approach (http://www.evidence-based-medicine.co.uk/ebmfiles/WhatisanICP.pdf; see Care Delivery Knowledge).

ROLE AND IMAGE OF THE NURSE

Although pre-registration nursing degrees have been available in a small selection of universities in the UK since the early 1960s, nursing has only relatively recently (1989) been accepted as a profession where all members should be educated within universities or higher education institutions (HEIs; United Kingdom Central Council for Nurses Midwives and Health Visitors 1986). Reasons for continuing to keep the apprenticeship work-based learning training model until the 1990s could be ascribed to the perceived public image of the nurse. According to Fealy & McNamara (2007) there is a particular and enduring set

Table 1.1 Selection of nursing theories/models

Focus of model/s	Name/year/place	Key idea	Practical application
Environment of care	Nightingale (1859) UK	Manipulation of external environment to heal the sick, e.g. ventilation, light, warmth, diet, cleanliness	Infection control in 19th century and applicable today with hospital acquired infections and safe environment issues Public health nursing
Dealing with patients' problems/needs	Henderson (1966) USA Roper Logan and Tierney (1980) UK	Patient has 14 basic needs Patient has 12 activities of living	Roper model widely used in nursing the physically ill in UK
Promoting independence/ self-care	Orem (1971) USA	Patient able to self-care and/or has self-care deficits	Nurse-led clinics and rehabilitation and elderly care in USA and in UK Used in children's nursing
Nursing as caring	Leininger (1978) USA Watson (1979) USA Benner (1984) USA	Caring is the core of nursing; is transcultural; is holistic; has 10 caring factors Expertise in caring developed through stages	Dealing with patients with diverse cultural needs; applied in critical care areas in adult and child to promote holistic care Assess clinical knowledge development in nurses in many practice settings (Benner)
Nursing as an interpersonal activity	Peplau (1952) USA	Nursing relationship with patients is therapeutic and nursing actions arise from this relationship	Main application in mental health nursing, psychotherapy
Patients as systems adapting to environment	Roy (1976) USA	Nurses help patients to adapt to illness and/or environment in physical, psychological and social ways	Led to development of 'nursing diagnosis'. Model adopted across an eclectic mix of adult nursing environments. Also used for child health care

of images of the nurse which provide a public argument against the notion of an 'educated' nurse. There is a view that mental work and manual work are opposites and that nursing should be a practical and commonsense occupation unworthy of academic study. Despite such views, the nursing profession is slowly becoming more visible within academia and more influential in the practice setting, with an acknowledgement that all nurses should be educated to degree level (European Federation of Nurses 2005; see also Contexts of Care).

Kalisch's recent work (Kalisch et al 2007) is significant in that it does show an improving image from those portrayed in the media during the 20th century (Kalisch & Kalisch 1986). It allows the profession to move on and continue to establish, maintain and consolidate its position as equal to other healthcare professions within the university setting and in the healthcare delivery arena. The scope of practice for professional nurses is expanding and role specialization and role autonomy are increasingly recognized.

Evidence-based practice

Kalisch et al (2007) reported on the results of a study of the image of nursing on the Internet utilizing content analysis methodology. A total of 144 websites were content-analysed in 2001 and 152 in 2004. Approximately 70% of the sites showed nurses as intelligent and educated and 60% as respected, accountable, committed, competent and trustworthy. Nurses were also shown as having specialized knowledge and skills in 70% (2001) and 62% (2004) of the websites. Doctoral-prepared nurses were evident in 19% of the websites in 2001 and this number doubled in 2004.

Reflection and portfolio evidence

Obtain a copy of a UK nursing journal which also includes job advertisements (e.g. *Nursing Times, Nursing Standard, Royal College of Nursing Bulletin*).

- Map the range and scope of nursing roles contained within the job adverts.
- Review the diversity of job titles and the image they portray.
- How many of the job roles advertised portray the nurse as the key clinical decision maker?
- Reflect on the range of choices available to you in future when you become a registered nurse in any of the branches of nursing.

PEOPLE AS RECIPIENTS OF NURSING CARE

All definitions, theories and models of nursing, whatever their origin, incorporate views of the patient/client as a recipient of care. The RCN (2003: 3) describes the nursing domain as focused on:

people's unique responses to and experience of health, illness, frailty, disability and health-related life events in whatever environment or circumstances they find themselves. People's responses may be physiological, psychological, social, cultural or spiritual, and are often a combination of all of these. The term 'people' includes individuals of all ages, families and communities, throughout the entire life span.

Throughout this textbook, the Subject Knowledge section of each chapter focuses on the knowledge underlying people's responses to health and illness by including information on physiological, psychosocial, cultural and spiritual needs and changes in health and illness. Your nursing programme will include an exploration of all these subject areas in some form within the curriculum.

Knowledge of the biological basis of practice is relevant in all branches of nursing, though application of that knowledge in practice will vary greatly depending on the care needs of people being nursed. Historically, when nursing was primarily described as taking place in an institution and focused on 'doing what the doctor ordered' to cure the patient, knowledge of the physical body in health and disease took priority (Rafferty 1996). With the development of nursing as a unique professional role offered in multiple contexts, the shift has been to re-focus on the knowledge needed for caring as opposed to curing. Although knowledge from the biosciences is still essential for safe nursing practice (Clancy et al 2000, Friedel & Treagust 2005), knowledge of the person's psychological, social, spiritual and cultural needs now tends to dominate the knowledge base of nursing.

It is important to note that knowledge disciplines studied in nursing are not unique to nursing. Other health and social care professions share the same knowledge base but will apply it in unique ways to suit their individual roles (Royal College of Nursing 2003). With the increasing complexity of people's health and social care problems, there is a growing need for all professions to collaborate more effectively in delivering patient/client centred care (Department of Health 2005). Professional teams are becoming more central to health care as evidence emerges that effective teamwork enhances the quality of patient care and healthcare consumers demand that healthcare professionals engage in effective partnerships (Illingworth & Chelvanayagam 2007).

Since 2000, the UK government has been encouraging universities to provide opportunities for students of health and social care courses to learn together (Department of Health 2000). Interprofessional learning is described by Barr (2005) as occurring when members (students) of two or more professions associated with health and/or social care engage in learning from and about each other (http://www.caipe.org.uk/). When completing your course, you may find that your university programme includes modules incorporating interprofessional learning in theory and practice throughout your course. You may also be participating in problem based learning activities that allow you to learn and work with students from other health and social care professions in providing collaborative solutions to patient case studies.

Shared partnership with people as clients and patients is being increasingly emphasized in a consumer led society (see Ch. 19). This requires genuine listening and respect for the contribution people make to their own health and/or recovery (Nursing and Midwifery Council 2008). People may have more choice in when and whom they access for health care and their expectations of the standard of care delivered is high. Patient led organizations and groups provide support at all levels and for a very large range of conditions (Binley's Handbook of Patient Groups 2008).

Reflection and portfolio evidence

Reflect on the range of patients/clients you cared for on your recent placements.

- What subject knowledge gained from your course was the most helpful to you in learning to provide nursing care?
- How did you cope with any deficits in your knowledge?
- List the other health or social care professionals also involved in providing care.
- Describe your perceptions of what knowledge these professionals have that is the same as your knowledge base and what might be different.
- Discuss your thoughts and findings with your peers and debate the advantages and disadvantages of participating in interprofessional learning.

CONTEXTS OF CARE

Throughout the 'first world', health care is predominantly purchased by people through contributions to insurance systems that will pay fully or proportionately for medical and hospital care when it is needed. In the developing world, health care is often delivered through voluntary organizations supported by worldwide charities. In the UK, the dominant system is through a state supported national health service. The following sections provide insights into the history and politics of the UK National

Health Service (NHS) before introducing the influence of globalization on the workforce and its impact on nursing worldwide.

The National Health Service

In the UK, the majority of nurses are trained by and, at some stage of their career, will work for the National Health Service (NHS). Established in 1948, the success of the NHS is measured by the successful treatment of illnesses and is influenced heavily by the medical model of working. In the beginning of the service, day-to-day NHS care was provided by general practitioners in the community, with more serious illnesses being referred to, and treated by, medical specialists in hospitals, either through the out-patient service or as an in-patient.

Funding for the NHS comes from general taxation and initially all services were non-means tested and free at the point of delivery, although as the service developed some charges were introduced, for example for prescriptions and for dental and optical care. It was at first expected that the cost of the NHS would fall as the medical profession treated the illnesses in the population. This did not happen, however. At its launch, NHS funding took 3.75% of the country's gross domestic product (GDP) but by 2000 this had risen to around 7% (Appleby 2005). Consequently, the cost and funding of the NHS has been questioned almost continuously since its inception.

The problem with the medical approach is that it is very effective at treating illnesses from which people can recover. Unfortunately, another group of people exist who suffer from long-term or chronic illnesses, and here the medical approach is less successful. The nature of these illnesses means that the sufferers will not recover from them fully and will continue to seek support from the NHS to manage their symptoms. Examples of long-term conditions include hypertension, arthritis, diabetes and obstructive pulmonary disease, some learning disabilities and long-term mental health problems as well as disabilities arising from other major conditions such as strokes. Long-term conditions tend to be more prevalent in older people and the UK has an ageing population, meaning that even greater demand is likely to be made on the NHS in the future. In this demographic context, to continue with the hospital centred NHS structure would be prohibitive on economic grounds so, following the implementation of the National Health Service and Community Care Act 1990, the provision of NHS care began to be transferred away from the hospitals and into the community. This enabled the use of informal (unpaid) carers at home, and in turn reduced the demand on expensive NHS staff and resources, and of course reduced the financial demand on the taxpayer. The role of the NHS consequently changed from being a provider of care to one that enables individuals, with their families, to care for themselves (for more information on this see Ch. 9, 'Stress, relaxation and rest').

The implications for hospital services in this latter period of the NHS's history were profound. The National Health Service and Community Care Act 1990 also introduced the marketplace philosophy into health and social care. Rather than being the natural provider of services for a community, hospital services now had to tender and compete for contracts for services which were negotiated with purchasers – community based general practitioners (GPs). The Health Act 1999 formalized this process, setting the foundations for the NHS to become a primary care led service. It also introduced National Service Frameworks (NSFs; see http://www.dh.gov.uk/en/Healthcare/NationalService Frameworks/index.htm for a complete list), which identify standards for the delivery of services and become targets that have to be achieved by the local health services. These are monitored and supervised by the Healthcare Commission and the Strategic Health Authorities (SHAs) which were introduced in *Shifting the Balance of Power Within the NHS* (Department of Health 2001). This change of emphasis on care commissioning and delivery – from a hospital based system to a community based system – was finalized in the *NHS Improvement Plan* (Department of Health 2004a), following which primary care services controlled 80% of NHS funding.

To enable community based services, contemporaneous legislation was introduced that focused on streamlining services and supporting carers. Throughout the history of the NHS there had been poor communication and conflicting working priorities between the NHS services and local authority provided social care services, to the detriment of community services overall. The *NHS Plan* (Department of Health 2000) and *Shifting the Balance of Power within the NHS* (Department of Health 2001) attempted to address some of the difficulties by introducing *partnership working*. In this system, health authorities and local authorities joined together to become one employer. Being a single organization it was hoped that this would lead to better targeting and consequently improved community services.

Because of the increasing demand placed upon informal carers, the government looked at ways to support them more fully. *Supporting People with Long Term Conditions: Liberating the Talents of Nurses who care for People with Long Term Conditions* (Department of Health 2005) introduced community matrons, whose role was to manage a caseload of people with chronic illnesses, and their carers, to help to prevent a deterioration in their condition, or if they did deteriorate, to help them to manage their problems at home rather than being admitted to hospital. Other legislation focused on supporting carers so that they could continue with their existing responsibilities as well as care for their relative (see Evolve 1.1 for list of legislation and a summary of its impact).

evolve
learning system

1.1 – A SUMMARY OF LEGISLATION TO SUPPORT CARERS

Objectives:
- List the main government Acts.
- Outline the main provisions between each Act/report.
- Be aware of the changing regulations surrounding provision within the Acts.

As a consequence of the change in emphasis in the NHS to community led services, many nurses working in hospitals are likely to find themselves concentrating on acute, fast-turnaround care, whereas nurses working in the community will be involved in various supportive schemes to either prevent people being admitted to hospital or to coordinate facilities that will enable their early discharge.

International influences

The delivery of nursing care in contemporary society is complex. Nursing can no longer be totally defined by geographical distance nor by region. Today health care is a global undertaking where there are worldwide influences. This section will briefly explore some key considerations.

The information highway

Today information about nursing is truly global. With the advent of the Internet and electronic library gateways, it is possible to retrieve evidence for care from a wide range of sources across the world. It is also possible to communicate via weblinks with nurses working in other countries and find out first hand about the experience of nursing globally. However, evidence should be considered with care. As well as the usual considerations associated with the evaluation of information and research (Cormack et al 2006, Parahoo 2006), there is a need to think about the application of evidence across cultures and contexts. Will the information from another culture transfer to your setting within the UK? Equally, will your knowledge of nursing from the UK transfer outwards to settings across the world?

The impact of migration, inward and outward

It is important to know more about international nursing today because there has been a massive increase in the movement of people across the globe over the last decade. Even if you decide that travelling or moving across the world is not for you, and do not migrate outwardly from the UK, you will encounter the impact of inward migration as people needing health and social care in the UK increasingly emanate from a diverse range of cultures and countries. Nurses also move to the UK to work, both from overseas countries and from the European Union (Nursing and Midwifery Council 2007).

The recruitment of nurses is not without some difficulties. While it is expected that individual nurses will move across the world for many reasons, including seeking experience or better conditions for themselves and their families or for work if jobs in their own localities are few, it is important to recognize that both in the UK and globally, the number of healthcare workers is insufficient to meet future demand. In fact in some countries the situation is critical, and this is frequently the case in areas where health care is needed most (e.g. sub-Saharan Africa). This has led the World Health Organization (WHO) to address the issue of a global workforce in nursing. WHO has made a number of recommendations, including the consideration of individual countries to develop a healthcare workforce for domestic need, and the recognition that recruitment of healthcare workers from disadvantaged countries by wealthy countries is unethical and leads to greater inequality (WHO 2006).

In the European Union (EU) there is a recognition that mobility and trade agreements between countries are beneficial as they enable development of wealth and economic growth. The Treaty of Lisbon (2007) is determining change within the EU towards greater economic collaboration. For nursing, it is the response of the universities to the Treaty of Lisbon which is likely to create the greatest impact. Universities across Europe are committed to the development of a European Higher Education Area by 2010. This is being achieved through the 'Bologna declaration' (Bologna Process 1999). There are many components in this complex process but the main ones include comparability of degrees and student experience, and mobility of qualifications. In the future it will mean that qualifications gained in the UK will have similar standards to those elsewhere in Europe and will be acceptable to employers. It should also mean that lifelong learning by individuals can be achieved across different countries. It is important also to recognize that nursing has an agreement from a professional perspective through the EU directive 2005/36/EC (European Union (EU) Parliament and Council 2005). This directive identifies the number of hours and type of experience student nurses must complete in order to register as a nurse responsible for the delivery of general care.

Electives and learning about internationalization

In order to be ready for this changing world, it is important that you take all opportunities to find out about global nursing and nursing in Europe. Universities are responding to this through the development of electives and exchange opportunities such as Erasmus (http://www.erasmus.ac.uk), and also through the development of shared work programmes with schools of nursing in other countries. The advent of video links and web based technology means that it is possible to talk about nursing with nurses from many other countries and even share lessons or conferences together. You can participate in European working through the Students' Union or through the RCN Association of Nursing Students who are members of the European Nursing Students Association (ENSA).

CARE DELIVERY KNOWLEDGE

The RCN definition of nursing refers to the 'use of clinical judgement in the provision of care' (Royal College of Nursing 2003: 3). In this section we will first look at the basis for clinical decision making in evidence-based practice before reviewing the organizational approaches in common use to manage the delivery of care. There is a brief overview of the scope for nursing practice in the different branches of nursing.

CLINICAL DECISION MAKING

In the delivery of nursing care in institutional settings, nurses are in constant contact with their patients over a 24-hour period. Any changes (physical and/or mental) observed in a patient's condition are first seen by the nurse; therefore clinical decision making is a key application of the nursing role. Nurses very often 'own' and manage the environment of care, ensuring that resources for care are available. A number of services are also 'nurse led' (e.g. tissue viability, diabetic care, 'first contact'), giving the nurse greater autonomy in decision making. However, the majority of decisions in day-to-day practice take place in a complex environment, in collaboration with a diverse healthcare team and in partnership with patients/clients who have complex needs (Gurbutt 2006).

Knowledge for decision making is obtained from many sources and has been described as both informative (i.e. acquired through the study of written knowledge) and intuitive/experiential (i.e. developed through experience and learning from that experience through reflective practice) (Schon 1991, Benner 2001, Banning 2008). The views and rights of patients/clients and the context of care are also key factors in clinical decision making. In the world of practice, all sources of knowledge are constantly interacting to inform day-to-day decisions in healthcare delivery. Registered nurses need to be able to describe how and why they came to particular decisions in the delivery of nursing care. As a learner in the practice setting you should be able to ask the nurse and other members of the

healthcare team about their decisions and thus learn from practice experience (Standing 2007).

Decision–making exercise

You are allocated to work with a registered nurse (RN) and a healthcare assistant in providing rehabilitation care to a group of 10 elderly people with complex care needs based on a mixture of mental and physical health problems. The RN managed and directed the care during the shift.

- Describe the RN's approach to organizing priorities in care giving during the shift.
- Under what influence or on what basis did he/she make decisions (try to obtain this information through reflective discussion at the end of the shift).
- Did you experience any changes in decisions over the period of the shift and what do you think influenced these changes.
- Decide how you could record what you had learned so that you could explain your understanding of the RN's decision making to another learner/peer group of learners.

There is an increasing emphasis on clinical decision making being more prescriptive as health care has to become more cost-effective and evidence based. Decisions of all healthcare professionals are now strongly influenced by protocols, clinical guidelines, clinical standards and benchmarks for best practice. Computer decision-support systems are used to make expert knowledge more widely available (Gurbutt 2006). Although clinical research evidence has strongly informed medical practice, the evidence-based healthcare movement is now accepted as a legitimate source for clinical decision making by all health professionals (Muir Gray 2001).

Sourcing and analysing the evidence

Decisions about groups of patients or populations are made by combining three factors: evidence, values and resources. If decisions are based on values and resources alone, then it is 'opinion based' decision making. The evidence base is produced by research and is the scientific factor in the decision-making process (Muir Gray 2001). Skills needed by any healthcare professional to practise evidence-based clinical decision making include the ability to do the following:

- define criteria for effectiveness, safety and acceptability
- resource the evidence
- assess the quality of the best evidence available at the time
- judge the reliability and validity of the evidence
- assess whether the results can be applied in the local situation (Muir Gray 2001).

Criteria for effectiveness and safety are now more often made available to practitioners through national and local guidelines (e.g. National Institute for Health and Clinical Excellence (NICE) guidelines) and are promoted through clinical governance in healthcare delivery (Swage 2003). Resourcing the evidence and making judgements on its quality is facilitated through the availability of centres of excellence in reviewing all the research evidence such as the Cochrane Reviews or the Centre for Evidence Based Nursing at the University of York or the Joanna Briggs Institute for Evidence Based Nursing (see annotated websites). The final decision is then based on whether results can be applied in the local practice setting and whether they are acceptable to the patient/client. In summary, core components of evidence-based healthcare include the integration of best research evidence with the clinical expertise of the healthcare professional, the resources available and the patient's values and choices (Pearson et al 2007).

Strauss et al (2005) refer to a hierarchy of evidence, starting at the base with the original research studies, followed by a systematic review of these studies to decide on evidence for best practice (Fig 1.1). These reviews are then summarized for ease of access and at the most sophisticated level can be incorporated into computer systems that would allow the practitioner to enter the patient profile and obtain a summary of the best evidence to help in the final decisions about care.

Learning how to make judgements about research-based evidence is obtained through the study of research methodologies which is a core component in all diploma/degree level courses in higher education (see Evolve 1.2).

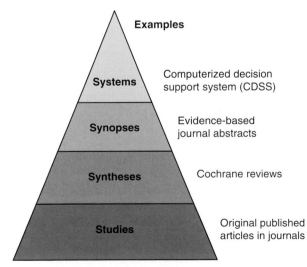

Figure 1.1 A hierarchy of evidence sources for clinical decision making (from Strauss et al 2005; by kind permission of Elsevier).

Evidence-based practice

Gerrish et al (2008) completed a cross-sectional survey of senior and junior RNs in two hospitals in England, using the Developing Evidence-Based Practice questionnaire ($n=598$). Findings revealed that while all respondents demonstrated confidence in accessing and using evidence for practice, they still relied heavily on personal experience and communication with colleagues. Senior nurses were more confident in accessing all sources of evidence and felt able to initiate change. Junior nurses perceived lack of time and resources as major barriers in implementing change, whereas senior nurses felt empowered to overcome these constraints.

1.2 – NURSING RESEARCH – AN OVERVIEW

- History and scope of nursing research in the UK.
- Overview of research methodologies.
- Application of research findings in practice.

Managing the delivery of nursing care

Systems for managing the delivery of nursing care continue to evolve over time. Although changes in these systems can be linked to the emerging role of the nurse as an autonomous practitioner, they are very strongly influenced by policy and politics of healthcare delivery. Table 1.2 describes the features of common nursing care delivery systems, some of which will still be observed in practice settings. As health care becomes increasingly more expensive, care management systems need to be seen to deliver quality and be cost-effective.

The focus is now on the efficient use of healthcare professionals with care needs being patient centred. The goal is the integration of all services to meet patients' needs, with all professions working collaboratively. The patient's journey through the health and social care system is a key driver for implementing new management systems. Interprofessional working is being promoted through the increasing use of integrated care pathways.

Integrated care pathways

An integrated care pathway (ICP) is a multiprofessional plan of care. It comprises detailed guidance for each stage in the care of a patient with a specific condition, stating what should be done, when it should be done and who should do it. It also predicts the type of response to any actions taken and by when the response should have

Table 1.2 Nursing care delivery systems

Title	Features	Application	Advantages	Disadvantages
Individual case method	Care for all needs of one patient	Private nursing in home Critical care	All patient's needs met quickly Close relationship with patient	Cost – very expensive
Task allocation method	Care divided into tasks with nurses allocated to particular tasks	Providing care in healthcare institutions particularly when shortage of staff	Very efficient way to deliver care. Staff competency matched to complexity of task so may be safer practice	Care of patient fragmented No identified nurse for patient. No accountability for nurse
Team care method	A RN as team leader manages the care of a group of patients. Team members plan and deliver care as a team	Commonly used system in all healthcare contexts including the community	All team members' capabilities are recognized; patient has one accountable nurse (team leader) with access to all others in the team	Requires good team leader and team spirit to succeed. May not be available 24 hours of the day
Primary nursing (primary nurse – PN)	One nurse cares for one group of patients with 24 hour accountability for planning their care. An associate nurse delivers the care when PN off duty	Popular in 1990s as the 'named nurse' in the UK Variable application in institutions but evidence of its application in community settings	Increased satisfaction for patients and nurses More professional system: PN plans and communicates with all disciplines	Intimidating for new graduates with less knowledge and experience Costly as many RNs needed to provide service

occurred. Any deviation from the plan is called a variance, which in turn forms the basis of the evaluation of the interventions. This provides the evidence for day-to-day monitoring and also forms part of the periodic auditing of pathways to ensure their effectiveness and safety.

Originating in North America in the 1980s, the use of ICPs began to grow in the UK during the 1990s, initially within the area of acute general medicine but more recently in all areas of health care.

There are many advantages to using ICPs. First, in the UK, they are developed using the latest evidence and reviewed regularly to ensure that they remain up-to-date. Because they are multiprofessional, this helps to ensure that the total package of care delivered by all professionals is based upon sound, contemporary information. Secondly, because all of the documentation is located in one place and available for all involved in the care to see, communication between professionals is clear – all of those involved in the care can see what is done, by whom and when. Thirdly, because time and resources are included in many pathways, it is possible to predict the demands on equipment and staffing. Ultimately this makes it possible to cost patient episodes. Indeed, this was a major impetus for their introduction in North America.

Interprofessional rivalry can sometimes be a problem in multiprofessional working (Gibbon et al 2002, Rees et al 2004). In many cases this originates from the negative attitudes of the staff involved. As ICPs require multiprofessional working, interprofessional rivalry could in effect sabotage their introduction. Logan (2003) and Hall (2001) reported that integrated care pathways enhanced multiprofessional working ; however, they noted that ownership was the key issue in their introduction. A top down approach was doomed to failure. If ICPs were to be introduced successfully, all who were to contribute to care, needed to be involved in developing the pathway.

Evidence–based practice

Allen & Rixson (2008) completed a systematic review of the impact of ICPs on providing an 'integrated service' for patients. The review focused on the care of adult patients who had suffered a stroke and included acute care, rehabilitation and long-term support – in hospital and community settings. ICPs were the intervention of interest and 'service integration' was the outcome. They critically appraised seven papers, representing five studies. Conclusions: ICPs can be effective: in ensuring that patients receive relevant clinical assessments and interventions in a timely manner; in improving the documentation of rehabilitation goals; in clarifying role boundaries and a shared understanding of the work. There is some evidence that ICPs may be effective in bringing about behavioural changes in contexts where deficiencies in service provision have been identified. None of the studies reviewed included an economic evaluation so that it remains unclear whether the benefits of ICPs justify the costs of their implementation.

The process of nursing

Regardless of which overall management system is in place, any health or social care professional working on a one-to-one basis with a patient/client will follow a pattern in their decision making on care delivery. This process follows the steps of a problem solving approach and has been termed 'the nursing process' (Carpenito-Moyet, 2005; Springhouse 2007). Similar to the problem solving approach, there are four/five stages to the nursing process; assess, plan, implement and evaluate. These are usually depicted as a cycle of events (Fig 1.2) as the evaluation stage leads back into a reassessment of care needs. A fifth stage can be added after assessment, usually labelled as 'nursing diagnoses' (more common in the USA). Throughout this book, in the Care Delivery Knowledge sections, many authors have chosen to follow the pattern of the nursing process in the layout of the information presented.

Health professionals use a variety of tools to make detailed assessments. When applied to the whole person these tools are designed to follow a particular approach to health care. For doctors their assessment tool kit is organized around physiological body systems; for physiotherapists their tools focus on mobility needs of the client. Nurses may use the particular tool integral to a nursing model, an example of which is an assessment based on the 12 activities of living outlined in the Roper, Logan and Tierney model of nursing (Holland et al 2003). Specific tools are also available for various parts and functions of the person, for example pain level assessment tools, oral care assessment tools, all of which are referred to in more detail throughout the chapters of this book. Integrated patient centred assessment tools, which can be used by all health professionals in a single care plan shared by all, including the patient as a partner in care, are now becoming more common. These are usually designed around a specific condition and treatment plan (see Integrated Care Pathways above).

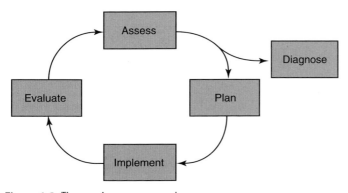

Figure 1.2 The nursing process cycle.

Delivering care to different client groups

The following section provides an overview of the scope of nursing practice in the four branches of nursing which are registered in the UK.

Nursing children and young people

Working with children and young people is a specific branch of nursing in the UK today. It is studied after the first-year common foundation programme and focuses upon the care of children, young people and their families. Children's nursing is based upon the philosophy that children are entitled to services which are sensitive to their requirements and designed and delivered around the needs of children and families (Department of Health 2004a). Children's nurses need to empower carers to manage their child's situation positively and proactively. There is a considerable amount of partnership working because the care of the child will be predominantly performed by their families or carers. Nursing care is planned around assessing the needs of children and families and of sensitive working, teaching and assessing carers in sharing the provision of care.

In the UK, there is increasing diversity in the needs of children and their families both from a social perspective and from a health one. Children's nurses work across healthcare settings. In the community they contribute to teams working within children's centres (Sure Start), providing health promotion, support and management of care. They also provide nursing for children who remain in the community rather than attend hospital care settings for treatment. Children's nurses still most commonly work in hospital settings in the UK, where children are acutely ill and cannot be managed at home. These children are frequently technologically dependent or require intensive treatment or surgery. Children's nurses therefore must learn a wide range of assessment and clinical skills. They need to know how to care for children at different ages and stages of development and they need to differentiate their care appropriately to meet individual needs.

In both the community setting and the acute hospital, standards for the care of children are focused around three main documents: the *National Service Framework for Children* (Department of Health 2004b) which determines the expectations of care for children and families; the Children Act (Office of Public Sector Information 2004); and the *Every Child Matters* initiative (Department of Education and Science 2003). *Every Child Matters* (2003) and the Children Act 2004 led to a radical change in child health care in the UK (see Evolve 1.3).

1.3 – STANDARDS OF CARE FOR CHILDREN

- The Children Act 2004.
- The *National Service Framework for Children* and its influence on your care.
- How you can use *Every Child Matters*.
- The common Assessment Framework and the vulnerable child.

Decision–making exercise

Jody is 3 years old, and does not want to take her medicine today. She says it tastes horrible and she does not like it at all. Sarah is 13 years old and is also refusing to take her medicine. Both have a temperature of 38 degrees Celsius. Both are of a stage of development which is commensurate with their chronological age.

- Decide how you would manage these two different situations.
- Would you treat them similarly or differently? What reasons do you have for your decisions?
- If they did refuse their medicines, what would the implications be for each one?

Adult nursing

Developing knowledge and skills to meet the needs of adults (those over 16 years) is the focus of the second and third year of an adult branch nursing programme. The scope of practice is very broad with healthcare delivery in multiple contexts. The demographics of an aging population and a policy shift to deliver more care in the community (Department of Health 2005) means a greater emphasis on developing nursing roles that are flexible and adaptable to changes in health care locally, nationally and internationally (see Subject Knowledge).

During your pre-registration programme, you will gain experience and knowledge during the first common foundation year of all branches of nursing. When completing your adult branch, you will gain practice learning experience in acute hospital care and in the community. Although the majority of time on your course may still be spent in learning in the hospital setting, the increasing focus on care in the community is being recognized by those responsible for developing pre-registration programmes with a commitment to more extensive placement experiences in the community. Table 1.3 outlines examples of the scope of current adult nursing roles in the community and Table 1.4 provides a selection of specialities and roles in the acute hospital setting.

The average time spent in gaining experience in each placement will vary between 6 and 12 weeks, with flexibility within some placements for students to gain observational

Table 1.3 Scope of adult nursing roles and placement experience in the community

Role title	Scope of role	Practice learning
Community RN	Delivers care in home within a district nursing team	District nursing team
District nurse (specialist registration)	Directs and manages a team delivering care in home	District nursing team
Practice nurse	Delivers care in GP practice setting	GP practice team
Community matron	Manages a case load of patients with long-term conditions across community and acute care settings	Community matron
First contact nurses	'First stop' health care advisors in NHS call centres or drop in centres	NHS call centres or walk in centres
Occupational health nurses	Health promotion and care for employees in industry and commercial sector	Factories, stores, NHS
Private nurse	Provides care to individuals in own homes for a fee	Private agency work
Prison nurses	Health promotion and care delivery within prisons	Prisons
Care home manager	Manages the care of elderly people in a community nursing home	Care homes
Health promotion nurses	Set up and deliver health promotion programmes in community	Health centres; rehabilitation centres/teams
Intermediate care team nurse	Member of a multiprofessional team for health and social care	Interprofessional learning with intermediate care teams

Table 1.4 Scope of adult nursing roles and placement experience in acute hospitals

Role title	Scope of role	Practice learning
Medical nursing	Care for patients with medical conditions especially cardiovascular and respiratory diseases	Areas and teams classified to deliver medical care
Surgical nursing	Care of patients requiring minor or major surgery	Day case surgery units, surgical wards, operating theatres and recovery areas
Elderly care nursing	Care of the older person with acute medical care needs	Areas classified for delivery of elderly and rehabilitative care; stroke units; day hospitals; day centres
Cancer care nursing	Care of people with cancer from diagnosis through to recovery and/or terminal care	Diagnostic centres; cancer care wards; specialist nurses; palliative care and hospice areas
Critical care nursing	Care of critically ill people	Units for: intensive care general/cardiac; high dependency; coronary care; burns; neurosurgical; accident and emergency care
Specialist surgery and medicine	Care of patients with orthopaedic, neurological, renal, gynaecological, genitourinary, eye and ear, nose and throat conditions	Specialist surgical and medical areas to include: outpatients and diagnostic centres; dialysis units; sexual health clinics

experience working alongside specialist nurses in the field and/or with other health professionals. It is important to remember to maintain a holistic approach to healthcare learning, as mental and physical health impact on one another. Insights and knowledge gained of care for children and adults and children with learning disabilities and/or mental health problems during the first year of a nursing programme are also important in adult branch nursing.

Mental health nursing

People can experience mental health problems at any stage of life and consequently mental health nurses will work with children, adolescents, adults and older people. Although some care is given in hospitals, most people receive care in their own homes and access mental health services at a local mental health centre, or will be visited by a member of the mental health team.

A good mental health nurse has a number of personal qualities that include an interest in working with people, good listening skills, a compassionate nature and a willingness to help people to develop skills that will help them to recover from their problems and return to their normal way of life. In addition to these skills you need the professional knowledge and skills that enable a nurse to understand a client's psychological, social and spiritual needs, as well as a robust understanding of the physiological aspects of the individual's problems and treatment.

Mental health nurses work closely with other members of the interprofessional team (which includes social workers, occupational therapists, psychiatrists, psychologists, physiotherapists and healthcare support workers). Assessing

and monitoring mental health problems is not as straightforward as assessing and monitoring physical illnesses, as the signs and symptoms are often not measurable. Mental health nurses therefore need to be confident in their professional ability and able to communicate effectively, both with the person suffering mental distress and with other members of the care team. Many mental health nurses will choose to specialize in an area of mental health following their initial registration, including substance misuse, child and adolescent psychiatry, cognitive behavioural therapy, forensic nursing, assertive outreach and crisis intervention. This enables the nurse to take additional training and develop a specialist career pathway.

Learning disabilities nursing

People with learning disabilities can struggle to cope independently with day-to-day life. It is the role of the learning disability nurse to support these individuals, and their families or carers, to enable the individual to live at home and be included within their local society and activities. Although most learning disabilities become apparent in childhood, they continue throughout adult life and learning disability nurses therefore work with clients and carers from all age groups.

As is the case with mental health nurses, most learning disability nurses work within the community, and this can involve working with people in their homes, in schools, in day centres or in residential care homes. In addition to personal qualities that include patience, understanding, compassion and excellent listening skills, learning disability nurses must acquire a good understanding of social inclusion and networking, as well as a sound knowledge of physiological conditions that may affect their clients. Learning disability nurses also need to develop skills of assertiveness as often they will be required to support their clients, both within society in general and sometimes within the care team.

Learning disability nurses work as part of a specialist interprofessional team which includes psychologists, social workers, occupational therapists, physiotherapists, teachers, speech therapists and healthcare support workers. Many people with learning disabilities have complex needs which can include physical and/or sensory impairments, mental health needs and challenging behaviour and these require the nurse to be able to provide a skilled assessment, care planning and intervention.

Once qualified, many learning disability nurses will go on to manage and lead teams of support staff. However, there are also many specialist career pathways available to learning disability nurses, such as challenging behaviour, sensory disability, education or management, many of which offer the nurse an opportunity of advanced education and training.

PROFESSIONAL AND ETHICAL KNOWLEDGE

Nursing has a claim to being a profession through fulfilling recognized requirements for professional status (UK Centre for the History of Nursing and Midwifery http://www.nursing.manchester.ac.uk/ukchnm/publications/bibliographies/nursingprofession/). These requirements are obtained through what is termed the professionalization process. Professions usually perform a service for the public and have the following characteristics:

- A distinct body of knowledge and skills that can be applied in practice.
- Formal education and training, usually 3 years or more in length with examinations to check knowledge and competence to practise in the profession.
- A regulatory body that has legal power to admit to and remove from a professional register.
- Members have ability and power to work autonomously and take responsibility for own standards of practice.
- Members must adhere to a formal code of conduct/ethics that governs their behaviour.

Throughout this textbook, authors refer to the professional standards and code of ethical conduct set by the nursing regulatory body in the UK (Nursing and Midwifery Council 2008; see also www.nmc-uk.org/) and also to legal issues as they are applied to the particular knowledge and skills being covered in the chapter. Here we will focus on autonomy and accountability in nursing and provide an overview of the legal and ethical principles that underpin nursing practice.

NURSING AUTONOMY AND ACCOUNTABILITY

Nurses, as professionals, should have the ability and power to work autonomously and take responsibility for their own standards of practice. Accountability for nursing standards is the other side of the coin from nursing autonomy and both can be enhanced or limited by the context in which care is delivered. According to Holland Wade (1999), accountability is the primary consequence of professional nurse autonomy, and empowerment of the nurse links work autonomy with professional autonomy, which leads to job satisfaction, commitment to the profession and the professionalization of nursing.

However, the delivery of health care in the 21st century is very much more focused on being patient centred, risk managed, quality assured and cost-effective. Accountability for the quality of health care delivered to people has become increasingly an organizational responsibility (Tiley & Watson 2005). Under the template of clinical governance, there is an increasing focus on ensuring team care and team accountability. This does not negate individual accountability for decisions made as a professional nurse and being held to account for those decisions.

Evidence-based practice

Rafferty et al (2001), asking the question as to whether teamwork and professional autonomy were compatible, conducted a postal questionnaire survey of 10 022 staff nurses in 32 hospitals in England to explore the relationship between interdisciplinary teamwork and nurse autonomy on patient and nurse outcomes and nurse assessed quality of care. Nursing autonomy was positively correlated with better perceptions of the quality of care delivered and higher levels of job satisfaction. Nurses with higher teamwork scores also exhibited higher levels of autonomy and were more involved in decision making. A strong association was found between teamwork and autonomy; this interaction suggests synergy rather than conflict. The researchers suggest that organizations be encouraged to promote nurse autonomy without the fear that it might undermine teamwork.

LEGAL AND ETHICAL BASIS FOR PROFESSIONAL NURSING PRACTICE

Continuing with the theme of autonomy, it is important to review its meaning in relation to patients' rights. The language of individual 'rights' is a key part of autonomy and has been embodied in law in the UK through the implementation of the Human Rights Act 1998 (arising from the Universal Declaration of Human Rights 1948/European Commission of Human Rights 1954) (McHale & Gallagher 2003).

Alongside a long list of human rights, the 'right to health' provides guidance for legal and ethical policy and practice in healthcare delivery. The enactment of the Human Rights Act 1998 has put patients' rights at centre stage and very much an issue that obtains publicity in the media on a regular basis. All areas of health care, where people are potentially more vulnerable due to their age, their health problems and/or the treatment options available, are potentially prone to scrutiny in relation to according human rights (McHale & Gallagher 2003 Box 1.1).

Respect for individual autonomy and human rights underpin the codes of ethics of health professions including the nursing profession (Nursing and Midwifery Council 2008). Nurses as autonomous practitioners are ethically and legally accountable for the delivery of nursing care. Ethical/moral decision making can be part of day-to-day practice for the nurse. Education and debate on the ethical principles underpinning the application of normative ethics – i.e. what kinds of action are right or wrong – are covered in nursing courses. Specific legal and ethical problems related to each chapter's subject area are included throughout this textbook.

There are five fundamental ethical principles that are relevant in healthcare practice (Beauchamp & Childress 2001). These are:

- autonomy
- beneficence
- truthfulness
- confidentiality
- justice and fairness.

Ideal ethical norms are incorporated into professional codes which influence the behaviour of practising nurses. Ethical dilemmas occur when the situations experienced in practice are less than ideal and decisions have to be made that reflect the best option available to all concerned, including the patient. Having to take or condone actions that contradict personal and professional ethical principles can cause considerable moral distress. Limited power or authority in an environment of care that makes it difficult to advocate for the patient may occur (Mallik 1997). However, the increasing power of the consumer and the legal protection of patients' rights at the heart of professional regulation make it increasingly important for all healthcare professionals to act always in the interests of their patients/clients (see Council for Healthcare Regulatory Excellence, http://www.chre.org.uk/; accessed May 2008).

A 'virtue ethics' approach, which is becoming increasingly integrated into the development of professional ethics, suits the service ideal of health and social care professions. It places an emphasis on the moral qualities ('virtues') of individual people and/or institutions. The focus is on the individual nurse as a moral agent within a community of practitioners who share a core moral purpose or 'service ideal'. Examples of virtues include: professional wisdom, care, respectfulness, trustworthiness, justice, courage and integrity (Banks & Gallagher 2008).

Reflection and portfolio evidence

Obtain a copy of the current nursing and midwifery Code of Practice (Nursing and Midwifery Council 2008; http://www.nmc-uk.org/).

- Review each statement in the Code and cross reference its content with the requirements of the Human Rights Act and ethical principles outlined above.
- Reflect on a week spent in your practice placement. How vulnerable were the patients? What made them vulnerable?
- How were they helped in making decisions about their care?
- What legal or ethical principles were subsumed in the decision making about care options?

Box 1.1 Key areas covered by the Human Rights Act (McHale & Gallagher 2003)

- Reproduction rights
- Consent to treatment
- Rights and mental health care
- Rights to privacy
- Rights to health information
- Allocation of resources
- Research and rights
- Rights at the end of life

LEADERSHIP AND CHANGE

As you will have noticed in this chapter, working in health care and being a member of the nursing profession is not a static process. Nurses work in a healthcare system that is constantly evolving in response to changes in health research, in society and in political ideology. Consequently, any profession, or individual professionals, unable to adapt to change will struggle to survive in this environment. On the other hand, those that are ready for innovation and change are more likely to succeed. It is appropriate therefore that nurses should not see change as a threat to stability but as an opportunity to develop, both personally and as a profession.

Allied to change is the concept of leadership. However, leadership in a large diverse profession must be considered in context. In the UK the Nursing and Midwifery Council (NMC) is charged with maintaining professional standards and leadership of the profession. It could be argued that the history of the NMC, and its predecessors the United Kingdom Central Council (UKCC) and the General Nursing Council (GNC), reveals limited evidence of proactive leadership and change. Similarly, while professional organisations such as the Royal College of Nursing may petition and influence some policy decisions, again, they have limited power to bring about change. This situation is common with most professions in health and social care and arises from the relationship between healthcare delivery and policy-making. As the agenda and funding of healthcare is controlled by central government, national leadership and change is difficult to achieve without support from policy and finance. Therefore, at a national level, leadership in nursing must be seen within the framework of the wider political agenda.

More direct leadership in nursing occurs locally and successful leaders are those that are aware of the contexts of care delivery and are able to act proactively. First of all, an individual needs to be effective in meeting the demands made upon them. It is easy in busy workplaces to become overwhelmed and in turn this can lead to reactive, rather than a more effective proactive way of working. Time management and stress management are essential skills to master (see Ch. 9, 'Stress, relaxation and rest').

It is useful to develop a career plan. It is likely that nurses will make several changes of direction in their career pathways during their working lives. Most nurses begin their careers working directly with clients. However, many go on to seek promotion in an area that they enjoy. This also increases their managerial responsibilities and affords them an opportunity to specialize and obtain further qualifications (Park et al 2007). The Knowledge and Skills Framework introduced in *Agenda for Change* (DH 2004c) helps individuals to plan their careers. However, they should also be aware of trends in their chosen area that are set by contemporary research and the direction of policy. This enables an individual nurse to engage with change proactively and in doing so, gradually provide direction and leadership for others.

PERSONAL AND REFLECTIVE KNOWLEDGE

LEARNING TO NURSE

When learning to be a nurse, there will be many approaches to how all course knowledge is presented to you within the university setting and how your time in practice learning is integrated in to the overall programme of study. The number of hours you spend on practice learning through having direct contact with patients/clients is stipulated by the Nursing and Midwifery Council and is currently set at 50% of your course time. There should be specific periods in each placement to allow you time to gain proficiency in the standards set by the NMC. Gaining these proficiencies are necessary for you to register as a qualified nurse (Nursing and Midwifery Council 2004: Standard 6).

During your course, knowledge may be presented to you from within different subject areas such as the biological sciences, the social sciences, philosophy, ethical and legal knowledge and nursing knowledge itself. Application of that knowledge to the delivery of patient/client care is then achieved through simulated case study work in a clinical learning laboratory and more importantly through the experiences you gain in the practice setting. This is sometimes called the 'front-loading' of core underpinning knowledge which can then be called upon to provide informed patient care. It is the traditional way in which knowledge is delivered within schools and universities and is often organized into modules which are assessed to give you credit points towards your diploma/degree.

An alternative approach is to integrate knowledge from all appropriately selected subject disciplines through providing students with individual patient/client case studies first. Groups of students are then encouraged to examine the case study and decide on what information they need to learn to deliver safe care. This approach has been termed variously: problem based learning (PBL; Barrows 2000); enquiry based learning (EBL) ; or enquiry focused learning (EFL). A PBL approach (the most common title used) to professional courses of study is promoted because it is expected to encourage students to be open-minded, reflective and critical and to participate more actively in their learning (Newman 2003). It is particularly useful in encouraging interprofessional learning with students from differing health and social care professions focused on the same case study, thus gaining an appreciation of the contributions of each profession to the overall care of the patient (Goelen et al 2006).

However, it may be that your programme of study offers a pragmatic mix of both the PBL and the traditional approach to encouraging your learning. This textbook acknowledges this pragmatic mixed approach through providing subject based knowledge related to all areas of patient needs where you as a nurse will be a key decision maker. At the same time it encourages you, through the many exercises scattered through the chapters, critically to review what is happening in reality in practice settings through self-reflection and follow-up discussion with your mentors, peers and lecturers.

REFLECTIVE LEARNING

An essential part of the learning process is the ability to reflect on what has been presented as theoretical knowledge and what you observe and assimilate through direct experience in the delivery of patient care (Dewey 1933). As a student you need actively to engage with all your experiences, whether in the classroom or in practice. Reflective learning requires a questioning approach where beliefs and ideas about an experience or a topic can be drawn out, examined, tested and then integrated with new approaches.

Authors writing about reflective learning focus particularly on learning from experience, using a structure to help you make your learning explicit (Kolb 1984, Boud et al 1985, Gibbs 1988, Schon 1991). All involve a process by which you move through a reflective cycle where you: return to and describe the experience/event; examine your knowledge and feelings about the experience; make sense of what is going on based on your current knowledge but also through seeking alternative views from those involved and/or your mentor/supervisor or through investigating new knowledge; decide what could be done differently if the event/experience should occur in the future. This type of learning requires active engagement with all stages of the reflective cycle and can potentially create tension and conflict as part of the process.

Experienced practitioners working alongside you in the practice setting have built up so much experiential knowledge of their work that they appear to make decisions based on intuition (Benner 2001). They may sometimes find it difficult to explain how they made these decisions. Schon (1991: 50) refers to this tacit knowledge as 'knowing-in-action' and associates it with 'the "art" by which practitioners sometimes deal with situations of uncertainty, instability, uniqueness and value conflict'.

However, practitioners may also be 'thinking on their feet' and if they are able to articulate their thinking and make a 'running commentary' (reflection-in-action) on how they are making decisions, this is very helpful for you as a student working alongside them. It then may be possible to re-visit events at the end of a shift and recall and recount what happened through reflection-on-action. Doing this together with your mentor is a powerful way of learning from practice experience (Jasper 2003, Bolton 2005, Bulman & Schuz 2008). You are generally encouraged to record your experience and learning in a personal portfolio.

KEEPING A PORTFOLIO OF LEARNING

Throughout your nursing course you will be encouraged to keep a record of your learning and development. It is important to develop your ability to write about and record your experiences and learning as a student because keeping an up-to-date professional portfolio is a requirement for pre-registration as a nurse (Nursing and Midwifery Council 2006). There are many resources available to provide guidance in organizing and maintaining an up-to-date portfolio, and relevant chapters in study skills books are a good starting point (Maslin-Prothero 2005).

It is likely to be a requirement of your course that you produce evidence in writing of your learning in practice for ongoing continuous assessment of your competence. This evidence needs to be gathered in a focused and systematic way to ensure accreditation of your knowledge and competence to meet professional standards. If the evidence you gather in your portfolio is assessed and graded, it will be important to read and follow any requirements set out by your course curriculum.

CASE STUDIES

In all the chapters in this book you will find four case studies, one related to each branch of nursing. In this introductory chapter, where we have focused on core underpinning knowledge for nursing practice, we have included a single family case study which will allow you to reflect on the knowledge presented and the questions raised by this chapter.

Family case study

Daniela is 25 years old and has recently come to England from Poland with her husband who is working as a hotel porter. Daniela is a registered nurse in Poland but though she wishes to do so in the near future, she is not working currently as she looks after Irina, 6 years old, and 2-year-old son, Henrik. They live in a small flat in the middle of a large town. During a visit to the practice nurse at the local surgery, it is observed that Daniela looks tired and stressed. Her English is limited but she manages to convey that she is feeling very alone and isolated, and that managing is difficult for her as she is used to having her friends and family nearby. Henrik appears well cared for but during the visit is demonstrating attention seeking behaviour.

- Map out the issues in this scenario.
- What range of health and social care professionals could potentially be involved in helping this family?

● Debate the professional accountability of the practice nurse in this first contact with the family.
● How can Daniela and the family best be supported and enabled to integrate into this country? Make a list of agencies who may be able to support the family.

● What may be the potential health risks to the family if support is not established?
● If Daniela wishes to work as a nurse in the UK, what steps does she need to take to become registered?

SUMMARY

This first chapter has introduced you to the knowledge base of key issues that underpin nursing practice in all branches of nursing. It has introduced you to:

1. Universal and UK definitions of nursing with an overview of the development and use of theories/models of nursing.
2. The history and politics of healthcare delivery in the UK with its potential impact on the changing role of the nurse.
3. The potential impact of globalization of the healthcare workforce with the advantages and challenges for future working as a nurse in a worldwide market place.
4. The ways of accessing and judging best evidence for clinical decision making in the delivery of quality nursing care.
5. Organizational systems in healthcare delivery that influence the way nurses work with each other and interprofessionally.
6. An overview of the scope of practice within each branch of nursing.
7. The underpinnings of professional and ethical knowledge to inform your approach to care in all contexts.
8. Ways of learning to be become a registered nurse that will encourage lifelong learning.

Annotated further reading and websites

Chambers R, Boath E, Rogers D 2007 Clinical effectiveness and clinical governance made easy, 4th edn. Radcliffe Publishing, Oxford

This is an easy to read textbook with clear instructions on how to access evidence and information on clinical audit and evaluation.

Gurgutt R 2006 Nurses' clinical decision making. Radcliffe Publishing, Oxford

A good introduction to the field of clinical decision making in nursing with a particular focus on outlining and reviewing studies related to nurses' decision-making capacity.

Key sites that will provide information related to: the regulation and education of the nursing profession in the UK (NMC); nursing union activity, policy and professional development of nurses (RCN); and policy and politics of healthcare delivery in the UK (DH) (all accessed May 2008):

Nursing and Midwifery Council: **http://www.nmc-uk.org/**
Royal College of Nursing: **http://www.rcn.org.uk/**
Department of Health: **http://www.dh.gov.uk/en/index.htm**

Joanna Briggs Institute: **http://www.joannabriggs.edu.au/about/about. php**

Established in 1996 in Adelaide, Australia, the Joanna Briggs Institute (JBI) is a nursing international collaboration focused on reviewing, dissemination and utilization of best practice evidence for health care. There are collaborating centres worldwide; examples in the UK include (all accessed August 2008):

● **http://www.rgu.ac.uk/nursing/research/page.cfm?pge=32496** Centre at Robert Gordon University in Scotland
● **http://www.joannabriggs.tvu.ac.uk/joannabriggs/** Centre at Thames Valley University in London
● **http://www.joannabriggs.edu.au/collab_ctrs/wales.php/** Centre for Wales in the University of Cardiff
● **http://pgstudy.nottingham.ac.uk/School/Research/additional.aspx? Id=65** Centre at University of Nottingham

http://www.jbiconnect.org/ (accessed March 2008)
Provides access to summaries of the latest evidence for practice from the Joanna Briggs Institute.

http://www.cochrane.org/ (accessed March 2008)
Cochrane Reviews provided access to the first worldwide systematic reviews of the effectiveness of healthcare interventions. It is a key site for accessing up to date information to support evidence-based practice and is referred to you by the majority of authors in this textbook.

http://www.york.ac.uk/healthsciences/centres/evidence/cebn.htm (accessed March 2008)
The Centre for Evidence Based Nursing at the University of York has been the leading centre in the UK for evaluating the implementation of evidence-based practice, particularly in NHS settings.

http://www.europeunit.ac.uk/bologna_process/index.cfm
This page offers information about the Bologna Process in developing a Europe-wide higher education area. Key parts of the Bologna Process include working towards the transferability of degree qualifications and opportunities for geographical mobility in study.

Journals

Worldviews on Evidence-based Nursing.

http://www.blackwellpublishing.com/journal.asp?ref=1545-102X&site=1 (accessed March 2008)
This is a series of journals by Blackwell Publishing, in press with four editions per year since 2004. There are many very useful articles examining the evidence base for nursing care worldwide.

References

Allen D, Rixson L 2008 How has the impact of 'care pathway technologies' on service integration in stroke care been measured and what is the strength of the evidence to support their effectiveness in this respect? International Journal of Evidence-Based Healthcare 6(1):78–110

Appleby J 2005 Economic growth and NHS spending. Health Service Journal 115(5937):23

Banks S, Gallagher A 2008 Ethics in professional life: virtues for health and social care. Palgrave Macmillan, Basingstoke

Banning M 2008 A review of clinical decision making: models and current research. Journal of Clinical Nursing 17(2):187–195

Barr H 2005 Interprofessional education today, yesterday and tomorrow. LTSN Centre for Health Sciences and Practice, London

Barrows HS 2000 Problem-based learning applied to medical education. Southern Illinois University School of Medicine, Springfield

Beauchamp T, Childress J 2001 Principles of biomedical ethics, 5th edn. Oxford University Press, Oxford

Benner P 1984 From novice to expert: excellence and power in clinical nursing practice. Addison Wesley, Menlo Park

Benner P 2001 From novice to expert, commemorative edn. Prentice Hall, Upper Saddle River, NJ

Binley's Handbook of Patient Groups 2008 Beechwood House Publishers, Basildon. Available online: http://www.binleys.com/Index.asp (accessed May 2008)

Bologna Process 1999 Available online: http://ec.europa.eu/education/policies/educ/bologna/bologna_en.html (accessed May 2008)

Bolton GE J 2005 Reflective practice: writing and professional development, 2nd edn. Sage, London

Boud D, Keogh R, Walker D 1985 Reflection: turning experience into learning. Kogan Page, London

Bulman C, Schuz S 2008 Reflective practice in nursing, 4th edn. Wiley Blackwell, Oxford

Carpenito-Moyet LJ 2005 Understanding the nursing process: concept mapping and care planning for students. Lippincott Williams & Wilkins, Philadelphia

Clancy J, McVicar A, Bird D 2000 Getting it right? An exploration of issues relating to the biological sciences in nurse education and nursing practice. Journal of Advanced Nursing 32(6):1522–1532

Cormack D, Gerrish K, Lacey A 2006 The research process in nursing, 5th edn. Blackwell Publishing, Oxford

Department for Education and Science 2003 Every child matters. Green Paper. Command number 5860. Available online: http://www.everychildmatters.gov.uk/publications (accessed May 2008)

Department of Health 2000, 2005 The NHS plan: a plan for investment a plan for reform. Department of Health, London. Available online: http://www.dh.gov.uk/en/Publicationsandstatistics/Publications/PublicationsPolicyAndGuidance/Browsable/DH_4112374 (accessed April 2008)

Department of Health 2001 Shifting the balance of power within the NHS. Stationery Office, London

Department of Health 2004a NHS improvement plan. Stationery Office, London

Department of Health 2004b National service framework for children, young people and maternity services: executive summary. Department of Health, London

Department of Health 2004c Agenda for change final agreement, December 2004. Stationery Office, London

Department of Health 2005 Supporting people with long term conditions: liberating the talents of nurses who care for people with long term conditions. Stationery Office, London

Dewey J 1933 How do we think? Heath, Boston

Dingwall R, Rafferty AM, Webster C 1988 An introduction to the social history of nursing. Routledge, London

European Federation of Nurses 2005 Available online: http://www.efnweb.org/version1/en/index.html (accessed May 2008)

European Union Parliament and Council 2005 Recognition of Professional Qualifications, Directive 2005/36/EC. EU Parliament and Council: Brussels, 7 September 2005

Fawcett J 2004 Contemporary nursing knowledge: analysis and evaluation of nursing models and theories, 2nd edn. FA Davis, Philadelphia

Fealy G, McNamara M 2007 A discourse analysis of debates surrounding the entry of nursing into higher education in Ireland. International Journal of Nursing Studies 44(7):1187–1195

Friedel JM, Treagust DF 2005 Learning bioscience in nursing education: perceptions of the intended and the prescribed curriculum. Learning in Health and Social Care 4(4):203–216

Gerrish K, Ashworth P, Lacey A, Bailey J 2008 Developing evidence-based practice: experiences of senior and junior clinical nurses. Journal of Advanced Nursing 62(1):62–73

Gibbon B, Watkins C, Barer D 2002 Can staff attitudes in team working in stroke care be improved? Journal of Advanced Nursing 40(1):105–111

Gibbs G 1988 Learning by doing: a guide to teaching and learning methods. Further Education Unit, Oxford Polytechnic, Oxford

Goelen G, De Clercq G, Huyghens L, Kerckhofs E 2006 Measuring the effect of interprofessional problem-based learning on the attitudes of undergraduate health care students. Medical Education 40(6):555–561

Gurbutt R 2006 Nurses' clinical decision making. Radcliffe Press, Oxford

Hall J 2001 A qualitative survey of staff responses to a pilot study in a mental healthcare setting. Nursing Times Research 6(3):696–706

Health Act 1999 Stationery Office, London

Health and Social Care Act 2001 Office of Public Sector Information, chapter 15. Available online: http://www.opsi.gov.uk/Acts/acts2001/ukpga_20010015_en_1 (accessed May 2008)

Henderson V 1960 Basic principles of nursing care. International Council of Nurses, Geneva

Henderson V 1966 The nature of nursing: a definition and its implications for practice research and education. Macmillan, New York

Holland K, Jenkins J, Solomon J, Whittam S 2003 Applying the Roper–Logan–Tierney model in practice. Churchill Livingstone Elsevier, Edinburgh

Holland Wade G 1999 Professional nurse autonomy: concept analysis and application to nursing education. Journal of Advanced Nursing 30(2):310–318

Human Rights Act 1998 Office of Public Sector Information, London

Illingworth P, Chelvanayagam S 2007 Benefits of interprofessional education in heath care. British Journal of Nursing 6(2):121–124

International Council of Nurses 1987 Position statement. International Council of Nurses, Geneva

International Council of Nurses 2002 The ICN definition of nursing. International Council of Nurses, Geneva

Jasper M 2003 Beginning reflective practice – foundations in health care. Nelson Thornes, Cheltenham

Kalisch PA, Kalisch BJ 1986 A comparative analysis of nurse and physician characters in the entertainment media. Journal of Advanced Nursing 11(2):179–195

Kalisch BJ, Begeny S, Neumann S 2007 The image of the nurse on the Internet. Nursing Outlook 55(4):182–188

Kolb D 1984 Experiential learning: experience in the source of learning and developing. Prentice Hall, New Jersey

Leininger M (ed) 1978 Transcultural nursing: concepts, theories and practices. John Wiley, New York

Logan K 2003 Indwelling catheters: developing an integrated care pathway package. Nursing Times 99(44):49–51

McHale J, Gallaher A 2003 Nursing and human rights. Butterworth Heinemann, Edinburgh

McKenna H, Cutliffe J, Slevin O 2008 Nursing models, theories and practice. Vital Notes for Nurses. Wiley Blackwell, Oxford

Mallik M 1997 Advocacy in nursing – perceptions of practising nurses. Journal of Clinical Nursing 6:303–313

Maslin-Prothero S 2005 Baillière's study skills for nurses and midwives. Elsevier, Edinburgh, section 3

Muir Gray JA 2001 Evidence-based healthcare: how to make health policy and management decisions, 2nd edn. Churchill Livingstone, Edinburgh

National Health Service and Community Care Act 1990 HMSO, London

Newman M 2003 A pilot systematic review and meta-analysis on the effectiveness of problem based learning. LTNS, London

Nightingale F 1859 Notes on nursing: what it is and what it is not. Harrison, London

Nolan P 1998 A history of mental health nursing. Nelson Thornes, Cheltenham

Nursing and Midwifery Council 2004 Standards of proficiency for pre-registration nursing education. Nursing and Midwifery Council, London. Available online: http://www.nmc-uk.org/aFrameDisplay.aspx?DocumentID=328 (accessed March 2008)

Nursing and Midwifery Council 2006 The PREP handbook. Nursing and Midwifery Council, London. Available online: http://www.nmc-uk.org/aFrameDisplay.aspx?DocumentID=1636 (accessed April 2008)

Nursing and Midwifery Council 2007 Statistical analysis of the register 1 April 2006 to 31 March 2007. Nursing and Midwifery Council, London

Nursing and Midwifery Council 2008 The code: standards of conduct, performance and ethics for nurses and midwives. Nursing and Midwifery Council, London

Office of Public Information 2001 Health and Social Care Act Part 4. Available online: http://www.opsi.gov.uk/ACTS/acts2001/ukpga_20010015_en_1 (accessed March 2008)

Office of Public Sector Information 2004 Children Act. Stationery Office, London

Orem DE 1971 Nursing: concepts of practice. McGraw-Hill, Scarborough, Ontario

Parahoo K 2006 Nursing research: principles, process and issues, 2nd edn. Palgrave Macmillan, Basingstoke

Park JR, Chapple M, Wharrad H, Bradley S 2007 Early nursing career experience for 1994–2000 graduates from the University of Nottingham. Journal of Nursing Management 15(4):414–423

Pearson A, Field J, Jordan Z 2007 Evidence-based clinical practice in nursing and healthcare: assimilating research, experience and expertise. Blackwell, Oxford

Peplau HE 1952 Interpersonal relations in nursing. Putnam, London

Rafferty AM 1996 The politics of nursing knowledge. Routledge, London

Rafferty AM, Ball J, Aiken LH 2001 Are teamwork and professional autonomy compatible, and do they result in improved hospital care? Quality in Health Care 10(Suppl. 2):ii, 32–37

Rees G, Huby G, McDade L, McKechnie L 2004 Joint working in community mental health teams: implementation of an integrated care pathway. Health and Social Care in the Community 12 (6):527–536

Roper N, Logan WW, Tierney AJ 1980 The elements of nursing. Churchill Livingstone, Edinburgh

Roper N, Logan WW, Tierney AJ 2000 The Roper–Logan–Tierney model of nursing: based on activities of living. Elsevier, Edinburgh

Roy C 1976 Introduction to nursing: an adaptation model. Prentice Hall, Englewood Cliffs

Royal College of Nursing 2003 Defining nursing. Royal College of Nursing, London. Available online: http://www.rcn.org.uk/__data/assets/pdf_file/0008/78569/001998.pdf (accessed March 2008)

Schon DA 1991 The reflective practitioner – how professionals think in action. Avebury, Aldershot

Springhouse 2007 Nursing care planning made incredibly easy. Springhouse Publications, Pennsylvania

Standing M 2007 Clinical decision-making skills on the developmental journey from student to registered nurse: a longitudinal inquiry. Journal of Advanced Nursing 60(3):257–269

Strauss SE, Scott Richardson W, Glasziou P, Haynes RB 2005 Evidence based medicine, 3rd edn. Churchill Livingstone, Edinburgh

Swage T 2003 Clinical governance in health care practice, 2nd edn. Butterworth-Heinemann, Oxford

Tiley S, Watson R 2005 Accountability in nursing and midwifery, 2nd edn. Blackwell Publishing, Oxford

Treaty of Lisbon 2007 Available online: http://europa.eu/lisbon_treaty/index_en.htm (accessed May 2008)

United Kingdom Central Council 1986 Project 2000: a new preparation for practice. United Kingdom Central Council for Nurses, Midwives and Health Visitors, London

UK Centre for the History of Nursing and Midwifery Available online: http://www.ukchnm.org/education/bibliographies/nursing-a-profession (accessed March 2008)

Watson J 1979 Nursing: the philosophy and science of caring. Little, Brown, Boston

Wimpenny P 2002 The meaning of models of nursing to practising nurses. Journal of Advanced Nursing 40(3):346–354

World Health Organization 2002 Strategic directions for strengthening nursing and midwifery services. World Health Organization, Geneva

World Health Organization 2006 Working together for health – the world health report. World Health Organization, Geneva

Chapter 2

Communication

Paul Crawford and Brian Brown

KEY ISSUES

SUBJECT KNOWLEDGE
- General models of communication
- The biological basis of communication
- Language acquisition
- Non-verbal communication
- Psychosocial factors influencing communication
- The role of culture in narratives of health and illness

CARE DELIVERY KNOWLEDGE
- Models for health communication approaches
- Interviewing and assessment
- Giving information, promoting health and teaching
- Communicating feedback
- Difficult communication
- Counselling and developing a therapeutic relationship

PROFESSIONAL AND ETHICAL KNOWLEDGE
- Professional and legal aspects of record keeping
- Confidentiality and access to records
- Complaints and communication
- Patient advocacy

PERSONAL AND REFLECTIVE KNOWLEDGE
- Reviewing the use of language in nursing
- Four case scenarios related to the four branches of nursing

INTRODUCTION

The ways in which people communicate have profound effects on those around them. It is over 50 years since Peplau (1952) took the first steps in redefining nursing as an interpersonal, interpretive process (Tilley 1999), providing one of the first manifestos for the study of nursing as a communicative process:

> *nurses – like other human beings – act on the basis of the meaning of events to them, that is, on the basis of their immediate interpretation of the climate and performances that transpire in a particular relationship. At the same time, the patient will act on the basis of the meaning of his illness to him. The interaction between nurse and patient is fruitful when a method of communication that identifies and uses common meanings is at work in the situation.*
> *(Peplau 1952: 283–284)*

The impact of this view of the nursing encounter has been profound and there has been an explosion of research and theory on communication processes in health care. Indeed, a recent search of the CINAHL® (Cumulative Index to Nursing and Allied Health) database yielded nearly 5000 citations in response to the terms 'nursing' and 'communication'. Consequently, it is important for practitioners to understand the major trends and topics in the study of communication, and to incorporate this knowledge within professional practice. It is clear that communication is a life-changing activity and very different results can emerge from the process of caring for others depending on how it is performed. Inadequate inter- and intraprofessional communication, as well as poor communication between staff and patients, has been consistently cited as a cause for concern by Ombudsman reports on the National Health Service (NHS) in the UK (Parliamentary and Health Service Ombudsman 2006). 'Communication is a cornerstone of the nurse–patient relationship. The power of effective nursing care is strengthened and enriched by good communication' (Sheldon et al 2006: 141).

This chapter addresses a variety of facets of the communication process in health care. The study of communication is a lifetime's work; the examples presented here demonstrate its importance in the life of an effective and compassionate practitioner.

OVERVIEW

Subject knowledge

In this section the theory and modes of communication are introduced. The biological basis of communication is outlined through describing the sensory organs and the interpretation of language and non-verbal signals in the brain. Insight into ideas about how and why human beings come to be language users is an important area to understand. Knowledge of the rich and versatile range of gestures, sounds and facial expressions which go to make up face-to-face communications is important for nurses. Finally, modes of communication that are used by health professionals to both care for, and control, clients are discussed.

Care delivery knowledge

There are various aspects to communication in care delivery, from questioning, interviewing and assessing patients to information giving, teaching and promoting health. At the heart of all communication should be general counselling skills and the means of developing a therapeutic relationship. In addition, care professionals need to keep accurate and appropriate records and need to be able to deal with a variety of communication difficulties. In performing these activities, however, it is important to consider how language can be used to comfort, socialize and establish roles as well as to restrict and punish individuals.

Professional and ethical knowledge

In this section, legal and ethical issues concerning record keeping are considered. The implications of good and bad record keeping are contrasted and the implications for service users, care workers and professionals are discussed. The quality of care that clients receive can depend on adequate communication so in the final section of this chapter, the nurse's role in client advocacy within this context is examined.

Personal and reflective knowledge

This chapter will enhance awareness of the importance of language in nursing and provide a basic understanding of what it takes to be a critical and sensitive communicator. This section helps you to reflect on the implications of issues raised within this chapter for your day-to-day practice. On pages 39–41 are four case studies, each one relating to one of the branch programmes. You may find it helpful to read one of them before you start the chapter and use it as a focus for your reflections while reading.

SUBJECT KNOWLEDGE

CONCEPTUALIZING COMMUNICATION: MODELS AND THEORIES

Communication is at the heart of all individuals' interpersonal lives – that is how they relate to others – and also their internal worlds of thoughts and feelings. Most people move freely in and out of these two realms of dialogue throughout their waking hours. Indeed, humans are always communicating – to themselves or to others. If they are not speaking, writing or gesticulating, then they are likely to be receiving messages from others. Thus, it is impossible to switch off communication since everything individuals do, even silence, sends out messages.

Reflection and portfolio evidence

Sit quietly for a few minutes and think about all the different kinds of communication going on around you.

- What do you hear, see, think and feel? As you do this, you will be experiencing the internal monologue of your own thoughts, and external verbal and non-verbal exchanges of other people. You will remind yourself that communication is the most important or central human activity.
- Extend this exercise by spending 5 or 10 minutes observing the kinds of communication that take place in your practice area. You may wish to repeat this activity at different times of the day or in different clinical situations. If applicable, record your findings in your portfolio.

In considering communication, the first task is to consider ways in which scholars have attempted to define and model the communication process. How people send and receive messages and the kinds of messages involved is complex. A number of scholars have tried to build models or metaphors of the communication process.

GENERAL MODELS OF COMMUNICATION

Early beginnings: the one–way flow

One of the oldest 'folk models' of communication sees it as a kind of conduit, where thoughts are translated into words and language transfers the thoughts bodily from one person to another. This began with Shannon & Weaver's (1949) model of communication, where an information source passes the message to a transmitter and the message then passes down a channel (originally, a telephone wire) and reaches the destination or recipient. This kind of thinking is also found in Lasswell's (1948) classic formula 'Who says what to whom in what channel with what effects'. These metaphors of communication tend to see communication as being rather like the transport of goods, services and people (Carey 1989). Examples of communication conceived upon this model include information sheets about drugs or illnesses, leaflets, pamphlets books and latterly websites where information is, hopefully, transmitted to the reader.

Communicating as a transaction: the two-way flow

In contrast to the one-way flow model, some researchers and theorists have proposed two-way or transactional models of communication (Ratzan et al 1996). Two-way communications are the preferred model in nurse–patient exchanges because they involve dialogue between sender and receiver where shared meaning and mutual understanding can be more easily developed. In other words, they involve a feedback loop (Kreps 2001). In health care, feedback is sometimes invited through questionnaires or given as part of teaching or supervision, but equally influential are the nods, smiles and 'uh-huh' sounds that people use during conversations.

Cognitivist models

These models of language emphasize how we process and interpret the information and explore how communication may be subject to psychological factors, hence the term 'cognitivist models'. Language is believed to be shaped by the individual speaker's intentions, mental representations, the neurological basis or 'hard-wiring' of their language faculties, and decoded in terms of the receiver's interpretative frameworks to make sense of any message (Chomsky 1993, Fodor 1998). Thus, in this model, any communication can be influenced by beliefs, values, assumptions and prejudices. Additionally, perceptual differences and distortions among individuals can affect communication. Any social event or situation will yield a variety of interpretations depending upon who perceives it. In this view the language is a window into the mind and what we say or write reflects a variety of preceding cognitive, emotional and neurological states. For example Reilly & Lambrecht (2001) argue that nurse–patient communication will improve if nurses develop an appreciation of patients' thoughts, feelings, situations and behaviour.

Contexts and intentions of communication

Another way of making sense of communication is to consider the context and purpose for sender and message,

following the Russian linguist Roman Jakobson (1960). In this tradition, theorists are also interested in how the context or circumstances in which individuals find themselves determines the meaning of any message. People are believed to engage in a good deal of 'recipient tailoring' to make the speech suit the situation (Brown & Fraser 1979).

Language as action: the theory of speech acts

All communication is a kind of action, that is, it has a purpose – promising, warning, threatening, praising, apologizing and so on (Searle 1979). Communication is fundamentally an activity; it is a way of doing things and getting others to do them. In Habermas's (1995) theory of communicative action, humans establish their persona or identity through communication with others. Sumner (2001) notes that these communicative actions in nursing can, if successful, lead to a sense of fulfilment and validation for client and carer. Hyde et al (2005) agree with Habermas that effective communicative action can make social processes such as nursing more empowering and democratic.

Language as a construction yard: co-constructing realities through language

In contrast to the above humanistic models of communication, there are other ways of conceptualizing the process of communication. To some students of communication in health care, language is a way of constructing reality in healthcare encounters. In this sense language is a kind of construction yard where versions of reality can be created (Potter 1996). As Fox (1993) demonstrated, a patient who has just undergone an operation may be in a great deal more pain than before the intervention, yet it is the job of the medical team to put a favourable gloss on this often unhappy situation. They do this by focusing on upbeat topics like the number of days until discharge, or until the stitches can come out.

This construction yard model of communication may sound abstract, but it is a useful way to think about the process of communication in nursing. For example, Bricher (1999: 453) describes how trust can be constructed between nurses and sick children. As one of her respondents said: 'I show them a photo of my dog and they realize … that you've got a backyard and a dog too, … not just this person that sticks suppositories up'. Within children's nursing, this focus can be particularly valuable. Trust is important in healthcare relationships (Sellman 2007); it enables treatments to be undertaken with a minimum of distress, and even when a distressing procedure is undertaken, the relationship can be quickly re-established.

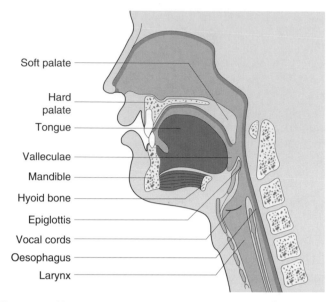

Figure 2.1 Normal anatomy of the head and neck (after Kristen Wienandt Marzejon, with kind permission; kristen@medartdesign.com).

So far this chapter has presented a variety of theories related to communication, and sketched out a number of different research approaches, demonstrating what language may do in health care. But how did human beings become technically competent as communicators in the first place?

THE BIOLOGICAL BASIS OF COMMUNICATION

Communication is founded in human anatomy and physiology. In speech, several parts of anatomy are involved: mouth, nose, pharynx, epiglottis, trachea and lungs (Fig. 2.1). These combine and relate to produce particular kinds of sound that make up the medium for conveying messages to others. But beyond direct speaking mechanisms, other parts of the body support and bring about communication. From the ears and eyes to complexes of muscles and the nervous system, individuals are able to do such things as type on a keyboard, write, or produce and receive a vast range of verbal and non-verbal messages. Moreover, this activity is facilitated by a variety of neurological processes. The next section examines these in more detail, beginning with a summary of mechanisms of speech.

Mechanisms of speech

To speak is to articulate sound by pushing air out of the lungs, through the trachea and into the larynx where vocal cords take up one of two positions. When the vocal cords are drawn together like a stiff pair of curtains, the air from the lungs has to push them apart, and this causes a vibration which can be experienced by placing a finger on the top of the larynx and producing sounds like [z]. Sounds made this way are described as 'voiced'. When the vocal cords are left apart, however, air passes silently to make 'voiceless' sounds such as [s] or [f]. In its journey onwards, the air passing through the larynx moves into the mouth and/or nose where sounds are formed by changing the shape of the oral cavity, notably with the tongue. Many of the sounds produced in this way form words, but a significant proportion form what have been termed 'guggles' or paralinguistic cues – expressions of surprise, support, 'um hmm', 'ah ha' and so forth which may be used to support and encourage a speaker or to indicate that a person wishes to interrupt. They are an informative part of the 'music' of conversation (Scherer et al 2002). Once sounds have been made, they must be perceived for communication to take place. In the ear, sound waves – a kind of 'compression wave' in the air – are converted into nervous impulses and enter the brain via the cochlear nerve. The basic anatomy of the ear is shown in Figure 2.2. Sound waves enter the ear via the pinna and outer ear canal and vibrate the eardrum or tympanum. This transmits vibration via the bones of the ear (the hammer, anvil and stirrup) to the cochlea, which is rich in nerve endings that are able to detect the minute deformations in the tissues caused by the vibrations and turn them into nerve impulses. These impulses then pass along the auditory nerve to the midbrain and then to the auditory cortex of the temporal lobes. The processing of sound into meaningful units of communication is not well understood, but it is

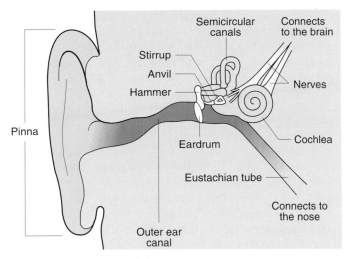

Figure 2.2 The anatomy of the ear.

possible that different brain cells or groups of cells specialize in the recognition of certain sounds.

Communication difficulties and disabilities

If the sensory processes themselves are impaired, this can lead to communication difficulties. There are a variety of techniques which can be used to compensate for these impairments. For example, as well as mechanical aids such as implants and hearing aids, deaf and hearing impaired people can use a number of strategies to communicating which rely on the hands. A variety of techniques such as sign language (Fig. 2.3) and finger spelling may be employed (http://www.british-sign.co.uk) to convey meaning. There are also a variety of aids to help visually impaired people communicate, including: glasses, Braille, large print, books and magazines on tape, dark lined writing paper or even a grooved writing board, through to electronic aids such as label readers or voice recognition phone diallers. One critical aspect of non-verbal communication is the interpretation of facial expressions of emotion, and children with learning difficulties have been found to be less accurate than non-disabled children in making such interpretations. As Bandura (1986) has pointed out, the ability to read the signs of emotions in social interaction has important adaptive value in guiding actions toward others.

Message interpretation in the brain

The ability to use language is located in the brain, and debate has ensued about the locality for this specific function. The role of Broca's area in the human brain in the production of speech and Wernicke's area in understanding the significance of content words in speech has been appreciated since the 19th century (Dronkers 2000; Fig. 2.4). These two areas are linked by a bundle of nerve fibres called the *arcuate fasciculus*. These two main areas have been studied closely in relation to various forms of brain damage and how such lesions affect language production. Damage to Broca's area is related to difficulty in producing speech, while damage to Wernicke's area is related to speech comprehension difficulties. In addition, a part of the motor cortex, close to Broca's area, controls the muscles that articulate the face, tongue and larynx – all key to language production – which when damaged also affect communication.

If a client were to hear a word and repeat it, this suggests a simple transmission of a word being heard and understood in Wernicke's area; this area transfers a signal via the arcuate fasciculus to Broca's area, where production of the word is set up with a signal being sent to the motor cortex to put it out in a physical form by moving particular muscles, etc. Yet there is evidence that a large number of different areas of the brain are used for the production of spoken utterances

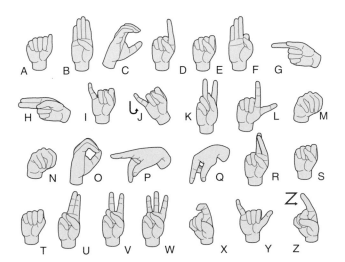

Figure 2.3 The alphabet in sign language.

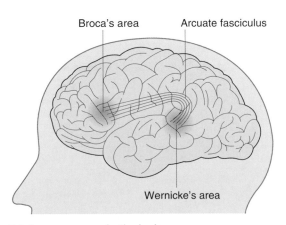

Figure 2.4 Language areas in the brain.

(Posner & Raichle 1997) and that different areas of the brain are activated for different aspects of speech. Hence, a rich variety of anatomical and physiological mechanisms and senses lie behind human communication, and scientists are still examining this complex phenomenon, just as they still have much to understand about consciousness itself. Thus, in contrast to a localized view of language functioning in particular parts of the brain, it appears that this human skill is wrapped up with interdependent aspects of brain function.

Sometimes people's predispositions may make them less likely to interpret cues in a particular way. For example those who are apt to be cynical or hostile are likely to misattribute happiness (Larkin et al 2002). Research has also revealed gender differences in the accuracy of decoding facial expressions of emotion, with males being less accurate than females (Pell 2002).

Language acquisition

It is extraordinary how children acquire language. As well as becoming competent users of a complex syntax, on average English-speaking children acquire a vocabulary of about 60 000 words by the age of 18. The early stages of children's communicative learning are outlined in Table 2.1. During peak vocabulary development periods during childhood this means learning a new word approximately every 2 hours. This has led some theorists, such as Chomsky (1976) and Pinker (1994), to suggest that there are somehow inbuilt – or as cognitive scientists sometimes say, 'hard-wired' – cognitive and neural structures that enable the grammar and lexicon to be learned so readily: in Chomsky's phrase, a 'language acquisition device'. This is debatable, however, and critics charge Chomsky and Pinker with paying insufficient attention to the sheer diversity of the world's languages, or with not considering how difficult it is to explain language

in evolutionary terms (Allott 2001). At the present state of knowledge, communication is far more than biology alone can explain, and to make sense of how communication has come to be employed we need to make sense of the evolution of cultural themes too (Oudeyer & Kaplan 2007).

Non-verbal communication

Much human communication is delivered through non-verbal channels or 'body language', and is not dependent on sound. Through gestures, postures and facial expressions, people convey rich vocabularies to others. Early attempts to study these phenomena identified about 20 000 different facial expressions (Birdwhistell 1970), which, when combined with gestures and movements yield about 700 000 different possibilities, which may or may not be meaningful (Pei 1997). Non-verbal communication involves a variety of issues (Patterson 1983). Some functions concern how an individual feels towards another person. That is, non-verbal communication may express feelings such as like or dislike; it can establish dominance or control; or it can be used to express intimacy, perhaps by touching and mutual eye contact. Non-verbal signals can be used to regulate interactions, for example by signalling the approaching end of an utterance or the desire to speak, or they may facilitate goal attainment, for example by pointing. Facial expressions add to this visual richness, especially through changes to the eyes and mouth. In interaction in contemporary Western cultures participants typically spend about 60% of the time gazing at one another and these gazes typically last about 3 seconds (Argyle & Ingham 1972). Mutual gazes take up 30% of the time, with the actual gaze lasting about 1 second (Kleineke 1986). The eyes often signal that a person is ready to speak or to end communication. The use of body space – how close people position themselves to others (proximity) – and the shape or posture they adopt affect how messages are sent

Table 2.1 Language development in children

Child's age	Communication development
0–4 months	Babies start to coo and produce vowel sounds. Will make sounds back when spoken to
6 months	Laughing. Will start to make consonant sounds like d, p and m
6–12 months	Laughing, smiling babbling. Multisyllable speech such as uh-oh, da-da. Points to objects of interest
12–24 months	Development of vocabulary – about 50 words by 18 months, or 100 by 24 months
2–3 years	Builds sentences such as 'doggy go home'. Acquires concepts such as 'in', 'under' or 'behind'
3–5 years	Development of vocabulary and syntactic ability (the grammatical arrangement of words). Can phrase requests. Sentences get longer. Working vocabulary of about 2300 words by the age of 5 and ability to comprehend 8000 words

and received. Whether individuals touch others, and how they do this, and what clothes they choose to wear signal messages such as status and bring yet more dynamics to communication. The issue of how well-attuned a healthcare professional is to the client's communicative preferences is therefore important. If healthcare professionals make decisions or communicate in a way that fails to account for clients' cultural beliefs and preferences, then the client's self-care, adherence to advice and overall outcome may well be poorer (Stewart et al 1999).

Decision-making exercise

Think of different styles of communication associated with different kinds of emotional tone. How would you speak and act if you were:

- Bullying?
- Nervous?
- Confident?
- Humorous?

Evidence suggests that people who are being abused would often like to talk to a health professional about it, but are unsure of how to broach the subject (McAfee 2001). Imagine that you had a client whose physical symptoms suggested that she came from an abusive family situation.

- How could you make it easier for her to disclose the problem? (Bear in mind that people in such a situation might not necessarily disclose this in response to a direct question.)
- Think about how you could use style of speech, vocabulary, delivery, facial expressions and gestures, or even the seating arrangements in the room to make it easier for the client.
- What systems should be in place to support you in dealing with this client?

Graphical communication

Drawing and graphical communication can be an important tool in the hands of nurses and their clients. Indeed, it may be especially useful when communicating with people from different language groups or with people who suffer sensory or communicative impairments. For example, there are cases of people who have been severely communication-impaired following a stroke but who have become functional communicators once more through drawing (Rao 1995). Some authors have also noted the way that drawings provide a useful window into the emotional lives of children who have suffered a traumatic event such as bereavement (Clements et al 2001, Wellings 2001).

PSYCHOSOCIAL FACTORS INFLUENCING COMMUNICATION

Communication takes place in a whole range of environments, involving people with a variety of identities and outlooks. Communication is affected by variables such as age, gender, social class, culture and ethnicity that can influence its content and style. Although this makes sense intuitively, it has been difficult reliably to identify specific markers or interpersonal differences in speech style (Hogg & Vaughan 2002), perhaps because people are extremely flexible and usually competent in several different speech styles. A person may be able to speak some version of the 'received pronunciation' (RP) or formal, official language in which a good deal of institutional business is done, yet at the same time, socially, may use a dialect or less formal language such as slang. The kind of language used, rules or laws of social behaviour, the social status and power relations of participants and the roles or life scripts that they have adopted may equally affect communication.

Decision-making exercise

Observe some interaction between consultant and nurse or nurse and patient. Look at the way they communicate. Observe who is in charge and note how this is manifested.

- How could you use this observation in your practice?
- For example, a patient adopting a 'sick role' may communicate in a very passive, dependent way. How would you counteract this tendency?
- If a consultant dominates a multidisciplinary team meeting, what might you as a nurse do to change the balance of power?

The speech style of a person in a powerless position tends to involve the use of features such as:

- 'intensifiers', e.g. 'very', 'really' and 'so'
- 'hedges', e.g. 'kind of', 'sort of', 'you know'
- rising intonation, which makes a declaration sound like a question
- polite forms of address (Lakoff 1975).

Power can be associated with the ability to interrupt and take control of the 'floor' in conversation (Reid & Ng 1999). Nearly 30 years ago, Zimmerman & West (1975) noted that 98% of interruptions were by men. More recently, although the situation has become more equitable, men are still more likely to interrupt, especially when interaction is studied in field settings and when there are more than three people present (Anderson & Leaper 1998).

Evidence-based practice

Interruptions can be considerably more than a nuisance. Individuals who interrupt a good deal may be doing this as part of the 'Type A' behaviour pattern, characterized by loud speech and frequent interruptions, as well as a rapid speech rate, hard-driving hurried behaviour, impatience and hostility. The Type A behaviour pattern has been associated with an increased likelihood of heart disease, originally by Friedman & Rosenman (1959), with the interest in speech styles being pursued by other researchers more recently (de Pino-Perez et al 1999, Zwaal et al, 2003). Indeed, Ekman & Rosenberg (1997) note that as well as rapid and aggressive speech, Type A behaviour is associated with more facial expressions of glare and disgust. Thus, communicative style can be a valuable clue that a person's lifestyle may be making them more vulnerable to illness (Zwaal et al 2003) and increasing their social isolation (Chen et al 2005). Friedman & Rosenman were cardiologists and their initial ideas were stimulated by noting that the edges of the seats in their consulting rooms wore away. Eventually they deduced that this was to do with the 'edge of the seat' stance of their impatient patients.

Gender differences in speech styles are not innate in any obvious sense, but reflect status differences in situations. We may anticipate changes in the pattern of gender differences as greater social, economic and occupational equality is achieved. In the meantime, Fairclough (1989) argues that nurses, among others, should be aware of 'how language contributes to the domination of some people by others' and suggests that being conscious of this 'is the first step towards emancipation' (Fairclough 1989: 1).

Awareness of language and communication thus involves an awareness of the diverse range of biological, personal and social factors that have an impact on the speech styles in use in health care. Becoming aware of these factors can enable nurses to work to change the situation to the benefit of clients and nurses themselves.

USING LANGUAGE IN HEALTH CARE

An individual's capacity for communication does not remain static, but changes over the lifespan, and adult communicators will be concerned with how to be efficient and effective communicators and avoid the pitfalls of communicating in limited, negative or harmful ways. The notion that language might be harmful is of particular importance in the context of health care, where the overriding premise is to promote human well-being (Crawford et al 1998).

Language, ideology and power

Nursing communication takes place in a context informed by wider political and economic directives, and involves communication with other healthcare professionals and patients. As such, it is caught in a web of powerful conceptions and ideologies of what society should be like, how it is constructed and what is important. According to Fairclough (1989), nursing is shaped by powerful ideologies of bureaucratic 'cost-effectiveness' and 'efficiency', and nurses' training tends to promote acquisition of communication or social skills 'whose primary motivation is efficient people-handling' (Fairclough 1989: 235). This may tempt nurses to communicate in a way which has more to do with economics, politics and the public image of the institution for which they work than with their profession's or their own value systems. The increasing conviction on the part of policymakers in the UK that there has been a power imbalance between patients and health care providers has led to a number of initiatives to try to ensure that patients' voices are heard. Of particular interest in the UK is the Commission for Patient and Public Involvement in Health (http://www.cppih.org), established in January 2003 as an independent public body, sponsored by the Department of Health, to ensure public involvement in decision making about health services. Across England there are over 400 Patient and Public Involvement (PPI) forums comprising volunteers in local communities who are involved in helping patients and members of the public to influence local healthcare delivery (Commission for Patient and Public Involvement in Health 2006). In an effort to strengthen the 'local voice' further, the UK government plans to replace these with Local Involvement Networks (LINks) (Department of Health 2006a). This reflects a belief on the part of policymakers that:

> NHS organisations, with their social care colleagues, need to have more effective and systematic ways of finding out what people want and need from their services. They need to reach out to those people whose needs are the greatest, to people who do not normally get involved and to people who find it hard to give their views.   (Department of Health 2006a: 11)

To ensure that voices are heard at an individual level, within the NHS there is the Patient Advice and Liaison Service (PALS; http://www.pals.nhs.uk/), which was introduced to 'ensure that the NHS listens to patients, their relatives, carers and friends, and answers their questions and resolves their concerns as quickly as possible' (Patient Advice and Liaison Service 2007). While the bodies involved and their jobs are dynamic and the sketch presented here simply represents the current situation at the time of writing, the focus on getting patients' needs taken seriously in the health services remains at the heart of policy and practice for the foreseeable future, and communication will play a central role in this process.

Telehealth and nursing

The American Telemedicine Association (2006) defines *tele-medicine* as 'the use of medical information exchanged from one site to another via electronic communications to improve patients' health status'. Telehealth covers a variety of activities in which information and communication technologies play a part. The term:

> is often used to encompass a broader definition of remote health care that may not involve clinical services. Video conferencing, transmission of still images, e-health including patient portals, remote monitoring of vital signs, continuing medical education, and nursing call centers are all considered part of telemedicine and telehealth.
>
> (Sorrells-Jones et al 2006: 42)

This can involve activities as simple as the use of the telephone to real-time monitoring of vital signs and online consultations. In the case of videolinks, a nurse can, for example, conduct an examination of a patient while at the same time being in audiovisual communication with other specialists who may assess the patient's problems remotely. In the UK, there is acknowledgement of the benefits of so called e-medicine, especially in rural areas where there may be isolated or elderly clients. However, barriers can be encountered, especially where there is limited training, or where providers baulk at the initial cost of setting up facilities and associated increases in workload (Richards et al 2005).

Kinds of talk in healthcare settings

Language can be a means of socializing a client into a particular kind of role, as a patient, a victim, as someone who is in pain or as someone who is incapable. There has been considerable research about the role of language styles and plot structures in enabling the roles of healthcare professionals and patients to be performed. Proctor et al (1996) studied how nurses in a trauma centre in a US hospital talked to injured patients. By video-taping interactions between nurses and patients in pain, the 'Comfort talk register' was identified, which included the following functions:

- *Holding on* was conducted through the use of phrases like 'Big girl', 'You're doing great', 'Count to three'. This served to praise, to let the patient know they can get through, to support, to instruct or distract the patient.
- *Assessing* involved 'How are you?' questions or giving the patient information – 'You're in the emergency room'. These involved getting information, explaining the situation or validating and confirming the patient's input.
- *Informing* were statements like 'It's gonna hurt' or 'We'll be inserting a catheter', i.e. warning the patient or explaining procedures.

- *Caring* included statements like 'Relax' or 'OK sweetie' or 'It does hurt, doesn't it?', i.e. reassuring, empathic or caring comments (Proctor et al 1996: 1673).

The authors suggest that because comfort talk is regularly used, it has a rhythmical, sing-song quality aimed at getting patients to endure the situation for longer. This highlights the importance of the style and content of communication in managing treatment.

The negative use of communication

As nurses deal with clients, some features of their language can be a source of complaint. Caregivers interacting with elderly clients have been observed using high-pitched baby talk, controlling institutional talk, short utterances, simple grammatical structures, interrogatives (questions) and imperatives (commands) (Ambady et al 2002). Moreover, there is some evidence to suggest that use of patronizing speech styles does not depend on the status of the patient – the confused are no more likely to be patronized than those who are alert and oriented. Rather, the speech style seemed to depend on the attitudes of the caregiver (Caporael et al 1983). The features of speech and non-verbal behaviour – for example high pitch, pats on the shoulder and expressions like 'That's a good girl' – are perceived by the elderly patients themselves as patronizing, and are seen as unfavourable by observers (Ryan et al 1994). It is important that those working with elderly people are aware of such behaviour and that instruction is incorporated into the education of caregivers (Ryan et al 1994).

Evidence-based practice

Anger in healthcare settings is a major problem. In the Healthcare Commission's NHS survey for 2006 (Healthcare Commission 2007a) 11% of staff had experienced physical violence and 26% had experienced bullying, harassment or abuse from patients or their relatives. Hollinworth et al (2005) note that there are many things that nurses can do to avert potentially angry responses.

To illustrate this let us consider a classic example from Albert Robillard (1996), a sociologist who suffers multiple disabilities arising from motor neurone disease, movingly describing the effects of patronizing talk. He illustrates people's responses to his anger at this kind of mistreatment thus:

> The response of my interlocutors to my visible anger ranges from 'I did not know you could hear', 'I didn't know you could think!', 'Most of my patients are stroke victims and have trouble understanding me' to 'Oh, I am sorry, I won't do it again.' Most react to my outburst by ignoring me, leading me to see the ignoral as a further documentary reading of my symptomatology by my interlocutor.

Continued

Hollinworth et al (2005) note fragmentary care from a variety of practitioners who may each seem ill prepared to deal with patients' problems. Also, practitioners who talk down to patients or who talk among themselves can contribute to feelings of exclusion on the part of patients and carers and may prompt an angry response. Equally, fear, physical illness and disability, confusion and pain may all present as anger.

Institutional care encourages dependency, by means of both open (overt) and secret or disguised (covert) strategies on the part of care staff (Ryan & Scullion 2000). Although the situation is changing slowly, being a 'good patient' traditionally involved being passive, compliant and docile. The language of the institution is thought to be more important in producing dependency than the disability itself. Moreover, despite the ethic of care in such institutions, the experience of being cared for is often profoundly dehumanizing:

> *Older residents must adapt to a new set of routines, expectations and rules, frequently compromising or abandoning their own lifetime preferences, habits and needs. Further, they must make these adaptations from the socially inferior or less powerful role of resident or patient.* (Ryan et al 1994: 238)

The role of language may be to offer comfort and to enlist clients in the rituals of health care in a way that will ultimately benefit them. It is important, however, to be aware of how language might just as easily patronize or incapacitate clients and place them in a position where they are disadvantaged.

THE ROLE OF CULTURE IN NARRATIVES OF HEALTH AND ILLNESS

Fundamental ideas about medicine are embedded in culture and language. Within the UK in the 21st century, most people think that they know what a sick person is. Everyday complaints like the common cold and gastrointestinal upsets have a set of symptoms that are expected to co-occur. However, history suggests that the way illness is defined depends a great deal on recent changes in patterns of sickness and health. Contemporary illnesses are different from those described in the 18th century – people no longer claim to suffer from 'seizures of the bowels' or 'rising of the lights'. Nevertheless, in all centuries, the coherence of an illness is an important part of the sufferer's experience of it. Concern with

narrative emerges from the everyday observation that when we find out about someone, we usually do so by means of a story that they tell or which someone else tells about them. These stories are important because they do not merely describe experience but constitute or make it. Nurses narrate both their own stories of care and the stories told to them by clients. This does not mean that the stories nurses tell are pure fictions, but much of what happens between nurses and patients is to do with narration. This idea has been developed in psychology, sociology, anthropology and in the study of medical and nursing activities and the experiences of clients.

Narratives also reflect the interests of the teller. For example, Hyden (1995) describes how in cases of domestic violence, male perpetrators favour words that emphasize purpose (why they acted as they did) whereas female partners emphasize agency (how they were beaten) and the physical and emotional consequences. This kind of storytelling reveals another important feature – the communicators are often at pains to manage their 'stake' and 'interest' in the piece. A critical comment about a patient may be prefaced with the claim 'I usually try to be on the patient's side, but . . .'. Everyday speech is littered with similar examples. Homophobic comments are often accompanied by statements like 'Some of my best friends are gay' or potential accusations of ethnic prejudice are headed off with 'I'm not racist but . . .'. In narratives of illness encountered by nurses, it is important to consider the role that culture has in helping to make sense of these phenomena. In European or North American white majority cultures, the degree of correspondence between the stories told by clients and professionals makes it easy to take signs, symptoms, syndromes and illnesses for granted. However, it is important to realize that if this cultural frame of reference is moved, the problems people express may seem at odds with dominant Western medical notions of health and illness.

CARE DELIVERY KNOWLEDGE

Much of nursing care delivery is about communicating in day-to-day spoken and written interactions with members of the healthcare team, patients and relatives. This might take place in such activities as assessment and care planning, information giving, teaching and health promotion, record keeping, dealing with communication difficulties and challenging communication, and in counselling and building therapeutic relationships. These areas will be explored further, but first, we must introduce models for communication approaches.

MODELS FOR HEALTH COMMUNICATION APPROACHES

A variety of theoretical models are available to guide nurses in reflecting and analysing communication. For example: the interpersonal relations model (Peplau 1952), client-centred therapy (Rogers 1951), the skilled helper (Egan 1974), six-category intervention analysis (Heron 1990) and the brief, ordinary and effective (BOE) model (Crawford et al 2006). Such models can be further investigated as commitment to continuing professional development, and as part of portfolio keeping. An excellent starting point for gaining a framework for therapeutic communication is Rogers's client-centred therapy which sets out 'to promote the growth, development, maturity, improved functioning and improved coping with life of the other' (Rogers 1951) through what he calls the core conditions in any helping relationship: acceptance (unconditional positive regard), empathy, and genuineness/congruence. This and other frameworks can be used to reflect upon communication exchanges and shape subsequent interactions.

Brief, ordinary, effective (BOE) model for communication in health care (Crawford et al 2006)

Recently, the brief, ordinary and effective (BOE) model (Crawford et al 2006) has been developed to help practitioners adapt their communication to busy health settings. Given demands on contemporary healthcare professionals and the limited time to carry out interventions it is crucial that practitioners use brief, ordinary and effective means of communication (Brown et al 2006, Crawford et al 2006). A key idea behind the model is that brief interactions can be bigger 'inside' than they appear from the 'outside' (the 'Tardis effect'). It challenges the view that communication can get in the way of healthcare encounters and offers an alternative to the more 'time-greedy' counselling models, calling for practitioners to adapt to task-dominated environments and utilize even momentary time slots to good effect. Such momentary and synchronous communication (that which takes place at the same time as completing other tasks) can create an emotionally supportive and communicative environment for patients and healthcare staff alike.

INTERVIEWING AND ASSESSMENT

Communication is particularly important in relation to assessment and planning care. In the UK, health and social care policy is increasingly focused on supporting people in their own homes rather than in hospital or nursing home environments. Good interprofessional communication is therefore vital to ensure a quality seamless service for the patient between home, health and social care organizations. Assessment, even with the very vulnerable or frail, should include the client as an active collaborator in the assessment process. The UK's Better Services for Vulnerable People agenda (Department of Health 1997a) has called upon local authorities to review their practice of multidisciplinary assessment of people with complex needs. Assessment should also provide care plans that help users achieve their personal goals (Department of Health 1998).

The assessment process

Despite technological advance, users and carers may have to repeat their stories to different health and social care professionals, facing various assessments with a limited coordination between agencies. This leads to separate assessment records being compiled with interview schedules peculiar to different professional groups (Health Committee 1999). However, there are increasing examples of interagency patient-held records which maximize the availability of a range of information to interested professionals, and also give the client a greater sense of ownership over their plan of care. In Children's Services specifically, the Common Assessment Framework (CAF) is emerging in response to such an identified need as a part of Every Child Matters (ECM) agenda (Department for Education and Science 2003). Nolan & Caldock (1996) suggest criteria for how the assessment process can be carried out (Box 2.1). The criteria in Box 2.1 are based on good communication and an acknowledgement of the central role of the client in the assessment process.

Reflection and portfolio evidence

In your practice placement, review the documentation and interactions that take place during the assessment of a patient/client.

- Reflect on how helpful the assessment process is in allowing the patient control over the subsequent plan of care.
- Review whether it is the approach of the individual professional that is of primary importance rather than the particular documentation used for assessment.
- Comment on the level of 'interprofessional' assessment achieved through the model in use.
- Record your findings in your portfolio.

GIVING INFORMATION, PROMOTING HEALTH AND TEACHING

The role of the nurse increasingly involves giving information, promoting health and teaching. As Hargie & Dickson (2004: 203) write: 'Giving adequate and relevant information

---

Box 2.1 Suggestions for the assessment process (from Nolan & Caldock 1996)

1. Empower both the user and carer – inform fully, clarify their understanding of the situation and of the role of the assessor before going ahead.
2. Involve the user and carer – make them feel that they are full partners in the assessment.
3. Shed your 'professional' perspective – have an open mind and be prepared to learn.
4. Start from where the user and carer are – establish their existing level of knowledge and what hopes and expectations they have.
5. Be interested in the user and carer as people.
6. Establish a suitable environment for the assessment which ensures there is privacy, quiet and sufficient time.
7. Take time – build trust and rapport and overcome the brief visitor syndrome; this will usually take more than one encounter.
8. Be sensitive, imaginative and creative in responding – users and carers may not know what is possible or available. For carers in particular, guilt and reticence may have to be overcome.
9. Avoid value judgements whenever possible – if such judgements are needed, make them explicit.
10. Consider social, emotional and relationship needs as well as practical needs and difficulties. Pay particular attention to the quality of the relationship between user and carer.
11. Listen to and value the user's and the carer's expertise and opinions, even if these run counter to your own values as a professional.
12. Present honest, realistic service options, identifying advantages and disadvantages and providing an indication of any delay or limitations in delivery of the service.
13. Do not make assessment a 'battle' in which users and carers feel they have to fight for services.
14. Balance all perspectives.
15. Clarify understanding at the end of the assessment, agree objectives and the nature of the review process.

---

and explanation can result in tangible benefits to patients in terms of reduced pain and discomfort, anxiety and depression, and earlier recovery ... It can also promote patient adherence to treatment regimes'. Poor explanations and information giving can result in patients forgetting key facts and may work against patient empowerment. We can adapt Silverman et al's (2005) identification of the process of providing the correct amount and type of information as follows:

- Assessing the patient's prior knowledge and wish for information.
- Signposting the kinds of information that will be given.

- Organizing information in a logical manner.
- Giving information in assimilable chunks and checking for understanding.
- Giving explanations and opinions at the right time.
- Using repetition and summarizing.
- Using visual methods of conveying information.
- Relating explanations to the patient's concerns and expectations.
- Asking what other information would be helpful.
- Encouraging the patient to seek clarification, ask questions.
- Picking up that the patient may be distressed by or over-loaded with information.

(Adapted from Silverman et al 2005: 147)

Providing information is at the heart of health promotion and has a number of aspects for nursing.

Health promotion not only encompasses a nurse educating an individual about his health needs, but also demands that the nurse play her part in attempting to address the wider environmental and social issues that adversely affect people's health (Mackintosh 1996: 14).

Despite this expanding role, there is little systematic evaluation of whether such activity has been effective. Nevertheless guidance can be offered based on existing knowledge about effective health communication and education:

- Determine individual learning styles, adopting a flexible approach to presentation of material to suit the learner.
- Establish and maintain effective learning environments. This means paying attention to when and where teaching takes place.
- Plan and structure learning activities. Where possible, it is best to set out learning objectives and outcomes for any teaching, paying attention to time limits and resources.
- Use appropriate resources to support learning. There are various resources available to enhance teaching, for example PowerPoint presentations, audiovisual materials, the Internet, and so on.
- Where possible provide handouts for any session, with suggested reading, and follow-up questions.
- It is desirable to undertake evaluations to determine whether the intervention is suitable for the client's needs and values, and aids their overall health (Whitehead 2003).

COMMUNICATING FEEDBACK

A key aspect of professional nursing is giving and receiving feedback. How we go about this process will either positively or negatively impact on our relationships with colleagues, our patients and their relatives. As Betts (1995) notes, the functions of feedback include promoting self-awareness by assimilating information about how others see us; providing new perspectives and options; reinforcing positive or productive behaviour; and motivating and valuing other people.

2.3 – COMMUNICATING FEEDBACK

Objectives:
- Components of feedback.
- A good environment for feedback.
- How to offer effective feedback.

DIFFICULT COMMUNICATION

In this section we consider the impact of communication difficulties, breaking bad news, and dealing with interpersonal conflict that might lead to aggression and violence.

Communication difficulties

Everyone experiences minor communication difficulties periodically. Take, for example, how sound production can be a problem when you have a sore throat, after receiving local anaesthetic at the dentist, or even when your mouth is very dry. Nurses may be called upon to work with clients with more serious communication difficulties. The nature of many illnesses is such that the client's ability to communicate is impaired, for example, and most obviously, in the case of loss of consciousness. Yet even under these circumstances, there are reports of people remembering conversations around them while they were apparently comatose or anaesthetized, thus highlighting the importance of ensuring that communication is appropriate. Disorders of speech may be due to problems with anatomical mechanisms for speech (*dysarthria*). A variety of speech and language problems arise when people suffer strokes or dementia, or have learning difficulties, sensory impairments and mental health problems, all of which may impair a person's communicative abilities. In strokes, for example, it is common for the sufferer's comprehension or expression of speech to be disturbed (*dysphasia*). Among clients who are conscious and attempting to recover communication ability, specific therapy may be undertaken by a speech therapist, but nurses will be the front-line carers. There are a number of reports in the literature of nurses being able to screen patients for difficulties with chewing, drinking and swallowing (Dumble & Tuson 1998, Cantwell 2000) which may require more specialist interventions and yield improvements in communication. The idea that communication is concerned with the reciprocal and mutually constitutive interactions between clients and their carers is important. According to Sundin et al (2001), identity is established through relationships, and the loss of a person's ability to communicate threatens their sense of self. Once people's communicative ability has been impaired, perhaps through a stroke, social relationships become much more difficult. In Sundin et al's (2001) study of the professional carers of people who had been disabled through stroke they detected a tendency to see the patients as fragile and vulnerable; at the same time it was felt to be important to support them in a way which sustained their dignity and did not make them feel even more disabled. Equally, important parts of the caring practice with these communication-impaired patients involved developing relationships, developing feelings of closeness and sensitivity often involving non-verbal communication. This was seen to be achievable by spending time with the patient as a companion, not necessarily just attending to the mechanics of care.

2.4 – COMMUNICATING WITH THE ANXIOUS/STRESSED, DEPRESSED OR CONFUSED PATIENT

Objectives:
- Key factors in assessment of anxious/stressed, depressed or confused patients.
- Skills for assessment of anxious/stressed, depressed or confused patients.
- Skills for communicating with anxious/stressed, depressed or confused patients.

Breaking bad news

Bad news is any information that a person does not wish to hear. Nurses are sometimes called upon to break bad news to patients and their loved ones. Bad news is often associated with a terminal illness such as cancer but is, in part, a perception of the client and is not always connected with life/death issues.

The following approaches should be taken when breaking bad news:

- Prepare all relevant information beforehand.
- Ensure privacy and non-interruption.
- Encourage the attendance of key relative/advocate.

- Summarize actions, interventions and progress to date.
- Seek out the person's current perspective.
- Use sensitive language and a sympathetic voice.
- Indicate that there is difficult news coming.
- Provide clear, steadily paced, chunk-by-chunk information (bad news).
- Empathize and be accepting of unique responses.
- Assess the person's reaction to the information.
- Provide honest yet sensitively delivered responses to questions.
- Support through appropriate touch and increased proximity.
- Allow the person to express anger, silence, passivity, withdrawal and loss of concentration (shutdown).
- Facilitate further exploration of issues, helping the person adapt to the news, make decisions and come to their own conclusions.
- Address concerns and emphasize your role in support/ further interventions.
- Consider and facilitate additional space and time for the individual and significant other to come to terms with the bad news at their own pace and without direction.

Dealing with interpersonal conflict

Interpersonal conflict can occur for a number of reasons, such as a person feeling offended, misunderstood, frustrated or blocked in some way in achieving their goals. Conflict may be displayed in verbal and non-verbal behaviour and lead to aggression or violence if unresolved. Since healthcare environments can be stressful, nurses need to possess the necessary skills to de-escalate and manage conflict situations and be able to apply local complaints procedures.

2.5 – DEALING WITH INTERPERSONAL CONFLICT

Objectives:
- Dealing with flashpoints and managing anger.
- What to do if you feel threatened.
- Managing telephone complaints.

COUNSELLING AND DEVELOPING A THERAPEUTIC RELATIONSHIP

This section examines some of the basic types and styles of communication needed for general counselling and building therapeutic relationships.

Listening and gaining rapport

In order to develop a therapeutic relationship with patients, it is vital to remember the finer aspects of courteous communication that are often taken for granted in daily life but are complained about bitterly when someone does not use them. For example, it is important to properly meet and greet clients in a respectful way. This may mean, for example, addressing them by a formal name such as 'Mrs Brown' and only using informal first name terms if invited to. For most clients brought up in a Western culture, an appropriate non-verbal performance should include facing the client with an open posture (not arms folded), leaning slightly towards them, with regular but not fixed eye contact, and maintaining a relaxed demeanour. By adopting such a stance and by attending to a person and actively listening in a genuine way to what they have to say (rather than thinking about what you are going to say next), or simply giving time to share your 'presence' with them, you will begin the process of gaining rapport or bonding with the client.

When listening to clients it is important to use an appropriate level of verbal prompts such as 'Yes', 'Go on', 'I see' or 'OK' and non-verbal prompts such as nodding, smiling, etc. These signal that you are interested in what they are saying. Again, avoid fiddling with objects while conversing, or looking away or over the patient's shoulder.

The process of gaining rapport will be further enhanced by demonstrating that you are a 'warm', authentic individual who is not going to judge in a negative fashion what they have to say, and that your attitudes and values are driven by 'unconditional positive regard' – you do not compromise or restrict your esteem or valuation of the patient even when their values, morals or behaviour do not agree with your own. Finally, fundamental to this whole process of gaining a client's trust and creating a therapeutic relationship, is empathy – attempting to enter into and understand what it might be like being a particular patient, in particular circumstances, in conversation with you.

Reflection and summarizing

One of the common ways that reflection on the content of what others say is facilitated is by paraphrasing. Rather than 'parrot-phrasing', in which what the other person said is merely repeated, paraphrasing involves restating in brief what was said in order to:

- Clarify whether they were heard accurately.
- Provide an opportunity to reflect on what was said (the content).
- Encourage further development of ideas or issues.

It is often also helpful to reflect back or acknowledge feelings or emotions that were expressed verbally and non-verbally during the conversation. This can deepen the sense of empathy and may help to review areas in the individual's life that need addressing. By summarizing the content of a conversation it is possible to draw together the key aspects of what was communicated. This can help to bring a shape to what may have been an unstructured discussion, and may lead to exploring possible solutions to problems. Once rapport is established, negotiating solutions can occur in a creative process of formulating new approaches or strategies, and where unhelpful thinking or behaviours can be challenged and reframed into a new, more helpful perspective.

Thus, a key aspect of assessing and probing for solutions occurs through questioning.

Questioning

The process of questioning is central to many aspects of communication. Although there are several forms of questions that can be used, these can be categorized into two major groups: open questions and closed questions. Closed questions are designed to obtain simple 'Yes' or 'No' responses. In contrast, open questions allow greater exploration of ideas and exchange of information. For example, if you ask a client, 'Are you in pain?' (closed question) the answer would usually be 'Yes' or 'No'. However, if you asked 'What is the pain like?' (open question) you would normally receive a longer account or response.

In asking questions, it is important to pay particular attention to topic areas that may be particularly sensitive and where questioning may come across as intrusive. Where topics are sensitive, for example in relation to sexual health or other potentially embarrassing areas of care, then issues of privacy and framing any questions in a suitably polite form need to be addressed. Asking too many questions, particularly in a quick-fire series, should be avoided as this can be uncomfortable and intrusive, particularly where rapport has not been fully established or developed. It may also be stressful, particularly if the individual is confused or anxious, and lacking in emotional warmth. Finally, it may come across as rude and increase frustration. Equally, it is best to avoid questions beginning with 'why' because this tends to suggest that judgement is being passed on what an individual has or has not done.

Closure

Ending a period of communication is as important as beginning one. In other words, attention needs to be paid to clarifying what has been discussed and decided upon in terms of any goals that have been set, and when further meetings will take place. In situations that occur over a longer period, such as counselling, clients may become dependent on the relationship and steps need to be taken to outflank this difficulty by setting out a clear contract of involvement from the start, indicating any time limitations and highlighting the desirability of preserving the autonomy and independence of the person throughout.

PROFESSIONAL AND ETHICAL KNOWLEDGE

Once interactions with clients have been undertaken, the next stage is to make some account of what has occurred. As well as providing information for day-to-day clinical care, records are important in resource management, self-evaluation, audits of performance, care, quality assurance and research (Currel & Wainwright 1996). The 1999 Audit Commission report *Setting the Record Straight: A Study of Hospital Medical Records* criticized the poor standard of NHS record keeping and strongly recommended that corrective action should be taken. Even though the nursing literature is full of exhortations to complete high quality records (Pennels 2002), there is good evidence that both doctors and nurses are not adhering to these criteria. The question thus arises of how policy makers, managers and practitioners are to improve the situation. Under the Clinical Governance agenda, audits are currently used to monitor performance and give advice on practice improvement (see Ch. 3, 'Safety and risk').

Evidence-based practice

Record keeping in clinical practice remains an area of concern despite several decades of education and encouragement for all practitioners to treat this area as a priority and keep adequate records. In 2005–6, 11% of the charges investigated by the Nursing and Midwifery Council related to failure to keep adequate records. Carpenter et al (2007) say that one of the problems is that clinicians write records as if they were just making a note for themselves rather than something that will be intelligible to colleagues. Equally, Owen (2005) notes that there are important barriers to record keeping, such as time constraints, staff shortages and the changing role of nurses, who are often taking on new roles and responsibilities. Nevertheless, record keeping is increasingly important as records may form part of the evidence in the event of complaint or investigation and are increasingly used as tools to monitor performance and as resources for research (Carpenter et al 2007).

PROFESSIONAL AND LEGAL ASPECTS OF RECORD KEEPING

Although record keeping is a vital facet of nursing there are problems surrounding the use of records. The patterns of care involved are complex and the record is only ever a partial account of what has transpired between client and nurse. In order to ensure the legal adequacy of records in the UK, the Nursing and Midwifery Council recommends:

- *a full account of your assessment and the care you have planned and provided*
- *relevant information about the condition of the patient or client at any given time and the measures you have taken to respond to their needs*
- *evidence that you have understood and honoured your duty of care, that you have taken all reasonable steps to care for the patient or client and that any actions or omissions on your part have not compromised their safety in any way*
- *a record of any arrangements you have made for the continuing care of a patient or client.*

The frequency of entries is determined both by professional judgement and local standards and agreements. You will need to exercise particular care and make more frequent entries when patients or clients present complex problems, show deviation from the norm, require more intensive care than normal, are confused and disoriented or generally give cause for concern. You must use your professional judgement (if necessary in discussion with other members of the health care team) to determine when these circumstances exist.

(Nursing and Midwifery Council 2002: 9)

Written communication is dictated by the nursing process of assessment, planning, implementation and evaluation. Despite having this framework, documentation is often problematic for nurses. Not only are they under pressure to record those nursing interventions that can easily be costed, but they must also adhere to the *Guidance for Records and Record Keeping* (NMC 2002), so as to demonstrate that their duty of care has been fulfilled. In contemporary health care, service planners have attempted to increase the productivity of record takers by introducing computer-aided documentation systems. Increasingly, information will be created, stored and disseminated electronically as work progresses towards implementation of the Electronic Patient Records (EPR) and Electronic Health Records (EHR) (Department of Health 2000). At the time of writing the UK's NHS is moving towards a greater use of electronic care records under the Connecting for Health initiative. At present so-called 'summary care records' are being created for patients and the addition of further information is undertaken with the knowledge and consent of the patient (Information Commissioner's Office 2007).

Reflection and portfolio evidence

How helpful are the following nursing entries in patient records: 'Slept well', 'Good appetite', 'Up and about', 'No complaints', 'No change', 'Resting comfortably'? Have a look through some nursing records of patients, perhaps even those that include entries made by you.

- Can you find other examples of 'weak' entries that provide little information?
- What factors are influencing the way nurses make entries in records?
- In your view, what kinds of records would be more useful?
- How might entries in nursing notes be improved?
- Record your findings in your portfolio.

The ideal is a record which is universally intelligible and follows a common nursing language. This has been developed in the ICN's International Classification for Nursing Practice (ICNP; International Council of Nurses 1999). This is a document designed to provide a common means of describing phenomena and activities in nursing and contains three elements, namely:

1. Nursing phenomena or nursing diagnoses.
2. Nursing actions or nursing interventions.
3. Nursing outcomes (Kisilowska 2001).

CONFIDENTIALITY AND ACCESS TO RECORDS

Williams et al (1993) observed that while the patient was becoming the centre of all NHS activity, the documentation of care had not developed in tandem to reflect this. Patient records are usually episode focused, provider based, and emerge in numerous different forms throughout their lifetime, even when describing a single experience of ill health. In the UK many records are kept about patients in a number of different places. An individual might have some records at the GP's surgery, some held by health visitors and district nurses, some at the hospitals they attend and other documentation relating to social services.

A further question concerns what kind of information from the record should be disclosed to different professional groups. The Caldicott Report, *Review of Patient Identifiable Information* (Department of Health 1997b), raised concerns about the general lack of awareness of confidentiality and information security requirements throughout the NHS at all levels. The Committee was also concerned at the NHS's ability to limit access to patient information to those who truly need to know. Consequently, NHS organizations have been charged with appointing so called 'Caldicott guardians' whose job is to support and champion responsible 'information governance' in their organizations. The principles laid down by the Department of Health (2006b: 1) specify that where confidential information is used, this should be justifiable, and only done when absolutely necessary. The minimum of information about identifiable patients should be used and access to personally identifiable information should be on a strict need-to-know basis.

Everyone working for or with the NHS who records, handles, stores or otherwise comes across patient information has a personal common law duty of confidence to patients and to his or her employer (Department of Health 2002). The duty of confidence continues even after the death of the patient, or after an employee or contractor has left the NHS. The duty of confidence to an employer regarding company/NHS trust information is included in the terms and conditions of the job and the contract of employment. Public breaches of confidentiality in relation to individual patients and/or of NHS trust information can result in disciplinary procedures being taken against the employee (as defined in the Data Protection Act 1998). The patient can take legal action against the individual within the remit of negligence in a 'duty of care' (McHale et al 1998). However, this duty of confidentiality is not absolute, and can be subject to an overriding public interest. This ruling is often applied to research findings where it is necessary to consider whether public interest in the research outweighs the duty of confidence, having regard to all the circumstances. Ethical permission must be sought for any research using patient records. Currently three areas have special regulations and include: those diagnosed with sexually transmitted diseases (including HIV and AIDS); information related to human fertilization; and information on abortions.

Patient access to records

The Access to Health Records Act 1990 permitted patients to have access to manual health records made after the Act came into force in 1991. The later Data Protection Act 1998 permits access to all manual health records whenever made, subject to specified exceptions. Although initially professional groups were unhappy with patient access on the basis of paternalistic arguments (e.g. lack of understanding by the patient, professionals being less candid in their reporting, gaining knowledge was not in the best interest of the patient), there is now recognition of the patient's right of access to his or her own records (McHale et al 1998). This is also contained in the Human Rights Act 2000. With the modernization agenda in the NHS, the climate has been reversed and the latest initiative, as part of partnership working, is to include the patient in all correspondence between a hospital consultant and the patient's GP – the 'Copy letters' project – and to allow patients to browse their own records on a computer terminal (NHS 2003).

COMPLAINTS AND COMMUNICATION

As society has become better informed, access to Internet information on health care has become more easily available, and consumer satisfaction has come to be regarded as a 'right' in Western democratic societies, there has been an inevitable rise in expectations of good quality health care. If not satisfied with the service offered, patients and patient groups will complain. The media have become involved and cases of negligence by any professional group now come under increasing public scrutiny (McHale et al 1998). Complaints against nurses are increasing (Beardwood et al 1999, Scott, 2001). In practical terms, at the time of writing there are agencies which will assist patients in making complaints. For example, the UK government set up the Independent Complaints Advocacy Service (ICAS) in 2003. This involves trained advocates with knowledge of the NHS complaints procedure, helping clients to understand whether they wish to pursue a complaint. Where necessary, advocates can support clients in doing so. The support offered ranges from helping the client with initial preparation through to 'attendance at resolution meetings and helping people with correspondence' (Department of Health 2005: 1).

The Nursing and Midwifery Council (2008: 2), in its Code of Conduct, emphasizes the need to communicate with patients and to share the information that they may need, and oversees complaints from the public, employers or the police; a complaint which is upheld can result in nurses being removed from the professional register. The NMC publishes reports from its professional conduct committee on its website and also the sanctions it has imposed upon nurses about whom complaints have been lodged. A recent report (2007) details an 18 month suspension against a nurse who shouted at patients, and who said 'I am going to put a nappy on you like a big baby because you are behaving like one'. The nurse was found to have shouted aggressively at patients' relatives and claimed he was too busy to attend to patients in pain (Nursing and Midwifery Council 2007). While nursing work may sometimes be frustrating and the demands may be heavy, such displays of ill temper can have a major effect on patients and relatives and increasingly are taken seriously by disciplinary bodies. Complaints about communication also make up the second most numerous category of complaint received by the UK's Healthcare Commission (Heathcare Commission 2007b), accounting for 16% of the complaints they reviewed in 2004–6.

While nurses can never guarantee the meanings of spoken or written words, they need to reduce the scope for misinterpretation and remain vigilant when considering the meanings of their own and other people's speech and writing. The power of language to construct the world in which we live makes it important for nurses to monitor healthcare language as it affects the lives of others. In writing, we should be concerned about how healthcare professionals represent those in their care and whether they linguistically 'incarcerate' or 'restrain' them by using judgemental words and phrases or by jumping to conclusions which might be untrue or might damage the client. For example, a GP's referral letter to a community mental health nurse described a client as a 'young prostitute' with an 'inadequate personality'. On visiting the client at home, the nurse found no evidence that she was either a 'prostitute' or 'inadequate', and she was merely complaining of tiredness (Crawford et al 1995). This incident highlights the often difficult issue of how to challenge communications which we feel are prejudicial, damaging or unethical. Rather, to fail to challenge in such a situation is to permit potential damage or harm to those for whom we stand as advocates. It is thus worth describing in a little more detail what it means to think of nursing as a process of advocacy.

PATIENT ADVOCACY

Advocacy has been linked to the nurse's role in the UK since the 1980s and is considered desirable because it furthers nursing's endeavours on behalf of patients (Grace 2001). The *Oxford English Dictionary* (1989: 194) defines an advocate as 'one who pleads, intercedes or speaks for or on behalf of, another: a pleader, intercessor, defender'. This definition emphasizes how the advocate may represent another through language. In the legal profession, the assumption is that a legal professional will be able to act solely and diligently on behalf of their client. Nurses, however, have a rather more ambiguous role. As Grace (2001) argues, there is little consensus as to what advocacy entails in nursing, as well as concern that nurses may use this role as a tool to serve their own self-interests and make themselves appear more professional (Mallik & Rafferty 2000). Nurses are sometimes in an awkward position when they do try to advocate on behalf of patients because they are often constrained by their employment situation, and 'rocking the boat' too much might result in personal and professional isolation or even job loss (Mallik & McHale 1995). Grace (2001) argues that rather than merely concentrating on the situation of patients in the immediate practice setting, nurses should embrace an advocacy role that includes broader issues of national health policy and funding. Not all policy makers are amenable to this kind of bottom-up persuasion, but it might be possible via more indirect routes, perhaps by mobilizing public opinion.

In addition, there are other frameworks for providing advocacy in health care. These include self-advocacy, agent advocacy and independent advocacy, all of which have a long tradition of providing support for clients in the mental health field, the disabled, people with chronic illnesses, the elderly, and ethnic minority groups accessing health care (Teasdale 1998). These pressure groups and individual agents are included in the current policy framework that established Patient Advice and Liaison Services (PALS) in all NHS acute trusts in the UK (Department of Health 2003).

In practice, when nurses are asked about their experiences of advocacy, those with an interest tend to see advocacy as strongly bound up with ideas about what it means to be a nurse and what a therapeutic relationship involves; indeed, nurses in Snowball's (1996) study held 'a philosophy of nursing which encompasses advocacy as a role responsibility both of professional practice and personal humanity' (Snowball 1996: 73). Moreover, in the same study there appeared an interest among the participants in working with other interested parties to promote patients' well-being, again highlighting the importance of communication, both inter- and intraprofessionally. However, in much research on advocacy the overall finding is that nurses tend to advocate at an individual level – concerned with the needs of particular patients – and not necessarily at the level of the whole organization or in terms of the resources which a society makes available for the clients of health services (Mallik 1997, Chafey et al 1998, Grace 2001).

PERSONAL AND REFLECTIVE KNOWLEDGE

AWARENESS OF THE USE OF LANGUAGE IN NURSING

Language enables you to describe and potentially transform aspects of your work. Progress and growth are positive outcomes of reflective practices, embodied in increased choices and increased professional awareness. By first reflecting critically on your own language you may gain the right, and indeed the skills, to challenge the language of others. Reflective practice, as championed by Schon (1983) and as discussed in the introduction to this book, is based on the belief that people can actually effect change through the raising of consciousness about their activities. The quality of your care will improve as you develop effective communication skills. For example, a nurse describes a particular piece of interaction in the following terms:

I said something like 'How are you doing Paul?' When he predictably answered 'Fine' I could easily have gone out the door and on with my work, but just by the way he answered I could tell he had much more to say. I asked Paul if he would like me to stay awhile and he replied that he would ... For almost an hour I just listened to Paul as he talked about his life, his achievements, the risks he had and hadn't taken and his hopes for his limited future ... When I stood up to go, his eyes met mine and we thanked each other in silence. *(Perry 1996: 9)*

This extract also shows some important things about caring work. Firstly, it is not wholly about catering to patients' physical needs; their desire for company and companionship may be especially important. Secondly, it highlights the importance of probing beyond the initial appearance of the interaction – the patient's assertion that he is 'fine' – to create an experience which is rewarding to both nurse and patient. This example highlights the value of communication in adding to a patient's quality of life. Often nurses cannot allocate an extended block of time for this kind of communication, but they should give as much time as possible to empathic communication and interaction during their working day.

CASE STUDIES INVOLVING THE USE OF LANGUAGE

The following examples highlight the role of language in health care. The questions aim to get you thinking about the centrality of language to different aspects of health care, from the initial description of health problems through to rehabilitation and therapy.

Case study: Adult

Margaret is 38 years old and is suffering from systemic lupus erythematosus (SLE), a disorder of the connective tissues primarily affecting women in their 30s and 40s. It may involve arthritis and problems with the kidneys, heart and brain. One day she opens up and begins to talk about her condition:

> If you have lupus, I mean one day it's my liver; one day it's my joints; one day it's my head, and it's like people really think you're a hypochondriac if you keep complaining about different ailments ... It's like you don't want to say anything because people are going to start thinking, you know, 'God, don't go near her, all she is ... is complaining about this'. And I think that's why I never say anything because I feel like everything I have is related one way or another to the lupus but most of the people don't know I have lupus, and even those that do are not going to believe that ten different ailments are the same thing. And I don't want anybody saying, you know, [that] they don't want to come around me because I complain.
>
> *(Adapted from Charnaz 1991: 114–115.)*

- How is Margaret making sense of her illness experience?
- What kinds of difficulties is she having in her working and social life?
- When you hear the term illness, what kinds of things does it make you think of? Does Margaret's account fit with your own ideas of illness?
- How could Margaret tell others about her condition in a way that might make her life easier?
- Try to write a few responses to Margaret and ask a mentor or peer to review these. For example, you may wish to focus on Margaret's account of how the illness has affected her notion of selfhood.

Case study: Mental health

Crystal is in his mid-40s and has been diagnosed as suffering from schizophrenia since his late teens. He lives in a hostel in the community and spends most of his day on the street. He has no friends and although he receives regular visits from a community nurse, he has failed to take his oral medication to control his symptoms. He experiences command hallucinations that tell him to actively waste other people's time. One morning he is overheard crying out 'Help me. The Time Wasters are coming to get me. They're going to tear me apart!' (Adapted from Crawford 2002.)

- Which of the following would be the best response and why?
  1. 'Don't worry about it. I'm sure they wouldn't do that.'
  2. 'I don't think that will happen. Do you fancy a cup of tea?'
  3. 'You must feel really frightened. Tell me more about these "Time Wasters".'
  4. 'Can you prove that these "Time Wasters" are coming to get you?'
- If you met Crystal for the first time how would you begin to build up rapport with him?

- What would you say to Crystal if you visited his flat and saw lots of tablets lying around on the floor?

Case study: Child

Donald is 12 years old and has been experiencing severe pain postoperatively. He is on a patient controlled analgesia (PCA) pump, but he still complains of pain to his mother. His mother is upset about this and is becoming frustrated because she does not understand how the pump works and does not feel able to seek further information from nursing staff. Each time nursing staff enter the room she complains that her son's pain is not properly controlled. During handover, she seeks out the nurses and tells them that Donald is in so much pain that he is crying loudly. One of the nurses tells her 'We'll go and see', to which the mother replies, 'Can't you take my word for it?' (Adapted from Simons et al 2001.)

- How might you communicate empathy for the mother witnessing Donald's pain?
- How might you go about educating and providing information for Donald and his mother?
- To what extent does the emotional state of Donald's mother make this kind of education difficult? How can we get round this problem?
- What weight should you attach to your own opinion about the level of pain Donald is experiencing, compared to that of Donald's mother, or Donald himself? How can you come up with a nursing strategy that satisfies everyone?
- Under what circumstances might you be sceptical of information provided by Donald's mother?

Case study: Learning disabilities

Janet is 16 years old, lives in a community residential unit and has a learning disability that means she is unable to give informed consent. According to staff, Janet needs to be chaperoned because she is young and attractive, very immature and adores being kissed and cuddled. In the past, this has led to difficult situations when Janet has struck up friendships with other people, and staff are concerned that she is not abused. (Adapted from Deeley 2001: 25; a further useful and evocative account of the sexuality of young women with learning difficulties and sexuality is provided by McCarthy 1999.)

- What sorts of difficulties over sexuality might a young woman in Janet's situation face?
- What ways are there of making the issue of sexuality and people with learning disabilities easier to talk about for staff and clients?
- What communication strategies would you use to foster more independence for Janet despite staff concerns for the need to chaperone her?

- How might you respond verbally and non-verbally to any show of affection by Janet?
- To what extent could a person in Janet's situation be empowered to make her own informed choices about relationships and sexuality?

- How might it be possible for you to help Janet avoid abusive and exploitative situations without being intrusive or over-controlling?

SUMMARY

This chapter has drawn together theoretical concepts relating to communication and applied this knowledge in relation to the practice of caring for individuals. It has included:

1. The biological theoretical basis of communication, models of communication, language acquisition and non-verbal communication.
2. Psychosocial and sociocultural factors influencing communication.
3. Consideration of factors influencing nurses' decision making in using communication in care delivery.
4. Professional and ethical dimensions of communication, the importance of maintaining records, issues of confidentiality and the role of the nurse as an advocate for the patient.
5. The use of communication in addressing and managing complaints and the dissatisfied client.

Knowledge illuminated within this chapter has been combined with evidence from other referenced sources and applied within a range of situations. Suggestions have been made for portfolio development in relation to the development of communication skills.

Annotated further reading and websites

Crawford P, Brown B, Bonham P 2006 Communication in clinical settings. Nelson Thornes, Cheltenham

This book will assist its readers to acquire a critical view of their use of language in professional practice. The authors synthesize theoretical studies and critical analysis of a wide range of examples of good and bad use of language, in order to guide nurses towards models of good practice.

Teasdale K 1998 Advocacy in health care. Blackwell Science, Oxford
An informative book on advocacy which outlines the advocacy frameworks in relation to all patient/client groups, such as self-advocacy, external advocacy and advocacy for special needs groups, as well as giving an overview of the development of patient advocacy as a nursing role.

http:/www.mhas.info/
Modernizing the Hearing Aid Services in the NHS is part of a government plan to upgrade the current service offered to patients in the UK. Targets have been set for the next 5 years and this new website provides up-to-date information on progress.

http:/www.ombudsman.org.uk
Provides the Parliamentary and Health Service Ombudsman's annual reports on the main areas of patient complaints, many of them related to failures in communication within healthcare teams.

http:/www.nmc-uk.org
As of mid-2008 the Nursing and Midwifery Council defined its functions as follows: 'The core function of the NMC is to establish standards of education, training, conduct and performance for nursing and midwifery and to ensure those standards are maintained, thereby safeguarding the health and wellbeing of the public.' It has taken over from the old UK Central Council and is concerned to promote good practice and to deal with complaints.

http:/www.dh.gov.uk/
The Department of Health has a useful website providing a good deal of information on policy and practice. Many documents can be downloaded free of charge, including reports, research, legislation and a great deal more.

http:/www.nhs.uk
The NHS website allows access to valuable information on all reports and guidelines related to services within the NHS that are referred to in this chapter. In addition, there is now a National Knowledge Service, accessible from the NHS main site.

References

Allott R 2001 The natural origin of language. Able, Hemel Hempstead

Ambady N, Koo J, Rosxenthal R 2002 Physical therapists nonverbal communication predicts geriatric patients' health outcomes. Psychology and Aging 17(3):443–452

American Telemedicine Association 2006 Defining telemedicine. Available online: http://www.americantelemed.org/news/definition.html (accessed 23 June 2006)

Anderson KJ, Leaper C 1998 Meta-analysis of gender effects in conversational interruption. Sex Roles 39(3–4):225–252

Argyle M, Ingham R 1972 Gaze, mutual gaze and proximity. Semiotica 6:32–49

Audit Commission 1999 Setting the record straight: a review of progress in health records services. Audit Commission, London

Bandura A 1986 Social foundations of thought and action: a social cognitive theory. Prentice-Hall, Englewood Cliffs

Beardwood B, Walters V, Eyles J 1999 Complaints against nurses: a reflection of 'the new managerialism' and consumerism in health care. Social Science and Medicine 48(3):363–374

Betts A 1995 Improving communication. In: Ellis RB, Gates RJ, Kenworthy N (eds) Interpersonal communication in nursing: theory and practice. Churchill Livingstone, Edinburgh, pp 59–70

Birdwhistell R 1970 Kinesics and context: essays on body movement communication. University of Pennsylvania Press, Philadelphia

Bricher G 1999 Paediatric nurses, children and the development of trust. Journal of Clinical Nursing 8:451–458

Brown P, Fraser C 1979 Speech as a marker of situation. In: Scherer KR, Giles H (eds) Social markers in speech. Cambridge University Press, Cambridge, pp 33–108

Brown B, Crawford P, Carter R 2006 Evidence based health communication. Open University Press, Maidenhead

Cantwell J 2000 Pressures, priorities and pre-emptive practice. Speech and Language Therapy (Winter):16–19

Caporael L, Lukaszewski M, Culbertson G 1983 Secondary baby talk: judgements by institutionalised elderly and their caregivers. Journal of Personality and Social Psychology 44(4):746–754

Carey J 1989 Communication as culture. Routledge, London

Carpenter I, Ram MB, Croft GP 2007 Medical records and record-keeping standards. Clinical Medicine 7:328–331

Chafey K, Rhea M, Shannon AM 1998 Characterisation of advocacy by practicing nurses. Journal of Professional Nursing 14(1):43–52

Charnaz K 1991 Good days, bad days: the self in chronic illness and time. Rutgers University Press, New Brunswick

Chen YY, Gilligan S, Coups EJ 2005 Hostility and perceived social support: interactive effects on cardiovascular reactivity to laboratory stressors. Annals of Behavioral Medicine 29(1):37–43

Chomsky N 1976 Reflections on language. Fontana, London

Chomsky N 1993 Language and thought. Moyer Bell, London

Clements PT, Benasutti KM, Henry GC 2001 Drawing from experience: using drawings to facilitate communication and understanding with children exposed to sudden traumatic deaths. Journal of Psychosocial Nursing and Mental Health Services 39(12):12–20

Commission for Patient and Public Involvement in Health 2006 Patient and public involvement forums' annual report 2005–06 national summary. Commission for Patient and Public Involvement in Health, London

Crawford P 2002 Nothing purple, nothing black. Book Guild, Lewes

Crawford P, Nolan P, Brown B 1995 Linguistic entrapment: medico-nursing biographies as fictions. Journal of Advanced Nursing 22:1141–1148

Crawford P, Brown B, Nolan P 1998 Communicating care: the language of nursing. Stanley Thornes, Cheltenham

Crawford P, Brown B, Bonham P 2006 Communication in clinical settings. Nelson Thornes Cheltenham

Currell R, Wainwright P 1996 Nursing record systems, nursing practice and patient care (protocol). In: Bero L, Grilli R, Grimshaw J (eds) Collaboration on effective professional practice module of the Cochrane database of systematic reviews. Cochrane Collaboration, Oxford, pp 47–61

de Pino-Perez A, Meizoso MTG Gonzalez RD 1999 Validity of the structured interview for the assessment of type A behaviour. European Journal of Psychological Assessment 15(1):39–48

Deeley S 2001 Professional ideology and learning disability: an analysis of internal conflict. Disability and Society 17(1):19–33

Department for Education and Science 2003 Every child matters. Green Paper. Command number 5860. Available online: http://www.everychildmatters.gov.uk/publications (accessed May 2008)

Department of Health 1997a Better services for vulnerable people, EL (97)62, CI(97)24. Department of Health, London

Department of Health 1997b The Caldicott Committee: report on the review of patient-identifiable information. Department of Health, London

Department of Health 1998 Partnership in action: new opportunities for joint working between health and social services – a discussion document. Department of Health, London

Department of Health 2000 Good practice guidelines for general practice: electronic patient records. Available online: http://www.doh. gov.uk/gpepr/ guidelines.pdf (accessed 24 May 2003)

Department of Health 2002 Statutory instrument 2002 no. 1438. The health service (control of patient information) regulations. Available online: http://www.doh.gov.uk/ipu/confiden/instrument.pdf (accessed 24 May 2003)

Department of Health 2003 Patient advice and liaison services. Available online: http://www.doh.gov.uk/patientadviceandliaisonservices/downloads.htm (accessed 24 May 2003)

Department of Health 2005 Independent Complaints Advocacy Service (ICAS): the first year of ICAS: 1 September 2003 – 31 August 2004. Department of Health, London

Department of Health 2006a A stronger local voice: a framework for creating a stronger local voice in the development of health and social care services. Department of Health, London

Department of Health 2006b The Caldicott guardian manual. Department of Health, London

Dronkers NF 2000 The pursuit of brain–language relationships. Brain and Language 71:59–71

Dumble M, Tuson W 1998 Identifying eating and drinking difficulties. Speech and Language Therapy Practice (Winter):4–6

Egan G 1974 The skilled helper: a model for systematic helping and interpersonal relating. Brooks Cole, Pacific Grove, CA

Ekman P, Rosenberg EL 1997 What the face reveals. Oxford University Press, Oxford

Fairclough N 1989 Language and power. Longman, Harlow

Fenton S, Sadiq-Sangster A 1996 Culture, relativism, and the expression of mental distress: South Asian women in Britain. Sociology of Health and Illness 18(1):66–85

Fodor JA 1998 In critical condition: polemical essays on cognitive science and the philosophy of mind. MIT Press, Cambridge

Fox NJ 1993 Discourse, organisation and the surgical ward round. Sociology of Health and Illness 15(1):16–42

Friedman M, Rosenman R 1959 Association of specific, overt behaviour pattern with blood and cardiovascular findings. Journal of the American Medical Association 169:1286

Grace PJ 2001 Professional advocacy: widening the scope of accountability. Nursing Philosophy 2:151–162

Habermas J 1995 Moral consciousness and communicative action. MIT Press, Cambridge

Hargie O, Dickson D 2004 Skilled interpersonal communication: research, theory and practice, 4th edn. Routledge, London

Health Committee 1999 Session 1998–1999: The relationship between health and social services. First Report, vol. 1. Report and proceedings of the committee. HMSO, London

Healthcare Commission 2007a The views of staff: key findings from the 2006 survey of NHS staff. Healthcare Commission, London

Healthcare Commission 2007b Spotlight on complaints: a report on second stage complaints about the NHS in England. Commission for Healthcare Audit and Inspection, London

Heron J 1990 Helping the client: a creative practical guide. Sage, London

Hogg MA, Vaughan GM 2002 Social psychology, 3rd edn. Prentice Hall, London

Hollinworth H, Clark C, Harland R 2005 Understanding the arousal of anger: a patient-centred approach. Nursing Standard 19(37):41–47

Hyde A, Treacy MP, Scott PA 2005 Modes of rationality in nursing documentation: biology, biography and the 'voice of nursing'. Nursing Inquiry 12(2): 66–77

Hyden M 1995 Verbal aggression as prehistory of woman battering. Journal of Family Violence 10:55–71

Information Commissioner's Office 2007 The Information Commissioner's view of electronic care records. Available online:

http://www.ico.gov.uk/upload/documents/library/data_protection/introductory/information_commissioners_view_of_nhs_electronic_care_reco%E2%80%A6.pdf (accessed 12 May 2007)

International Council of Nurses 1999 International classification for nursing practice, beta version. International Council of Nurses, Geneva

Jakobson R 1960 Closing statement: linguistics and poetics. In: Sebeok TA (ed) Style in language. MIT Press, Cambridge, pp 350–377

Kisilowska M 2001 Reorganized structure and other proposals for the ICNP development. International Nursing Review 4:218–233

Kleinke CL 1986 Gaze and eye contact: a research review. Psychological Bulletin 100:76–100

Kreps G 2001 The evolution and advancement of health communication inquiry. In: Gudykurst B (ed) Communication yearbook, vol. 24. Sage, Thousand Oaks, pp 231–253

Lakoff R 1975 Language and woman's place. Harper & Row, New York

Larkin KT, Martin RR, McClain SE 2002 Cynical hostility and the accuracy of decoding facial expressions of emotions. Journal of Behavioural Medicine 25(3):285–293

Lasswell H 1948 The structure and function of communication in society. In: Bryson L (ed) The communication of ideas. Harper & Row, New York, pp 37–53

McAfee RE 2001 Domestic violence as a women's health issue. Women's Health Issues 11(4):371–376

McCarthy M 1999 Sexuality and women with learning disabilities. Jessica Kingsley, London

McHale J, Tingle J, Peysner J 1998 Law and nursing. Butterworth Heinemann, Oxford

Mackintosh N 1996 Promoting health: an issue for nursing. Quay, Dinton

Mallik M 1997 Advocacy in nursing: perceptions of practising nurses. Journal of Clinical Nursing 6(4):303–313

Mallik M, McHale J 1995 Support for advocacy. Nursing Times 91(4):28–30

Mallik M, Rafferty AM 2000 Diffusion of the concept of patient advocacy. Journal of Nursing Scholarship 32(4):399–404

National Health Service 2003 IT questions and answers. Available online: http://www.nhs.uk/nhsmagazine/primarycare/it_qa.asp (accessed 24 May 2003)

Nolan M, Caldock K 1996 Assessment: identifying the barriers to good practice. Health and Social Care in the Community 4(2):77–85

Nursing and Midwifery Council 2002 Guidelines for records and record keeping. Nursing and Midwifery Council, London

Nursing and Midwifery Council 2007 Scott Armstrong. Fitness to Practise. Annual Report 1 April 2005 to 31 March 2006. Available online: http://www.nmc-uk.org/aFrameDisplay.aspx?DocumentID=3134 (accessed 25 November 2007)

Nursing and Midwifery Council 2008 The Code: standards of conduct, performance and ethics for nurses and midwives. Nursing and Midwifery Council, London

Oudeyer P-Y, Kaplan F 2007 Language evolution as a Darwinian process: computational studies. Cognitive Processing 8(1):21–35

Owen K 2005 Documentation in nursing practice. Nursing Standard 19(32):48–49

Oxford English Dictionary, 2nd edn. 1989 Clarendon Press, Oxford

Parliamentary and Health Service Ombudsman 2006 Making a difference: annual report 2005–6. Stationery Office, London

Patient Advice and Liaison Service 2007 What is PALS and what does PALS offer? http://www.pals.nhs.uk/cmsContentView.aspx?ItemID=932 (accessed 12 May 2007)

Patterson ML 1983 Nonverbal behaviour: a functional perspective. Springer, New York

Pei M 1997 The story of language, 2nd edn. Lippincott, Philadelphia

Pell MD 2002 Evaluation of nonverbal emotion in face and voice: some preliminary findings on a new battery of tests. Brain and Cognition 48(2–3):499–504

Pennels C 2002 The importance of accurate and comprehensive record keeping. Professional Nurse 17(5):294–296

Peplau H 1952 Interpersonal relations in nursing. Putnam, New York

Perry B 1996 Influence of nurse gender on the use of silence, touch and humour. International Journal of Palliative Nursing 2:7–14

Pinker S 1994 The language instinct. Morrow, New York

Posner MI, Raichle ME 1997 Images of mind. Scientific American Library, New York

Potter J 1996 Representing reality. Sage, London

Proctor A, Morse JM, Khonsari ES 1996 Sounds of comfort in the trauma centre: how nurses talk to patients in pain. Social Science and Medicine 42(12):1669–1680

Rao PR 1995 Drawing and gesture as communication options in a person with severe aphasia. Topics in Stroke Rehabilitation 2(1):49–56

Reid SA, Ng SH 1999 Language, power and intergroup relations. Journal of Social Issues 55:119–139

Reilly CE, Lambrecht ME 2001 The cognitive model: interventions for improved patient–provider communication. Journal of Psychosocial Nursing and Mental Health Services 39(6):32–39

Richards H, King G, Reid M 2005 Remote working: survey of attitudes to eHealth of doctors and nurses in rural general practices in the United Kingdom. Family Practice 22:2–7

Robillard AB 1996 Anger in the social order. Body and Society 2(1):17–30

Rogers CR 1951 Client-centered therapy: its current practice, implications, and theory. Houghton Mifflin, Boston

Ryan AA, Scullion HS 2000 Family and staff perceptions of the role of families in nursing homes. Journal of Advanced Nursing 32(2): 626–634

Ryan EB, Meredith SD, Shantz GB 1994 Evaluative perceptions of patronizing speech addressed to institutionalized elders in contrasting conversational contexts. Canadian Journal on Ageing 13(2):236–248

Scherer KR, Banse R, Wallbott HG 2002 Emotion inferences from vocal expression correlate across languages and cultures. Journal of Cross Cultural Psychology 13(1):74–92

Schon T 1983 The reflective practitioner. Basic Books, New York

Scott H 2001 Complaints about nurses are on the increase. British Journal of Nursing 10(13):828

Searle J 1979 Speech acts: an essay in the philosophy of language. Cambridge University Press, London

Sellman D 2007 Trusting patients, trusting nurses. Nursing Philosophy 8:28–36

Shannon CE, Weaver W 1949 The mathematical theory of communication. University of Illinois Press, Champaign

Sheldon LK, Barrett R, Ellington L 2006 Difficult communication in nursing. Journal of Scholarship in Nursing 38(2):141–147

Silverman J, Kurtz S, Draper J 2005 Skills for communicating with patients, 2nd edn. Radcliffe Press, Oxford

Simons J, Franck L, Roberson E 2001 Parent involvement in children's pain care: views of parents and nurses. Journal of Advanced Nursing 36(4):591–599

Snowball J 1996 Asking nurses about advocating for patients: reactive and proactive accounts. Journal of Advanced Nursing 24:67–75

Sorrells-Jones J, Tschirch P, Liong MS 2006 Nursing and telehealth: opportunities for nurse leaders to shape the future. Nurse Leader 4(5):42–58

Stewart AL, Napoles-Springer A, Perez-Stable E 1999 Interpersonal processes of care in diverse populations. Millbank Quarterly 77(3):305–339

Sumner J 2001 Caring in nursing: a different interpretation. Journal of Advanced Nursing 35(6):926–932

Sundin K, Norberg A, Jansson L 2001 The meaning of skilled care providers' relationships with stroke and aphasia patients. Qualitative Health Research 11(3):308–321

Teasdale K 1998 Advocacy in health care. Blackwell Science, Oxford

Tilley S 1999 Altschul's legacy in mediating British and American psychiatric nursing discourses: common sense and the 'absence' of the accountable practitioner. Journal of Psychiatric and Mental Health Nursing 6:283–285

Wellings T 2001 Drawings by dying and bereaved children. Paediatric Nursing 13(4):30–31

Whitehead D 2003 Evaluating health promotion: a model for nursing practice. Journal of Advanced Nursing 41(5):490–498

Williams JG, Roberts R, Rigby MJ 1993 Integrated patient records: another move towards quality for patients. Quality in Health Care 2(2):73–74

Zimmerman DH, West C 1975 Sex roles, interruptions and silences in conversations. In: Thorne B, Henley N (eds) Language and sex: differences and dominance. Newbury House, Rowley, pp 105–129

Zwaal C, Prkachin KM, Husted J 2003 Components of hostility and verbal communication of emotion. Psychology and Health 18(2):261–273

Chapter 3

Safety and risk

Kevin Rowan

KEY ISSUES

SUBJECT KNOWLEDGE
- Exploration of the concept of internal and external environments
- Basic human requirements for life
- Hazards to human safety
- Psychological and social concepts of risk
- Risk concepts in health care
- Environmental and occupational safety
- Health promotion in relation to safety

CARE DELIVERY KNOWLEDGE
- Safety of the individual
- Learning from incidents and 'near misses'
- Safe systems of care
- Risk assessment
- Planning and implementing a strategy for risk management
- Safe equipment and safe substances
- Implementing strategies for a safe environment

PROFESSIONAL AND ETHICAL KNOWLEDGE
- Interprofessional working
- Upholding the law and maintaining standards
- Statutory requirements
- Professional requirements
- The consent process
- Ethical dilemmas in risk management

PERSONAL AND REFLECTIVE KNOWLEDGE
- Case studies applying principles of safety and risk in branches of nursing

INTRODUCTION

A safe environment is something many of us take for granted. Florence Nightingale highlighted the importance of ensuring that patients were safe when she stated in her instructions to nurses, *Notes on Nursing* (Nightingale 1860), that nursing should 'Do the patient no harm'. She also offered advice on the design of hospital wards in an attempt to ensure an optimum environment for hospital patients (Nightingale 1863). Over 140 years later, the Department of Health, in conjunction with the National Patient Safety Agency, has reiterated Florence Nightingale's ideal, while recognizing that 'no harm' may be optimistic. The report *An Organisation with a Memory* (Department of Health 2000), which was the outcome of an expert group on learning from adverse events in the National Health Service, has become one of the building blocks of safety and risk management in the NHS in the UK. This report was preceded by a US report entitled *To Err is Human: Building a Safer Health System* (Institute of Medicine 2000), which had a major influence on the development of safety within health care, both in the USA and internationally. However, to view the promotion of a safe environment as simply something nurses can do for their patients is simplistic. This perspective alone fails to recognize the sociological components of maintaining a safe environment, that is the need for patients (and nurses) to be aware of potential threats to health within their personal environments and to behave in a safe manner. Nursing has a responsibility to understand and promote both the concept of maintaining patient safety in care environments and the notion of safe patient behaviour through health promotion.

Risk management, i.e. the effective identification and response to risk, can be considered to be a component of Clinical Governance. Clinical Governance was introduced to the NHS in 1997 in the document *The New NHS: Modern, Dependable* (Department of Health 1997). The concept was then developed in 1998, through a consultation document on quality in the NHS entitled *A First Class Service* (Department of Health 1998). In that document, Clinical

Governance is defined as: 'a system through which NHS organizations are accountable for continuously improving the quality of their services and safeguarding high standards of care by creating an environment in which excellence will flourish.'

In some ways, Clinical Governance was merely a renaming and collation of a number of initiatives designed to (directly or indirectly) improve the quality of clinical care in the NHS, such as clinical audit, risk management, continuing professional development, etc. However, it did impose new requirements, which involved the application of far greater structure and rigour to such initiatives than was previously the case. Looking back, more than 10 years on, it is fair to say that clinical quality is higher up the agenda than ever before, though whether this can be attributed primarily to the Clinical Governance initiative as opposed to, for example, wider societal pressure is open to debate.

Although patients have always featured as a prime concern with regard to health and safety, the safety of nurses at work has not always received the same attention. The last century saw many legislative attempts at improving the health of the worker in society, though many people, including health service workers, were not given legal protection while at work until the last decade or so. For many, the establishment of the Health and Safety at Work etc. Act 1974 was the first opportunity for ensuring safe working premises and practices. The NHS became subject to the new law but avoided the need for implementation because of Crown immunity. After well publicized incidents of poor standards, this immunity was finally lifted by the NHS (Amendment) Act 1986.

Today, the provision and maintenance of an optimum environment for both patients and healthcare staff is a major concern. Laws, regulations, local procedures and policies at European, national and local levels offer guidance for safe practice. Nurses have a responsibility to ensure that the workplace is a safe place for themselves and their patients. Some nurses, in particular occupational health nurses and those who represent unions with regard to health and safety, have additional responsibility to ensure that the workplace is a safe place for all employees.

This chapter explores issues in the provision of a safe environment for patients and carers. It presents a broad overview, since other chapters in this book contain sections that focus on specific areas of safety such as handling and moving (see Ch. 6), infection control (see Ch. 5) and medicines (see Ch. 10). Food safety is addressed under nutrition (see Ch. 8) and stress arising from multiple external environmental sources is explored under stress, relaxation and rest (see Ch. 9). The functions and maintenance of the body in dealing with environmental threats are addressed under homeostasis (see Ch. 7).

OVERVIEW

Subject knowledge

The concept of 'environment' and the meanings of internal and external environment are explored. Threats to safety that are either part of the natural world or human-made are outlined. In relation to psychosocial knowledge, our interaction with the world around us is considered and there is discussion about the basic human needs for maintaining safety and well-being. Behavioural issues are addressed, with a particular reference to factors that may compromise safety. These factors include theories of risk behaviour and individual and societal non-compliance in maintaining a healthy environment.

Care delivery knowledge

Ways to facilitate an optimum environment for patients are explored in relation to the planning of safe care for the individual as well as the need to minimize hazards in the care environment. Emphasis is placed on risk assessment and on incident and 'near miss' reporting and investigating, as the key components of effective risk management.

Professional and ethical knowledge

This section touches on interprofessional team working but addresses in more depth the requirement for nurses to maintain professional and statutory requirements. There is a review of the many external agencies that set standards for the management of risk in the NHS today. Consideration is given to some ethical dilemmas within risk management which may provide a stimulus for further discussion and deliberation.

Personal and reflective knowledge

Throughout the chapter you will be encouraged to apply information reflectively through exercises and by considering examples. In this final section case studies from the four branches of nursing help you reflect further and apply the knowledge you have gained. You may find it helpful to read one of these before you start the chapter and use it as a focus for your reflections while reading.

SUBJECT KNOWLEDGE

BIOLOGICAL

A SAFE ENVIRONMENT

It is important to clarify what is meant by the 'internal' and 'external' environments, for it is within these domains that threats to well-being and safety take place. Although both have potential dangers for human life and well-being, they are discretely different, both in the likely risks to safety and in the way in which threats may be managed.

For the purposes of this chapter, the internal environment can be described as the functions and workings of the human body. The body's ability to maintain a homeostatic (stable) internal environment is essential to well-being (see Ch. 7). The essential consideration of the internal environment in relation to health and safety is concerned with its interaction with the external environment and the effects which may result. The external environment is the world surrounding the human body. In order to function, the human body has essential requirements, which must be met externally. Conversely, the actions of individuals can influence the safety and ambience of the external environment for all who live in it. Both environments are highly dependent upon one another for their own maintenance.

Basic needs of human life

The basic requirements of living are well known. Physiological needs include:

- air
- water
- food
- shelter.

Without these basic needs, higher order psychological needs such as belonging and esteem cannot easily be achieved (Maslow 1970). Over many thousands of years of development, however, an increasingly complicated way for meeting basic needs has developed. This has resulted in our modifying the external environment to suit our needs.

Table 3.1 illustrates how individuals interact within the external environmental system. It demonstrates how components essential for life support are taken from the external environment and how the two environments interact through activities of living. Waste and residues are contributed to the external environment as a by-product of human existence.

Throughout life activities, individuals may find threats to safety, both to and from the external environment. These are also summarized in the categories outlined in Table 3.1.

POTENTIAL HAZARDS IN MEETING BASIC REQUIREMENTS FOR LIVING

Air

The air that we breathe usually contains 21% oxygen and 78% nitrogen, with the other 1% being made up of trace gases such as carbon dioxide, xenon and neon. If the oxygen concentration were to drop below 16%, anoxia would develop resulting in effects on the brain and other body

Table 3.1 The environmental system (adapted from Purdom & Walton 1971)

Life support	Activities	Residues and waste
Air	Home	Solids
Water	Work	Liquids
Food	Recreation	Gases
Shelter	Transportation	

Environmental hazards

Type	Example	Type	Example
Biological	Animal Insect Microbiological	Psychological	Stress Boredom Anxiety Discomfort Depression
Chemical	Poisons and toxins Allergens Irritants	Sociological	Overcrowding Isolation Anomie
Physical	Vibration Radiation Forces and abrasion Humidity		

functions. If the oxygen level decreased further to 6%, life could not be sustained and immediate loss of consciousness results from exposure to a zero oxygen atmosphere.

Air can also act as a vehicle for microorganisms, allergens, waste gases and dust, all of which enter the body via the lungs (Harrington & Gill 1992). These pollutants may cause damage or illness if present in sufficient quantity or if an individual develops an allergic response to them. Air quality is particularly compromised in large urban areas when the temperature rises and there is little wind movement. Threats to health have been acknowledged in the increasing rates of respiratory disease, especially in young children (Brunekreef et al 1997, Clancy et al 2002, Karol 2002). There is evidence to suggest that children exposed to lead in exhaust fumes arising from the increased use of the car in our society have exhibited symptoms (such as decreased intelligence) consistent with the expected neurological sequelae identified in those with high levels of lead exposure via other sources such as contaminated drinking water (Maas et al 2002).

Water

Life for individuals without water can be measured in days, but it is not only individuals who suffer if water is in short supply. A civilization cannot develop or prosper without sufficient water to grow crops, develop industries or establish communities for people to live in. Water for human consumption must be clean and free from toxins and microorganisms.

In developing countries and in areas affected by war or disaster the greatest risk to the population may be contamination of the drinking water, resulting in life-threatening infections such as cholera and amoebic dysentery. In developed countries, most residents have access to water purification systems that have been in place for many decades (Ineichen 1993). Preoccupation with contamination of water supplies among the wealthier population in the UK has spawned a large water bottling industry. This development in the provision of water for drinking, however, is not without problems, as it is not suitable for everyone. Small babies cannot physically manage the increased mineral content found in many bottled waters due to renal immaturity. Care is required in educating parents about the provision of water for consumption by infants and young children.

In nursing, there are occasions when water must be sterile. This is especially important when water is being used for the preparation of feeds for those who are immunosuppressed as a result of illness. Infants require sterile feeds because they have not developed resistance to infective organisms. Sterile water is also essential where water is used to irrigate wounds or in the preparation of medication via infusion, to protect patients from absorbing harmful contaminants.

Food

For dietary provision to be considered safe, it must be free from contaminants such as harmful bacteria (e.g. *Salmonella, Escherichia coli*) or diseases (e.g. bovine spongiform encephalopathy) (Irani & Johnson 2003) which may be passed to humans. Additionally, food should be in adequate supply, and this is not always the case in the developing world or in some instances in developed countries such as the UK. Within nursing, providing adequate nutrition for clients is important to promote healing and recovery. Health promotion is also important to prevent malnutrition and obesity.

Decision-making exercise

What information about 'sterile' feed preparation would you need to offer Julie, a new mother, who wishes to bottle-feed her baby?

- How would she ensure that the feeding implements are sterile?
- How would she ensure that the water she is using is safe for her baby?
- Where would you obtain information to give to Julie?

Although the main impact of nutrition on health is discussed in greater detail in Chapter 8, it is important to recognize that modern systems for developing food sources need to be monitored closely. Contamination of food at any stage in the external food chain processing will be a potential threat to the well-being of the internal environment.

Shelter

Shelter is essential for survival, providing protection from excessive heat and cold, from the weather and from other environmental hazards. However, shelter should be safe for the resident and should not itself be contributory to disease. These two aspects are surprisingly difficult to achieve within the home and institutional setting.

Evidence-based practice

Poor housing has been linked to poor health. Specifically, Howden-Chapman et al (2007) showed that insulating existing houses led to a significantly warmer, drier environments, resulting in improved self-rated health, reduced self-reported wheezing, days off school and work, and visits to general practitioners as well as a trend for fewer hospital admissions for respiratory conditions. On a more general note, the World Health Organization's Regional Office for Europe has undertaken a large study to evaluate housing and health in seven European cities. Survey tools were used to obtain information about housing and living conditions, health perception, and health status from a representative sample of city populations. Preliminary results reported in 2003 revealed important potential links between housing and health (Bonnefoy et al 2003). The completed study will likely generate recommendations about mental health and housing; poverty, housing, and health; noise and health; allergies and housing; perceptions of housing conditions and associated perceptions of health; and immediate-environment conditions and health status.

Care institutions are often work settings and there is an increasing interest in how the design of individual workplace buildings can have an effect on the health of the individual workers within the building (Raw & Goldman 1996). Sick building syndrome (SBS) has been linked to a group of symptoms developed by people in certain buildings, notably office blocks. Symptoms of SBS include physical and behavioural problems such as irritation of the eyes, nose, throat and skin, headaches, lethargy and lack of concentration. Features of the buildings that appear to cause problems are associated with air conditioning systems, office layouts, windows and light, furnishings and decorations (Raw & Goldman 1996).

ENVIRONMENTAL HAZARDS

As shown above, an individual's basic needs can be threatened by insufficiency or excess or poor management leading to the occurrence of identified hazards to health such as food poisoning or respiratory illness. Potential hazards in the environment may be naturally occurring or result from human-made conditions, including the production of wastes and residues. Production of waste is unavoidable within communal societies and with modern technology and the production of consumer goods. Safe waste removal and disposal strategies are of vital importance to the survival of a community. Within nursing the type of waste is different from that produced domestically or industrially because of its clinical nature. Sharps and dressings need to be treated separately from paper and glass because of the risks to health associated with cross-infection. Policies for the safe disposal of clinical waste and environmental policies ensure the safe disposal of clinical and non-clinical waste in care settings. Apart from waste products, other hazards can seriously compromise the safety of the internal and external environments. They may be categorized into the following five groups:

- biological
- chemical
- physical
- psychological
- sociological.

Biological hazards

Biological hazards are concerned primarily with the entry of disease-producing infectious agents into the body, thus causing a risk to the stability of the internal environment. Such organisms include bacteria, viruses and fungi as well as parasites, which may additionally carry harmful pathogens.

Chemical hazards

Chemical hazards are not new: the gaining of knowledge by our predecessors into which plants were safe to eat and which liquids were safe to drink must have been fraught and littered with many accidents. Even though our ancestors may not have known the finer physiological details of any particular poison, they would have learnt to avoid it. Chemical agents may be synthetic or derived from natural substances and can affect the internal or the external environment beneficially or detrimentally. The most important consideration related to chemical hazards is regarding knowledge about the substance and the judicious application of this knowledge in using chemical substances safely and effectively. It is important to consider the impact of improper use or exposure to substances by patients.

Landrigan & Garg (2002) describe the potential chronic effects of toxic environmental exposure on children's health. Children have unusual patterns of exposure to environmental chemicals, and they have vulnerabilities that are quite distinct from those of adults. Increasingly, children's exposure to chemicals in the environment is understood to contribute to the causation and exacerbation of certain chronic, disabling diseases in children including asthma, cancer, birth defects and neurobehavioral dysfunction. The protection of children against environmental toxins is a major challenge to modern society (Landrigan & Garg 2002). There is also a nursing role in the management and education of the public in maintaining a safe home environment for themselves and their families.

Physical hazards

Physical hazards are all around us and may cause disease, disability or fatality, and are manifest in many different ways. Certain dusts can be dangerous to the internal environment if they are inhaled and then absorbed, while other powders can be used therapeutically in the form of inhalers. Temperature in the external environment can also be a physical hazard. Extreme external temperatures can lead to a loss of the internal homeostatic balance (see Ch. 7). Contact with an extreme hot or cold source can cause extensive physical damage (burning) and, potentially, death.

Electromagnetic radiation, which includes X-rays, ultraviolet and infrared light and microwaves, can cause skin burns, an elevation in temperature and fatality with prolonged exposure. Understanding the dangers related to uncontrolled exposure to these radiations is vital for nurses since controlled ionizing radiation such as X-rays and gamma rays can also be used beneficially to produce radiographic pictures and in the treatment of neoplastic disease (cancer).

Human inventions such as equipment and machinery can cause accidents as well as offering intended benefits. Modern machinery, including all nursing equipment, is continually being made safer as it is evaluated through use. Equipment that is used inappropriately or without regard to the manufacturer's instructions may provide a hazard to safety, even if it is functioning correctly technically. In the community, everyday machinery such as motor vehicles, drills or gardening equipment can be dangerous if not used appropriately.

Accidents

The above hazards are associated with a risk of accident or an undesirable interaction between the internal and external environment. The risk may be higher if an individual is unable physically to meet the demands of the world in which he or she is living, for example an elderly frail individual may be more likely to fall, or a small child may tumble while trying to reach an object from a high shelf. Additionally, accidents may occur if individuals are unable to appreciate the effects of their behaviour, either because of their stage of cognitive development or because of their disease process. Such examples would include a baby who becomes burned as a result of pulling a cup of hot tea from a nearby table onto herself because she is too young to understand the hazard associated with such contact with extremes of heat. Another example is an individual with senile dementia who wanders out into a busy road and is knocked down by a car because he is confused about his environment.

Some accidents can be prevented if carers are aware of hazards and can offer health and safety education. Patients need to clearly understand the outcomes of risky behaviour and the implications that may arise. This requires imaginative education for the most vulnerable groups, to communicate information in a way that can be easily understood and accepted.

PSYCHOSOCIAL

PSYCHOLOGICAL AND SOCIAL HAZARDS

Psychological and social hazards are closely linked to human interactions with the environment. The next section explores the influence of psychosocial factors in the promotion of a safe and healthy environment.

There are many ways in which individuals strive to understand risks in their daily lives and many factors influencing how they may act in the light of such perceptions (Bloor 1995). Fallowfield (1990) suggests that quality of life, and therefore ultimately perceived health and well-being, is directly related to the quality of the environment in which life exists. The environment must also satisfy physiological, psychological and sociological needs. Fallowfield (1990) further identifies four areas where the perception of life quality is paramount:

- psychological – related to the perception of mental well-being
- social – related to involvement in social activities
- occupational – related to functional ability to achieve work (paid or voluntary)
- physical – related to pain, comfort, sleep, physical ability.

These areas are useful for exploring factors associated with determining life quality. However, it should be remembered that the way you view something may be very different from the way another person perceives it. Culture, social class, gender, age, level of education and emotional state should be acknowledged. Toxic effects from drugs and general level of health are also important. Finally, there may be differences in the perception of priorities between patients and their carers. A knowledge of these differences can be critical in facilitating the provision of appropriate care.

PSYCHOLOGICAL STRESS

Stress can alter an individual's perceived environment, which can ultimately become hazardous. The main issues associated with psychological stress and its effects on the internal environment are addressed elsewhere (see Ch. 9). However, it is important to consider how the effects of stress on an individual can impact on his or her immediate external environment.

RISK PERCEPTION

Risk perception is different from the knowledge of a danger, as it does not necessarily cause people to worry. Risk perception may result from the personal orientations that guide an individual to make commitments consistent with one specific political culture and inconsistent with others. At the same time cultures may select those individuals who support their way of life. Individuals may choose what to fear in supporting their preferred way of life (Royal Society Study Group 1992). For example, a religious sect propounding a particular set of beliefs may attract new members who are sympathetic to the views of that sect. Gabe (1995) identifies that in this sense risk cannot be objectively 'measured', but must be viewed as a social construct. This draws from the original anthropological work by Douglas (1966), which addressed questions about why different cultures select different risks for particular attention using beliefs to rationalize behaviour. Given that such interpretations of risk perception are valid, then points of cultural difference are extremely important in nursing. If a patient has different social expectations and selects different risks from the nurse's social expectation then a true assessment could be difficult and treatment could fail to meet the expectations of both parties. There may even be open conflict between the patient and health professional. For instance, Jehovah's Witnesses can present a challenge because they may refuse to receive blood transfusions. Where patients are severely ill and unable to give informed consent to treatment or where children require urgent blood transfusion, nurses may then face moral dilemmas in respecting the cultural beliefs of such individuals while acting in their best interest to maintain their safety.

Finally, individuals may react differently in different environments. A perception of risk and a knowledge of danger are important in the care setting because patients may rely on the nurse to protect them (Simpson 1991). Those who are particularly vulnerable include:

- Children and people with a learning disability, who may not perceive risks to their well-being as they are unable to understand them.
- People with a mental health problem whose perception of danger may be reduced as the result of their illness or because of the treatment they are receiving.
- People who are critically ill and unable to determine dangers.

Within the hospital setting most patients are away from their known environment and are therefore unable to perceive risks in what amounts to an 'alien' environment. It is the responsibility of the nurse to ensure that individuals are aware of hazards wherever possible and are protected by either their own action or action on their behalf by the nurse. The nurse's role is to ensure the safety of the environment by assessing the potential risks and facilitating action for change.

Risk – the possibility of injury or loss – must be in the minds of all who deliver health care, in every clinical episode and in the planning of all healthcare delivery. The roots of risk management lie in risk assessment and implementation of ensuing preventative action and in the reporting, analysis, investigation and prevention-planning of incidents. Therefore, there are two aspects to risk management: one is forward looking, trying to identify issues and circumstances with the potential to go wrong, and act before they do go wrong. The other is backward looking, trying to learn from incidents by thoroughly investigating the causes and aiming to prevent recurrence.

A key principle in both the *To Err is Human* and the *Organisation with a Memory* reports was that when things do go wrong, the most likely and accurate underlying causes are related to 'systems failures' rather than the failures of individuals. It is of course possible that incidents where safety has been compromised are due to reckless or thoughtless actions by individuals, but evidence from research into 'human factors' (the study of all aspects of the way humans relate to the world around them) predominantly points to individuals being as much victims of failings within the design of systems and processes than the causes of such failings. The National Patient Safety Agency (NPSA) in the UK, which was established as a result of the *Organisation with a Memory* report, promotes the principle of systems failures being at the heart of most incidents in much of its work.

PSYCHOSOCIAL HAZARDS IN THE WORK ENVIRONMENT

So far, there has been an emphasis upon individual responsibility within personal environments, with some discussion about people's behaviour when interacting within the healthcare environment. It is, however, important to recognize that the organization has influence in creating a healthy environment. According to Cox & Griffiths (1996: 128) a 'safe' environment might be relatively easy to define, but perceptions of a 'healthy' work environment are usually narrowly focused on physical threats to health. These authors argue that healthy work can be defined as 'work that does not threaten but which helps maintain and enhance physical, psychological and social well-being'.

A 'hazard' has been defined as an event or situation that has the potential to cause harm (Cox & Griffiths 1996). Besides physical hazards referred to in the previous section, the International Labour Organization (1986) has defined psychosocial hazards arising from interactions between job content, work, organizational, management and environmental conditions, and the employee's competencies and needs. Those interactions that can be defined as hazardous influence the health of employees through their 'perceptions' and 'experiences' of these conditions (International Labour Organization 1986, Cox et al 1995). Exposure to psychosocial hazards in particular is often chronic and cumulative, except when a particular acute, traumatic incident occurs. Table 3.2 outlines the common psychosocial hazards associated with the work environment and the conditions that define the potential level of hazard for the individual employee.

The synergistic nature of the physical and psychosocial hazard in the work environment is also important. Interactions can occur between the different types of hazard and their consequent effects on the health of the individual (Levi 1984). Stress in the workplace, from whatever cause, may inadvertently lead to risk taking behaviour by the individual worker.

MANAGEMENT OF HAZARDS AND DANGERS

When dealing with safety issues in the workplace environment, there have been three common approaches (Landy 1989):

1. The 'engineering' approach assumes that by modifying the environment or the equipment used, safety can be enhanced and accident rates reduced. Modifying the environment should include both physical and psychosocial factors.
2. In the 'person psychology' approach the psychologist attempts to identify particular individual characteristics that might lead a worker to be more accident-prone or to take risks. Within this particular approach the focus is on training programmes that will highlight individual behaviour and attempt to influence change in unsafe behaviour.
3. The 'industrial–social' approach makes the assumption that unsafe behaviour is linked to group motivation. Individual motivation is linked with conditions in the

Table 3.2 Psychosocial hazards in the work environment (from Cox & Griffiths 1996)

Category	Conditions
Content of work	
Job content	Lack of variety or short work cycles, fragmented or meaningless work, underuse of skills, high uncertainty
Workload and work pace	Work overload or underload, lack of control over pacing, high levels of time pressure
Work schedule	Shift working, inflexible work schedules, unpredictable hours, long or unsocial hours
Interpersonal relationships at work	Social or physical isolation, poor relationships with superiors, interpersonal conflict, lack of social support
Control	Low participation in decision making, lack of control over work
Context of work	**Pages 127–143**
Organizational culture and function	Poor communication, low levels of support for problem solving and personal development, lack of definition of organizational objectives
Role in organization	Role ambiguity and role conflict, responsibility for people
Career development	Career stagnation and uncertainty, underpromotion or overpromotion, poor pay, job insecurity, low social value of work
Home–work interface	Conflicting demands of work and home, low support at home, dual career problems

environment that might support unsafe behaviour, for example it might be that taking risks is considered the 'macho' thing to do or that safe behaviour takes a lot more energy than careless behaviour. The focus in this approach is to try and change group behaviour so that people prefer safe practices (Landy 1989).

These approaches can be applied to reduce risks and promote health in other environments besides the workplace. Although health promotion approaches (Naidoo & Wills 2000) recognize the multiple factors that influence the health status of an individual, they often focus on changing individual behaviour. When exploring 'how' individuals may change their behaviour to avert hazards to their external or internal environment, nurses must also be aware about 'why' individuals behave the way they do. They must also be aware that individuals may not carry out stated intentions (Ajzen & Fishbein 1980). The nurse's role in health education and promotion of safety is thus reliant upon the patient's willingness to listen, understand and comply with the information he or she is being offered. Health professionals must present information in a way that is appropriate to the patient's needs and sensitive to the patient's likely reaction if it is to be successful.

The main factors influencing an individual's response to health advice include:

- readiness
- motivation
- maturity
- level of education (Akinsola 1983).

Readiness

Human beings will only respond positively when they are physically, socially and psychologically ready to respond. For instance, the parent of an acutely ill 2-year-old child may not be ready to learn what caused the child's illness until the physical condition of the child improves; or elderly patients may be reluctant to mobilize independently in hospital because the floor is too slippery or they are unsure of the ward layout.

Motivation

To gain a better patient outcome, patient involvement and active participation are essential. Motivation requires an explanation about the importance of treatment and the use of equipment. Teaching patients with newly diagnosed diabetes mellitus to test their own blood sugar and to give their own insulin will mean that they can regain their self-esteem by being independent. Gaining someone's involvement in his or her treatment requires the individual to have some insight into the illness. This can be difficult if the nature of the illness affects perception, as in some mental illnesses in which the individual has no insight, or if there is apathy due to low self-esteem.

Maturity

Because of differences in the maturity of individuals, carers need to be able to choose their words carefully so as not to either patronize clients and relatives or use words and concepts that are inappropriate. Careful consideration also has to be given to people with learning disabilities or to adolescents who appear physically more mature than their chronological age. Although they may appear adult, their perceptions and experiences and understandings may be limited. Initiatives such as 'A campaign with street cred' (Lowery 1996) have successfully targeted teenagers with asthma, aiming information and support directly at the adolescent age group in order to resolve risk-taking problems associated with poor compliance.

Theories of risk taking are of interest to psychologists and health educators alike because they can help to explain major barriers to the effective provision of healthcare advice. Campaigns to encourage individuals to stop smoking or to reduce the number of people drinking and driving are two examples where individuals may be aware of the risk to safety in their own (and others') environment, but still persist in risk-taking behaviour.

CARE DELIVERY KNOWLEDGE

Risk management in nursing falls within two main remits: firstly the safety of the individual patient or client and secondly, in partnership with the multidisciplinary team, ensuring safe systems of care.

PATIENT SAFETY

There is a need to assess individual patients in relation to their own safety and the safety of others. This is an essential part of nursing care. The need for cognitive understanding of risk and physical compatibility within the environment has already been illustrated in relation to accidents in the community and these features are equally applicable in the care setting. In caring for children these two considerations are particularly important. For clients with learning disabilities, assessment of individual ability and understanding is essential as it cannot be assumed that an individual will behave consistently with someone of a similar chronological age. Nurses in mental health have to assess and plan care for their patients ensuring the safety of the patient and other patients within the care setting, and their own personal safety. Nurses are also becoming involved in ensuring that patients who are released into the community do not pose a hazard to themselves or anyone else (Noak 1997). Finally, in caring for adults, there is a need for all of the above, because adult individuals develop to different stages of maturity both physically and psychologically, and the effects of disease can impair individual ability to maintain a safe environment.

Ensuring patient safety while receiving care is ultimately an employer's responsibility in all settings, but nurses have a direct role in implementing safe care for patients who bring individual perceptions to the care setting. Fear or anxiety may mean a patient is not willing to comply with planned care procedures regardless of how happy they may have appeared with the negotiated plan. For example, a patient

with a stroke may not like the hoist used to transfer him or her from the bed to the chair. There will always be dilemmas about how patients should receive intervention that is appropriate and safe. Discussing interventions with the patient can air anxieties, and in this case finding a different lifting system that the patient would feel happier with could be safer for all concerned.

Generally, the nurse identifying a risk must ensure that action is taken. Further investigation may reveal that the problem has already been recognized and a solution is being sought; a policy decision may be required; or the solution may have cost implications and the money has yet to be found. The nurse has a responsibility to establish the current position and if necessary to facilitate change for improvement. Change must be implemented with the co-operation of all staff to ensure maximum benefit. If working with managers and staff to resolve a risk to the patient is ineffective, then advice may be required from outside agencies with a remit for the facilitation of health and safety at work. A safe policy for practice should exist and be readily available for most of the procedures that a nurse will perform with a patient.

Evidence-based practice

The 2007 National Confidential Enquiry into Patient Outcome and Death (NCEPOD) report on emergency admissions (National Confidential Enquiry into Patient Outcome and Death 2007) highlighted the need for early decision making by doctors with the most appropriate skills and knowledge based on the clinical needs of the patient. The key findings of the report were that:

- 7.1% of cases had an initial assessment that was assessed by the NCEPOD advisors as poor or unacceptable.
- 6.8% of patients did not receive adequate clinical observations, both in type and frequency.

One recommendation was that a clear physiological monitoring plan should be made for each patient commensurate with their clinical condition. This should detail what is to be monitored, the desirable parameters and the frequency of observations, and be so regardless of the type of ward to which the patients are transferred. The report also highlighted, within its case studies, that in some cases nursing handover was poor.

A LEARNING ENVIRONMENT

It is vital that we learn from events where things have gone wrong. There is a variety of terminology used within the risk management arena, with terms such as incident, adverse event, accident, etc. all being used by different organizations to describe the same thing. It is recognized that such variation can cause confusion and act as a barrier to learning. To attempt to introduce some international uniformity in the area of patient safety the World Health Organization's World Alliance for Patient Safety has launched a project to develop an international classification for patient safety. This project, 'Taxonomy for Patient Safety', aims to define, harmonize and group patient safety concepts into an internationally agreed classification. This will help elicit, capture and analyse factors relevant to patient safety in a manner conducive to learning and system improvement. The classification aims to be adaptable yet consistent across the entire spectrum of health care and across cultures and languages (World Health Organization 2006).

Events where things have gone wrong will be referred to as 'incidents'. Hospitals are encouraged to have a single process for the reporting and managing of all incidents, whether involving staff (for example, a needlestick injury) or patients. The value of structured local investigation into the causes of incidents and of learning from incidents reported nationally and internationally is now well recognized. Nurses and health workers, in all settings, have a duty to report any act or omission arising during health care that could have led or did lead to unintended or unexpected harm, loss or damage. Not all incidents lead to harm as in many cases actions or circumstances prevent harm, even though a system or process has failed to work as it should have done. Such incidents are invaluable as tools that provide 'free lessons' and should not be wasted. The person who notices the incident should complete an incident report at the time and not assume someone else will do so. It is important that the reporting system is entirely separate from the disciplinary process, except when an event has involved malicious or criminal activity or where it was part of an activity which contravened the individual's professional code of conduct.

Reporting incidents allows safer systems of care to be developed. New guidelines, care pathways, policies or additional training can be introduced in response to incidents, to reduce future risk of errors. As incident report forms are disclosable in the event of litigation or external inquiry, it is vital to ensure details are accurate and factual without apportioning blame or giving opinions.

Examples of incidents involving patients include the following:

- delay in diagnosis or wrong diagnosis
- administration of the wrong drug or incorrect quantity of the right drug
- patient falls.

Most hospitals apply a grading system to incidents, to allow differentiation between those incidents that require a full and detailed investigation and those that in themselves do not warrant such a detailed investigation but should be considered en masse with similar incidents over a particular period, to identify patterns or trends. The grading system usually involves a matrix with a choice being made on a fixed point scale of how likely the incident is to recur and what the potential consequences could have been. Such grading systems were adopted from the grading of risks (i.e. they were forward looking), but they have been of use in differentiating between incidents (i.e. backward looking events). Some trusts ask the person reporting the incident to make a judgement on the likelihood of recurrence and the potential consequences. Others request that only those with particular levels of authority make this judgement.

Trusts are required to provide incident data, including the degree of actual harm to the patient, as part of their submissions to the National Reporting and Learning System (NRLS), with the options being no harm, low, moderate, severe and death (National Patient Safety Agency 2003). The NPSA uses the information reported to the NRLS to provide feedback reports to individual trusts. These highlight key themes from the pattern of reports from that trust, in relation to the national pattern of reporting. Such feedback reports are not available publicly, but sample reports, using real data but for a fictitious 'Anytown' organization, are available via the NPSA website, at http://www.npsa.nhs.uk/nrls/patient-safety-incident-data/feedback-reports/sample-reports-benchmarking/.

Additionally, the NPSA publishes anonymized national data reports from the NRLS (National Patient Safety Agency 2007a). The NPSA uses NRLS data to identify trends and patterns in patient safety, and in providing solutions to problems. Publications include a *Patient Safety Bulletin* (National Patient Safety Agency 2007b), and reports such as *Safer Care for the Acutely Ill Patient: Learning from Serious Incidents* (National Patient Safety Agency 2007c).

In addition to reporting aggregated incident data to the NPSA, certain specific incidents are required to be reported to national agencies, including the following:

- The Health and Safety Executive, for work-related deaths, major injuries or over-three-day injuries, work related diseases and dangerous occurrences (near miss accidents). Such reports are required under the Reporting of Injuries, Diseases and Dangerous Occurrences Regulations 1995 (RIDDOR).
- The Medicines and Healthcare products Regulatory Agency (MHRA), for side-effects (adverse drug reaction) from a medicine; incidents involving a medical device; and serious adverse events and serious adverse reactions related to blood and blood components (as required by the UK Blood Safety and Quality Regulations 2005 and the EU Blood Safety Directive).

In most NHS trusts, reporting to external agencies, including submissions to the NPSA NRLS, is usually carried out by a corporate department though direct reporting from frontline staff is possible.

Investigation of incidents

All staff should fully cooperate with incident investigations, otherwise limitations will be placed on the learning to be gained. Root cause analysis (RCA) is the NPSA's preferred method of investigating incidents. It is a technique pioneered outside health care but in recent years has begun to be adapted for use within health care. Root cause analysis (RCA) is a retrospective review of an incident to identify what happened, how it happened and why it happened. 'Root causes' are the fundamental issues which have led to an incident happening. There are a number of techniques to assist in conducting a root cause analysis. The NPSA has an Incident Investigation and Root Cause Analysis Toolkit available via its website (National Patient Safety Agency 2006).

 3.1 – ROOT CAUSE ANALYSIS

Objectives:
- To determine a definition of root cause analysis.
- To identify the steps in the process of root cause analysis as determined by the NPSA.
- To apply the process of root cause analysis in practice.

SAFE SYSTEMS OF CARE

The second remit for nurses in risk assessment is more general and interprofessional and relates to the care environment. The outcome of risk assessment must be the identification and implementation of risk management strategies to ensure that particular risks are eliminated or adequately controlled. However, there is evidence that accidents do happen and that many result from the failure of control systems, such as policy failure, deficient working practices and inadequate communication, as well as poorly defined responsibilities and staff working beyond their competence.

RISK ASSESSMENT

Nurses need to know what the risks are and develop appropriate control systems. Risk assessment is not a 'once and for all' activity; it must be revised as changes occur such as new equipment, revised systems of work and different approaches to patient care.

Defining a risk

Before carrying out the risk assessment, a distinction must be made between 'hazard' and 'risk'. You will have already seen that a hazard can be defined as something with the potential to cause harm (Cox and Griffiths 1996). A risk can be defined as the likelihood that the harm from a particular hazard is realized. The relationship between risk and hazard can be illustrated by the use of glutaraldehyde, which is a hazard in nursing. The risk of industrial asthma resulting from inhalation of glutaraldehyde is high if it is used in areas without adequate ventilation and personal protective clothing (i.e. inappropriately). However, with effective ventilation and a defined safe system of work, the risks associated with glutaraldehyde can be reduced, although it still remains a hazard.

PLANNING AND IMPLEMENTING A STRATEGY FOR RISK MANAGEMENT

Planning care relates to the promotion of a safe environment for clients. There are two levels to planning: firstly, planning care in relation to the safety of the individual client, and secondly, planning daily work in relation to controlling of risks or hazards in the environment.

Issues in planning related to patients

The need for a hospital admission may bring about physical hazards associated with the strangeness of the environment and an unknown ward layout. Patients may demonstrate anxiety and an unnatural response as a result of their situation. The nurse should identify and address these problems when making the assessment of a client's needs and in negotiating a safe and acceptable plan of care. Talking with the patient about how best to address his or her needs is an important starting point, since compliance with a safe plan for care is critical. An example could relate to a hospital 'no smoking' policy. If a client usually enjoys cigarettes at home and will not entertain giving up smoking in hospital, it is not helpful to include in the nursing care plan that smoking is prohibited. For the client, this may lead to anger and frustration and potential non-compliance, either overtly or covertly. In a setting where there are inflammable substances (such as oxygen) this can create a serious risk both for the client and all others in the vicinity. It is safer to negotiate a plan with the client which agrees where cigarettes can be smoked safely, also ensuring that the client is able to gain access to this area. Information can also be given about the hazards of smoking in no-smoking areas, and there may be an opportunity for health education, leading to a reduction in smoking.

Reflection and portfolio evidence

In your next practice setting, look at a patient's plan of care. Take a particular note of any assessment that includes areas where safety may require interprofessional care planning.

- What measures would you plan for this patient?
- How do your ideas compare with those of the care team?
- Have both psychological and physical safety issues been addressed?
- Has the plan been updated to incorporate any changes in the patient's situation?
- Record your findings as a 'managing risk case study' in your portfolio.

Risk and hazard control in the care setting

The key questions in identification of risk (Roberts 2002) are:

- What can go wrong?
- How frequently can it go wrong?
- What would be the effect?
- What can be done to stop it happening?

Risk management provides a framework for the assessment, analysis, prioritization, treatment and review of risks. A register of identified risks should be compiled in every area. This should include the date the risk was identified, the risk itself, the impact (consequence) the risk would have, the chance (likelihood) of the risk happening and the risk score (consequence × likelihood). In addition, the register should also provide information on the person assigned as responsible for the risk, what action needs to be taken to minimize the risk, what residual risk (if any) remains and the continuing monitoring action plan. Risk registers in healthcare organizations are usually coordinated by a corporate department.

Decision-making exercise

Managers opened an acute mental illness admission ward on the fourth floor of a general hospital to replace the admission facility of the local psychiatric hospital, which was due to close. The ward was previously used as an acute surgical ward and there were numerous cubicles and several exits; the windows opened without restriction and were not glazed with safety glass. Shortly after the ward opened, the managers were surprised by the occurrence of a number of suicides.

- How might a risk assessment have identified potential hazards in this situation?
- Using methods of hazard control, how could you address the hazards of poor observation from cubicles, exits and windows?

- Find out what the National Patient Safety Agency's position is on suicides achieved through hanging from non-collapsible shower rails.
- What measures should be taken to prevent this? Are these measures applicable to all healthcare settings? If not, how would you ensure the safety of 'at-risk' patients?

Safe equipment

In order to ensure an optimum working environment for nursing, it is important that all equipment in use is well maintained and all practices are safe and without risks to health as outlined by Section 2(2)(a) of the Health and Safety at Work Act 1974. This is a general requirement, defined by the Health and Safety at Work etc. Act as including machinery, equipment and appliances used at work, as well as the establishment of safe systems or practices while working.

In caring for clients, nurses use a wide variety of equipment. The following criteria apply to the way in which all equipment is used:

- Equipment must meet all the current health and safety standards.
- Equipment must be regularly inspected and serviced.
- The system of work must be safe.
- Repair and maintenance operations must have a safe system of work identified.
- Personal protective equipment should be provided if required.

A safe system of work needs to be identified for repair and maintenance operations themselves and this can have implications for nurses. For instance, the safe decontamination of equipment before maintenance must be specified. This may be especially important in areas where equipment has been used with clients carrying infectious organisms. At a simple level working with children for instance, this may mean that there should be a procedure for cleaning toys safely after a child who has an infection such as diarrhoea and vomiting has used them, before checking their safety for offering to another child. It also implies the appropriate cleaning of equipment or even rooms after use by patients.

Managing safe handling and storage of substances

Within nursing practice, handling of potentially hazardous substances may be a regular occurrence. Issues related to the safe handling of substances are addressed in Section 53 of the Health and Safety at Work Act and are developed further by the Control of Substances Hazardous to Health (COSHH) Regulations 1988 and 2002.

COSHH Regulations 1988 and 2002

This was the most significant piece of health and safety legislation after the Health and Safety at Work etc. Act 1974. It applies to all work where people (including nurses) are exposed or liable to be exposed to substances hazardous to health. The regulations give both a general description of the types of substances that are hazardous to health and a specific list of materials currently regarded as hazardous. There are 19 regulations, which include key duties such as assessment and training and a related Approved Code of Practice is given for each regulation.

Any 'substance' should be regarded as hazardous to health in the form in which it occurs in the work activity, whether or not its mode of causing injury to health is known and whether or not the active constituent has been identified. A substance hazardous to health is not just a single chemical compound but also includes mixtures, for example of compounds, microorganisms or allergens. The Approved Code of Practice further defines what is hazardous. Among the key points are that:

- Different forms of the same substance may present different hazards, for instance when a solid is ground into dust.
- Impurities may create hazards.
- Fibres of a certain size or shape can be hazardous.

There is also a summary of duties of employers under the COSHH Regulations, which states that the employer must:

- Assess the risks.
- Assess the steps needed to meet the regulation.
- Prevent or at least control exposure.
- Ensure controls are used to monitor exposure.
- Provide health surveillance.
- Examine and test control.
- Inform, instruct and train employees and non-employees (Brewer 1994).

The storage of substances on a ward or unit should follow the principles of 'good housekeeping' to improve safety. This may mean storing glass bottles on the back of a low shelf to avoid breakages, or keeping the stock of substances to a minimum to avoid stock expiring and the dangers of major spillages. There should be procedures and policies in relation to the handling of substances and these should be readily available.

PROFESSIONAL AND ETHICAL KNOWLEDGE

INTERPROFESSIONAL WORKING

Initiatives to minimize risk are best formulated and actioned through a team approach. However, all members of healthcare teams may not necessarily share the same interests, values, beliefs and reasons and may not support the same objectives. This can be a significant hurdle to the implementation of any risk reduction strategy. Whilst there is sometimes resistance to change, the nature and reasons for resistance need to be understood and respected, encouraging shared ownership. Nurses must work with their health colleagues, valuing and sharing the expertise that each profession brings to patient care, to achieve successful changes in practice and improve quality and safety of health care.

Reflection and portfolio evidence

- Find out what method of reporting patient safety incidents is used in the healthcare setting in which you are working.
- Using a standard report, try writing an incident report about a patient for whom you have been caring, imagining that the patient has been given intravenous antibiotics intended for a different patient.
- Record your findings in your portfolio.

UPHOLDING THE LAW AND MAINTAINING STANDARDS

There are many laws that relate to the provision of health care and in addition there are professional and patient standards, regulations, rules, guidelines and expectations, which all govern the way health professionals must work. Some of the laws, for example the National Health Act 1977 and the Health Act 1999, impose upon carers a duty of quality. Case law also sets ever-increasing standards of care in a climate which requires increasing patient involvement. Key issues for nurses are statutory requirements and professional requirements. Local policies and guidelines are often formed on the basis of these requirements and therefore serve to assist health professionals in meeting the standards of care required of them.

Evidence-based practice

Gershon et al (1995) surveyed 1716 American care workers about their compliance with universal safety precautions. They found that compliance varied according to activity, but was overall strongly correlated to several key factors, including perceived organizational commitment to safety and perceived conflict of interest between the workers' need to protect themselves and the need to provide care for their patients. Risk taking personality, perception of risk, and knowledge and training were also noted to be influential factors.

Statutory requirements

Statutory requirements are laid down in legislation as Acts of Parliament. The key legislation that governs the way all health professionals must work is the Health and Safety at Work Act 1974. This Act aims to secure the health, safety and welfare of persons at work and to protect members of the public from risks that might be created by the work of others. European Union (EU) Directives (nicknamed the 'six-pack'; Box 3.1) came into force in 1993 and the Management of Health and Safety at Work Regulations 1999 form the legal framework for health and safety in the UK today. It is a criminal offence to fail to discharge any of the duties laid down in the Act and subsequent regulations, whether by intention or neglect. It is therefore vital that all nurses familiarize themselves with both the Act and subsequent regulations.

One set of regulations, the Reporting of Injuries, Diseases and Dangerous Occurrences Regulations (RIDDOR), is of particular importance in relation to incident reporting. Accidents and incidents covered by the regulations must be reported directly to the Health and Safety Executive, using a statutory reporting form. This is usually the responsibility of a designated person (e.g. the health and safety officer or risk manager) but the legal requirement for this highlights the necessity for nurses to ensure all incidents are reported in a timely manner.

Decision-making exercise

The following scenario could be used for a debate between two teams, one team representing the plaintiff and one the employer.

You are the defendant in a court case based on the Health and Safety at Work Act 1974, after you received a back injury from slipping on a wet floor. Although the floor dryer was broken and had been sent for repair, the cleaners did possess warning cones to advise employees about wet floors. There were none in evidence on the day that you slipped. The onus of proving that an employer has not fulfilled the statutory obligation by being 'reasonably practicable' is placed on the defendant (i.e. you). The court would then have to decide what is or was reasonable or practicable in your case.

● Decide how you could convince a court that the employer had broken the law.

Professional requirements

The UK Nursing and Midwifery Council (NMC) requires nurses to maintain a safe environment for their patients. This is illustrated within the Code of Professional Conduct

---

Box 3.1 The 'six-pack' regulations for health and safety: UK interpretations of the EU Directives

Management of Health and Safety at Work Regulations 1992
Manual Handling Regulations (Health and Safety Executive) 1992
Workplace (Health, Safety and Welfare) Regulations 1992
Health and Safety (Display Screen Equipment) Regulations 1992
Provision and Use of Work Equipment Regulations 1992
Personal Protective Equipment (PPE) at Work Regulations 1992

(Nursing and Midwifery Council 2008), which states that 'You must work with colleagues to monitor the quality of your work and maintain the safety of those in your care', and also that 'you must act without delay if you believe that you, a colleague or anyone else may be putting someone at risk'. Professional requirements are the standards required of all health professionals and can be used to regulate activities, to discipline individuals and increasingly, in the assessment of professional liability and medical negligence. Negligence can be defined as breaching a duty to use reasonable care and causing an injury to another. Compensation for injury (which may be psychological as well as physical) as the result of the action of a health professional is usually pursued through the civil law but may also come under the jurisdiction of the criminal courts. It is incumbent upon all health professionals and the health provider to have a duty of care to every patient.

External agencies and standards

In terms of risk management, numerous external agencies set their own standards and requirements, with which healthcare providers must demonstrate compliance. The agencies discussed below, and the standards they set, form the basis of the way risk is managed in the NHS.

Standards for Better Health

The Department of Health issued the *Standards for Better Health* in July 2004 and updated it in 2006 (Department of Health 2006a). The standards describe the level of quality that healthcare organizations are expected to meet in terms of: 1) safety; 2) clinical effectiveness and cost-effectiveness; 3) governance; 4) patient focus; 5) accessible and responsive care; 6) care environment and amenities; and 7) public health. These seven areas are known as 'domains'. In each of the domains the individual standards fall into two categories:

- Core standards – which bring together and rationalize existing requirements for the health service, setting out the minimum level of service patients and service users have a right to expect.
- Developmental standards – which signal the direction of travel and provide a framework for NHS bodies to plan the delivery of services which continue to improve in line with increasing patient expectations.

The specified standards for better health form a key part of the performance assessment by the Healthcare Commission. There are 24 core standards but some have been split, resulting in 44 separate components. Each financial year healthcare organizations are required to make a public declaration of how they have performed in relation to each standard. The organization can state that a particular standard has been 'met' or 'not met', or that it has 'insufficient assurance' that the standard has been met, which means that it lacks the necessary evidence to support a clear assessment. Many of the standards relate to safety and risk. Some standards are of direct relevance as they all fall within the 'safety' domain and have been included within an Evolve presentation for your further reading (see Evolve 3.2).

3.2 – STANDARDS FOR BETTER HEALTH

Objectives:
- To identify the key specific standards for achievement of safety for health trusts as identified within the above documents.
- To consider how these can be used in personal nursing practice.

Healthcare Commission

The Healthcare Commission is the independent inspection body for both the NHS and independent health care. In England, they are responsible for assessing and reporting on the performance of both NHS and independent healthcare organizations to ensure that they are providing a high standard of care. In Wales, their role is more limited and relates mainly to working on national reviews that cover both England and Wales, as well as their annual report on the state of health care. The Commission has a number of functions, which it summarizes as 'Inspecting, informing, improving' (Healthcare Commission 2005).

Care Quality Commission

The Care Quality Commission will combine the Commission for Social Care Inspection, the Healthcare Commission and the Mental Health Act Commission (Department of Health 2007). The intention is that the Care Quality Commission will apply a consistent approach to regulation for all types of services through a new registration regime requiring providers of health services and adult social care to be registered. It will also take rapid action against any organization that puts patients or users of services at risk. The government's stated plan is that the Care Quality Commission will be established in October 2008 and will take on responsibility for the regulation of health and adult social care in April 2009 – working towards full implementation of the new registration system from April 2010.

NHS Litigation Authority (NHSLA)

The NHS Litigation Authority (NHSLA) is a Special Health Authority which was established in 1995 to administer the Clinical Negligence Scheme for Trusts (CNST) and thereby provide a means for NHS organizations to fund the cost of clinical negligence claims. In addition to dealing with claims when they arise, there is an active risk management programme to help raise standards of care in the NHS and hence reduce the number of incidents leading to claims. Towards the end of 2004/5 the board of the NHSLA determined that it should develop its existing standards to produce a single set of risk management standards for each type of trust incorporating organizational, clinical and non-clinical/health and safety risks. There is therefore now a single set of risk management standards for each type of NHS healthcare organization: acute, ambulance, mental health and learning disability, and primary care trusts.

There are four levels of compliance with the NHSLA standards: 0, 1, 2 and 3, with level 3 being the maximum that can currently be achieved. Level 0 organizations must be assessed on an annual basis until such time as they achieve level 1. Level 1 organizations must be assessed against the standards at least once in any 2-year period. Level 2 and 3 organizations must be assessed against the standards at least once in any 3-year period.

There are five standards, each with 10 criteria (Table 3.3). The NHSLA issues separate clinical (CNST) standards against which maternity services are assessed where these are provided by the organization. Starting in 2007/8 these standards will be revised, with formal assessments against the new standards due to begin in April 2009. The maternity standards will continue to be clinical only.

Table 3.3 Standards and criteria (National Health Service Litigation Authority 2008)

Standard	1	2	3	4	5
Criterion	Governance	Competent and capable workforce	Safe environment	Clinical care	Learning from experience
1	Risk management strategy	Corporate induction	Secure environment	Patient identification	Incident reporting
2	Policy on procedural documents	Local induction of permanent staff	Child protection	Patient information	Raising concerns
3	Risk management committee(s)	Local induction of temporary staff	Vulnerable adults	Consent	Complaints
4	Risk awareness training for senior management	Supervision of medical staff in training	Moving and handling	Clinical record-keeping standards	Claims
5	Risk management process	Risk management training	Slips, trips and falls	Transfer of patients	Investigations
6	Risk register	Training needs analysis	Inoculation incidents	Medicines management	Analysis
7	Responding to external recommendations specific to the organization	Medical devices training	Maintenance of medical devices and equipment	Blood transfusion	Improvement
8	Clinical records management	Hand hygiene training	Harassment and bullying	Resuscitation	Best practice – NICE, NCEs and national guidance
9	Professional clinical registration	Moving and handling training	Violence and aggression	Infection control	Best practice – NSFs and high level enquiries
10	Employment checks	Supporting staff involved in an incident, complaint or claim	Stress	Discharge of patients	Being open

Essence of Care

The *Essence of Care* initiative, launched in February 2001 and revised in 2003 (National Health Service Modernisation Agency 2003), provides a tool to help practitioners take a patient-focused and structured approach to sharing and comparing practice. It has enabled healthcare personnel to work with patients to identify best practice and to develop action plans to improve care. This resulted in benchmarks originally covering eight areas of care (continence and bladder and bowel care; personal and oral hygiene; food and nutrition; pressure ulcers; privacy and dignity; record keeping; safety of clients with mental health needs in acute mental health and general hospital settings; and principles of self-care). Since then, further benchmark areas have been added (communication; promoting health; care environment). Many of the Essence of Care benchmark indicators are related to safety and risk.

The National Audit Office (NAO)

The National Audit Office scrutinizes public spending on behalf of Parliament. They audit the accounts of all central government departments and agencies as well as a wide range of other public bodies, and report to Parliament on the economy, efficiency and effectiveness with which they have used public money. They also report to Parliament on the value for money with which these bodies have spent public money. In 2005, the NAO published a report entitled *A Safer Place for Patients: Learning to Improve Patient Safety*. The report made a number of recommendations targeted at the Department of Health, the NPSA, the Healthcare Commission, and NHS trusts in general. The NAO report prompted a review, commissioned by the Chief Medical Officer, of the issues raised. This review resulted in a further report, *Safety First: A Report for Patients, Clinicians and Healthcare Managers* (Department of Health 2006b). This report highlighted the need to build on the progress that has been achieved in addressing the patient safety agenda to refocus efforts to enable clinicians and healthcare organizations to deliver safe health care. Fourteen recommendations were made which together signalled a new national approach. This is likely to have significant impact on the role of the NPSA, and the future use of the NRLS.

Decision-making exercise

You are at work when the fire alarm sounds. The fire doors shut automatically.

- What would your action be?
  Staff and visitors continue to go through the doors and do not respond to the alarm.
- How would you deal with this situation?

  You are advised by the fire officer that the ward should be evacuated. While you are making arrangements for evacuation a patient has a cardiac arrest.

- What would be the priority? The patient who has arrested or the other patients?
- What action would you need to take in both cases?
- What questions may you need to ask (a) at the time? (b) afterwards?

THE CONSENT PROCESS

Gaining patient consent to treatment is a process largely overseen within risk management, and the NHS Litigation Authority in the Clinical Negligence Scheme for trusts sets out standards of good practice. An overview of the consent process is therefore included within this chapter. In 2001, the Department of Health introduced guidance documents on consent, as well as a 'model' consent policy and consent forms (Department of Health 2001). These are required to be adopted in all NHS trusts. This has the advantage of ensuring that the transient population of health professionals is familiar with consent procedures and documentation in every NHS hospital in the UK. Consent is a patient's agreement for a health professional to provide care and must be 'informed', meaning that the patient must give agreement based on a sound understanding of the nature and consequences of the care offered, or indeed the consequences of not agreeing. For consent to be valid, the patient must:

- be competent (mentally able) to take the particular decision
- have received sufficient information to take it
- not be acting under duress.

While a patient must agree to every act of nursing care this can usually be a verbal agreement whereas for significant procedures it is essential for health professionals to document clearly both a patient's agreement to the intervention and the discussions that led up to that agreement. Consent to treatment of children and adults who lack mental capacity is complex and requires specialist knowledge. For guidance on this and for further information health professionals should consult the *Reference Guide to Consent for Examination or Treatment* (Department of Health 2001), also available on the Department of Health website, the address of which is listed at the end of this chapter.

ETHICAL DILEMMAS IN RISK MANAGEMENT

The government seeks to meet its objective of standardizing quality in health care through Clinical Governance. The Department of Health states as the official view that Clinical Governance is necessary to overcome regional variations in the quality of health care. One of the functions of NICE is to develop the standardization of treatments throughout the UK. Evidence-based guidelines on the most appropriate treatments for a range of medical conditions are drawn up by NICE, which bases its recommendations on cost as well as on clinical effectiveness. While the government's objective is to end the so-called 'postcode' prescribing lottery, Harpwood (2001) points out that NICE, as a public body, is subject to the Human Rights Act 1998 and must therefore not act in a manner that is incompatible with the rights in the European Convention on Human Rights. She comments that it might be possible for an individual who believes that a NICE recommendation has denied him the right to life-saving treatment to bring a challenge under the Act. This might prove an interesting ethical and legal challenge.

Following the tragic events at Bristol Royal Infirmary, where there was found to be an unacceptably high mortality rate in paediatric cardiac surgery, the Bristol Inquiry made many recommendations (see annotated website). The inquiry sought to identify any professional, management and organizational failures and to recommend action to safeguard future patients. 'Whistleblowing' is the term given to raising concerns about the professional competency of colleagues. As a result of the inquiry, NHS trusts are being encouraged to require employees to pass on such information and must establish mechanisms of protection for those that do. Many trusts are therefore establishing 'raising concerns' policies which allow concerns to be expressed in a confidential manner. There are ethical dilemmas surrounding whistleblowing, for while it is essential that incompetent or unsafe health professionals are prevented from doing harm, policies may be open to abuse by aggrieved or malicious members of staff. In addition, it may prove very difficult to afford career protection to a person who in good faith reports a concern about the practice of a colleague.

PERSONAL AND REFLECTIVE KNOWLEDGE

Within the scope of your role, it is important to maintain your own health and safety and promote that of your patients and clients. Occupational health departments provide support for all workers and should be accessed for advice whenever you have concerns about your own health. Risk and safety are everybody's business. It can be argued that the most crucial role for the nurse is as set out in the Nursing and Midwifery Council's (2008) Code of Professional Conduct: to act to identify and minimize the risk to patients and clients and above all else, as Florence Nightingale said, 'Do no harm'.

CASE STUDIES APPLYING PRINCIPLES OF SAFETY AND RISK

Case study: Mental health

Jeremiah Jacobs is 62 years old. He has lived in a large rural hospital for the mentally ill for the last 30 years and is diagnosed as having moderate learning disabilities and schizophrenia. Jeremiah remains in a long-term care facility because as yet no appropriate community facility has been found. In the hospital where he lives many patients have been moved into community homes and wards have been closed. The hospital is now a small facility where all clients are well known by the resident staff. Jeremiah enjoys sitting on the main ward corridor trying to trip passers-by up. As everyone knows him, they know to keep out of tripping distance. One day a visitor comes into the hospital and is tripped up by Jeremiah. The visitor sustains a number of bruises and sues the hospital.

- Do you think the visitor will be successful in her claim?
- Who was responsible for ensuring the visitor's safety?
- Which section of the Health and Safety at Work Act 1974 may be referred to in this case?
- Decide how you could have prevented this situation from arising.

Case study: Adult

Mrs Smith is a 95-year-old woman who has arrived at the accident and emergency department after a fall at her home. She had been found by neighbours after crying out for some hours. On arrival in hospital Mrs Smith is cold and in pain and appears confused. She is to have a radiograph of her femur as a fracture is suspected. A nurse takes Mrs Smith to the radiography department and then goes on a coffee break. Mrs Smith attempts to get off the trolley while left alone in the radiography department and falls again.

- Using the information gained from this chapter write down the questions that you think should be asked, in the event of an inquiry into the incident. For example, did the nurse inform the radiographer that the patient was there? If not, why not? If yes, why was there no one with her?
- Were the trolley sides up or down? What system of work is there for transferring patients from the accident and emergency department to the radiography department? Is there one? Was it followed?

Case study: Child

As a school nurse you are attempting to reduce the number of home accidents among schoolchildren. This means that you plan to attend the children's school and talk to a group of 5–7-year-olds about the types of accidents that may occur in the home.

- What factors may influence the way in which you help to ensure that the children can participate actively in their own risk assessment and hazard management?
- Decide on a plan of action that could help get the safety message across to this group.
- Who is ultimately responsible for ensuring your safety while you are visiting the school to talk to the children? Which section of the Health and Safety at Work Act 1974 would apply in this instance?

Case study: Learning disabilities

Benny Wong is a 25-year-old Chinese man with moderate learning difficulties. He is unable to care independently for himself and tends to be noisy and aggressive at times. Benny's parents are elderly and although they have been caring for him at home they have recently been finding him an increasing challenge. Benny has now been accepted into a community home which provides full-time care for a few clients with learning disabilities. For Benny the move is a great change since he is used to living with his Chinese-speaking parents in a quiet house in a small village where he is well known to the community. His new home is in a suburban estate close to a main road.

- Using the principles of risk assessment, identify the hazards that may be a problem for Benny in his new home.
- Try to decide what the main safety risks are for Benny.
- Now decide what strategies may be appropriate for tackling the risks that you have identified.
- Finally, identify what barriers may need to be overcome in making Benny safe in his new home.

SUMMARY

This chapter has sought to draw together the concepts of a safe environment and safety for the individual. It has included:

1. Basic human needs and the problems that might arise from a lack of or substandard level of achievement of these needs.
2. An overview of the hazards that might be encountered in the environment and the risks associated with the effect of these hazards.
3. Examination of ways that health professionals might seek to reduce the likelihood of materialization of risk for their patients.
4. Principles of careful risk management, both proactive and reactive, that are applicable to all healthcare settings, demonstrated by case study exercises in the four branches of nursing.
5. An insight into health and safety, thereby including health workers in the wide context of risk.
6. The current and rapidly evolving agenda for patient safety in the UK, which is based on the need to prevent occurrence and recurrence of adverse healthcare events.
7. A brief overview of the consent process.

Annotated Further Reading and Websites

http://www.dh.gov.uk/en/Publicationsandstatistics/Publications/PublicationsPolicyAndGuidance/DH_4005475
The Essence of Care: Patient-focused Benchmarking for Health Care Practitioners, on the Department of Health website.

http://2007ratings.healthcarecommission.org.uk/homepage.cfm
http://www.npsa.nhs.uk
The Healthcare Commission website highlights the activities of the National Patient Safety Agency (NPSA), which is dedicated to analysing reports on incidents and near misses among NHS patients, introducing preventative measures and bringing the patient safety movement to a national level.

http://www.nhsla.com/home.htm
NHS Litigation Authority (NHSLA) website.

www.mhra.gov.uk/home/idcplg?IdcService=SS_GET_PAGE&nodeId=5
The Medicines and Healthcare products Regulatory Agency (MHRA) website.

http://www.bristol-inquiry.org.uk
This provides useful reading on the Bristol Inquiry and lessons learned, which might be said to have generated the emphasis on risk management in the UK today.

www.dh.gov.uk/consent
This site gives information about the consent process, the reference document, *Reference Guide to Consent for Examination or Treatment* and the Department of Health model consent policy and forms.

www.nice.org.uk
The National Institute for Health and Clinical Excellence website publishes current guidelines on best practice in a variety of clinical fields.

www.rospa.org.uk
The website of the Royal Society for the Prevention of Accidents (RoSPA). This is a useful site if you wish to research accident statistics for project work.

References

Ajzen I, Fishbein M 1980 Understanding attitudes and predicting social behavior. Prentice Hall, Englewood Cliffs

Akinsola HY 1983 Behavioural science for nurses. Churchill Livingstone, Singapore

Bloor M 1995 The sociology of HIV transmission. Sage, London

Bonnefoy XR, Braubach M, Moissonnier B, Monolbaev K, Röbbel N 2003 Housing and health in Europe: preliminary results of a pan-European study. American Journal of Public Health 93(9): 1559–1563

Brewer S 1994 Royal College of Nursing safety representatives' manual. Royal College of Nursing of the UK, Southampton

Brunekreef B, Janssen NA, De Hartog J et al 1997 Air pollution from truck traffic and lung function in children living near motorways. Epidemiology 8(3):298–303

Clancy L, Goodman P, Sinclair H et al 2002 Effects of air pollution control in Dublin, Ireland: an intervention study. Lancet 360 (9341):1210–1214

Control of Substances Hazardous to Health (COSHH) Regulations 1988 HMSO, London

Control of Substances Hazardous to Health (COSHH) Regulations 2002 HMSO, London

Cox T, Griffiths A 1996 Assessment of psychosocial hazards at work. In: Schabracq MJ, Winnubst JAM, Cooper CL (eds) Handbook of work and health psychology. John Wiley, Chichester, pp 127–143

Cox T, Griffiths A, Cox S 1995 Work-related stress in nursing: managing the risk. International Labour Organization, Geneva

Department of Health 1997 The new NHS: modern dependable. Department of Health, London

Department of Health 1998 A first class service: quality in the new NHS. Department of Health, London

Department of Health 2000 Organization with a memory. Department of Health, London

Department of Health 2001 Reference guide to consent for examination or treatment. Department of Health, London

Department of Health 2006a Standards for better health (updated) April 2006. Department of Health, London

Department of Health 2006b Safety first: a report for patients, clinicians and healthcare managers. Department of Health, London

Department of Health 2007 The future regulation of health and adult social care in England: response to consultation. Department of Health, London

Douglas M 1966 Purity and danger: an analysis of concepts of pollution and taboo. Routledge, London

Fallowfield L 1990 The quality of life: the missing measurement in healthcare. University College London Press, London

Gabe J 1995 Medicine, health and risk: sociological approaches. Blackwell, Oxford

Gershon RRM, Vlahov D, Felknor SA et al 1995 Compliance with universal precautions among healthcare workers at three regional hospitals. American Journal of Infection Control 23(4):225–236

Harpwood V 2001 Negligence in healthcare: clinical claims and risk. Informa, London

Harrington JM, Gill FS 1992 Occupational health, 3rd edn. Blackwell, Oxford

Health and Safety (Display Screen Equipment) Regulations SI 2792 1992 HMSO, London

Health and Safety at Work Act 1974 HMSO, London

Healthcare Commission 2005 About the Healthcare Commission. Healthcare Commission, London

Howden-Chapman P, Matheson A, Crane J et al 2007 Effect of insulating existing houses on health inequality: cluster randomised study in the community. British Medical Journal 334(7591):460

Ineichen B 1993 Homes and health: how housing and health interact. Spon, London

Institute of Medicine 2000 To err is human: building a safer health system. Committee on Quality of Health Care in America, Institute of Medicine, National Academy Press, Washington, DC

International Labour Organization 1986 Psychosocial factors at work: recognition and control. International Labour Organization, Geneva

Irani DN, Johnson RT 2003 Diagnosis and prevention of bovine spongiform encephalopathy and variant Creutzfeldt–Jakob disease. Annual Review of Medicine 54:305–319

Karol MH 2002 Respiratory allergy: what are the uncertainties? Toxicology 181–182:305–310

Landrigan PJ, Garg A 2002 Chronic effects of toxic environmental exposures on children's health. Journal of Clinical Toxicology 40(4):449–456

Landy F 1989 Psychology of work behaviour, 4th edn. Brooks Cole, Pacific Grove

Levi L 1984 Stress in industry: causes, effects and prevention. International Labour Organization, Geneva

Lowery M 1996 A campaign with street cred to target teenagers with asthma. Nursing Times 92(42):34–37

Maas RP, Patch SC, Parker AF 2002 An assessment of lead exposure potential from residential cutoff valves. Journal of Environmental Health 65(1):9–14, 28

Management of Health and Safety at Work Regulations SI 2051 1992 HMSO, London

Management of Health and Safety at Work Regulations 1999 No. 3242. HMSO, London

Manual Handling Operations Regulations SI 2793 and Guidance on Regulations L23 1992 HMSO, London

Maslow AH 1970 Motivation and personality, 2nd edn. Harper & Row, New York

Naidoo J, Wills J 2000 Health promotion: foundations for practice, 2nd edn. Baillière Tindall, Edinburgh

National Audit Office 2005 A safer place for patients: learning to improve patient safety. HMSO, London

National Confidential Enquiry into Patient Outcome and Death (NCEPOD) 2007 Emergency admissions: a journey in the right direction? Available online: http://www.ncepod.org.uk/2007report1/Downloads/EA_report.pdf (accessed 8 August 2008)

National Health Service Litigation Authority 2008 NHSLA Risk management standards for acute trusts. Available on line: http://www.nhsla.com/NR/rdonlyres/A0BF6746-FDE4-4081-9BBE-4E3BF572E9E4/0/NHSLARiskManagementStandardsforAcuteTrusts2008V15Finalwebsite.doc (accessed 6 October 2008)

National Health Service Modernisation Agency 2003 Essence of care: patient-focused benchmarks for clinical governance. National Health Service Modernisation Agency, London

National Patient Safety Agency 2003 NRLS service dataset (document NSD001). Available online: http://www.npsa.nhs.uk/EasysiteWeb/getresource.axd?AssetID=6286&type=Full&servicetype=Attachment (accessed 6 October 2008)

National Patient Safety Agency 2006 Learning through action to reduce infection October 2006. Available online: http://www.npsa.nhs.uk/EasysiteWeb/getresource.axd?AssetID=5926&type=Full&servicetype=Attachment (accessed 6 October 2008)

National Patient Safety Agency 2007a National reporting and learning system data summary, issue 5, 1 April to 30 June 2007. Available online: http://www.npsa.nhs.uk/EasysiteWeb/getresource.axd?AssetID=5578&type=Full&servicetype=Attachment (accessed 6 October 2008)

National Patient Safety Agency 2007b Patient safety bulletin, issue 4, August 2007. Available online: http://www.npsa.nhs.uk/EasysiteWeb/getresource.axd?AssetID=6263&type=Full&servicetype=Attachment (accessed 6 October 2008)

National Patient Safety Agency 2007c Safer care for the acutely ill patient: learning from serious incidents. Available online: http://www.npsa.nhs.uk/patientsafety/alerts-and-directives/directives-guidance/acutely-ill-patient/(accessed 6 October 2008)

Nightingale F 1860 Notes on nursing: what it is and what it is not. Harrison, London

Nightingale F 1863 Notes on hospitals, 3rd edn. Longman Roberts & Green, London

Noak J 1997 Assessment of the risks posed by people with mental illness. Nursing Times 93(1):1–8

Nursing and Midwifery Council 2008 The Code: standards of conduct, performance and ethics for nurses and midwives. Nursing and Midwifery Council, London

Personal Protective Equipment (PPE) at Work Regulations SI 2966 1992 HMSO, London

Provision and Use of Work Equipment Regulations SI 2932 1992 HMSO, London

Purdom P, Walton XY 1971 Environmental health. Academic Press, London

Raw G, Goldman L 1996 Sick building syndrome: a suitable case for treatment. Occupational Health 48(11):388–392

Reporting of Injuries, Diseases and Dangerous Occurrences Regulations SI 2023 1985 (amended 1995) HMSO, London

Roberts G 2002 Risk management in healthcare, 2nd edn. Witherby, London

Royal Society Study Group 1992 Risk analysis perception and management. Royal Society, London

Simpson GC 1991 Risk perception and hazard awareness as factors in safe and efficient working: report for the Commission of the European Community. British Coal Corporation, Eastwood

Workplace (Health, Safety and Welfare) Regulations SI 3004 1992 HMSO, London

World Health Organization 2006 World Alliance for Patient Safety project to develop an international patient safety event classification: the conceptual framework of an international patient safety event classification. World Health Organization, Geneva

Chapter 4

Resuscitation and emergency care

Roderick Cable and Helen Swain

KEY ISSUES

SUBJECT KNOWLEDGE
- Early detection and the prevention of collapse
- Resuscitation guidelines
- The collapsed adult
- The heart and ventricular fibrillation
- The chain of survival
- The collapsed child
- Common causes of sudden collapse in children and adults, with particular reference to altered anatomy and physiology

CARE DELIVERY KNOWLEDGE
- Assessment, prevention of collapse and management of resuscitation
- Knowledge of the 2005 Resuscitation Guidelines

PROFESSIONAL AND ETHICAL KNOWLEDGE
- Role of the professional nurse in the emergency situation
- Legal issues relating to emergency interventions
- Ethical dilemmas surrounding resuscitation
- Reactions to sudden trauma and death

PERSONAL AND REFLECTIVE KNOWLEDGE
- Applying theory to practice through reflective and decision making exercises
- Expanding your knowledge through identified research based evidence
- Case studies to consolidate your knowledge (you may find it helpful to read one of the case studies on p. 85 before you start the chapter and use it as a focus for your reflections)
- Assessment of your own practice through specifically designed checklists

INTRODUCTION

When the new student nurse is first identified as 'a nurse' by their home community everyone appears to make a mental note, so that when an emergency occurs friends and relatives know where to turn for help. This general principle appears to apply equally to all nurses, including those who have specialized in diverse areas of practice, as many members of the public only recognize the traditional general nurse, and all nurses are expected to fill this role. How the nurse fulfils their role in the emergency situation when called to help as 'a nurse' has many implications. While it is important to begin by addressing the nursing knowledge needed to support the provision of resuscitation and emergency care, this chapter also focuses upon issues surrounding how the nurse might participate in emergency. Although remaining mostly in the same order to others in the book for convenience of reading, some components of psychosocial knowledge can be found within the section on professional knowledge. This is because many elements of the two sections are combined in this subject, needing to be considered together. This also allows for logical consideration of physical emergency care. It is, however, important to move through the chapter to remind yourself about the implications of participating in care at the same time as determining how you might do this and what types of knowledge you might need.

SUBJECT KNOWLEDGE

UNDERLYING PRINCIPLES OF EMERGENCY PHYSIOLOGY

Please revise the homeostatic mechanisms described in Chapter 7 before continuing with the following section.

Before considering the practicalities of resuscitation, it is important to have an understanding of the potential mechanism of sudden collapse so that a more logical approach can be made. The Resuscitation Council Guidelines (2005) have a basic assumption which is worth mentioning: that is, *the most common cause of non-traumatic sudden pulseless collapse in adults is cardiac in origin*, and more specifically ventricular fibrillation (VF), which will be described further in the next section. 'Collapse' can be defined as 'a potentially reversible, sudden and unexpected loss of normal consciousness' (sometimes this follows a period of deterioration). In infants and children, as we will see later, the situation is usually different, hence there is a different set of guidelines for them. The primary cause of non-traumatic collapse in children is classically of respiratory origin.

THE CARDIAC COLLAPSE

The heart and ventricular fibrillation

The heart is a four-chambered organ situated centrally and slightly to the left in the chest, behind the sternum (Figs 4.1 and 4.2).

A characteristic of cardiac muscle is its ability to contract in the absence of any external stimulation. This independent mechanism is coordinated by a unique electrical system within the heart, which results in a coordinated contraction of the heart muscle. This is sinus rhythm (Fig. 4.3) – a regular, coordinated cardiac rhythm producing a palpable pulse.

Reflection and portfolio exercise

Figure 4.3 is a representation of the normal electrical activity of the heart as measured by skin electrodes and a cardiac monitor. This is an electrocardiograph or ECG.

Referring to a physiology textbook, explain the pattern in relation to the way the electrical activity coordinates cardiac muscle contraction. Remember that this is only an indication of electrical activity and it does not necessarily relate directly to mechanical function.

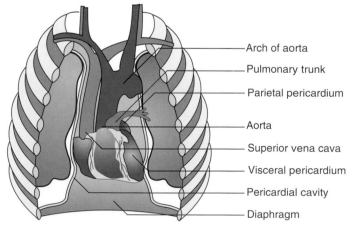

Figure 4.1 Location of the heart (adapted from Montague et al 2005, with kind permission of Elsevier).

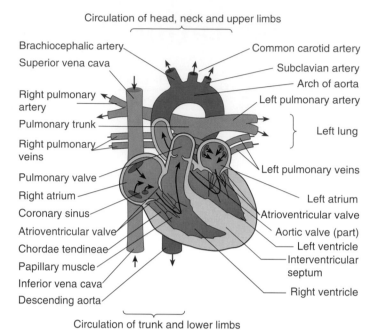

Figure 4.2 Structure of the heart and the direction of blood flow (from Montague et al 2005, with kind permission of Elsevier).

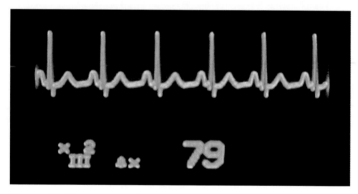

Figure 4.3 Normal sinus rhythm.

When the normal electric conduction system in the heart fails because of ischaemic heart disease (IHD), instead of stopping 'dead' (known as asystole; Fig. 4.4), each muscle fibre independently contracts and relaxes, giving the heart a shivering appearance: this is ventricular fibrillation (VF; Fig. 4.5). Although the heart is active there is no effective pumping action, therefore the collapsed individual will have no pulse and will quickly lose consciousness.

The significance of VF is the relative simplicity of treatment – passing an electric discharge over the heart (known as defibrillation) will often terminate a chaotic rhythm and (hopefully) allow a return to a spontaneous rhythm. The key factor in the success of the process of defibrillation is time. The longer the delay between the onset of VF and treatment by defibrillation, the worse the outcome.

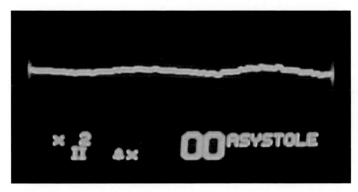

Figure 4.4 Asystole.

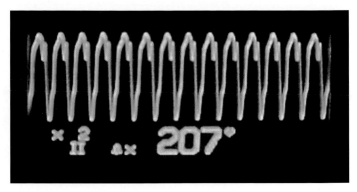

Figure 4.6 Pulseless ventricular tachycardia.

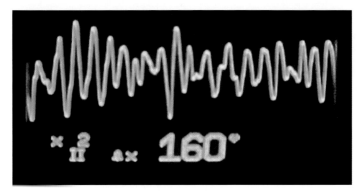

Figure 4.5 Ventricular fibrillation.

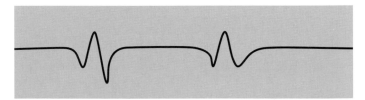

Figure 4.7 Pulseless electrical activity.

While the patient is in VF there is no coronary circulation and therefore no myocardial oxygenation, so the patient deteriorates rapidly. It is unlikely that basic life support (BLS) resuscitation is very efficient in maintaining an effective coronary circulation. It does, however, buy the patient time until further help is available.

During VF the lack of oxygen supply to the cardiac muscle results in the VF activity becoming less 'strong' or 'coarse' with time and eventually decaying to asystole.

Asystole (Fig. 4.4) is the classic 'straight line' (which, if you look carefully, is not really straight) on the cardiac monitor that is frequently used in films and TV soaps. Asystole indicates no apparent cardiac electrical activity and commonly occurs as a result of prolonged hypoxia or another significant illness. In practice, apparently well patients do not usually suddenly collapse into asystole as presented by the media.

The third rhythm (and the second requiring defibrillation) is pulseless ventricular tachycardia (with an emphasis on the word 'pulseless'). Within normal limits, as the heart rate increases, so does the cardiac output (rate × stroke volume); however, at very high pulse rates stroke volume will drop due to inadequate time for the heart to refill. As the heart rate increases a patient will initially become dizzy (cerebral hypoxia) and will show progressive symptoms of collapse as the blood pressure falls. Ultimately the patient will present as a cardiac arrest even though a connected electrocardiograph (ECG) will show a very rapid ventricular rate (Fig. 4.6).

Pulseless electrical activity (PEA) is the fourth rhythm associated with cardiac arrest (Fig. 4.7). In this situation, the nurse will see a rhythm on the cardiac monitor which is normally expected to be associated with a cardiac output, but no palpable carotid pulse is found on examining the patient. Essentially, the electrical conduction system within the cardiac muscle is functioning but there is no associated cardiac output (hence PEA). It is most often found in hospital patients after a period of deterioration. In the simplest situation, when a patient has lost most of the circulating blood volume, the heart will continue to work while it is still oxygenated, but no significant amount of blood will be circulated. There are several causes of PEA, including hypovolaemia (fluid loss, including bleeding and dehydration), severe pneumothorax (collapsed lung), hypothermia (low body temperature) and electrolyte imbalance in the blood and intracellular fluids. All these situations occur in adults and children, so both groups can present with PEA.

THE CHAIN OF SURVIVAL

The ideal survival scenario from ventricular fibrillation was first described by Cummins et al (1991) in the 'chain of survival' concept, further updated by the Resuscitation Council (UK) (2005), indicating the links required (Fig. 4.8). Following these stages can help guide you through the emergency situation. However, you will need further skills training to become competent in all aspects:

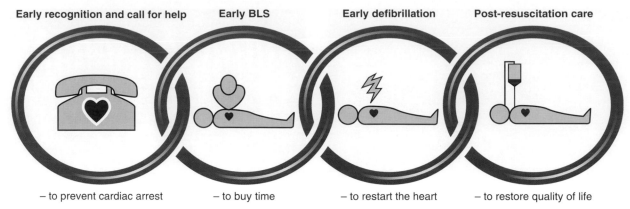

Early recognition and call for help	Early BLS	Early defibrillation	Post-resuscitation care
– to prevent cardiac arrest	– to buy time	– to restart the heart	– to restore quality of life

Figure 4.8 The chain of survival (Resuscitation Council 2005).

- Early recognition and help identifies the significance of preventing the collapse and ensures that defibrillation time is as short as possible.
- Early BLS slows deterioration.
- Early defibrillation (when appropriate) is the key to reversing the situation.
- Finally the provision of post-resuscitation life care to stabilize the patient and promote recovery.

As the VF scenario is potentially so treatable, this is the target of the adult resuscitation guidelines. Conveniently, all other medical emergencies are also reasonably managed by these guidelines.

THE COLLAPSED CHILD: DOES AGE MATTER?

Sudden collapse can occur in any victim of any age. Consideration must be given to the changes in anatomy and physiology between birth and adulthood as this requires a different approach in resuscitation skills (see Evolve 4.1).

The causes of collapse in infants (under 1 year old) and children (1–8 years old) are usually respiratory problems and resulting hypoxia rather than the cardiac problems found in adults, as degenerative heart disease is not common in children (Nadkarni et al 1997). This is due to the growing respiratory system, see below. Cardiac failure in children and infants rarely occurs as an initial problem and is usually linked to congenital cardiac abnormalities.

℮volve
learning system

4.1 – COMPARING PHYSIOLOGICAL DIFFERENCES ACCORDING TO AGE

- The normal physiological parameters of children and adults.
- Different physiological responses of children and adults to emergency and traumatic situations.
- How you can use this information in identifying potential emergency situations in your practice.

Evidence-based practice

The National Audit of Paediatric Resuscitation (NAPR) Study records out-of-hospital cardiopulmonary events (Resuscitation Council 2006); by July 2006 the sample stood at 642. The findings are as follows:

Cardiac	27%
Respiratory	25%
Trauma	12%
Sudden infant death syndrome (SIDS)	9%
Drowning	5%
Threatened airway	5%
Fitting	1%
Other	16%

This suggests the amalgamated figure of respiratory events exceeds those of a cardiac nature. However, events leading up to the cardiac and respiratory situations were not recorded so the actual cause is not clear.

The greatest mortality during childhood occurs in the first years of life. Causes include congenital problems, prematurity and infection due to the immature immune system. Sudden infant death syndrome (SIDS) remains the main cause of death in infants aged between 1 month and 1 year, although the guidelines on positioning infants have reduced this number considerably (Department of Health 1992, Coyne 1996, SIDS 2008). In children over 1 year of age, trauma is the most frequent cause of death (Child Accident Prevention Trust 2008). Choking is the third most common cause of childhood death; the Child Accident Prevention Trust (CAPT; 2008) states that in 2005, 16 children under 15 years of age died as a result of choking, and 12 children under 5.

Children who have had an out-of-hospital cardiac arrest and arrive in accident and emergency departments not breathing and pulseless have a poor outcome due to the brain damage resulting from lack of oxygen. There are

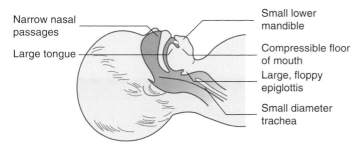

Narrow nasal passages

Large tongue

Small lower mandible

Compressible floor of mouth

Large, floppy epiglottis

Small diameter trachea

Figure 4.9 The upper airway in the infant (from Advanced Life Support Group 2005).

three potential outcomes of child arrest: survival, survival with neurological insult or death (Advanced Life Support Group 2005).

The respiratory system (Fig. 4.9) in children continues to develop until approximately 8 years of age. Therefore the following points need to be considered in emergency care:

- Infants tend to breathe only through their nose until the age of 3 months, which adds to the problems of resuscitation as the nasal passages are small.
- The tongue is very large and collapses into the oropharynx easily, thus blocking the airway.
- The lower mandible is small in comparison to the large tongue, which further exacerbates the problem of airway obstruction.
- The diameter of the trachea increases threefold by puberty – the trachea is approximately the same size as the child or infant's little finger, thus increasing the resistance to air entering and leaving the lungs.
- The epiglottis is floppy and will easily occlude the airway.

The following additional anatomical characteristics should also be borne in mind:

- The cartilaginous rings of the trachea are soft and easily compressed.
- Respiration depends upon movement of the diaphragm as the intercostal muscles are not fully developed and therefore abdominal respirations are observed until at least 6 years of age.
- The left ventricle of the heart does not develop its characteristic thick muscular wall until about 6 months of age, and this affects how well blood circulates around the body because of the limited power of each contraction.
- The basal metabolic rate and oxygen consumption in infants are much higher than in adults resulting in increased heart and respiratory rates, and therefore they are much more prone to hypoxia and resulting neurological damage.

The BLS guidelines are thus based on maintaining oxygenation rather than restoring normal cardiac rhythm. However, without oxygen an infant or child will soon become bradycardic (i.e. have a slow pulse rate) and this will quickly progress to pulselessness.

CARE DELIVERY KNOWLEDGE

ACTION IN AN EMERGENCY SITUATION

Personal safety of the rescuer

The personal safety of the rescuer is an obvious priority, so it is important always to look carefully at any situation before 'diving in'.

There is never a situation when to consider personal safety first is wrong. Potential hazards can include electricity, gas, fire, water, or a casualty holding a double-barrelled shotgun! While one concern might be that time spent looking carefully at the situation could be 'wasted', in fact it only takes about the same time as putting on a pair of disposable gloves, which is probably a good thing to be doing (if they are available) while thinking. Another health and safety consideration is infection control. Although there is much concern in this area regarding first-aider safety, there is little current evidence that this is a great problem as long as the usual universal precautions are followed, for example wearing gloves when handling body fluids (see Ch. 5 on infection control for more information).

Much concern has been raised about the possibility of a rescuer catching the human immunodeficiency virus (HIV) while carrying out mouth-to-mouth resuscitation. At the time of writing the authors of this chapter have heard of no such cases. However, there are other infections that pose a potentially greater risk. Barrier devices (simple protective devices which can be placed on the patient's face) for use with mouth-to-mouth resuscitation need to be considered by the individual rescuer. In order to make use of such devices, it is essential to be well practised in their use on a mannikin first. The pocket mask (Fig. 4.10) is especially useful, as an oxygen supply can be added to the mask, increasing the percentage of oxygen delivered to the casualty from less than 20% to up to 50%, so making the whole process much more efficient.

Reflection and portfolio exercise

Refer to Chapter 5 on infection control and other literature on HIV and its mode of spread.

- List the potential airborne infections that might be a risk to rescuers.
- Review the effectiveness of any methods at present available to reduce risk to the first-aider.
- Review the potential for preventive immunizations from those organisms of high risk.
- Regarding the potential 'risk' of mouth-to-mouth breathing in resuscitation, would you socially kiss a new friend without demanding an HIV screen?

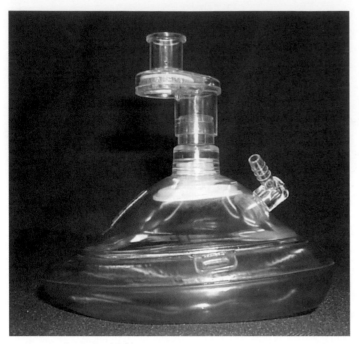

Figure 4.10 A face mask.

applies where you work (some smaller hospitals with limited internal emergency support may use the UK 999 system).

Assessing help required and establishing priorities

An important consideration at the early stage is to ask whether the situation can be realistically managed or whether help is needed now, soon or not at all. In the most extreme situation, that of a multiple casualty incident, there are two basic choices: either jump in and save a few lives while others are dying or choose to obtain a general overview of the situation and then call 999 to ensure the most appropriate response by the emergency services. Evidence from previous disasters shows that this initial stage is crucial to the overall organization of the incident. Reports of any of the British disasters usually discuss this area of management (further information regarding emergency planning can be found at the website of the Department of Health – see section on websites at the end of the chapter).

A call for help must include sufficient information to allow the emergency services coordinator to produce a full and adequate response (i.e. it is important to know the number and nature of the casualties). If this information is not accurately provided it will be up to the first emergency services vehicle to fulfil this role, resulting in a further delay. Clearly if a bystander is available this role can be delegated, but confirmation that the call has been made must be ensured.

Most acute hospitals have an emergency team who provide internal emergency support, for example the cardiac arrest or critical care outreach team. The UK NHS national internal emergency number is 2222, but check that this

ASSESSING THE CRITICALLY ILL PATIENT

The early detection and prevention of collapse

Survival from the pulseless collapse remains poor despite advances in the science of resuscitation and hence there is increasing interest in preventing cardiac arrest and in the determination of risk factors.

Hodgetts et al (2002) point out the potential advantages of a designated emergency team to attend to deteriorating patients prior to a cardiac arrest. Often it is fairly difficult to quantify events such as 'nurse concern' which occur prior to the eventual collapse; the most important observation for nurses is the routine measurement of respiratory effort and rate.

Recognition of the critically ill victim follows a quick assessment process focusing on the physical assessment of the victim by the healthcare professional. This assessment can be found in the advance life support (ALS) manuals for both adults and children. This simple process formulates the information regarding the victim in a format that is clearly understood by nursing and medical staff.

The general ABC approach is described well in the BLS guidelines which will follow later in the chapter. After this initial assessment, a more comprehensive assessment can be undertaken.

For the acutely ill or injured patient an ABCDE approach is taken. There are many versions of this approach, targeting different levels of expertise (notably Smith et al 2002). The principles are that ABCDE identifies the priorities in order of significance, each major problem being managed before moving on to the next stage. However, if there is a need to deal with a priority, the whole examination should be continued, completed and repeated, as soon as possible.

The ABCDE (and potentially FGH) assessment

The process described below follows an 'ABC' quick approach followed by a more detailed (and potentially slower) 'ABCDEFGH' approach; this has been found to be helpful for less experienced healthcare staff.

The initial ABC quick approach focuses on the primary assessment to identify whether the patient requires immediate resuscitation, followed by a more detailed approach if this is not required.

Conscious?

An initial general assessment of the patient's consciousness level should be made by calling to them and gently shaking the shoulder (depending on potential injuries). The following assessment can then be undertaken:

Airway (A)

General issues will be considered first, and then variations to this process for specific situations.

The unresponsive casualty may not breathe unless he or she has a patent airway. Although it is not physically possible to swallow the tongue, this phrase is often used to describe the relaxed tongue dropping into and blocking the posterior pharynx. The manoeuvres described aim to relieve this obstruction. When opening the airway, the position of the lower jaw is at least as important as the head tilt (Fig. 4.11), especially the need to realign it into its normal functional position with the upper and lower

teeth on the same plane. (NB: Remember the specific needs of infants discussed in the physiology section earlier.)

A brief simultaneous look into the mouth may show food debris (and hence a risk of airway obstruction) or other airway abnormality.

An additional manoeuvre is the jaw thrust (Fig. 4.12). The idea for this is to bring the lower jaw upwards – along with the jaw will come the attached tongue, thus clearing it from the airway. This is an especially important manoeuvre if the casualty has a potential neck injury, in which case it can be used alone without the head tilt manoeuvre (Fig. 4.11), which could cause further damage.

Breathing (B)

Airway opening must be maintained when assessing breathing. While assessing breathing, the patient could be making a purposeful respiration, have gasping/agonal (uncoordinated) breathing or not breathing at all.

Observation should be of the chest wall in older children and adults, whereas for children under 6 years the focus should be on the abdomen as the diaphragm is the dominant respiratory muscle. The healthcare professional should be aware of the normal respiratory rates for infants, children and adults. The significance of gasping and agonal breathing is that it indicates that there is lack of control of breathing and this is inadequate to maintain normal oxygen levels; therefore it is treated as not breathing.

Ultimately, the rescuer needs to decide whether the patient's breathing is adequate – if it is not, then support is required.

Circulation (C)

When checking the circulation, the only appropriate pulse to initially check is the carotid pulse, as the peripheral pulses are unreliable indicators in the collapsed patient (they can disappear as a result of normal blood pressure homeostasis). In order to prevent uncertainty when the rescuer is anxious and adrenaline levels are high, the carotid pulse is best felt via anatomical landmarks rather than by

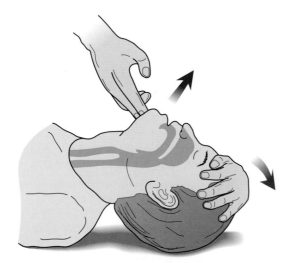

Figure 4.11 Head tilt.

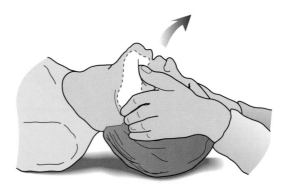

Figure 4.12 Jaw thrust.

guesswork. On the patient's neck the trachea and the sternomastoid muscle should be palpated. The fingers should be placed in the trough between these two structures in the mid-neck region and pressure exerted by the tips of the fingers until they reach the bottom of the trough (Fig. 4.13). This should be performed on the side nearest the first-aider to avoid occluding the trachea. When practising this exercise, it is essential to press on one side only, or fainting may be caused as a result of reducing blood flow to the brain; equally the rescuer should not press too hard as this will stop the blood flow if the blood pressure is low.

Handley et al (1997) comment that the practice of the pulse check may be a less than reliable technique, especially by lay first-aiders, and perhaps the expression 'look for signs of a circulation', which includes a more general assessment of circulation as well as a pulse check, is more appropriate.

If unsure and the patient appears effectively 'dead', the rescuer should commence chest compressions. Because time is very limited this needs to be undertaken quickly. There is no evidence that 'inappropriate' chest compressions stop the heart and if you review the approach of advanced life support, chest compressions are used to initially support the heart which has recently restarted.

In infants, because of the short neck, the initial pulse assessment is made using the brachial artery, which is found just medial (towards the centre of the body) to the biceps tendon in the antecubital fossa (the front of the elbow).

Disability (neurological) (D)

Although the Glasgow Coma Scale is generally used in hospital, it is time-consuming to apply and requires regular practice; a faster and more straightforward system is the AVPU system (Box 4.1), which is widely used in pre-hospital care. The rescuer simply records the patient's best response.

Box 4.1	AVPU	
A	Alert	Patient fully responsive, eyes are open without prompting
V	Voice	Patient drowsy, eyes only open to command
P	Pain	A painful stimulus (applying a finger squeeze to the trapezius muscle) is required to elicit a response from the patient
U	Unresponsive	No response

If the patient is in pain an assessment can be made here (see Ch. 11, pp. 256–257, for pain assessment structures).

Exposure (environment) (E)

The patient should be fully examined from top to toe to detect any physical injuries or abnormalities. The patient's temperature should be recorded here.

F, G and H

These are not found in traditional systems and integrate into the above but they may be useful reminders for the less experienced rescuer.

Function (F)

Pertaining to limb injuries (which are often involved). Is there a peripheral circulation? (Can a peripheral pulse be found, are the fingers/toes warm?) Has the patient normal sensation and is there a full range of movements?

Glucose (G – included in D with other systems)

Low blood glucose (hypoglycaemia) is a relatively common cause of altered consciousness or behaviour and should be investigated. And while we are on the subject of the patient's concurrent health problems – do they have any other health related conditions?

History (H)

If the assessment is still unclear, revisit the history of the incident (mechanism of injury) and find out how the patient has been in the previous day/hours to see if there are any other clues.

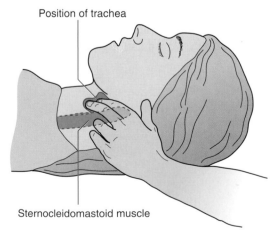

Position of trachea

Sternocleidomastoid muscle

Figure 4.13 Locating the carotid pulse. List the possible signs of a circulation, other than a pulse check.

4.2 – ASSESSING THE CRITICALLY ILL PERSON

You will learn the knowledge and skills needed to:
- Conduct a two stage systematic assessment of your collapsed patient.
- Write notes on the assessment.

Outreach teams and medical emergency teams (MET)

A driver for enhancing the skills of ward staff regarding recognition of critically ill adults was the Department of Health's report *Comprehensive Critical Care* (2000). Many trusts have taken this development on board as the evidence supports the proposed changes. Priestley et al (2004) found a significant difference in mortality before and after the implementation of a critical care outreach service for adult in-patients. Tibballs et al (2005) found that with the implementation of a medical emergency team, the risk of ill children having a cardiopulmonary arrest on the ward was reduced and the number of calls from nurses requesting an assessment of the child increased. A critical component of outreach and MET is knowing when they should be called. This has led to the development of early warning systems for both adults and children. Use Evolve 4.3 to find out more.

4.3 – REVIEW OF ASSESSMENT – BRINGING IT ALL TOGETHER

Objectives:
- Conduct your own assessment.
- Review your practice against set criteria.
- Learn about early warning systems and paediatric early warning systems(EWS and PEWS).
- Report the assessment for your portfolio.

INTERVENTION

Resuscitation guidelines

The aim of the BLS guidelines is to produce an accurate and rapid diagnosis, ensure appropriate help is summoned and limit the effects of hypoxia (lack of oxygen).

In resuscitation, a consistent approach to care is critical, that is, there should be the same management by everyone from scouts to consultant cardiologists. A truly international approach has been a target of the resuscitation training bodies for many years. The European Resuscitation Council (ERC) integrated the work of many countries and the International Liaison Committee on Resuscitation (ILCOR) presented advisory statements on resuscitation in order to develop a global approach (ILCOR 1997). These guidelines were further developed to include North America in 2000. Updated guidelines were released in 2005 (check http://www.resus.org.uk for further updates).

The term 'guidelines' is used to allow for adaptation according to individual circumstances, as 'rules' might discourage 'necessary' variations. Despite many potential causes there are only two main approaches to resuscitation and these are based upon the physiological development of individuals across the lifespan (i.e. the adult and the infant).

There may need to be variation from the guidelines if there is a specific reason for the collapse. Examples would be differences in resuscitation techniques for an infant who has stopped breathing, as opposed to an adult who has had a heart attack. It is therefore important to be able to make decisions and to have knowledge of the differences in resuscitation techniques for an infant as opposed to an adult.

Some variations also occur between the guidelines for the public and those for a trainee healthcare professional (that's you). The emphasis for public training is on a relatively simple approach which can be easily remembered. Education and training for healthcare professionals allows a more comprehensive approach.

The following section highlights interventions for collapse and resuscitation.

The unconscious patient

If you have established that the patient is unconscious but with adequate breathing and circulation, the recovery position is called for and is suitable for all ages. Although it will not totally protect the airway and lungs from stomach contents it will reduce the risk of death from aspiration (inhaling vomit).

Once the patient is on their side, ensure their airway is open and limbs are positioned comfortably. Undertake a comprehensive reassessment while waiting for further assistance.

Primary respiratory arrest

Choking (foreign body airway obstruction, FBAO)

A nurse may face airway obstruction in almost any area of practice. It is essential that nurses can perform procedures to alleviate choking quickly and efficiently, to reduce the risk of death.

A typical situation might arise at meal times (and play times with children). In all cases it is probably the context which will alert a nurse to the potential of airway obstruction as it is unlikely that the obstruction will be visible during a brief airway check. Typical signs of complete obstruction are:

- hand held to the throat
- 'silent' attempts at coughing
- salivating
- distress
- rapid onset of cyanosis.

With partial obstruction, stridor (a snoring sound usually on inspiration), hoarseness, 'whispering' voice and coughing may be observed.

Management of choking in the adult

If the individual still has some respiratory effort, just helping the casualty empty the mouth may prevent the situation deteriorating further. This may be especially important for individuals with swallowing difficulties such as the elderly stroke patient or the young physically disabled person.

Figure 4.14 shows the current recommendations for the management of choking in the adult (European Resuscitation Council 2005).

Recent evidence has demonstrated that the most effective technique in increasing airway pressure and hence 'blowing out' obstructions is the 'chest thrust' (as per chest compression) (Langhelle et al 2000). This has been implemented in the management of the unconscious patient and also makes the management procedure easier to remember.

The Heimlich manoeuvre or abdominal thrust (Fig. 4.15) aims to push the diaphragm upwards to increase the pressure in the chest cavity and so push or squeeze the object out of the trachea. If successful, the object will be ejected with some force.

Management of choking in the infant or child

The risk of choking is higher in infants and children than in adults because the upper airway is narrower and the swallowing reflex is not as well coordinated. The upper airway should be observed carefully during the initial assessment. Obstruction of the airway is not anticipated until the chest will not inflate. Only then is the choking procedure commenced. However, if choking is witnessed initially, the choking procedure should be started immediately.

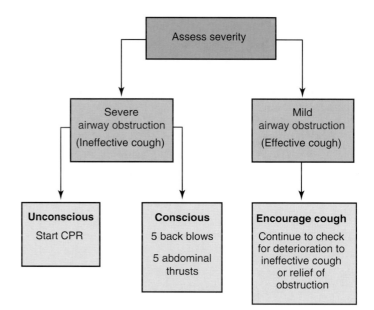

Figure 4.14 Basic airway management of choking in the adult (from Resuscitation Council (UK) Guidelines 2005).

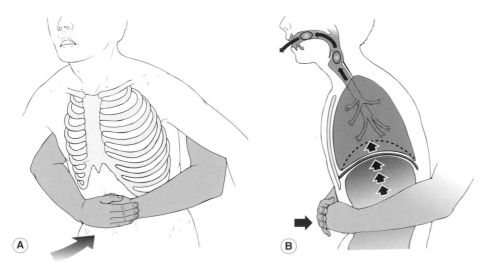

(A)

(B)

Figure 4.15 The Heimlich manoeuvre used if a patient is choking. (A) Stand behind the patient and clasp your hands over their mid-abdomen. (B) Apply a sharp movement to compress the abdomen. Repeat as necessary. (Courtesy of Nottingham Health Authority.)

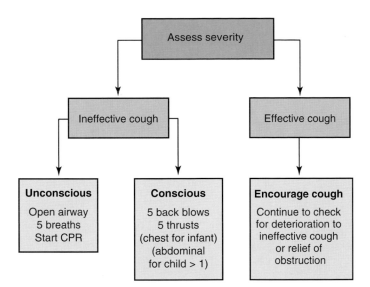

Figure 4.16 Dealing with choking in the infant or child (from Resuscitation Council (UK) Guidelines 2005).

The Resuscitation Council (UK) (2005) has produced guidelines for the management of choking in infants and children (Fig. 4.16). The differences between the two age groups are linked to the immaturity of the liver and disconnection of the spleen from the back of the abdomen in the younger age group when the Heimlich manoeuvre (abdominal thrust) is used. Therefore *this manoeuvre should be avoided at all costs in babies* and replaced by the chest thrust as indicated. Chest thrusts are performed in the same manner and place as chest compressions but are carried out more rapidly.

Decision-making exercise

Your friend and her 6-year-old daughter are visiting you. You and your friend go into the kitchen to prepare coffee and leave the child playing happily in the sitting room. The child is eating sweets recently bought by her mother on the way to visit you. Suddenly the child rushes into the kitchen, distressed and unable to speak.

- What will your first action be?
- What health promotion advice may be given to your friend to prevent an accident occurring again in the future?

Mouth–to–mouth ventilation

Should the rescuer be required to ventilate the patient's lungs, the key is 'low pressure' ventilation. In the unconscious casualty, the oesophageal sphincters may not be tightly closed so relatively slow (and low pressure) ventilations are required. The harder and faster you blow, the more air will enter the stomach, and hence the risk of regurgitation increases.

Unconscious patients are unable to vomit. However, they can passively regurgitate their stomach contents into the upper airway, so ventilating too hard is also to the detriment of the rescuers. According to Baskett et al (1996), 400–600 mL of air per ventilation is required for adults, and one-tenth of this volume (i.e. 40–60 mL) for infants. As far as the judgement of ventilation volumes are concerned in reality, as long as there is some chest or abdominal lift with each ventilation, it is likely to be adequate.

Healthcare staff commonly use a pocket mask (see Fig. 4.10), which removes the need for direct patient contact. An additional advantage of the pocket mask is the ability to add supplementary oxygen.

Altered airway anatomy

This is currently a relatively uncommon situation, but is on the increase as a result of reconstructive surgery following treatment for neoplasms (cancers) in the region of the throat. It is therefore probably good practice to include an inspection of the patient's throat down to the suprasternal notch. The management of the situation is exceptionally easy: ventilation should take place using the alternative orifice (Fig. 4.17).

Primary cardiac arrest

This is the most likely event to occur in adults. The 'chain of survival' indicates that basic life support should be performed until a defibrillator is available; however, if there is a defibrillator on hand it should be used immediately.

Chest compressions

The two major theories regarding chest compressions are the cardiac theory and the thoracic pump theory. Robertson & Holmberg (1992) consider that neither of these is actually proven. It is likely that chest compression moves blood by a combination of:

- directly squeezing the heart between the sternum and the spine (cardiac pump theory)
- generally increasing the intrathoracic pressure (thoracic pump theory).

This forces blood out of the heart and chest, with the venous valve system ensuring a unidirectional flow.

As with ventilations, efficiency is related to rate and timing. Theoretically the faster the rate the greater the output, assuming a constant stroke volume (the volume of blood filling the ventricles). In practice, as the compression rate increases, the stroke volume may be falling because

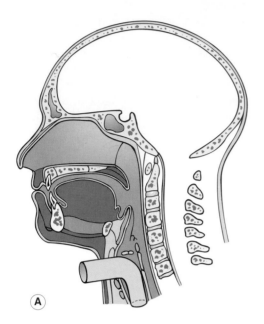
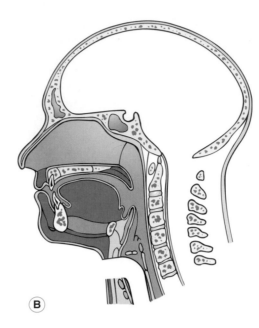

(A)

(B)

Figure 4.17 Altered anatomical upper airway. (A) Temporary artificial airway. (B) Permanent artificial airway (laryngostomy).

the venous return to the chest and heart is reduced, so that the actual rate is a compromise between these factors. To make the best use of the rate remember that the relaxation phase is at least as important as the compression phase, so leave adequate time between compressions to allow thoracic and ventricular refill before the next compression.

Combining ventilations and compressions

Debate continues regarding the most effective combination. In an adult a ratio of 30 compressions to 2 ventilations is used, as it appears to take a number of compressions to 'build up' a circulatory pressure before blood actually flows. This is only changed to continuous compressions once the patient has been intubated (a secure airway tube normally inserted by an anaesthetist), when higher airway pressure can be used.

In paediatrics this ratio would result in inadequate oxygenation; hence a ratio of 15 to 2 is used.

The rescuer's hands are placed two-thirds of the way down the sternum (public training recommends slightly higher up because of the risk of pressing on the stomach). The adult chest is compressed by a depth of 4–5 cm (⅓ of the chest diameter in infants and children because of the increased flexibilty) at a rate of 100 compressions per minute (note that this is the rate not the expected number of compressions in any given minute. Care should be taken to ensure the chest is fully released between each compression to allow refill. To aid practice, a useful 'pacing' metronome can be found online at: http://www.metronomeonline.com.

Even with the most competent rescuer, survival is not good without advanced help arriving rapidly.

Evidence-based practice

Lack of oxygen (hypoxia) caused by a static circulation to vital organs takes various lengths of time to take effect. Lungs can withstand long periods of hypoxia, the liver 1–2 hours, the heart and kidneys 30 minutes, and the brain 4–6 minutes (Newbold 1987). Therefore the effect and efficiency of compressions is very important.

The blood flow that occurs as a result of chest compressions is only about 25% of normal, and cerebral blood flow only 15% of normal, and this is assuming good quality chest compressions (Jackson 1984, Mackenzie 1964). Therefore delaying cardiac chest compressions for up to 5 minutes can result in no cerebral blood flow because of the pathological changes such as stasis of deoxygenated blood in the large veins (Lee 1984).

Defibrillation

Advisory defibrillation should be taught and competency tested within the pre-registration education of all nurses and doctors. The Chief Nursing Officer states within her 10 key roles for nurses that they should: 'Carry out a wide range of resuscitation procedures including defibrillation' (Mullally 2001).

There still appears to be some reluctance by nurses to undertake this role. Current opinion varies, from nurses being worried about the potential legal implications of nurse defibrillation and hence resistance to carrying it out to widespread implementation across health trusts. It is worth pointing out to hesitant nurses that the government used the example of defibrillation by nurses as normal practice for adult branch nurses as far back as their 1997 recruitment campaign advertisement.

In the hospital setting, nurses are in an ideal position to carry out early defibrillation and make a significant contribution to reducing the death rate from ischaemic heart disease. In the pre-hospital environment, defibrillation by volunteers is now widespread.

One of the most significant developments in defibrillator technology has been the advisory external defibrillator (AED). The AED system will analyse a patient's cardiac rhythm and indicate if the patient requires defibrillation or not. In use, it is simply a matter of connecting two large electrodes to the patient and following a '1, 2, 3' approach in terms of operation where '1' is on, 2 is 'analyse' (determine the rhythm) and 3 is 'fire' (defibrillate).

Since the mid-1990s community based defibrillation has rapidly expanded. In the UK AEDs are commonly found in such places as shopping centres, railway stations and leisure centres. Some acute NHS trusts have been slower to respond to the idea of 'first responder' defibrillation and defibrillation has been delayed until the arrival of the cardiac arrest team. Generally it is expected the first person to aid a collapsed patient (commonly a nurse) will use a defibrillator if appropriate.

Experience with the use of AEDs on children is limited and the subject of current research. It is considered that it is safe to defibrillate a child from the age of 8 years old, with a standard AED using attenuated leads (Atkins et al 2001). Luckily it is rare that defibrillating an infant is required, especially outside paediatric critical care areas.

Reflection and portfolio exercise

During your practice placements review the availability of resuscitation equipment. This is usually a significant part of your orientation to any new practice setting.

- Check whether there is a defibrillator available and how it is operated.
- Review the local policies about when, how often, and by whom resuscitation equipment is checked.
- Discuss with your practice supervisor which members of the multidisciplinary team are allowed to perform more advanced procedures after the initial resuscitation phase (BLS).
- How is resuscitation dealt with in primary healthcare settings and by individual community nurses? The documents *The Health of the Nation* (Department of Health 1991) and *Targeting Practice, The Contribution of Nurses, Midwives and Health Visitors* (Department of Health 1993) clearly identify national targets to reduce the death rates from coronary heart disease (CHD).

- Debate the role of the nurse in helping to meet *The Health of the Nation* targets for CHD.
- Consider the impact on the adult mortality figures of training sufficient numbers of the public to instigate BLS. How could the specialist nurse become involved in training members of the public?

Reflection and portfolio exercise

You will need access to an infant and junior resuscitation mannikin for this exercise. Using the marking grids in the chapter test your skills in BLS for infants and children following the guidelines. Ideally, ask another student to assess your skills, and remember the real situation may last a long time, so demonstrate your skills over at least 5 minutes.

A potential controversy is the issue of priorities. Pause, and reviewing information given previously in this chapter, decide which of the following is more important: the patent airway or immobilization of a potential fracture of the cervical spine? Think for a few moments about how you might open the airway of a patient who has suffered a neck injury.

Figures 4.18 and 4.19 show the healthcare professional versions of the adult basic life support checklist and the infant/child basic life support checklist.

RESUSCITATION IN A HEALTHCARE SETTING

Although the relative efficiency of BLS is not good (somewhere in the region of 20% of 'normal' cardiac output), it is a significant part of the chain of survival; it buys time and must not be forgotten, especially in high-technology settings. We have already identified the significance of defibrillation in adults and airway care in children – so what are the other interventions of resuscitation?

Many devices are available to increase the patency of the patient's airway during the resuscitation process. The most useful for nurses is the Guedel airway, but this requires accurate measurements to ensure the correct size is selected. These are obtained by measuring the Guedel airway alongside the jaw, the flange of the airway level with the incisor teeth and the distal part of the airway level with the corner of the jaw. In children over 5 years of age and in older age groups, the airway is inserted upside down and turned over in the mouth to hook over the back of the tongue. If the child is under 5 years of age inserting anything into the airway should be avoided unless you have been specially educated.

With a patent airway, another early consideration is the addition of supplementary oxygen. All suddenly collapsed

Checklist		Achieved	Comment
Considers own safety	**(Safe)**		
Checks responsiveness (shout and gentle shake)	**(No response)**		
Shouts for help	**(None appears)**		
Brief airway check			
Opens airway (head tilt, chin lift)			
Checks breathing (look, listen and feel for up to 10 seconds)	**(Absent/inadequate)**		
Phones for ambulance/hospital team (0.5 if not immediate)			
Check for 'signs of circulation' including carotid pulse (preferably simultaneously with the breathing if a second rescuer is present)	**(Pulse=0)**		
Commences chest compressions (30, counting out loud)			
Correct postion for compression (centre of lower half sternum)			
Correct depth (4–5 cm and full release)			
Correct compression rate (100/minute)			
Opens airway (head tilt, chin lift)			
Performs 2 effective mouth-to-mouth ventilations			
1 second inflation time, NOT hyperventilating patient			
Successfully readjusts airway if fails to ventilate (score 1 if all effective)			
Continues; 30 compressions to 2 effective ventilations			
Maintains correct position for compressions and correct compression rate			
Continues effective resuscitation (training target = 5 cycles/2 mins)			

Figure 4.18 Adult basic life support checklist.

patients will benefit from the administration of additional oxygen. It is likely that the patient's respiratory function or cardiac function will be reduced, therefore increasing the oxygen saturation of the available circulation will be in the best interests of the patient. There are, however, two commonly expressed concerns by nurses regarding oxygen delivery.

1. Oxygen is a prescription medication and therefore a physician's signature is required before administration. Local oxygen administration policies should be read carefully to identify emergency patient group directives. When a patient is suffering from acute hypoxia, for example sudden chest pain, shortness of breath and blood loss, they will always benefit from higher oxygen administration during the acute phase.
2. Another concern expressed by nurses relates to administering oxygen to patients with chronic obstructive pulmonary disease (COPD). Very rarely a patient with hypoxic respiratory drive will stop breathing when given high concentrations of oxygen. All acutely ill patients on emergency oxygen must be closely observed and this will therefore be noticed early. Even patients who are normally hypoxic will suffer adverse effects with further hypoxia. The care and management of patients with COPD is a complex issue which you should study further and it should be remembered that the above only relates to acute emergency situations. This also applies to children.

Many different types of oxygen administration devices are available, for all ages e.g. Venturi-based face masks, nasal cannulae and non-rebreathing (trauma) masks. Investigate what is available in your clinical area and how they function.

When the patient is not spontaneously breathing, administration of oxygen can be by a self-inflating bag

Checklist		Achieved	Comment
Considers own safety	(Safe)		
Checks responsiveness (gently stimulate and shout)	(No response)		
Shouts for help	(None appears)		
Checks and opens airway (minimal head tilt, chin lift)			
Checks breathing (look, listen and feel)			
Commences mouth-to-mouth/nose ventilation			
Successfully readjusts airway if fails to ventilate (score one if all effective)			
Performs a total of 5 effective ventilations			
Check for signs of circulation including pulse check	(Less than 60/min with poor perfusion)		
Correct postion for compression (centre of lower half sternum)			
Commences chest compressions (15)			
Effective depth (1/3 chest depth)			
Performs 2 effective ventilations			
Continues 15 compressions to 2 ventilations			
Correct rate (100/minute)			
Continues for one minute			
Definitive help (999/2222) if not previously summoned			
On return from summoning help – cotinue unless signs of life noted			
Recommences effective resuscitation (training target = 10 cycles/2 mins)			

Figure 4.19 Infant/child basic life support checklist.

(bag/valve/mask). These bags are available in different sizes to suit the infant, child or adult patient. This piece of equipment has useful features such as a pop-off valve to prevent over-inflation, and it can be used without a continual gas flow. It is important to select a face mask that covers the nose and mouth comfortably and creates a good seal so that the victim can receive adequate ventilation. It is also important that the user ensures patient chest movement occurs when the bag is squeezed.

Fluids

To ensure the blood can carry oxygen to the vital organs of the body, it is essential to ensure that there is enough blood volume. Administration of intravenous fluids is required, and in the case of children, intraosseously (via the bone marrow). The body has compensatory mechanisms, which means that in response to physiological stress there will be an attempt to conserve oxygen and so blood. This results in the blood vessels vasoconstricting in the limbs, and hence the patient's hands and feet feel cold. The heart rate will increase as a response to ensure the blood carries oxygen quickly to the vital organs and removes waste products such as carbon dioxide. Blood may be lost through bleeding or may move into a different body compartment therefore depleting the volume in the systemic circulation, and this will eventually lead to hypotension. Note that hypotension is a late sign of deterioration.

Drugs

The use of drugs during the resuscitation process has been a controversial topic over the years and it is only recently that objective research studies have started. Although there are potentially many drugs that might be required during a cardiac arrest, the three most commonly used drugs are adrenaline, atropine and amiodarone

Adrenaline appears to improve BLS by increasing oxygen uptake and delivery to the cardiac muscle (it does, however, unfortunately also increase the demand).

Atropine is used in the bradycardiac (or asystolic) patient to block the inhibitory affect of the parasympathetic nervous system (via the vagus nerve). Amiodarone is an anti-arrythmic drug. For further information read an up-to-date drug handbook such as the British National Formulary (http://www.bnf.org/bnf/).

Because of the very poor circulation associated with basic life support all intravenous drugs are followed by a bolus of 20 mL normal (isotonic) saline to send the drug into the central circulation.

For all three drugs identify the following:

- The indications for their use (and when they are used in the resuscitation algorithm).
- Their actions.
- Their potential side-effects.
- Typical adult and child doses.

SPECIFIC CONSIDERATIONS IN EMERGENCY CARE

There are specific considerations to be made in any individual situation but the most important relates to the use of ABC. However, there are particular considerations in trauma care and in pregnancy which merit further development (see Evolve 4.4).

4.4 – SPECIFIC CONSIDERATIONS IN EMERGENCY CARE

- Issues specific to pregnancy.
- Issues in trauma first aid.
- Immobilizing the neck combined with jaw thrust.
- Application of issues to a practice setting.

LEGAL, PROFESSIONAL AND ETHICAL ISSUES SURROUNDING RESUSCITATION

THE 'DUTY OF CARE' TO A NEIGHBOUR AS A MEMBER OF THE PUBLIC

In the UK there is no legal duty of care to a 'neighbour', which may be anyone and not just a physical neighbour. In practice, this means anyone can walk past an accident or step over a collapsed person in the street. Although a legal duty of care does not exist, there is, however, a moral duty towards fellow human beings that must be considered.

In the British legal system, the two major divisions are criminal law and civil law. Entering a patient's house without consent may be trespass, which is a civil offence, and in some cases may be a criminal offence. Touching a patient without consent might be considered to be assault, and inappropriate treatment of a patient might result in accusations of actual bodily harm. It is no wonder that nurses worry about being sued. However, one of the major considerations in criminal law is the 'intent' and 'motive' that is associated with the act. Both 'intent' and 'motive' are very complex legal issues and it would be advisable to consult a legal text to investigate these further. The courts will consider a situation where the intent when aiding an individual is to do harm in a very different light to a situation where the rescuer is trying to help. It appears more likely that the first-aider would be involved in a case related to civil law, and most probably that of negligence where the patient has suffered additional harm due to the actions of a first-aider.

Tingle (1991) undertook a major review of the situation regarding nurses, first aid and the law. One of his major considerations was that 'legal action against Good Samaritan acts is a remote possibility'. These premises are supported in good discussion by the UK Resuscitation Council found on their web pages at http://www.resus.org.uk.

It is important to remember that although there is no duty to care for everyone, if an injured person is already 'under the care' of the potential first-aider's employer, the first-aider then has a duty to care for them. As Tingle (1991) points out, 'a nurse could not leave a fallen patient but could leave a witnessed accident'. Although there is no immediate legal duty of care to the witnessed accident, once the nurse has presented herself as a nurse to help 'a duty of care' exists.

When undertaking emergency care for individuals 'in the care' of an employer – for example a National Health Service trust – if anything goes wrong it is more likely that the individual will sue the employer than the employee. This is likely to be the case for a nurse who is the 'designated' first-aider as described in the first aid regulations of the Health and Safety at Work Act (Health and Safety Commission 1981). Outside this situation the first-aider is 'on their own' and it seems reasonable that every nurse should have some personal indemnity insurance to cover them in such circumstances. Personal indemnity insurance is often part of a 'package' a nurse receives if they join a union or professional organization. Such an option appears to be sensible and is strongly encouraged by the Nursing and Midwifery Council. Equally, informed consent should be sought when possible.

It can be concluded, then, that as a member of the public there is no legal duty to help a stranger. The previous Nursing and Midwifery Council (2004) placed this responsibility on all nurses in its Code of Professional Conduct in the code stating: '(8.5) In an emergency, in or outside the work setting, you have a professional duty to provide care.' The 2008 code of conduct (Nursing and Midwifery Council 2008) maintains this: 'You must make the care of people your first concern, treating them as individuals and respecting their dignity' and 'work with others to protect and promote the health and wellbeing of those in your care, their families and carers, and the wider community'.

The Code provides a clear mandate for all nurses that goes beyond the legal responsibilities and indicates that nurses must always act in the manner of the Good Samaritan.

ETHICS OF RESUSCITATION

Much has been written about the ethics of resuscitation, the definitive document being *Decisions Relating to Cardiopulmonary Resuscitation* by the Royal College of Nursing, the UK Resuscitation Council and British Medical Association (Royal College of Nursing 2007).

The issue of whether actively to resuscitate an individual or not is a difficult one to address. However, it must be remembered that the final decision should be in the patient's interest, respect the individual's desires as far as possible, and consider the value of human life.

'Living wills' or 'advanced directives' are sometimes used by patients to identify their wishes, with respect to end-of-life decisions. In England and Wales, advance decisions are covered by the Mental Capacity Act 2005. Further details can be found in the Royal College of Nursing, UK Resuscitation Council and the British Medical Association document (Royal College of Nursing 2007).

Reflection and portfolio exercise

Using *Decisions Relating to Cardiopulmonary Resuscitation* (Royal College of Nursing 2007; available on the web at rcn.org.uk and http://www.bma.org.uk) and the Mental Capacity Act (2005), investigate the issue of informed consent for:

- Children (Department of Health 2001).
- The unconscious adult.
- The individual with learning difficulties.
- Those with mental health problems.

Cross-refer to Chapter 13 on End of Life Care and your ethico-legal textbooks.

EDUCATION AND TRAINING FOR RESUSCITATION

As developing resuscitation skills 'on the job' is inappropriate, a number of nationally recognized courses have been developed to provide these skills. St John Ambulance and the British Red Cross undertake excellent first aid training that develops individual skills in core BLS.

For more advanced training in cardiac collapse the multiprofessional courses of the Resuscitation Council (UK) are considered to be the 'gold standard' – the advanced life support (ALS) course for adults, and for dealing with children, the paediatric advanced life support (PALS) course. As all participants are assessed at the same level regardless of profession they support the concept that a team can be the clinically most appropriate person, be that a nurse or a doctor. Finally, for those more interested in the trauma approach, there is the advanced trauma nursing course (ATNC). All of these courses are usually residential as they last 2–4 days and are regularly advertised in the nursing press.

All first aid and resuscitation skills require regular practice. Under local regulations, yearly updates may be mandatory in your areas of practice. Simulations set up in the work area can be either practical or 'talk through' and can be completed on a regular basis to keep skills fresh and up to date. Working as a team is especially important, so these exercises should be undertaken with as many members of the regular team as possible.

PERSONAL AND REFLECTIVE KNOWLEDGE

The public appears to expect nurses to help in emergency situations and therefore nurses should be able to deal with the initial management of any physical emergency until more specialist staff are available. The practice of first aid and resuscitation carries legal risks. A basic understanding of the legal and professional basis of nursing practice helps to decide how to practise safely. Nurses should not be over-worried when helping out at the scene of an emergency as long as they proceed with caution according to a well-tested plan and only undertake those interventions that are 'necessary'. It also appears to be reasonable that nurses have some form of personal indemnity insurance cover.

Resuscitation is primarily a practical skill that requires a fairly wide knowledge base. As a practical skill, the ability to use it decays with lack of use. Simulation exercises need to be a common feature of the updating process.

Nurses are obliged to become involved in emergency care, if not by law then by the Nursing and Midwifery Council. It is necessary that all nurses receive instruction and updating in emergency care to fulfil this role.

Overall, a cautious intervention by nurses in emergency situations is to encouraged. The well-tested plan of action at any emergency is that described in the *First Aid Manual* of the voluntary first aid organizations (British Red Cross/St Andrew's Ambulance Association/St John Ambulance 2006). The Resuscitation Council (UK) reviews and updates its guidelines based on evidence gathered from the increasing number of research studies in the field of resuscitation. These should be adhered to by all healthcare personnel in any team involved in the resuscitation process.

LEARNING TO LEARN FROM CRITICAL EVENTS

Throughout this chapter there are some reflective exercises for your portfolio. In the practice setting, it is important to learn from critical events such as those described in this chapter. Get into the habit of thinking about your actions and identifying both the positive points and those that you could improve on next time.

During healthcare education and training programmes, students will receive practical BLS training. The checklists earlier in the chapter can be used for updating and revising such skills. These are specially designed for adult, infant and child resuscitation situations.

PSYCHOSOCIAL CONSIDERATIONS

The cardiopulmonary arrest situation is stressful for those observing or resuscitating the patient. This section highlights some issues, but do turn to Chapter 9 on stress, Chapter 13 on death and dying and Chapter 12 on aggression for further background reading.

Situational life crisis

The main focus in this section is on the impact of sudden collapse and death on individual family members and on society as a whole, particularly in the case of major disasters. The effects on members of the healthcare team of failure to achieve a successful resuscitation are also considered.

The term 'situational life crisis' used by Wright (1996) defines how intensive periods of psychological, behavioural and physical disarray through loss and grief can challenge a person's existing coping mechanisms. If not addressed through crisis intervention (Caplan 1964), mental health problems may arise later.

Box 4.2 The six determinants of grief (Parkes 1975)

Determinant
Mode of death
Nature of the attachment
Who was the person?
Historical antecedents
Personality variables
Social variables

Parkes (1975, cited by Wright 1996) identified six different determinants or predictors of grief (see above), the most significant being the mode of death (Box 4.2). Sudden death through trauma creates images of suffering and injustice for the grieving relatives, producing feelings of anger and guilt. These feelings may be directed towards the relatives themselves by thoughts of 'I should have been there' to blaming others: 'The emergency services were just not quick enough.' Anger may be compounded if monetary compensation becomes an issue at a later stage as the deceased is often seen as devalued (Wright 1996).

The relatives

The most difficult issue for relatives to grasp is the fact their loved one, who may have recently been fit and healthy, is now dead. This can be distressing when a child is involved and parents' emotions can increase if one or both parents were not present at the time of death. Reactions of relatives can vary from denial, to guilt, blame and anger. Wright (1996) found relatives identified two emotions when a loved one has died suddenly:

- loss of control over their lives
- powerlessness and helplessness to support, prevent or intervene.

The needs of relatives at this time have been identified by many authors on this subject (Cook 1999, Wright 1996), and Jurkovich et al (2000) found that similar results in their study, where they asked what the bereaved relatives required, confirmed these needs (Box 4.3).

Witnessing the resuscitation of a loved one is fraught with uncertainty exacerbated by lack of understanding. Rattrie (2000) and Meyers et al (2000) found that health professionals supported the relatives' need to be present during a resuscitation attempt, nurses more so than doctors. However, this also had more implications for further staff development and the need for a specialist clinician to

Box 4.3 Needs of relatives in the event of a sudden death

Perceived needs (Cook 1999, Wright 1996)
For information
Time – with their relative, for questions, to talk, to express fears and feelings
Siblings – to be honest and involve them
Health professionals – for support, listening, sharing and time
Social support – from family and friends
Spiritual support – minister/ hospital chaplain, carry out rites such as baptism, blessing and anointing
Physical support – food, drink, rest – caring and anxiety are exhausting

Relatives' stated needs (Jurkovich et al 2000)
Caring attitude
Clarity of message
Privacy
Ability to answer questions
Sympathy
Time for questions
Autopsy information
Clergy available
Direction after death
Location of conversation
Timing of conversation
Rank/seniority of news-breaker
Follow-up contact
Attire of news-giver

support the relatives. Other issues include consent by the victim and harm of witnessing the resuscitation by the relatives. Consent is covered by the fact that resuscitation is usually an emergency event and there is evidence of increasing use of living wills. The involvement of relatives by being in the resuscitation room, seeing that everything is being done and not being separated from their loved one, may offset the reaction of anger and decrease the legal risks of harm of the relatives due to the situation. The Royal College of Nursing has issued guidelines to support staff involved with relatives who find themselves in such a situation (Royal College of Nursing 2002).

Evidence-based practice

Wright (1996), in his book on sudden death, cites a study undertaken by Hanson & Strawser (1992) in which they survey the feelings of 47 family members who were present during the resuscitation of their relatives. Adjustment to the death was found to be easier than if they had not been with the patient according to 76% of respondents, and 64% felt that their presence was valuable to the dying person. Most respondents felt that the dying person had heard them express their love and say their goodbyes.

It has been noted that presence at resuscitation aids the grieving process and it should be an option in as many situations as possible, bearing in mind that it can cause difficulties for the healthcare professionals who may be undertaking invasive procedures in order to save the patient (Zoltie et al 1994).

Decision-making exercise

John O'Neill, a 14-year-old boy with a mild learning disability, sustained a head injury in a fall from a tree at the day centre he attended. He was rushed to hospital by ambulance and his mother was called at her workplace. There was difficulty in getting information to his father as he was a long-distance lorry driver. John's mother arrived at the accident and emergency department just as John began to show difficulty in breathing. The A&E team were beginning the process of intubation and ventilation. John's mother wished to be present and became increasingly agitated and aggressive when denied entrance to the emergency room.

- Debate what the particular issues are for each person in the situation including John and what might be the long-term effects on the family.
- What strategies could be developed by the staff of the A&E department to cope with a similar situation should it arise in the future?

Decision–making exercise

John, a community psychiatric nurse, has been visiting 50-year-old Mohan Khan in his home weekly for the past 3 months. Mohan had become very depressed after he had been forced to take an early retirement offer when the company he was working for cut staff costs. Mohan's wife and two children and the local Sikh community had given him as much support as possible, but despite this and medication and counselling, Mohan has become steadily more withdrawn. On his regular Monday visit John could not get into the house and had to call Mohan's wife at the factory where she worked. On gaining entry as advised by Mohan's wife, John found Mohan collapsed in the bathroom with obvious signs of having slashed his wrists.

- Decide on the immediate steps that John should take to provide basic life support.
- When Mohan's wife arrives, how should John direct her activities?
- How might this family react to the immediate situation?
- Decide what strategies John may have to use to support Mohan and his family if he survives this suicide attempt (see also Ch. 9).

The healthcare professional

Wright (1996) states that the cost of caring in crisis situations can physically and emotionally drain staff and suggests several different ways in which staff can support each other. These include debriefing and mutual support, re-education, activities outside work and a change of situation (see also Ch. 9 for further discussion on coping with stress).

Debriefing

Feelings of stress and anxiety can easily arise after a 'failed' resuscitation attempt. As long as the attempt has been conducted reasonably, 'failure', as it is often perceived, is more often due to the underlying pathology in the patient than the inadequacies of an effective resuscitation attempt. Debriefing after traumatic events such as a resuscitation are important, not just to improve the efficiency of the next attempt, but also to ensure that staff are not left with feelings of self-blame. This can be done through a critical incident technique. The important rule to remember for debriefing is that you are there to support each other and that it should be confidential. A traumatic resuscitation

attempt is not something you can just walk away from without any follow-up.

Re-education

We all become used to our own ways and it is necessary to address our knowledge to develop our skills further. Attending teaching sessions, seminars or conferences can lead to new ways of tackling this stressful situation.

Life outside work

Maintaining leisure time away from the area allows the thought processes to rest and the person to look at life differently. It is also important for the workforce as a team to socialize away from the stressful situations in the clinical areas.

Change of environment

Many professionals find that a change from a clinical area, even if only a temporary one, not only relieves the stress but also allows a development and improvement in skills in other areas.

Post–traumatic stress disorder

Post-traumatic stress disorder (PTSD) was first described in the USA by Durham et al (1985) and involves the long-term distressing emotions that have been experienced by ancillary medical and rescue workers such as the police and firemen in response to a major disaster event. This disorder has been highlighted in recent years after major disasters such as the Hillsborough football stadium disaster, the mass shooting of children in Dunblane in Scotland in 1996 and the events of 11 September 2001.

According to Wright (1996), sufferers of PTSD may:

- During an initial phase experience denial with a lack of awareness of the severity of the event.
- During an intermediate stage seen as a phase of confrontation and disorder start to experience signs of stress such as sleeplessness, nightmares and hypersensitivity to noise and become more easily angry and irritable.
- During the final phase, readjust and recover and regain control of their life, becoming more hopeful and less dependent on others.

Early recognition of the possibility of PTSD now leads to the provision of support in the form of counselling in a major disaster situation in an attempt to prevent the syndrome, while debriefing continues to play an important role for many years after the event. The ongoing difficulties for the victims of the Hillsborough disaster demonstrate this.

Reflection and portfolio exercise

Gibson (1991), in her book *Order from Chaos: Responding to Traumatic Events*, has produced a helpful guide to the topic based on her experiences in Belfast, Northern Ireland. Much has been written about the complex process of helping individuals after traumatic and stressful events. If you undertake a literature search in this area, look under 'post-traumatic stress reaction'.

- Reflect on how you would react if the rescuers in a traumatic event received more monetary compensation for PTSD than the actual relatives of the victims of the disaster. Decide how this crisis situation should be sensitively handled immediately.
- Along with your peer group, debate the legal and moral issues involved in the above dilemma.

CASE STUDIES IN EMERGENCY CARE

The following case histories use the content of the chapter to reflect on situations you may need to address in your particular field of nursing in the future. Completing them will help you consolidate your learning so far.

Case study: Learning disabilities

Remember the 30-year-old woman (Linda) with profound learning disabilities who was a passenger in one of the two cars involved in a crash (see p. 70)? Linda was the back seat passenger in one of the cars and when you came on the scene she was screaming loudly. This lady needs to come to terms with such a traumatic event and coping strategies need to be developed to help her in the future. Obviously, Linda needs to understand how the events happened and, in some ways, most importantly of all, realize that it was an accident and no one's fault.

- Reflect on and identify some of the feelings Linda may have experienced immediately following and subsequent to the accident.
- Review again how you would have prioritized her particular care within the life-threatening scenario of the car crash.
- Linda's father recovered from his chest and head injuries, but is concerned that his daughter's needs were ignored by the rescuers. He intends to sue for negligence. Decide on the type of

defence you will have in law should there be a civil case for damages.

Case study: Child

You are on a practice placement in a local school for children with special needs. Jennifer, a 4-year-old child with cerebral palsy, is found collapsed by the dinner table at school. As the only 'nurse' present you are immediately called upon by the teacher in charge to help.

- What is your first action?
- Your attempts at expired air respiration fail. What should you assume?
- After several cycles of the choking procedure a piece of meat is retrieved from Jennifer's mouth, but she is still not breathing. What should you do now?
- Rehearse practically what you have decided to do using a mannikin and self-assess your performance using the checklist for resuscitation of children.

Case study: Mental health

James is a 17-year-old client who has been admitted to an acute mental health ward with manic depression. He tells you that he has taken 50 of his lithium carbonate and haloperidol tablets over the last 10 minutes and states that he wants to die. He makes it very clear that he does not want to be treated.

- Consider whether you would undertake active resuscitation should he collapse in your presence.
- What immediate actions would you take if he did collapse?
- Reflect on and debate with your peers the ethical and legal issues involved in this particular situation.

Case study: Adult

You are having an evening out with a friend. While walking home you have come across a middle-aged man slumped against a wall who has been vomiting profusely. He smells strongly of alcohol and is barely rousable.

- Consider how you might approach this situation.
- Should his condition deteriorate, how would you carry out mouth-to-mouth ventilations and still protect your own safety?
- It is later discovered that this patient has hepatitis B. What additional actions might you now have to take to protect yourself in the long term?

SUMMARY

This chapter has drawn together theoretical concepts relating to resuscitation and emergency care. It has applied knowledge in relation to the practice of caring for individuals in emergency situations. It has included:

1. The causes of cardiopulmonary arrest and the physiology of care giving in relation to airway management and chest compression.
2. Knowledge for the assessment and care of individuals in situations of collapse, choking or resuscitation.
3. The professional and ethical considerations which must be taken into account in life-threatening situations.
4. The legal considerations facing nurses in relation to resuscitation and emergency care.

Annotated further reading and websites

Resuscitation Council (UK) 2005 Guidance on resuscitation. Resuscitation Council (UK), London. Available online: http://www.resus.org.uk (accessed 1 September 2008)

The algorithms contained in the guidelines, including basic and advanced adult and paediatric life support, are available online as separate single-page documents for easy reference.

Tingle J 1991 First aid law. Nursing Times 87(35):48–49

A common sense review of British law as it relates to the nurse as a first-aider.

British Red Cross/St Andrew's Ambulance Association/St John Ambulance 2006 First aid manual, 8th edn. Dorling Kindersley, London

The authorized manual of the voluntary aid societies.

Wright B 1996 Sudden death: a research base for practice, 2nd edn. Churchill Livingstone, Edinburgh

This is an excellent book on the psychological impact of sudden death of a loved one (adult or child) on families, based on the research and experience of its author as a clinical nurse specialist in crisis care. The book also deals with the effects of crisis management on healthcare staff and makes very useful suggestions for staff support and training.

Guidelines

http://www.resus.org.uk
Resuscitation Council (UK). UK specific guidelines and discussion of the implementation in the UK.

http://www.erc.edu
European Resuscitation Council. Contains the overall European guidelines and supporting information.

http://www.hse.gov.uk/
Health and Safety Executive. Contains UK accident figures and information regarding accident prevention.

Emergency planning

http://www.dh.gov.uk/en/Managingyourorganisation/Emergencyplanning/index.htm
Emergency planning guidance for the National Health Service.

Training/further information

http://www.bbc.co.uk/health/first_aid/
Interactive first aid training from the BBC.

http://www.acls.net/
Supporting information for cardiac life support (USA, includes quizzes).

http://www.rospa.co.uk
Royal Society for the Prevention of Accidents. Statistics and information regarding accident prevention.

http://www.trauma.org
Information supporting the management of trauma patients. See also the 'moulage' section for interactive exercise.

http://www.laerdal.co.uk/
Laerdal Medical, suppliers of emergency care equipment, most notably 'microsim', a software based interactive training system.

Patient support information

http://www.bhf.org.uk
British Heart Foundation. Health promotion regarding the prevention of heart disease.

http://www.bcpa.co.uk
British Cardiac Patients Association. Support site for patients suffering from heart disease.

Defibrillation

http://www.medical.philips.com/
Phillips Healthcare, a supplier of resuscitation equipment. Contains many useful educational resources.

References

Advanced Life Support Group 2005 Advanced paediatric life support: the practical approach, 4th edn. Blackwell Publishing, Oxford, p 9

Atkins DL, Bossaert LL, Hazinski MF et al 2001 Automated external defibrillation/public access defibrillation. Annals of Internal Medicine 37:S60–S67

Basic Life Support Working Party of the European Resuscitation Council 1992 Guidelines for basic life support. Resuscitation 24(2):103–110

Baskett P, Nolan J, Parr M 1996 Tidal volumes which are perceived to be adequate for resuscitation. Resuscitation 31(3):231–234

British Red Cross/St Andrew's Ambulance Association/St John Ambulance 2006 First aid manual, 8th edn. Dorling Kindersley Limited, London

Caplan G 1964 Principles of preventative psychiatry. Basic Books, New York

Child Accident Prevention Trust 2008 Child accident facts. Available online: http://www.capt.org.uk (accessed 9 August 2008)

Cook P 1999 Supporting sick children and their families. Baillière Tindall, London

Coyne I 1996 Sudden infant death syndrome and baby care practices. Paediatric Nursing 8(10):16–18

Cummins RO, Ornato JP, Thies WH et al 1991 Improving survival from sudden cardiac arrest: the 'chain of survival' concept. Circulation 83(5):1832–1847

Department of Health 1991 The health of the nation. HMSO, London

Department of Health 1992 Back to sleep: reducing the risk of cot death. HMSO, London

Department of Health 1993 Targeting practice: the contribution of nurses, midwives and health visitors. HMSO, London

Department of Health 2000 Comprehensive critical care. Department of Health, London

Department of Health 2001 Seeking consent: working with children. Available online: http://www.dh.gov.uk/en/PublicHealth/Scientificdevelopmentgeneticsandbioethics/Consent/Consentgeneralinformation/index.htm (accessed 20 August 2008)

Durham TW, McCammon SL, Allison EJ 1985 The psychological impact of disaster on personnel. Annals of Emergency Medicine 14:7

European Resuscitation Council 2005 Basic life support: guidelines 2005. Available online: http://www.resus.org.uk/ (accessed 9 August 2008)

Gibson M 1991 Order from chaos: responding to traumatic events. Venture Press, Birmingham

Handley AJ, Becker LB, Allen M et al 1997 Single rescuer adult basic life support: an advisory statement from the Basic Life Support Working Group of the International Liaison Committee on Resuscitation (ILCOR). Resuscitation 34(2):101–108

Hanson C, Strawser D 1992 Family presence during cardio-pulmonary resuscitation: Foote Hospital's 9 year perspective. Journal of Emergency Nursing 18(2):104–106

Health and Safety Commission 1981 First aid at work. The Health and Safety (First-Aid) Regulations 1981. Approved Code of Practice and Guidance L74. HSE Books, London. Available online: http://www.hse.gov.uk/firstaid/legislation.htm (accessed 18 August 2008)

Hodgetts T, Kenward G, Vlachonikolis I, Payne S, Castle N 2002 The identification of risk factors for cardiac arrest and formulation of activation criteria to alert a medical emergency team. Resuscitation 54(2):125–131

ILCOR 1997 The ILCOR advisory statements. Resuscitation 34(2):97–149

Jackson RJ 1984 Blood flow in the cerebral cortex during CPR with dogs. Annals of Emergency Medicine 13:657–659

Jurkovich GJ, Pierce B, Pananem L et al 2000 Giving bad news: the family perspective. Journal of Trauma, Injury, Infection and Critical Care 48(5): 865–873

Langhelle A, Sunde K, Wik L et al 2000 Airway pressure with chest compressions versus Heimlich manoeuvre in recently dead adults with complete airway obstruction. Resuscitation 44(2):105–108

Lee SK 1984 Effect of cardiac arrest time on the cortical cerebral blood flow generated by subsequent standard CPR in rabbits. Resuscitation 17(2):105–117

Mackenzie G 1964 Haemodynamic effects of external cardiac compression. Lancet i:1342

Meyers TA, Eichorn DJ, Guzzetta CE et al 2000 Family presence during invasive procedures and resuscitation: the experience of family members, nurses and physicians. American Journal of Nursing 100(2):32–43

Montague SE, Watson R, Herbert RE (eds) 2005 Physiology for nursing practice, 3rd edn. Elsevier, Edinburgh

Mullally S 2001 The NHS plan: a guide for nurses, midwives and health visitors. Department of Health, London. Available online: http://www.dh.gov.uk/en/Publicationsandstatistics/Publications/PublicationsPolicyAndGuidance/DH_4007776 (accessed 18 August 2008)

Nadkarni V, Hazinsiki MF, Zideman D et al 1997 Paediatric life support. Resuscitation 34(2):115–127

Newbold D 1987 Critical care: the physiology of cardiac massage. Nursing Times 83(25):59–62

Nursing and Midwifery Council 2004 Code of Professional Conduct. Nursing and Midwifery Council, London

Nursing and Midwifery Council 2008 The Code: standards of conduct, performance and ethics for nurses and midwives. Nursing and Midwifery Council, London

Parkes CM 1975 Bereavement: studies of grief in adult life, 2nd edn. Penguin, Harmondsworth

Priestley G, Watson W, Rashidian A et al 2004 Introducing critical care outreach: a ward-randomised trial of phased introduction in a general hospital. Intensive Care Medicine 30:1398–1404

Rattrie E 2000 Witnessed resuscitation: good practice or not? Nursing Standard 14(24):32–35

Resuscitation Council (UK) 1997 CPR '97: annual scientific symposium, Brighton, England, April 1997. Resuscitation Council (UK), London

Resuscitation Council (UK) 2000 The 2000 resuscitation guidelines for use in the United Kingdom. Resuscitation Council (UK), London. Available online: http://www.resus.org.uk (accessed 9 August 2008)

Resuscitation Council (UK) 2005 Resuscitation guidelines 2005. Available online: http://www.resus.org.uk/ (accessed 9 August 2008)

Resuscitation Council (UK) 2006 National audit of paediatric resuscitation (NAPR) study. Available online: http://www.resus.org.uk/pages/naprinfo.htm (accessed 18 August 2008)

Robertson C, Holmberg S 1992 Compression techniques and blood flow during cardiopulmonary resuscitation. Resuscitation 24(2):123–132

Royal College of Nursing 2002 Witnessing resuscitation. Royal College of Nursing, London

Royal College of Nursing 2007 Decisions relating to cardiopulmonary resuscitation: a joint statement from the British Medical Association, the Resuscitation Council (UK) and the Royal College of Nursing. Royal College of Nursing, London. Available online: http://www.rcn.org.uk/__data/assets/pdf_file/0004/108337/003206.pdf (accessed 18 August 2008)

SIDS 2008 Foundation for the Study of Infant Deaths guidelines. Available online: http://www.sids.org.uk (accessed 9 August 2008)

Smith GB, Osgood VM, Crane S 2002 ALERT – a multiprofessional training course in the care of the acutely ill adult patient. Resuscitation 52:281–286

Tibballs J, Kinney S, Duke T, Oakley E, Hennessy M 2005 Reduction of paediatric in-patient cardiac arrest and death with a medical emergency team: preliminary results. Archives of Disease in Childhood 90:1148–1152

Tingle J 1991 First aid law. Nursing Times 87(35):48–49

Wright B 1996 Sudden death: a research base for practice, 2nd edn. Churchill Livingstone, Edinburgh

Zoltie N, Sloan J, Wright B 1994 Observed resuscitation may affect a doctor's performance. British Medical Journal 309:404

Chapter 5

Infection prevention and control

Rachel Peto

INTRODUCTION

The prevention of spread of disease caused by infection is fundamental to all nursing care, and is an essential part of all health care in hospital and community settings. With the rise of healthcare associated infections, all healthcare professionals have a key role to ensure that infection control procedures and practices are implemented, both to prevent patients from acquiring an infection and to protect healthcare staff from infection (Wilson 2006).

Infectious diseases have been a threat to health and well-being since human life began, with outbreaks of infection over the centuries often generating great fear in people. Just over 100 years ago the science of microbiology was born when the relationship between disease and microorganisms was discovered by Louis Pasteur. In Britain, major infectious diseases kill only a small number of people compared to the past, but across the world the diseases of HIV/AIDS, tuberculosis and malaria account for millions of deaths each year (World Health Organization 2004).

Today, despite modern healthcare having saved countless lives, infectious diseases remain a massive global threat. Alongside the emergence of new diseases such as AIDS, variant Creutzfeldt–Jakob disease and severe acute respiratory syndrome (SARS), there has been the re-emergence of old diseases such as tuberculosis (Wilson 2006).

In the UK there are two particular infection control challenges in hospital care which cause deaths, impede recovery and make frequent headline news: the increasing number of healthcare associated infections (HCAI) and antibiotic resistant bacteria. Most notably these infections are caused by meticillin(methicillin)-resistant *Staphylococcus aureus* (MRSA), often described as a 'superbug', and *Clostridium difficile*. Infection prevention and control in the community is a key service within public health. As with hospitals, MRSA and *C. difficile* are being increasingly noted within the community as patients are discharged from hospital with these infections (Lawrence and May 2003).

Infection prevention and control must be a priority for all healthcare staff and should underpin quality clinical practice across all areas of health care. With the current challenge to both hospital and community staff of increasing antimicrobial resistance, healthcare staff can no longer rely on treating organisms with antibiotics; instead healthcare staff need to concentrate again on the basics – proven infection control procedures.

Nurses of all branches have a role to play with their specific patient or client groups. Whether nursing in an institution (hospital or nursing home) or in the community (individual homes, health centres or shared housing), nurses must recognize the sources and modes of spread of infectious microorganisms and understand how to apply evidence-based practice to prevent and control infection.

OVERVIEW

This chapter aims to provide you with an understanding of what infection prevention and control means for individual people (sick or well) and their carers (health professional or informal family and friends), whether this care is in a home or community setting or in a hospital or institution.

Subject knowledge

This section introduces the biological aspects of infection, including the four main groups of microorganisms (bacteria, viruses, fungi, protozoa), routes, modes of spread and sources of physiological and physical control.

The complex psychosocial issues related to the prevention and control of infection are considered, with particular reference to the influence of personal and group behaviour, attitude and culture. Epidemiology and its importance in the identification and control of infection, with particular reference to health promotion, is included.

Care delivery knowledge

A range of nursing practices is explored using a problem solving approach of assessment, planning, implementation and evaluation. Both standard precautions (Royal College of Nursing 2005) and specific practices to prevent and control infection are considered.

Professional and ethical knowledge

Professional accountability is highlighted with specific sections on ethical and political issues. The roles of the infection control team in the hospital and the environmental health team in the community are considered.

Personal and reflective knowledge

Throughout the chapter there are decision-making exercises and suggestions for reflection and portfolio evidence. Case studies related to each branch of nursing are included

here to encourage reflection upon practices you have observed and material you have learned from this chapter.

SUBJECT KNOWLEDGE

BIOLOGICAL

CLASSIFICATION OF INFECTIVE AGENTS

An infection is caused by the invasion of a person's immunological defences by microorganisms that actively cause harm to body tissues (Wilson 2006). Bacteria, viruses, fungi and protozoa are the four main groups of organisms capable of causing disease (Box 5.1). Protozoa are not commonly encountered in the healthcare environment today (Wilson 2006).

Bacteria are the most common cause of HCAI with viruses considered to be the most common condition in the community, e.g. influenza, common cold. However, not all microorganisms cause infection or disease. Many live quite harmlessly in soil, water, air; and in alcohol and cheesemaking (yeasts). Some bacteria are vital in the production of antibiotics.

Microorganisms capable of causing disease are called pathogens, but the presence of a pathogen does not necessarily mean that an infection will ensue. The surface of the body is densely populated by a wide variety of microorganisms and every day the intestinal system excretes millions of microorganisms. Pathogens that live on their host in a specific body site without causing harm are called commensals and are often described as the normal flora of the body. They only become pathogenic and cause an infection when transferred to an abnormal body site. For example, MRSA is commonly found to be colonized in the nasal mucosa and can live there harmlessly, but organisms from the nose can be easily transferred to other body sites, such as wounds, therefore in some instances it is recommended that patients are decolonized prior to surgery to prevent surgical wounds becoming infected with MRSA (Wilson 2006).

SOURCES OF INFECTION

Bacteria

Bacteria are unicellular organisms that evolved millions of years ago. They are visible under the high magnification of an ordinary light microscope using an appropriate stain. Surrounding the bacterial cell is a membrane made up of proteins and phospholipids and surrounding the membrane is a hard cell wall, which gives the organism its shape.

Bacteria are most commonly classified by their shape (Fig. 5.1) and their response to a laboratory reaction when

Box 5.1 Common organisms and infections and diseases they cause

Organism	Infections and diseases
Bacteria	
Gram positive	
Staphylococcus aureus	Wound infections, pneumonia, osteomyelitis, food poisoning
Staphylococcus epidermidis	Wound infection, associated with invasive plastic and metal devices, e.g. IV cannulas
Streptococci (group A)	Streptococcal throat, impetigo, rheumatic fever, scarlet fever
Streptococci (group B)	Urinary tract infection, wound infection, meningitis
Streptococcus pneumoniae	Pneumonia, bronchitis, meningitis, otitis media
Enterococci	Urinary tract infection, wound infection
Mycobacterium tuberculosis	Tuberculosis
Clostridium tetani	Tetanus
Clostridium difficile	Diarrhoea, hospital acquired gastrointestinal infections
Listeria	Premature delivery, septicaemia and meningitis in neonates
Gram negative	
Neisseria gonorrhoea	Gonorrhoea, pelvic inflammatory disease, conjunctivitis, infective arthritis
Neisseria meningococcus	Meningococcal septicaemia
Pseudomonas	Wound infections, chest infections
Legionella	Chest infection, legionnaires' disease
Escherichia coli	Wound infections, urinary tract infection, pelvic inflammatory disease
Salmonella	Food poisoning
Acinetobacter	Urinary tract infection, wound infections, respiratory infections
Campylobacter	Diarrhoea, gastroenteritis
Helicobacter pylori	Gastritis, gastric ulcers
Chlamydia	Trachoma, non-specific urethritis in males
Viruses	
Hepatitis A	Infectious hepatitis
Hepatitis B	Serum hepatitis
Hepatitis C	If chronic – liver disease and cirrhosis
Herpes (type 1)	Cold sores, sexually transmitted disease
Herpes (type 2)	Genital lesions
Human immunodeficiency	Acquired immunodeficiency syndrome (AIDS)
Enterovirus	Poliomyelitis
Epstein–Barr	Glandular fever
Virus-like prions	Creutzfeldt–Jakob disease (CJD)
Fungi	
Candida albicans	Vaginal thrush, urinary tract infection
Tinea	Athlete's foot, ringworm
Protozoa	
Trichomonas vaginalis	Sexually transmitted disease in women
Plasmodium falciparum	Malaria
Entamoeba	Amoebic dysentery

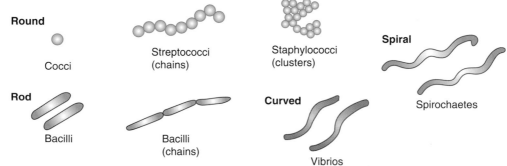

Figure 5.1 Bacterial classification according to shape.

treated with a dye called Gram's stain. The response is determined by a chemical present in the bacteria's cell wall. Bacteria are termed *gram positive* if they stain blue/purple and *gram negative* if they fail to take up the stain and remain the red colour of the counterstain.

Wilson (2006) states there are four main groups of bacteria: gram positive cocci and bacilli and gram negative cocci and bacilli, with other important groups including acid-fast bacilli, spirochaetes and atypical bacteria (see Box 5.1).

MRSA is an example of a gram positive coccus, and as with all bacteria has the potential to cause a whole range of infections including those of the lungs, wounds and urinary tract. More detail regarding specific bacteria, including the increasing problem of antibiotic resistance and methods used to prevent the spread of infection, are included in the Care Delivery section of this chapter.

Some bacteria have the ability to form spores to allow them to survive for longer when environmental conditions are not suitable for their cells to multiply. An example of this is *Clostridium difficile*, responsible for antibiotic-associated infections of the gastrointestinal tract.

Viruses

Viruses are not cells but minute particles consisting of genetic material and protein. Each virus is a piece of nucleic acid that is protected by a protein coat or lipid membrane. Viruses are not usually defined as a living organism, and instead of growing and dividing like cells, they infect cells. For example, the human immunodeficiency virus (HIV) infects human T cells of the immune system; while viruses that cause the common cold attach themselves to the epithelial cell membrane and invade the cell, releasing new virus particles and destroying the host cell. Viruses are extremely small and can only be seen with a high-powered electron microscope. Unlike bacteria, most viruses are very fragile and cannot survive outside a living cell for very long. Viruses are fairly resistant to disinfectants, such as chlorhexidine, which are unable to penetrate the protein coat or lipid membrane.

There are many viruses (see Box 5.1), of which a number, primarily those transmitted by blood and body fluid, are of particular importance for nurses and other healthcare workers. They are referred to in some detail within the Care Delivery section of this chapter.

Prions

Prions – virus-like agents – are abnormal proteins that contain no nucleic acid. They are unique among microbes and appear to cause disease by replacing normal proteins on the surface of host cells and then gradually compromising their function. The main prion disease in humans in the UK is Creutzfeldt–Jakob disease (CJD), although scrapie, a prion disease in sheep, has been known for centuries. CJD is associated with the destruction of brain tissue. In 1996 a new form of CJD was found called variant CJD (vCJD) which generally affects young people under the age of 30. These cause a range of unusual neurological symptoms and it is likely that such cases are linked to exposure to bovine spongiform encephalitis (BSE) (Wilson 2006). Prion proteins are highly resistant to conventional methods of decontamination, including heat and many chemical disinfectants.

Fungi

Fungi have a more complicated structure than bacteria and contain a nucleus. They are either branch shaped (e.g. mushrooms) or form buds (e.g. yeasts). There are over 700 000 species but few are pathogenic (see Box 5.1).

Candida, the yeast that is responsible for causing thrush, destroys the normal bacteria of the area it infects, namely the mouth, large bowel and vagina. The most common, *C. albicans*, causes vaginal thrush. *Tinea* is a fungus that produces a superficial infection. It is responsible for athlete's foot, causing a painful and irritant rash in the folds of skin, most commonly between the toes. Deeper fungal infections are more common in hot climates.

Protozoa

Protozoa are microscopic single-celled animals (see Box 5.1), and although unusual in the UK, they are very common in other parts of the world. Associated with poor sanitation, UK cases are often acquired from abroad. Two pathogens found in the UK are *Cryptosporidium*, a water borne pathogen which is a common cause of gastroenteritis in children under the age of 5 years, and *Trichomonas vaginalis*, a sexually transmitted infection which causes a foul-smelling, green–yellow vaginal discharge (Wilson 2006). Malaria, caused by the protozoon *Plasmodium falciparum*, remains an endemic disease in many parts of the African, Indian and Asian continents. Although malaria does not occur in the UK, nearly 2000 cases are reported in travellers returning to the UK each year (Health Protection Agency 2005); it can be easily avoided by taking antimalarial medication and other precautionary measures. Neither *Trichomonas* nor malaria poses any risk of cross-infection in hospitals. A third protozoon, *Toxoplasma gondii*, is a parasite that lives in the intestine of cats, cysts of which are released in their faeces. These parasites can remain alive in soil and it is possible for humans to become infected by either handling cat faeces or contaminated soil. People at particular risk are women in early pregnancy when the infection can cause foetal death or brain damage.

GROWTH REQUIREMENTS OF LIVING ORGANISMS

All living organisms require nutrients: water, oxygen, light, temperature and a suitable pH to grow and thrive (Box 5.2). It is necessary to understand the growth requirements of organisms so that infection control measures can be based on scientific principles, not on rituals. For example, most bacteria that cause HCAI, such as *Pseudomonas*, are not demanding and will readily multiply in any warm moist environment. Others – anaerobic bacteria – require little or no oxygen and are able to flourish deep in the body. Unlike bacteria, viruses depend on living cells for their replication and therefore need an environment that will maintain them.

Box 5.2 Environmental requirements to support the growth of organisms	
Water	Most organisms require water
	Bacteria require a moist external environment to thrive and multiply
	Spore-forming bacteria can live without water
	Some organisms die rapidly on drying (e.g. *Candida*, *E. coli*)
Oxygen	Aerobic bacteria require oxygen
	Anaerobic bacteria require no oxygen to survive, e.g. *Clostridium*
	Others require it when available, e.g. *Streptococcus*, *Staphylococcus*
Food	All organisms require food, e.g. organic matter – *Clostridium*, undigested food stuffs – *E. coli*
	Food can include inorganic matter, e.g. bed linen, work surfaces soiled with body secretions
Temperature	Organisms require a certain range of temperature
	Some can survive in extremes, e.g. some viruses are resistant to boiling water
	Cold temperature prevents bacterial growth
Light	Organisms can thrive in dark environments, e.g. in body cavities
	Ultraviolet light kills some types of bacteria
pH	Acidity determines the viability of organisms
	Most prefer a slightly alkaline environment with pH 5–8
	Some thrive in a high pH, e.g. bacteria in alkaline urine
	Most organisms cannot tolerate the acid environment of the stomach

TRANSMISSION OF INFECTION

A series of interconnecting events has to take place for an individual to acquire an infection. This is called the 'chain of infection' (Fig. 5.2). All microorganisms require a reservoir where they live and multiply, which may be in the environment, in a person or in an animal. To cause an infection, microorganisms need to find a way to enter the human body – a portal of entry – and in order to spread to another person they require a way to leave the body – a portal of exit (Box 5.3). Once the microorganisms have left the body in excretions and secretions, they are important sources of infection and may spread by a number of different routes.

These routes are categorized into airborne, direct contact and indirect contact (Table 5.1). A common example of the indirect route is the faecal–oral route of transmission by which food is indirectly contaminated by unwashed hands, and this remains a common cause of disease. Some diseases spread by a specific route while others might spread by more than one route. For example, if you sneeze the tiny droplets from the nose will become airborne, but if you then put your hand up to your nose as you sneeze the droplets will come into contact with your hand. If you did not then wash your hands you could pass it on by indirect contact to the next object you touch. For this reason it is important that all healthcare workers have an understanding of appropriate infection prevention and control measures (see Care Delivery section).

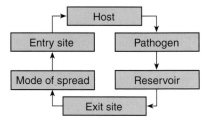

Figure 5.2 Chain of infection.

Box 5.3 Portals of entry and portals of exit of pathogens	
Respiratory tract	Inhalation and exhalation
Gastrointestinal system	Ingestion and excretion
Skin and mucous membrane	Inoculation
Reproductive system	Sexually transmitted
Urinary tract	Sexually transmitted and excretion
Blood	Congenital and trauma

Table 5.1 Routes of spread of infection

Route of spread	Source	Example
Airborne	Human	Bedding, skin scales, coughing, sneezing, talking
	Aerosols	Nebulizers, humidifiers, showers, cooling towers
	Dust	Sweeping, dusting, building work
Direct contact	Human	Hands, uniform, sexual contact
	Food	Hands, equipment, uncooked food
	Fluids	Disinfectants, antiseptics, blood, body fluids, water
	Insects	Flies, mosquitoes
	Animals	Cows, pigs
Indirect contact	Inanimate objects	Bedpans, bedclothes, needles, washbowls, surgical instruments

The sources of microorganisms causing infections or diseases can be classified as either:

- endogenous (or self-infection) which refers to microorganisms that exist harmlessly in one part of a person's body but become pathogenic when transferred to another site
- exogenous (or cross-infection) which refers to microorganisms that do not originate from the patient but are transmitted from another source.

Reflection and portfolio evidence

Think back to a patient during a placement who had either a MRSA or *Clostridium difficile* infection.

- Using the chain of infection (see Fig. 5.2) – consider the ways that their particular infection might have entered the body, the potential reservoir(s) and exit site(s).
- Reflect upon the specific practices that are required to be undertaken by staff to prevent the spread of infection to staff and other patients.
- Discuss your answers with a member of staff and record your findings in your portfolio.

The host

The patient or host is the final link in the chain (see Fig. 5.2) and is the most common reservoir or source of microorganisms in hospital departments, particularly their body secretions, excretions and skin lesions. A person who acquires microorganisms does not necessarily develop an infection; they may simply act as a source but be a risk to other susceptible patients. These patients are sometimes called 'carriers' as they carry infections around and transfer them to other patients.

The hepatitis B virus and the meningitis bacterium (*Neisseria meningitidis*) are two examples of microorganisms present in carriers. There are between 2% and 10% of those infected who fail to completely eliminate the virus and continue to carry it in their blood (Wilson 2006). Similarly many people are unknowingly carriers of *N. meningitidis* bacteria in their respiratory tract; they show no symptoms but can pass the bacteria on to other susceptible people.

Antimicrobial resistance

Prior to the introduction of antibiotics death from sepsis was common and until recently many infections could be successfully treated despite the increasing problems of resistance to antibiotics. While few microorganisms show resistance to all antibiotics, there are key pathogens which pose significant problems in healthcare settings in the UK. These include MRSA and multidrug-resistant *Mycobacterium tuberculosis* (Wilson 2006). A number of factors are considered to play a key role in the increasing resistance of antimicrobials, including the unnecessary and inappropriate use of antibiotics (Wilson 2006).

Staphylococcus aureus, a gram positive coccus, is an important cause of infection in both hospitals and the community, and remains the commonest cause of wound infection, after either accidental injury or surgery (Department of Health 2005b). Today, owing to this bacterium's remarkable ability to adapt to the presence of antibiotics, approximately 90% of hospital strains and 50% of community strains are resistant to penicillin. Today MRSA occurs worldwide with strains usually resistant to two or more antibiotics (see Evolve 5.1 for more detailed information).

5.1 – METICILLIN(METHICILLIN)– RESISTANT *STAPHYLOCOCCUS AUREUS* (MRSA)

- Definition and history of MRSA.
- How MRSA affects people.
- Prevention and control of MRSA.
- Screening for MRSA.
- Management of MRSA.

Resistance to drugs originally used to treat tuberculosis has occurred since streptomycin was first used in the 1940s. Treatment regimens were then devised using a second drug to destroy resistance to the first drug. Today treatment now requires a combination of three or four drugs for at least 6 months. A World Health Organization report has indicated resistance to the four first-line drugs in 35 countries (Lawrence & May 2003). In England, Wales and Northern Ireland, a report covering the years 2002–5 showed 8.7% had a resistance to one or more of the first-line drugs (isoniazid and rifampicin), and 0.9% were multidrug-resistant (Health Protection Agency 2006a). Of particular concern worldwide is HIV related drug-resistant tuberculosis, with infection more likely to become active or a latent infection more likely to reactivate. The poor absorption of drugs and interactions with other drugs makes the treatment of tuberculosis in HIV-positive patients much more complicated.

CONTROLLING THE SPREAD OF INFECTION

Both physiological and physical systems of control can be used in the prevention of infection. For such control the chain of infection (see Fig. 5.2) needs to be broken.

In the past the isolation of patients has been a recognized way to prevention. But since the 1980s and the rise in bloodborne infections a universal approach is for staff to use blood and body fluid precautions regardless of infectious status – i.e. a risk assessment approach. As there is a particular need to prevent the spread of MRSA, 'source isolation', with its aim to prevent the transfer of microorganisms from infected patients, has been recognized as a significant measure in the prevention of its spread (Coia et al 2006). Please access Evolve 5.2 for more information on isolation care.

---

evolve

5.2 – ISOLATION CARE

- General principles of care.
- Management of source isolation.
- Management of protective isolation.

Physiological controls

The body's immune system resists the invasion of microorganisms and protects against foreign material. The first line of defence is the non-specific or passive immune response. Body systems play unique roles providing anatomical and physical barriers against the invasion of pathogens (Table 5.2).

The body's specific or active immune response involves innate (non-specific) immunity and acquired immunity. Innate immunity is provided by genetic and cellular factors and can be influenced by age, nutritional status and any underlying disease. Active immunity results when the host develops antibodies following immunization. The active

Table 5.2 Non-specific immune response

Route of spread	Source	Example
Skin	Layers of skin	Mechanical and waterproof barrier
	Sebaceous glands	Secrete sebum – bactericidal properties
		Fatty acid kills bacteria
Eyes	Tears	Lysozyme – digests and destroys bacteria
	Eyelashes	Blinking reflex protects cornea from injury
Mouth	Mucosa	Mechanical barrier
	Saliva	White blood cells destroy bacteria
Stomach	Gastric secretions	High acidity destroys bacteria
Duodenum	Bile	Alkaline pH inhibits bacterial growth
Small intestine	Lymphatic tissue	Destroys bacteria
	Rapid peristalsis	Prevents bacteria from remaining in intestine
Nostrils	Hairs	Trap inhaled particles and microorganisms
	Turbinal bones	Trap inhaled particles and microorganisms
Pharynx and nasopharynx	Tonsils	Lymphoid tissue traps inspired particles
Respiratory tree (except alveoli)	Cilia	Beat mucus and particles away from lungs
	Mucus	Traps particles during inhalation
	Lung tissue	Isolates focus of infection
Vagina	Secretions	Acid pH inhibits bacterial growth
Urethra	Male length	Prevents migration of bacteria to bladder
Urine	Flushing action	Washes away microorganisms

immune system is made up of two types of white blood cells:

- B lymphocytes, which produce antibodies.
- T lymphocytes, which attack cells invaded by microorganisms.

Lymphocytes have memory cells and if they encounter a particular antigen – a response that may trigger an immune response – they become active and respond by producing large numbers of specific lymphocytes and create an antibody to fight the invading microorganisms.

The body also acquires immunity artificially, through immunizations. Vaccines have been developed since the 19th century, after Edward Jenner demonstrated in 1796 that human beings could be protected from smallpox by inoculation with a similar virus that caused cowpox in cows. Vaccines are given to stimulate the production of antibodies; this induces a specific immune response, but without causing the actual disease.

The ability for people to resist and fight infection varies widely and can depend upon many factors, such as age, nutritional status and previous exposure to vaccinations and organisms. Young children with an immature immune system and the elderly with a diminished immune response are both at particular risk.

Physical stress from disease or major surgery are also recognized as important factors when assessing a patient's individual risk of acquiring an infection. Today there are increasing numbers of patients who have or are recovering from illnesses that have caused them to become immuno-compromised. They are therefore at much greater risk of acquiring infections. Patients include those with HIV/AIDS, and those who have had an organ transplant, received chemotherapy for cancer, or had multiple episodes of antibiotic treatment when very young.

Physical controls

Decontamination is the collective term used to describe the three important physical processes of cleaning, disinfection and sterilization. Inadequate decontamination has been cited as being responsible for outbreaks of infection in hospital (Wilson 2006).

The choice of decontamination method depends on the level of risk the item poses as a source of infection and the toleration of the method of decontamination (Lawrence & May 2003). The emergence of infections such as HIV, CJD and hepatitis C has seen an increased focus on decontamination procedures and policies, with particular attention paid to the potential of medical equipment to transmit such infections. An EU Directive (93/42EEC) prevents the reuse of single-use items by healthcare staff, and national standards for the provision of decontamination processes (NHS Estates 2003) ensures that all reusable medical devices are decontaminated to an acceptable standard.

CONTROL IN RELATION TO RISK

The decision as to whether an item requires cleaning, disinfection or sterilization depends upon whether it carries a low, medium or high risk of causing infection to the patient or client. The use of all disinfectants is regulated by the Control of Substances Hazardous to Health (COSHH) Regulations (Department of Health 2002) which requires employers to carry out a full risk assessment of products to be used and provide staff with appropriate information and training (Royal College of Nursing 2005).

Low risk

Cleaning – the physical removal of microorganisms and organic matter on which they thrive – is considered appropriate for equipment or practices that are considered low risk (Box 5.4). After cleaning, any article should have fewer microorganisms on it, but the dry method might simply redistribute the microorganisms into the air, while the wet method might distribute and increase the microorganisms through the use of contaminated articles such as mop heads and cloths or contaminated water. Approximately 80% of microorganisms are removed during the cleaning procedure, with drying equally important to prevent any remaining bacteria from multiplying (Wilson 2006). While cleaning alone may be an adequate method of decontamination, it is also an essential preparation for items requiring disinfection or sterilization.

Medium risk

Disinfection – the destruction of vegetative microorganisms to a level unlikely to cause infection – reduces the number of viable microorganisms but may not inactivate some bacterial spores (Lawrence & May 2003). It is associated with equipment that may come in close contact with mucous membranes but is not used for invasive procedures (see Box 5.4). Pathogens remaining after disinfection may pose an infection risk to particularly susceptible patients, for example those receiving cytotoxic (chemotherapy) therapy.

The two main methods of disinfection are heat and chemicals (see Box 5.4). Heat is the preferred method for disinfecting articles (e.g. surgical instruments) as it is more penetrative and easier to control than chemicals. Chemical disinfection may be required if heat is unsuitable, for example skin disinfection and heat sensitive items such as fibreoptic endoscopes. The choice is complex and requires a working knowledge of the disinfectants available and the make-up of the article that requires disinfecting (see Box 5.4).

High risk

Sterilization is the complete destruction or removal of all living microorganisms including bacterial spores (Lawrence & May 2003) and involves the use of heat, gas, chemicals or

Box 5.4 Physical systems of infection control

Low risk

Cleaning	Dry	Mechanical action to loosen and remove large particles but may increase airborne count of bacteria up to tenfold
		Does not remove stains
		Sweeping redisperses bacteria in dust and larger particles
		Dry mops may be specifically treated to attract and retain dust particles
		Vacuum cleaning should not increase airborne counts of bacteria
		Expelled air from machine should not blow dust from uncleaned surfaces back into the air
		Dry dusting increases the air count of dust and bacteria and recontaminates cleaned surfaces
	Wet	Water containing detergents or solvents to dissolve adherent dirt and dust
		Dispersal of microorganisms into the air is less likely
		Cleaning fluids may grow bacteria due to contamination
		Damp dusting is less likely to disperse bacteria into air
		Need to rinse after cleaning with detergent to prevent build-up of detergent film
		All surfaces need to be dry before use to prevent contamination from bacterial growth

Medium risk

Disinfection	Heat	80°C for 1 minute or 65°C for 10 minutes kills vegetative organisms
		Steam heat is most effective, e.g. autoclave
		Damage relates to time and temperature
		Disinfection at a lower temperature for a longer time is possible for heat-sensitive equipment
	Chemical	Phenolics, e.g. Stericol, Hycolin, widely used for disinfecting inanimate objects
		Not active against bacterial spores or some viruses
		Toxic, unsuitable for living tissue until thoroughly rinsed
		Chemicals should not be used for food preparation or storage surfaces
		Hypochlorites (bleach), e.g. Milton, Sanichlor, mainly used for environmental disinfection, active against many microorganisms including viruses
		May corrode metals and bleach fabrics
		Chlorhexidine is used clinically, should not be used to disinfect inanimate objects
		Active against gram positive cocci (*S. aureus*), less active against bacilli and spores, little virucidal activity
		Inactivated in the presence of soap
		Alcohol (70% ethyl or 60% isopropyl) is rapidly active against vegetative bacteria, poor sporicidal
		Acts rapidly – useful surface disinfectant for physically clean surfaces, e.g. trolley tops, injection sites, hands
		Evaporates rapidly to leave a dry clean surface
		Peracetic acid (Nucidex) rapidly kills bacteria, fungi and viruses within 10 minutes. Has a strong smell and needs to be used in an area with exhaust ventilation
		Goggles and gloves should be worn
		No adverse health effects known

High risk

Sterilization	Heat	Autoclaves sterilize using moist heat – steam at an increased pressure (134°C) for 3 minutes
		Suitable for most metal instruments, plastics, glass, fabrics
		Sterilizing ovens use dry heat, 160°C, for 45 minutes, 190°C for 60 minutes
		Heat distortion can occur, materials may become brittle or scorched
	Gas	Ethylene oxide is very toxic and requires careful control of temperature, humidity, gas concentration and pressure
		Used to sterilize manufactured goods
	Chemicals	Used when heat or other methods are not possible or reliable sterilization is difficult
		Grease, proteins (blood, tissue) or air will prevent fluids coming into contact with all surfaces
		Prolonged immersion times are required to kill bacterial spores
	Irradiation	Gamma rays are used industrially, e.g. for disposable plastics after packaging
		Repeated irradiation causes plastics to become brittle
		Is expensive and uneconomical to use in hospital

irradiation (see Box 5.4). Items requiring sterilization are described as being high risk to patients. Sterilization is recommended for all instruments and equipment used during invasive procedures (for example intravenous (IV) cannulas, surgical instruments, urinary catheters). As with disinfection, the choice of method used depends upon the item being sterilized (see Box 5.4).

OTHER METHODS OF INFECTION PREVENTION AND CONTROL

Other methods of control include hand hygiene, waste disposal and personal hygiene. These will be discussed in detail in the Care Delivery section. It is now recognized that an unclean clinical environment may contribute towards infection rates (Royal College of Nursing 2005). To assist with this important aspect of infection prevention and control, several pieces of guidance, including a resource to assist in training and setting standards (*The NHS Healthcare Cleaning Manual*, NHS Estates 2004), are available to promote the cleanliness of hospitals. Since the implementation of the Health Act (Department of Health 2006a), all NHS bodies have a duty to provide and maintain a clean healthcare environment.

Individual susceptibility to infection

Individual susceptibility varies enormously and can be caused when a person's immunity is impaired. Particular groups of patients are known to be at a greater risk (Table 5.3). The Third Prevalence Survey of HCAI in acute hospitals showed that in 2006 one in seven (7.6%) of patients in UK and Ireland had an infection or were being treated for an infection that they did not have on admission to hospital (Hospital Infection Society 2006). The cost to the National Health Service has previously been

Table 5.3 Patients at greatest risk of infections

Group	Examples
Extremes of age	Very young and elderly
Critically ill	Patients in intensive care, multiple injuries
Chronically sick	Patients with heart and respiratory disease
Surgical patients	Abdominal surgery, trauma
Patients with underlying diseases	Patients with diabetes mellitus, malignancy
Immunosuppressed	Patients on steroids or chemotherapy; transplant patients

approximately £1000 million per year (National Patient Safety Agency 2004). While it is acknowledged that not all HCAI are preventable, the 2005 Lowbury lecture stated that globally 10–70% are preventable (Hambraeus 2006).

Decision-making exercise

Identify some of the equipment you have used for moving and handling patients, e.g. sliding sheets, hoist slings.

- How were they cleaned?
- Were they cleaned between patients?
- Do you consider these items to be low, medium or high risk in terms of transmission of infection?
- Discuss your decision with your mentor/educator in terms of current practice observed on your placement area/s.

Although hospital patients are considered to be at an increased risk due to cross-infection between staff and patients, individuals being cared for in their own homes still remain at risk, especially where they have wounds or urinary catheters in situ.

It is important to recognize not only the causal relationship and influence of physical sources and controls of infection and disease, but also the complex psychosocial issues that can be involved.

PSYCHOSOCIAL

BEHAVIOUR

Behaviour is influenced by personal beliefs and attitudes. In the past disease and infections were normally perceived as being outside an individual's own control. For example, in the 19th century, dirty water was associated with infections and diseases such as cholera and typhoid, but it was perceived to be the responsibility of the government to prevent and control such infections (Lawrence & May 2003). Today many psychological, social and emotional factors are acknowledged as being particular influences, with the relationship between individuals and their lifestyle choices recognized as potential causes of infection and disease (Lawrence & May 2003). For example, the practice of sharing blood-contaminated needles and injecting equipment has resulted in the spread of bloodborne viruses (Department of Health 2002); and the practice of unprotected sex despite national campaigns to persuade young people of the benefits of using condoms is still resulting in a rise of newly diagnosed sexually transmitted infections (STI) in genitourinary clinics (Health Protection Agency 2007b).

However, many other groups and individuals also have a particular risk of developing life-threatening diseases and are often ignorant or unaware of them, for example people living in communal or shared accommodation.

An important aspect of health behaviour is compliance, the extent to which behaviour coincides with medical or health advice. An example of poor compliance is the failure of healthcare staff to carry out good hand hygiene (Randle et al 2006, Whitby et al 2006), despite knowing how to carry it out (Hambraeus 2006).

Evidence-based practice

For healthcare staff, it is now recognized globally that non-compliance of a hand hygiene policy is a worldwide problem, with one reason being cited as 'nobody else does'. Studies into reasons for non-compliance were surprisingly similar for two quite different healthcare settings, neonatal nurses in Russia and first-year medical students in London (Hambraeus 2006).

An area where change in health behaviour has occurred amongst parents has been over the importance of immunizations and attending baby clinics, in particular over the issue of whether the combined mumps, measles and rubella (MMR) vaccination increases the risk of autism. To date (2007) there has been no research published to back up the initial claims (BBC News 2007), but the decrease in uptake of the triple vaccine has already shown an increase in numbers of reported measles cases. The infection prevention and control perspective is that the risk associated with getting the disease itself, for example measles, is far greater. But it is important that parents are listened to when social customs and religious practices conflict with the education that is being put forward by the health visitor.

People with mental health problems such as depression may not need hospitalization, but may have poor motivation and self-esteem and little desire to care for themselves. This can result in food poisoning leading to gastroenteritis as a result of being unable or incapable of storing, preparing and cooking food adequately, and fungal and bacterial infections of the skin as a result of poor personal hygiene.

The carer of a person with a learning disability might need to take extra care and pay extra attention to ensure that behaviour and practices do not increase the risk of infection.

Reflection and portfolio evidence

Reflect upon a placement where you have cared for a person with a learning disability. Observe how any basic infection control practices such as handwashing before meals and after using the toilet were encouraged and carried out.

- In what ways did staff teach and encourage the clients to undertake such practices?
- If such basic infection control practices were not carried out, how might you go about implementing them in a similar practice setting.
- Record your findings and ideas in your portfolio.

CULTURAL BEHAVIOUR

Behaviour adopted by particular ethnic, cultural and religious groups can put them at a greater risk of infection and disease. Examples include the eating of raw or undercooked foods by some Far Eastern cultures, the prohibition of contraceptives including condoms by religious groups, and the non-seeking of treatment by men because it is considered unmanly or weak.

Occupation might also increase the risk of infections and diseases, for example those who have worked in a coal mine or with asbestos have a greatly increased risk of developing chest infections and life-disabling and life-threatening lung diseases in later life.

Smoking as a cultural behaviour has over the years received a great deal of attention in the media regarding its effect on the smoker's health as well as on those who are in close contact with the smoker. For example, babies and children who live with parents who smoke have a greater risk of developing recurrent chest infections and asthma (Arshad et al 2005).

Behaviour, attitudes and practices do change, but this can only happen by influencing individuals and groups. This might be by education in the form of knowledge and understanding, by observation of people, peer groups and organizations, and from outside influences.

One example of how culture can cause infection and deaths is that of the outbreak of avian influenza (bird flu) in China, where the practice of living in very close proximity to their hens was considered normal.

Increasing international travel for holidays and business has seen an increase of particular infections, such as hepatitis A, where cultural differences in water and food hygiene in underdeveloped countries are the main cause. During the 1980s, mass media education about safe sexual practices resulted in a dramatic reduction of HIV infections among homosexual men, although numbers among heterosexuals did similarly decline. The outcome of past behaviour is now known to take many years, for example the recent increase in numbers of cases of hepatitis C dates from 1960s behaviour, namely the sharing of needles to take drugs.

Certain customs and rituals, despite being considered infection prevention and control risks, are still widespread among particular cultural groups. Examples include the practice of religious circumcisions on Jewish baby boys in their own homes and female circumcisions of young and teenage girls from certain African, Arabian and Far Eastern countries. Again the media have highlighted these practices as being dangerous and an infection risk (BBC 2007).

EPIDEMIOLOGY

The term 'epidemiology' is derived from the Greek and means 'studies upon people' (Lawrence & May 2003), and is often used to describe the study of disease and ill health in human populations. Incidence and distribution of disease can be assessed to provide data for the control and eradication of disease. Epidemiological studies can be small (micro) or large (macro) in scale. They involve determining an understanding of how infections and diseases spread and who may be at risk or susceptible to the infection. Risk factors might be physical (for example infective organisms) or psychosocial (for example behavioural, such as smoking or eating raw food). The risk to the individual is partly determined by estimating the experience of the whole population.

To measure the occurrence of a disease within a population two rates are commonly used: a prevalence rate, which measures the number of infections present at a particular time, and an incidence rate which measures the number of new infections that occur in a population. Within a population a disease that is always present at a static level is described as endemic, but if the numbers with the disease significantly increase above the normal endemic level, it is described as being an epidemic. MRSA is now considered to be endemic in many UK hospitals (Coia et al 2006).

Epidemiologists provide healthcare workers with data to enable planning of the particular health needs and services of a community. Outbreaks of infections are common in both institutional and community care. However, whereas an outbreak of an infection in a hospital ward or nursing home is usually on a micro scale, outbreaks of infections in the community are usually on a macro scale, at times involving hundreds of people. The influenza virus is a common cause of a macro scale infection. In a bid to try and control influenza epidemics, people over the age of 65 years and those considered at particular risk are offered free influenza immunizations.

An increasing concern to the community is the numbers of refugees and asylum seekers coming to the UK. One effect is that some of the diseases that might be endemic in their country of origin may be uncommon in the UK, which may cause a delay in diagnosis, because health professionals are unaware of some imported conditions (Lawrence & May 2003). However, the rate of infectious diseases among migrants in Britain is low (Health Protection Agency 2006b), although the majority of newly diagnosed patients of HIV, TB and malaria are born outside the UK.

HEALTH PROMOTION

Health promotion is an important aspect of infection prevention and control. This can be on a small scale, such as teaching a group of patients or ward staff, or large scale, involving large groups or entire communities.

Specific groups and individuals have already been noted in this chapter as being at particular risk from infections due to their behaviours, attitudes and beliefs. For these people, health promotion attempts to prevent and control infection either to themselves or to others. The attitudes and behaviours of the health professionals carrying out such health promotion are important. Whether it is meeting a group of drug addicts to discuss the risk of sharing needles or talking to a particular cultural or religious group about child immunizations, health professionals need to be aware of their own personal beliefs, traditions and practices. Often health professionals who are not specifically specialized in infection prevention and control nursing are involved. For example, promoting the importance of immunizing babies to prevent and control potential life-threatening diseases is usually undertaken by health visitors, while community psychiatric nurses usually advise drug addicts about the importance of using sterile needles and not sharing them with others.

An example of a recent health promotion is the 'clean-yourhands' campaign (National Patient Safety Agency 2004) which involved healthcare staff and was in direct response to increasing national concerns to have cleaner hospitals and lower the rates of infection. It was a bid both to get healthcare staff to disinfect or wash their hands between each patient contact and to empower patients to check that staff had decontaminated their hands before attending to them (Department of Health 2004a, National Patient Safety Agency 2004). Evidence from one of the six acute trusts that piloted the campaign indicates that this health promotion campaign has already had an improvement in hand hygiene compliance (Randle et al 2006).

The aim of this section has been to enable you to examine and consider some the important biological and psychosocial aspects of infection control. You should by now be more aware of the relevance of the sciences surrounding infection control so that you can apply them to the more practical nursing issues examined in the next section.

CARE DELIVERY KNOWLEDGE

The prevention and control of infection is largely founded on nursing practice, and to help the healthcare professional there is a wealth of research based studies on specific infection control practices, for example hand hygiene agents (Sickbert-Bennett et al 2004), as well as systematic reviews of evidence, for example for the correct usage and wearing of gloves (Pratt et al 2007).

USING A PROBLEM SOLVING APPROACH TO INFECTION CONTROL

The four stages of the nursing process (a problem solving approach) – assessment, planning, implementation and evaluation – are used here to present care delivery knowledge and practice.

ASSESSMENT

Assessment involves the gathering of information, its analysis, and the determining of actual and potential problems. Within infection control, the two terms *clinical audit* and *surveillance* have become synonymous with assessment. This involves visits to clinical areas by infection prevention and control nurses to risk assess the needs of specific patients or to undertake surveillance of an outbreak of a specific infection, as well as healthcare workers undertaking clinical audits of their own clinical area and practices.

For an individual with an infection, an assessment requires an in-depth analysis of the:

- source and site of infection
- causative organism
- route of spread
- associated risk to other patients and healthcare
- severity of risk, including general and specific risk factors (Box 5.5).

From all this information an assessment of the degree of risk can be made followed by the planning and immediate initiation and implementation of preventive measures such as isolation of the patient or wearing protective clothing (e.g. gloves).

Box 5.5 General and specific risk factors for infection

General	Specific
Age of patient	Type of invasive procedure
General health	Present medication
General hygiene	Surgery
Mental state	Pressure sores
Nutrition	
Mobility	
Continence	

Reflection and portfolio evidence

Consider a client with whom you have been involved in providing care. Reflecting upon this client's specific health problems:

- Assess the general and specific risk factors for infection (see Box 5.5) that you think apply.
- Present your findings to your mentor and discuss the preventive actions that need to be planned into the delivery of care.
- Record your findings in your portfolio and summarize your learning.

Regular infection prevention and control audits provide a formal check that infection control measures are being routinely adhered to in patient care areas. In an audit of a hospital ward all areas are inspected, including the treatment room and the ward kitchen. Areas are checked for general cleanliness and specific infection prevention and control measures. Specific audits would highlight the availability and correct use of a sharps bin in the treatment room, and the presence and correct use of a food refrigerator thermometer. Results of these clinical audits and surveillances of HCAI (Hospital Infection Society 2006) facilitated the development of national evidence based guidelines (see Implementation section) (Pratt et al 2007).

PLANNING

Planning can only commence when the organism, site of infection and mode of spread have all been identified. It involves the prioritizing of goals of care and can be divided into those that will prevent, control and reduce endogenous and exogenous infection. As the patient's condition improves or deteriorates, priorities may change.

This stage might also include the planning of the working environment, for example the design of new wards and departments needs to ensure that hand hygiene facilities are located in appropriate places. However, research still indicates that despite the provision of easily accessible hand hygiene products, compliance remains low, and needs to include an associated behavioural modification programme to increase handwashing compliance (Whitby et al 2006).

IMPLEMENTATION

Implementation involves putting into practice evidence-based and appropriate infection control practices to reduce the risk of cross-infection and self-infection to patients, visitors and healthcare personnel.

Safe practice should ensure that the chain of infection (see Fig. 5.2) is broken, thereby preventing the transmission of pathogens to potential sites of infection. Reservoirs of infection can be eliminated, sites of entry and exit controlled, and modes of spread minimized by actions such as safe disposal of body fluids, wearing protective garments, effective hand hygiene and aseptic procedures, especially when handling an invasive device.

Government action plans for cleaner hospitals and lower rates of infection (Department of Health 2004a) and the Code of Practice embodied in the 2006 Health Act (Department of Health 2006a), have put the responsibility back on to the hospital staff to implement evidence based guidelines and protocols with the aim of reducing HCAI.

The implementation of practices requires both adequate resources and clear communication between the patient and all those involved with their care. It is therefore important that the patient and all those who visit, either socially or professionally, are kept well informed of all infection control practices.

STANDARD PRECAUTIONS

Standard Precautions, originally called Universal Precautions, have been recognized since the end of the 1980s as an effective means of reducing HCAI and protecting healthcare staff, patients and the public (Gammon & Gould 2005). This comprehensive approach promotes the use of barrier precautions to ensure that everyone, healthcare staff and public alike, are prevented from becoming contaminated from bloodborne infections. Standard Precautions embrace the notion that all blood and body fluids are potentially infectious and therefore such practices are to be used with all patients at all times, regardless of whether they are known to have a blood or body fluid infection.

The principles of Universal Precautions have been developed into Standard Precautions for preventing HCAI. One set of published guidance is *Good Practice in Infection Prevention and Control* published by the RCN (2005) as part of their 'Wipe it out' campaign on MRSA, in which 11 precautions are identified. One argument for implementing such precautions is that they protect staff from known and unknown diseases and the patient from acquiring an infection.

Reflection and portfolio evidence

In relation to the practice of Standard Precautions, reflect upon a recent placement, and your care of a number of specific patients:

- Consider the rationale for when you wore gloves, a plastic apron, eye protection, or undertook the antiseptic method of handwashing.

- Decide which of these practices were undertaken to prevent you from becoming infected and which were to prevent the patient from getting an infection.
- Record your findings in your portfolio.

PRINCIPLES OF INFECTION CONTROL

It is now widely acknowledged that there are a number of specific practices, including the isolation of specific patients, that are key to both the prevention and control of infection. Incorporating the Royal College of Nursing (2005) *Good Practice in Infection Prevention and Control* and *epic2* guidelines (Pratt et al 2007), this next section will specifically look at the following Standard Precautions:

- hand hygiene
- safe management of healthcare waste, sharps and linen.
- wearing of personal protective equipment
- maintaining a clean environment
- aseptic technique
- personal care.

Patient isolation is an important part of caring for patients with an infection, for example MRSA, but according to Coia et al (2006) such isolation will be dependent on the facilities available and the associated level of risk (see Evolve 5.1 for a specific presentation on Isolation care and action to be taken on the outbreak of an infection).

Hand hygiene

The important role of handwashing in preventing the transmission of disease was demonstrated most convincingly as early as 1847 by Semmelweiss (Boyce & Pittet 2002) and it remains the single most important infection prevention and control procedure to prevent cross-infection (Wearmouth 2004, Royal College of Nursing 2005, Hambraeus 2006).

The aim of hand hygiene is to remove physical dirt and substantially reduce the number of bacteria to a level below that needed to establish infection when transferred to a susceptible patient. The precise number of bacteria needed is not known, but factors such as the virulence of the bacteria, the health and age of the patient, and any disruption to the body's natural defence to infection (for example from catheters, intravenous lines) affects the outcome (Royal College of Nursing 2005).

Bacteria, as microorganisms, are either 'transient' or 'resident', depending upon how long they coexist on the body (Lawrence & May 2003). Transient bacteria, which are normally responsible for HCAI and are often found on the hands of healthcare staff, survive and multiply for only a relatively short time on the body – a few hours, days or weeks – until they are removed. Resident bacteria colonize hair follicles and sebaceous glands, which are found in the deeper crevices of skin and under nails; they persist and may require more prolonged cleaning and disinfection. Thorough hand hygiene using soap and water, antiseptic solutions or alcohol hand rubs are all considered to be appropriate methods to remove and destroy transient and resident microorganisms. Despite much research over the years highlighting the importance of hand hygiene, it is still strongly recognized that the frequency of or lack of adequate hand hygiene is due to many factors (Box 5.6).

The government-led initiative in 2004 to tackle hospital infections included a national campaign to promote hand cleaning (Department of Health 2004a). Following a pilot study in six acute trusts, the 'Clean-your-hands' campaign led to the installing of an alcohol hand rub 'at the point of care' across all NHS acute trusts in England and Wales from April 2005 (National Patient Safety Agency 2004).

The choice of method of hand hygiene has been much debated, but the World Health Organization's (WHO) (2005) *Guidelines on Hand Hygiene in Health Care (advanced draft)* now provides a global consensus on the recommendation that an alcohol hand rub should be used in all clinical situations unless hands are visibly dirty. However, it is now recognized that alcohol hand rubs are not effective against *Clostridium difficile* spores and therefore soap and water needs to be used as the most effective method (Department of Health 2007a). Table 5.4 provides a brief summary of the methods of hand hygiene which are expanded upon in the Evolve 5.3 presentation of handwashing.

℮volve *learning system*

5.3 – HAND HYGIENE

- Three methods of hand hygiene used in health care
- When to use each type
- Effective techniques of:
  - Handwashing with soap and water
  - Use of alcohol rubs.

Cross-reference with Evolve 14.1 – Soap and the Skin.

Evidence-based practice

Randle et al (2006) completed a small study in one acute hospital in the UK to evaluate the success of the 'Clean-your-hands' campaign. Following multiple methods of educational input, data were collected from three time periods: at the start, middle and end of a six month period. In total 56 episodes of 20-minute observations were completed. The results showed an increase in compliance with handwashing from 32% to 63% at the end of the 6 months. Usage of alcohol rub placed near patients increased by 184%.

Decision-making exercise

When next out on a clinical placement watch and make a note of when the different methods of hand hygiene (soap and water, alcohol hand rub) were used by staff (and yourself).

- Note what you had done or were about to do that made you use soap and water or alcohol rub.
- Try to determine whether the hand hygiene was to protect yourself or to protect the patient.
- Review whether the decisions you made were correct through referring back to the research based evidence and through discussion of your findings with your practice mentor/educator.

Box 5.6 Factors that influence handwashing

Products	Lack of soap
	Irritation caused by soap and towels
	Not liking soap or handrub
	Harsh products
	Hard or harsh non-absorbent towels
Facilities	Lack of handwash basins
	Inaccessible handwash basins
	Antiquated facilities
	Lack of mixer taps
	Extremes of water temperature
	Number and position of sinks and soap dispensers
Time/staff	Too busy
	Not enough time
	Not enough staff

Safe management of healthcare waste, sharps and linen

Healthcare waste

Each year healthcare settings produce thousands of tons of waste and it is imperative that it is disposed of safely and correctly. In the community, safe disposal is becoming an increasing problem as more clients receive nursing care in their own home.

In hospitals and the community all healthcare waste has to be 'clinically and specifically assessed by the producer at

Table 5.4 Methods of hand hygiene

Method	Technique	Example of procedures
Routine hand hygiene	Soap and water or alcohol hand rub	Before: entering and leaving the ward/department Between: caring for different patients or between different care activities for the same patient After: removing gloves Before: preparing and eating food After: visiting the toilet, helping a patient with toileting, handling
Hand disinfection	Soap and water followed by alcohol hand rub	Before: any procedure involving high-risk patients, all procedures requiring an aseptic technique, e.g. dressing, catheterization After: contact with infected patient
Surgical handwashing	Anti-microbial agent for first wash, may be followed by alcohol hand rub	Before: surgery and aseptic technique for invasive procedures

the time of production for medicinal waste, chemical properties and infectious properties' (Department of Health 2006b: 22–23). This document, *Safe Management of Healthcare Waste*, requires the producer to determine whether the waste is:

- infectious clinical waste
- hazardous waste
- offensive/hygiene waste
- dangerous for carriage

and it is required to be segregated into suitable colour-coded packaging, for example:

- yellow – for waste which requires disposal by incineration
- black – for domestic (municipal) waste to a landfill site
- yellow/black – offensive hygiene waste to landfill site
- purple – cytotoxic and cytostatic waste which requires incineration.

All blood spillages may expose healthcare workers to bloodborne viruses and other pathogens. It is recommended that a hypochlorite solution containing a high concentration of chlorine-releasing compounds is used, especially for large spills of blood (Wilson 2006). Chlorine-releasing granules that absorb and contain the spill are preferable to a liquid that adds to the volume of spillage. In the home, the use of detergent and water with a disposable cloth is recommended as hypochlorites bleach carpets (Lawrence & May 2003).

Handling and disposal of sharps

The disposal of all sharps is the personal responsibility of the user, and irrespective of the care setting. Under the Health and Safety at Work Act 1974 all care workers have a responsibility to prevent injury to others, and this must include the safe disposal of sharps. Studies show that many of the injuries taking place could be prevented.

The safe use and disposal of sharps forms part of *epic2: National Evidence-Based Guidelines for Preventing Healthcare-Associated Infections in NHS Hospitals in England* (Pratt et al 2007) and must form part of an overall disposal of clinical waste strategy to ensure the protection of staff, patients and visitors from exposure to bloodborne pathogens (Damani 2003). Needlestick injuries, despite education input, still continue to occur (National Audit Office 2005), with improvements in surveillance techniques being recommended. However, obtaining accurate figures for sharps injuries is difficult as many staff fail to report injuries (Cutter & Jordan 2004).

'Sharps' are items that could cause a puncture wound or cuts and include:

- needles
- syringes with needles attached
- broken glass ampoules
- scalpel and other blades
- infusion sets (the sharps parts) (Department of Health 2006b).

All sharps are required to be disposed of into a sharps container which conforms to the UN3291 and BS7320 standards for sharps containers (Wearmouth 2004). They are colour coded with the colour depending upon how the waste should be treated and disposed of (Department of Health 2006b). The treatment of all sharps injuries must always be followed up properly. The role of occupational health departments is discussed later in this section under Personal Care.

Linen

The regulations surrounding the handling and washing of laundry in hospitals are based on Department of Health guidance (National Health Service Executive 1995) which requires hospital linen to be categorized using a national colour code for laundry bags and standards in the laundry for heat disinfection (Wilson 2006). In order to minimize the risk of cross-infection to workers who handle linen, the guidance states that infected linen should be sealed in a white water-soluble or soluble-stitched bag and placed in a red outer bag. This means that the handlers can then place the water-soluble bag directly in the washing machine without opening it. Infection among laundry workers who handle soiled linen is rarely reported (Damani 2003); it is the inadvertent disposal of objects, including sharps, that is the cause of injuries.

Requirements for water temperature vary between hospital and home. A hot-water wash with a water temperature of 71°C for a minimum of 25 minutes is recommended (Damani 2003), but studies have also shown that lower water temperatures can reduce contamination if appropriate amounts of detergents and bleach are controlled (Damani 2003). The temperatures used in the drying and ironing are also recognized as important for reducing microorganisms.

Personal protective equipment

Personal protective equipment (PPE) is primarily used 'to protect staff and reduce any opportunity for the transmission of micro-organisms in hospitals' (Pratt et al 2007: S19). Over the past 20 years there has been a trend to reduce the inappropriate wearing of aprons, gowns, and masks due to the lack of evidence that they prevent HCAI. Today decisions whether to wear PPE should be based upon an individual patient risk assessment of both the related patient care activity or intervention, as well as relevant health and safety legislation, e.g. the Personal Protective Equipment at Work Regulations (Health and Safety Executive 1992). For example, a nursing activity where there is no direct contact with blood or body fluids, such as taking a pulse or blood pressure, would not require the use of protective clothing. Conversely, an activity that may result in the contamination of hands or uniform, such as helping a patient with a commode or emptying a catheter drainage bag, would require the use of gloves and a plastic apron. It should be remembered that the use of protective equipment must not be considered in isolation to other practices, and in particular to hand hygiene.

The most common items of protection include: gloves, plastic aprons, masks and eye protectors. However, if worn incorrectly (e.g. if gloves are only washed between each care activity, rather than being changed), protective items will not prevent the transmission of organisms (Pratt et al 2007). Other protective clothing such as shoes, hats and gowns are generally restricted to use within operating theatres.

Although the use of protective clothing may be important, it must not be forgotten that such protection can be very alarming to the public. Therefore care needs to be taken in explaining the rationale for protective clothing to both the client and their relatives.

Over the years a number of studies have examined the cross-infection risk that nurses' uniforms pose, and all recognize that such uniforms do become contaminated with organisms and recommend that plastic aprons be worn to reduce levels of contamination to uniforms (Nye et al 2005) (see also the section on uniforms under Personal Care).

Gloves

Gloves have been identified and used by healthcare staff as an everyday part of clinical practice since the 1980s. Expert opinion (Clark et al 2002) identifies two main indications for their use:

1. To protect the hands of staff from contamination with organic matter and microorganisms.
2. To reduce the risk of cross-infection to both patients and staff.

It is therefore imperative that gloves are worn for:

- any practice that involves the handling of blood and body fluids, including procedures such as the emptying of urinary catheter bags and the handling of dirty linen, soiled dressings, colostomy bags and incontinence pads
- any aseptic invasive procedure.

The increased usage of gloves has seen a corresponding increase in reports of latex allergies (Health and Safety Executive 2007). Common symptoms include itchy skin rashes, itching eyes and nose, wheezing and asthma. People with other allergies such as hay fever may be more sensitive to latex. Latex-free gloves (e.g. nitrile) and clinical products are now commonly available and used in many hospitals and care settings. It is advisable that staff who show symptoms of latex sensitivity or allergy should attend an occupational health unit for further advice.

There is a wealth of evidence-based literature available regarding the correct selection, usage, and wearing of gloves including the *epic2 National Evidence-Based Guidelines for Preventing Healthcare-Associated Infections in NHS Hospitals in England* (Pratt et al 2007) (see Evolve 5.4 for more details).

 5.4 – GLOVES

- Reasons for using gloves
- Types and choices of gloves
- Correct application, removal and disposal of gloves
- Risks of glove wearing

Aprons

The wearing of plastic aprons has been recommended for many years; however, it has yet to be established that there is a direct association between contaminated uniforms and HCAI (Pratt et al 2007).

The most recent evidence-based national guidelines (Pratt et al 2007) recommend that disposable aprons must be worn when:

- close contact with the patient, materials or equipment is anticipated

or

- there is a risk that clothing may become contaminated with pathogenic microorganisms or blood, body fluids, secretions or excretions, with the exception of perspiration.

Pratt et al (2007: S21) also advocate that plastic aprons/gowns should be worn as 'a single-use item, for one procedure or episode of patient care, and then discarded and disposed of as clinical waste'.

Masks

Masks are rarely worn today outside the operating theatre. Pratt et al (2007) found no robust experimental studies that demonstrated that the wearing of facemasks by healthcare staff protected patients from HCAI during wound dressings or invasive medical procedures as part of a routine ward procedure.

Facemasks may be used to protect the wearer from inhaling minute airborne respiratory particles; however, specialized respiratory equipment is recommended to be worn for the care of certain patients, such as those with active multiple drug resistant pulmonary tuberculosis, as the ordinary surgical facemask is not effective in filtering out the very small respiratory particles (Pratt et al 2007).

Today the main rationale for wearing a surgical facemask in the operating theatre is to protect the healthcare team from splashes of blood and body fluids on to the mucous membranes of the mouth.

Evidence-based practice

A Cochrane Review of all the randomized controlled trials and quasi-randomized controlled trials compared the use of disposable surgical masks with the use of no mask. Two trials met all the inclusion criteria.

This review concluded that it is 'unclear whether wearing surgical facemasks results in any harm or benefit to the patient undergoing clean surgery' (Lipp and Edwards 2006).

Eye protection

Studies show that eye protection offers protection against the physical splashing of infected substances and should be worn for any activity where there is a risk of blood or body fluids splashing on to the face, eyes or mouth and discarded immediately after use (Royal College of Nursing 2005). Special glasses, goggles or visors should be used in all high risk environments, such as an operating theatre, as well as during other high risk procedures such as obstetrical procedures and dentistry. Eye guards also offer protection against splashes of the chemicals that are used in the sterilization and disinfection of endoscopes and other surgical instruments (Damani 2003).

Other protective clothing

Other items of protective clothing have traditionally involved the wearing of gowns, hats and overshoes. Over the years studies into operating theatre practice have produced conflicting evidence over whether the wearing of disposable hats and theatre footwear have any effect on the reduction of surgical-related infections with some research showing that the wearing of overshoes can actually increase, rather than decrease floor colony counts of bacteria.

Gowns

Gowns should be worn where the risk of potential contamination from blood and blood products is very high. Research over the last 20 years has consistently shown that operating gowns made from non water-repellent materials such as cotton do not prevent fluid penetration, and indicate that they may not protect either patient or surgeon from the transmission of infection.

The use of gowns and their role in the prevention of cross-infection on the wards is questionable. A small study by Grant et al (2006) concluded that the contribution made by gowns on the wards of a small community teaching hospital in the prevention of MRSA transmission was small.

Maintaining a clean environment

A dirty clinical environment is recognized by the RCN (2005) as a factor which contributes towards rates of infection. Cleaning removes dust and dirt which may contain large numbers of microorganisms and organic matter from faeces, blood and bodily fluids. The NHS Cleaning Manual (NHS Estates 2004) is a useful resource to assist in the training of staff and setting standards. Unannounced inspections by the Healthcare Commission in 2007 found dirty commodes in corridors and cluttered sluices difficult to keep clean (Guardian 2007), which can contribute to an increase of MRSA and Clostridium difficile infections.

Aseptic technique

The 'aseptic technique' has been actively identified as an important aspect of infection prevention and control, and was pledged in the Winning Ways report (Department of Health 2003) to be one of the actions that clinical teams must consistently demonstrate at a high standard. Further government documents continue to support the need for high standards (Department of Health 2005c, Preston 2005).

An 'aseptic technique' aims to prevent microorganisms on hands, equipment and surfaces being transmitted to wounds and other susceptible sites (Preston 2005). Two examples of where an aseptic procedure is required are urinary catheterization and setting up an intravenous infusion. The method and equipment for a specific procedure may vary, but the principles of asepsis remain the same (access Evolve 5.5 for Aseptic technique).

Over the last 10 years there has been a move away from an aseptic towards a clean technique when dealing with some chronic wounds. This technique adopts all the same aims as an aseptic technique, but may use clean rather than sterile gloves, and non-sterile solutions such as tap water for irrigation (Joanna Briggs Institute 2006). For wound care, current evidence indicates that all wounds need to be assessed on an individual basis and that for some patients, wound cleansing can be modified.

Evidence-based practice

A Joanna Briggs Institute review evaluated 14 randomized clinical trials to determine the best solution for wound cleansing, including tap water vs no cleansing; normal saline vs no cleansing and tap water vs normal saline.

It recommended that potable tap water could be used to cleanse chronic wounds, for example leg ulcers, if no normal saline was available, and boiled and cooled water could be used in the absence of normal saline or tap water deemed suitable for drinking (Joanna Briggs Institute 2006).

The principles of an aseptic technique should include:

- suitable hand hygiene
- selection and preparation of sterile packs, equipment and solutions
- the appropriate use of gloves
- maintaining a sterile field (throughout the procedure)
- application of appropriate dressing.

evolve learning system

5.5 – ASEPTIC TECHNIQUE

- Principles of aseptic technique.
- Appropriate hand hygiene.
- Equipment and solutions.
- Use of gloves.
- Appropriate dressings.
Cross-reference with wound care in Ch. 15, 'Skin integrity'.

Decision-making exercise

Observe a practice that requires the use of an aseptic technique.

- Consider the principles stated in the section on aseptic technique and decide whether they were upheld, for example which hand hygiene procedure was undertaken?
- At the end of the observation decide whether any of the principles were breached, for example did the nurse touch something that was not sterile, such as the trolley?
- Review the potential consequences in relation to infection control.

Personal care

Attention to personal care and health is very important in the prevention of infection. Staff carrying an infection may increase the risk to patients, particularly the young, the old and those who are acutely ill.

Occupational health departments have a vital role in infection prevention and control and liaise closely with both hospital and community infection control teams. Occupational health staff are able to provide confidential professional advice and specialist support and counselling. Under the *The Code: Standards of Conduct, Performance and Ethics for Nurses and Midwives* (Nursing and Midwifery Council 2008), registered nurses are personally accountable for their own actions to protect and support the health of individual patients.

Transmission of infection between staff and patients is well recognized, and Damani (2003) identifies three measures that should be available to protect healthcare staff:

- Immunization – all healthcare staff need to be immunized against all vaccine-preventable diseases, which should include hepatitis B.
- Education and training – appropriate education and training must be provided as part of a healthcare worker's orientation, and needs to be reinforced through regular updating.
- Reporting of accidents or illness – one of the commonest infections frequently passed between staff and patients is gastrointestinal, usually with symptoms of diarrhoea and vomiting. It is vital that staff seek advice from the occupational health department and do not return to work until symptom free for 48 hours.

Healthcare workers may also be symptom-free carriers of infections such as MRSA, hepatitis virus B and C. In the past staff have been implicated in outbreaks of MRSA and therefore if a healthcare worker has any suspicions that they have been infected or might be a carrier, it is imperative that they seek advice.

Uniforms

Personal care must also include the care of any uniform worn while caring for patients and clients. The issue of staff wearing a clean uniform every day and the need for appropriate laundering of them has been much debated; with Perry et al (2001) demonstrating that uniforms progressively become contaminated during clinical care. However, no study has demonstrated that the microorganisms have transferred from a uniform to patients in the clinical situation (Wilson et al 2007). To help the development of NHS policies the Department of Health (2007b) have put together an evidence base on the wearing and laundering of uniforms.

Evidence-based practice

Despite much evidence and agreement by hospitals that healthcare staff uniforms should be changed daily, the lack of provision of sufficient uniforms has been an issue for many years.

Nye et al (2005) circulated 170 questionnaires to infection control teams in the UK. From 86 (51%) responses representing 101 NHS acute trusts, only 47% provided adequate uniforms to allow a clean uniform per shift, and 65% did not launder uniforms; 91% of staff stated they laundered their uniforms at home due to lack of or inadequate on-site changing facilities.

The study recommended that minimum standards are required to be set for the provision of uniforms, laundering and changing facilities.

Skin care

The care of hands is a particularly important aspect of personal care for all healthcare staff. Particular attention must be paid to any breaks in the skin of hands which may be in direct contact with the patient with possible skin infections being caused by bacteria or fungi (Wilson 2006). Waterproof dressings should always be used to cover all cuts, abrasions and lesions. Staff with dermatological conditions that cause areas of skin to become broken should assess very carefully whether they are putting themselves at risk from contamination with blood and body fluids. Such staff should seek advice from the occupational health department.

Expert opinion now recognizes that poor hand hygiene techniques and the detergent base of hand wash preparations are associated with skin damage, and encourages staff to regularly use an emollient hand cream after washing hands before a break or going off duty and when off duty (Pratt et al 2007).

Bloodborne infections

There is much concern amongst healthcare staff regarding the three high risk infections of hepatitis B, hepatitis C and HIV. Under European law employers are required to offer free hepatitis B vaccinations to all clinical staff at risk from infection. It is vitally important that the full course of vaccinations is completed and the blood levels of immunity are checked following the course. For a few people full immunity is not achieved and again occupational health departments need to be involved to provide ongoing help and advice regarding increased levels of risk due to reduced immunity status. Guidelines are in place which set out a healthcare worker's rights to return to work following infection by hepatitis B (Department of Health 2004b).

EVALUATION

Evaluation involves measuring the effectiveness of infection control practices, with surveillance, the collecting and analysis of data, and feedback of results being central to detecting infections.

The *Winning Ways* report (Department of Health 2003) identified 'active surveillance' as one of seven action areas to reduce HCAI and within the Matron's Charter part of the *Action Plan for Cleaner Hospitals* (Department of Health 2004a) patients were identified as having a part to play in the monitoring and reporting on standards of cleanliness. National mandatory surveillance is now part of the work undertaken by the Health Protection Agency which produces quarterly data on hospital acquired infection (Health Protection Agency 2007a). This will be discussed in more detail within the next section.

PROFESSIONAL AND ETHICAL KNOWLEDGE

PROFESSIONAL ISSUES

Professional issues are clearly stated in the nurses' and midwives' Code of Conduct (Nursing and Midwifery Council 2008), with every registered nurse, midwife and specialist community public health nurse personally accountable for their own practice. When used in the context of infection control, sections of the Code show that nurses have several areas of direct responsibility:

- cooperate within teams
- keep skills and knowledge up to date
- act without delay if you believe that you, a colleague or a patient may be putting someone at risk.

In the prevention and control of infection, nurses have the responsibility to educate and inform others, including both the patient and their family. Nurses have to demonstrate a wide range of infection control practices as well as the knowledge to enhance a patient's general or specific resistance to infection. Professional responsibility requires the nurse to remain up to date with new practices, made available through guidelines, policies and legislation. Legislation laid down in the Health and Safety at Work Act 1974 states that while the employer has responsibility to ensure protective clothing is available for use, all employees have a personal responsibility to use and wear the protective clothing provided.

Interprofessional working is important in order that all members of the team adhere to evidence-based practices. National guidelines are increasingly the work of multiprofessional teams (Pratt et al 2007) and need to be both up to date and easily accessible for teams to refer to and use in their practice. Local protocols and guidelines require regular monitoring and management to ensure that they are current and in line with new national and European legislation.

An important area of personal responsibility is that of self-care. All healthcare workers should ensure that they are self-protected from infections through immunizations and know where they can get advice and guidelines regarding practice (see previous section, Personal Care).

Acting as an advocate, particularly for vulnerable groups, is important. Some patients and clients may be particularly vulnerable to infections, but be unaware of the issue themselves. In this situation the nurse must be able to speak up and ensure that the care being given will not put the individual or group at risk from infection. For example, a child or a person with a learning disability may not recognize the importance of washing hands after using the toilet or before eating a meal. Therefore the carer needs to ensure that this is done, thereby protecting the patient or client from a gastrointestinal infection.

ETHICAL ISSUES

Personal care by nurses to prevent infection is also an ethical issue. The declaration of personal health status by nurses and other healthcare workers is an important debatable ethical issue. By not declaring a particular illness, a nurse could be putting a patient at risk from an infection. For example, if a nurse is known to be HIV-positive and is applying for a job in an acute care unit such as an operating department, it might be argued by some that the nurse is potentially putting patients and staff at risk. Others would argue that as long as the nurse is aware of the importance of the potential causes of cross-contamination of blood and blood products and upholds good infection control practices, patients and staff would not be at risk. The only infection prevention and control risk would be if the member of staff performed exposure prone procedures.

The role of the occupational health department is both to ensure the health and safety of healthcare staff and to protect patients from healthcare staff with illness and infection. But nurses also have an ethical responsibility to provide an honest health declaration, which may mean that for a minority of staff it might be difficult to secure a job because of a specific condition.

Confidentiality is an ethical issue in infection prevention and control for both staff and patients; for example a patient with an infection may wish to keep it confidential and not inform family and friends. However, the ethical debate over whether the patient is putting those they come into close contact with at risk requires examination. This issue is commonly seen with HIV infection or in other sexually transmitted diseases. The ethical dilemma is patient confidentiality versus the potential risk of infecting their close contacts, such as a sexual partner or carers.

POLITICAL ISSUES

Infection prevention and control has, since 2000, become an important item on the political agenda, particularly in relation to HCAI and the uncleanliness of hospital wards. A number of important national documents clearly state the roles and responsibilities of all healthcare staff (Department of Health 2003, 2004a; Royal College of Nursing 2005). Yet, despite these, and some key changes in working practice, such as the introduction of an alcohol hand rub by every bed, cases of HCAI continue to rise (Health Protection Agency 2007a), and the state of patient care environments continues to concern staff and the public.

All healthcare settings are required to uphold many local guidelines, practice protocols and policies, which are derived from national guidelines and documents, for example the disposal of clinical waste, where the national guidelines state the colour coding of bags for clinical waste, and the methods by which rubbish must be handled and disposed of (Department of Health 2006b).

Policies and guidelines can be considered expensive, and in the past some managers and staff may have disregarded or only partially implemented them. Now, under the HAI Code of Practice within the Health Act (Department of Health 2006a), all NHS bodies have a legal duty to have in place appropriate core policies and protocols applicable to infection prevention and control. However, national action plans such as *Towards Cleaner Hospitals and Lower Rates of Infection* (Department of Health 2004a), the launch of *Saving Lives* (Department of Health 2005a) which provided tools and resources for NHS organizations, and the Health Act (Department of Health 2006a) have all placed a much greater responsibility on the management of all NHS organizations.

Documents regarding the specific infection prevention and control healthcare needs in the community, including nursing homes, have also been published (National Institute for Health and Clinical Excellence 2003, Department of Health 2006c).

Infection prevention and control is set to stay on the political agenda, but with the Department of Health clearly stating its commitment to reducing HACI (Department of Health 2006a), high standards of infection prevention and control are the goal.

Immunization programmes are also commonly subjected to political pressure and media coverage. On the one hand government is encouraging the uptake of this important but expensive infection control measure, both for the elderly and the very young. Some parents, without clear guidelines and understanding of what constitutes safer practice, might see the government sponsored health promotion campaigns for immunizations for all babies as part of a political agenda. An example of how the government is trying to help parents make such an informed choice is an MMR information pack developed by the Department of Health (2004c), available on the internet.

Other areas of infection prevention and control are also subject to mandatory national standards to ensure the environment is safe for the total population. For example, the control of sewage, the provision of clean safe water, and the removal of household rubbish and waste are all central to a clean environment. However, the provision of these services is also determined by finance. Even though central to the control of infection for individuals and large populations, they require large financial input by local and national government. The cost of infection, if an outbreak of disease occurred due to widespread water contamination, would be enormous. It is politically and ethically correct that such environmental control on water contamination is maintained and monitored regularly for compliance (see also Ch. 3, 'Safety and risk').

ROLE OF THE INFECTION PREVENTION AND CONTROL TEAM

Infection prevention and control teams under the overall leadership of the Department of Health are important at national, regional and local level both in hospitals and the community. At national level there is the Health Protection Agency, which provides surveillance reports, policy expertise and investigates outbreaks of infection and epidemics. At regional level directors of public health coordinate health protection activities. At local level health and local authorities work together to address infections and diseases in the community with hospital based teams dealing with HCAI (Department of Health 2006a).

A hospital infection control team has traditionally been made up of a director of infection prevention and control (DIPC), an infection control doctor, usually a microbiologist, and infection control nurses and other members of staff with a special interest and knowledge of infection control.

The *Winning Ways* report (Department of Health 2003) identified that a key action to help tackle HCAI was to introduce a director of infection prevention and control (DIPC), recognizing that tackling HCAI could not be left to clinical staff alone. This report, and other developments such as the Health Act (Department of Health 2006a) and the establishment of the Healthcare Commission, have resulted in the need to review the role of the DIPC. A Department of Health (2007c) letter to all DIPCs set out the future development of the DIPC role.

The hospital infection control team has a key role in ensuring that wards and departments take specific isolation precautions when infections are reported. In the community such decisions would be made by the community infection control team, which is part of public health within a primary care trust.

To encourage team working many hospitals have ward and department based nurses who have a specific interest in infection control (infection control link practitioners (ICLPs), who are able to provide a very important link between the ward and infection control team in the education of staff and upholding good practice at clinical level. In many hospitals there are very robust ICLP groups who meet on a regular basis for educational updates and specific training, and have the responsibility to ensure that knowledge and best practice is maintained by healthcare staff.

PERSONAL AND REFLECTIVE KNOWLEDGE

This chapter has considered some of the important issues concerning infection control, a fundamental principle that must underpin all nursing practices. Although the prevention and control of infection are commonly perceived as issues that only affect the hospital patient and healthcare professionals caring for them, this chapter has demonstrated that they are increasingly important aspects of care in the community and issues that affect all, irrespective of age. Failure to prevent or control an infection may seriously affect the health of an individual or fail to ensure the health and safety of the healthcare worker.

Based on your practice experience and knowledge gained from this chapter, review your own personal practice at home and at work in relation to the prevention of infection to yourself and others. Completing the following case studies will also help you to consolidate your learning.

CASE STUDIES RELATED TO INFECTION PREVENTION AND CONTROL

Case study: Adult

Ivy Brown is 78 years old, and 6 weeks ago fell and fractured her left hip. Following surgery Ivy's wound became infected with MRSA and has been very slow to heal. Ivy is now at home and managing to care for herself with the help of carers and her family, but her daughter is very worried that they will also become infected when caring for her.

You are on a community placement and are due to visit Ivy with the district nurse to change her wound dressing.

- What specific infection prevention and control factors would you need to consider when dressing the wound ?
- What specific precautions would you need to take when tending to a wound which is infected with MRSA ?
- How would you dispose of the dressings and dressing pack used?
- What advice could you give to Ivy's daughter to assure her that family and carers are not at risk of becoming infected with MRSA?

Case study: Child

Emma Davis is 2 years old. She has been admitted to hospital with severe diarrhoea and vomiting. According to her mother she has been unwell for 2 days. She is complaining of abdominal pain and needs rehydration. The nurse admitting Emma decides that in order to protect the other children on the ward she must be nursed in a side room.

The staff nurse has asked you to be involved with Emma's care.

- How would you explain to Emma's mother the reason why she must be nursed in a single room?
- What is the risk of this infection to yourself, Emma's mother, other staff and other patients?
- Basing your care on the five specific infection prevention and control practices discussed in the section Nursing Knowledge, how you would go about assessing, planning and implementing your care for Emma?

Case study: Mental health

Richard Crosby is 46 years old. He was divorced 8 years ago and his wife cares for their two children aged 14 and 12 years. Over the years Richard has had several episodes of mild depression, but has managed to hold down a job. Three years ago he was made redundant from his job as an electrician and since then has only had some casual work. Until recently he has been living in a flat, but was made homeless when a fire destroyed it and all his belongings. At first Richard started to sleep rough on the streets, turning to alcohol as a way of escaping from his financial problems and homelessness. He is now living in a hostel for the homeless. One of the staff members has just discovered that Richard has started to use drugs and some used needles and syringes have been found under his mattress. You are a student on placement with a community psychiatric nurse (CPN) who has been asked to see Richard.

- Taking into account his alcohol ingestion and apparent use of intravenous drugs, what are the specific needs and actual problems Richard has in relation to his health?
- Using Box 5.3, outline the ways Richard might be putting himself and others at risk of infections.

The CPN decides that Richard needs to understand more about the particular risks of infection he and others around him face.

- Basing your health education session upon the modes of spread (airborne, direct and indirect), what are the main infection control measures you think should be included in this talk?

Case study: Learning disability

Kevin Roberts is 19 years old and has a mild learning disability. For the last 10 years he has been attending mainstream school and is now living in his own flat. Currently he has a job in a local supermarket where he helps to stack shelves in the dairy section. Kevin has some support from his mum who lives in the next street and his sister takes him to do his weekly shopping. Recently concern

has been expressed by his employers regarding his personal hygiene. When they visited his flat to discuss this with him they noted that the kitchen was disorganized and dirty.

You are a student nurse on placement with the community learning disabilities team (CLDT) and have just taken a referral from Kevin's sister. Outbreaks of food poisoning are not uncommon among people with learning disabilities living alone for the first time.

Using the chain of infection shown in Figure 5.2 as your framework, consider how Kevin might be putting his own health at risk.

Consider how you would explain to Kevin the importance of washing up, and keeping his flat clean.

- Identify some of the particular situations throughout the day when Kevin would need to remember to wash his hands.

SUMMARY

This chapter has sought to draw together all the knowledge needed to promote and maintain infection control. It has included:

1. Information on the different microorganisms capable of causing infections, their modes of transmission, the environment in which microorganisms thrive, and the body's response to infection.
2. An outline of physiological and physical methods to control the spread of infection linking these to levels of risk posed by the infection source.
3. A description of different behaviours, attitudes, beliefs and practices towards risk taking in relation to infection control.
4. An insight into the discipline of epidemiology and the importance of health promotion.
5. An overview of standard precautions and information on specific infection control practices in: hand hygiene; disposal of healthcare waste, sharps and linen; wearing personal protective equipment; maintaining a clean environment; aseptic technique; and personal care.
6. A presentation of the professional, ethical and political influences on the requirements for infection control.
7. An outline of the roles and responsibilities of infection control teams in hospitals and the community.

Annotated further reading and websites

Lawrence J, May D 2003 Infection control in the community. Churchill Livingstone, Edinburgh

This is an excellent, community focused book which provides the reader with a depth and breadth of infection control issues in very diverse

community settings, including nurseries and schools, health centres, dental practices and prisons, as well as useful information regarding tattooing and body piercing, and the needs of travellers, the homeless and refugees.

Pratt R, Pellowe C, Wilson, JA et al 2007 epic2: National evidence-based guidelines for preventing healthcare-associated infections. Journal of Hospital Infection 65(Suppl. 1):S1–S64

These multiprofessional guidelines, commissioned by the Department of Health, have been developed after a systematic and expert review of all the available scientific evidence. They update and supersede the previous guidelines on this topic published in January 2001.

Wilson J 2006 Infection control in clinical practice, 3rd edn. Baillière Tindall, Edinburgh

A really comprehensive textbook. This 3rd edition addresses the many problems of healthcare associated infections related to clinical practice, and in particular the role of handwashing which is highlighted throughout the book.

http://www.hpa.org.uk

The Health Protection Agency is an independent body that protects the health and well-being of the population. It is an excellent website which provides a comprehensive understanding of many infectious diseases and hazards involving chemicals, poisons and radiation. It is updated almost daily.

http://www.his.org.uk

The Hospital Infection Society runs an excellent site, aimed at providing information to those interested in hospital acquired infections. It is linked to the Journal of Hospital Infections and other relevant sites, as well as making available reports and guidelines from working parties supported by HIS.

http://cochrane.co.uk

The Cochrane Library provides comprehensive research and literature reviews on a range of infection control subjects, e.g. surgical wounds, handwashing, infectious diseases. Published four times per year, each issue contains all existing reviews plus an increasingly wider range of new or updated reviews.

http://www.npsa/nhs.uk/
As part of the NHS, the National Patient Safety Agency collects, analyses, and prioritizes data on patient safety incidents in the NHS in England and Wales. They also provide confidential advice and support to the NHS in situations where performance of doctors causes concerns. It is a really useful website to read the results of confidential enquiries, including patient outcome and death.

References

Arshad SH, Kurulaaratchy RJ, Fenn M et al 2005 Early life risk factors for current wheeze, asthma and bronchial hyperresponsiveness at 10 years of age. Chest 127(2):502–508

BBC 2007 Female circumcision. Available online: http://BBC.co.uk/religion/ethics/femalecircumcision (accessed 9 January 2008)

BBC News 2007 Q&A: The MMR debate. Available online: http://www.bbc.co.uk/news (accessed 30 January 2008)

Boyce JM, Pittet D 2002 Guidelines for hand hygiene in health-care settings. In: Morbidity and mortality weekly report 2002. Guideline for hand hygiene in health care settings. Centers for Disease Control and Prevention 51(RR16). Available online: http//:www.cdc.gov/mmwr/ (accessed 30 January 2008)

Clark L, Smith W, Young L 2002 Protective clothing: principles and guidance. Infection Control Nurses Association, London

Coia JE, Duckworth GJ, Edwards DI et al 2006 Guidelines for the control and prevention of MRSA in healthcare facilities. Journal of Hospital Infection 635:S1–44

Cutter J, Jordan S 2004 Uptake of guidelines to avoid and report exposure to blood and body fluids. Journal of Advanced Nursing 46(4):441–452

Damani N 2003 Manual of infection control procedures. Greenwich Medical Media, London

Department of Health 2002 Control of Substances Hazardous to Health. HMSO London

Department of Health 2003 Winning ways. HMSO, London

Department of Health 2004a Towards cleaner hospitals and lower rates of infection: a summary of action. HMSO, London

Department of Health 2004b Hepatitis B infected health care workers and oral antiviral therapy. HMSO, London

Department of Health 2004c MMR information pack. Available online: http://www.dh.gov.uk/en/Publicationsandstatistics/Publications/PublicationsPolicyAndGuidance/DH_4078380 (accessed 30 January 2008)

Department of Health 2005a Saving lives. Available online: http://www.dh.gov.uk (accessed 30 January 2008)

Department of Health 2005b A simple guide to MRSA. Available online: http://www.haringeypct.nhs.uk/foi/foi_docs/4955_simple_guide%20to%20mrsa.pdf (accessed 30 January 2008)

Department of Health 2005c Chief Nursing Officer. Hospitals must spread best practice on reducing MRSA. Department of Health, London. In: Preston RM 2005 Aseptic technique: evidence-based approach for patient safety. British Journal of Nursing 14(10):541–546

Department of Health 2006a The Health Act 2006. Code of Practice for the prevention and control of healthcare associated infections. Available online: http://www.dh.gov.uk/en/Publicationsandstatistics/Publications/PublicationsPolicyAndGuidance/DH_4139336 (accessed 30 January 2008)

Department of Health 2006b Health Technical Memorandum 07-01. Safe management of healthcare waste. Available online: http://www.dh.gov.uk/en/Publicationsandstatistics/Publications/PublicationsPolicyAndGuidance/DH_063274 (accessed 30 January 2008)

Department of Health 2006c Infection control guidance for care homes. Available online: http://www.dh.gov.uk/prod_consum_dh/groups/dh_digitalassets/@dh/@en/documents/digitalasset/dh_4136384.pdf (accessed 30 January 2008)

Department of Health 2007a Saving lives: high impact intervention no 7. Care bundle to reduce the risk of Clostridium difficile. Available online: http://www.archive.official-documents.co.uk/document/cm43/4386/4386.htm (accessed 30 January 2008)

Department of Health 2007b Uniforms and workwear. Available online: http://www.dh.gov.uk/en/Publicationsandstatistics/Publications/PublicationsPolicyAndGuidance/DH_078433 (accessed 30 January 2008)

Department of Health 2007c Further 'Winning ways' for directors of infection prevention and control. Available online: htpp//:www.dh.gov.uk/publicationsandstatistics/Lettersandcirculars/ (accessed 30 January 2008)

Gammon J, Gould D 2005 Universal precautions – a review of knowledge, compliance and strategies to improve practice. Journal of Research in Nursing 10(5):529–547

Grant J, Ramman-Haddad L, Dendukuri N et al 2006 The role of gowns in preventing nosocomial transmission of methicillin-resistant Staphylococcus aureus (MRSA): gown use in MRSA control. Infection Control and Epidemiology 27(2):191–194

Guardian 2007 Health inspectors find hospital in breach of hygiene code. Guardian, 9 July 2007:9

Hambraeus A 2006 Lowbury lecture 2005: infection control from a global perspective. Journal of Hospital Infection 64:217–223

Health and Safety Executive 1992 Personal Protective Equipment at Work Regulations. Health and Safety Executive, Leeds

Health and Safety Executive 2007 About latex allergies. Available online: http://www.hse.gov.uk/latex/about.htm (accessed 8 May 2007)

Health Protection Agency 2005 Malaria deaths prompt health warning to 'Winter sun' travellers. Available online: http://www.hpa.org.uk/news/articles/press_releases/2005/051209_malaria.htm (accessed 30 January 2008)

Health Protection Agency 2006a Recent trends in tuberculosis 2006. Available online: http://www.hpa.org.uk/publications/PublicationDisplay.asp? PublicationID=62 (accessed 30 January 2008)

Health Protection Agency 2006b Migrant health. Infectious diseases in non-UK populations in England, Wales and Northern Ireland. A baseline report. Available online: www.hpa.org.uk/publications/2006/migrant_health/default.htm (accessed 30 January 2008)

Health Protection Agency 2007a Quarterly reporting infectious diseases. Available online: www.hpa.org.uk/infections/publications (accessed 30 January 2008)

Health Protection Agency 2007b Sexually transmitted infections. Available online: http://www.hpa.org.uk/publications (accessed 30 January 2008)

Hospital Infection Society 2006 Third prevalence survey of HCAI in acute hospitals. Results for England. Available online: http//:www.his.org.uk/ (accessed 30 January 2008)

Joanna Briggs Institute 2006 Solutions, techniques and pressure in wound cleaning. Best Practice 10(2):1–4. Available online: http://www.Joannabriggs.edu.ac/pubs/best_practice.php (accessed 30 January 2008)

Lawrence J, May D 2003 Infection control in the community. Churchill Livingstone, Edinburgh

Lipp A, Edwards P 2006 Disposable surgical facemasks for preventing surgical wound infection unclean surgery [Review]. Issue 4. The Cochrane Library. Available online: http://www.thecochranelibrary.com (accessed 30 January 2008)

National Audit Office 2005 Needlestick injuries in healthcare workers still occurring (press release). Available online: http://www.hpa. org.uk/hpa/news/articles/press_releases/2005/ 050125_needlestick.htm (accessed 30 Jan 2008)

National Health Service Estates 2003 National standards – local delivery. Strategy for modernizing the provision of decontamination services. HMSO, London

National Health Service Estates 2004 The NHS healthcare cleaning manual. HMSO, London

National Health Service Executive 1995 Hospital laundry arrangements for used and infected linen. HMSO, London

National Institute for Health and Clinical Excellence 2003 Infection control. Prevention of health-care associated infection in primary and community care. Available online: http://www.nice.org.uk (accessed 30 January 2008)

National Patient Safety Agency 2004 Patient safety alert. 04 Clean hands to help save lives. Available online: http://www.npsa.nhs.uk/ advice (accessed 30 January 2008)

Nursing and Midwifery Council 2008 The Code: standards of conduct, performance and ethics for nurses and midwives. Nursing and Midwifery Council, London

Nye KJ, Leggett VA, Watterson L 2005 Provision and decontamination of uniforms in the NHS. Nursing Standard 19(33):41–45

Perry C, Marshall R, Jones E 2001 Bacterial contamination of uniforms. Journal of Hospital Infection 48:238–241

Pratt RJ, Pellowe CM, Wilson JA et al 2007 epic2: National evidence-based guidelines for preventing healthcare-associated infections in NHS hospitals in England. Journal of Hospital Infection 65(Suppl. 1): S1–S64

Preston RM 2005 Aseptic technique: evidence-based approach for patient safety. British Journal of Nursing 14(10):541–546

Randle J, Clarke M, Storr J 2006 Hand hygiene compliance in healthcare workers. Journal of Hospital Infection 64:205–209

Royal College of Nursing 2005 Good practice in infection prevention and control. Royal College of Nursing, London

Sickbert-Bennett EE, Weber DJ, Gergen-Teague MF et al 2004 The effects of test variables on the efficacy of hand hygiene agents. American Journal of Infection Control 32(2):69–83

Wearmouth P 2004 Cleanliness matters. Nursing Standard 18(44) (Suppl.)

Whitby M, McLaws M-L, Ross MW 2006 Why healthcare workers don't wash their hands: a behavioral explanation. Infection Control and Hospital Epidemiology 27:484–492

Wilson J (ed) 2006 Infection control in clinical practice, 3rd edn. Baillière Tindall, Edinburgh

Wilson JA, Loveday HP, Hoffman PN, Pratt RJ 2007 Uniform: an evidence review of the microbiological significance of uniforms and uniform policy in the prevention and control of healthcare-associated infections. Report to the Department of Health. Journal of Hospital Infection 66:301–307

World Health Organization 2004 Malaria and HIV interactions and their implications for public health policy. Available online: http://www. who,int/malaria/html (accessed 30 January 2008)

World Health Organization 2005 Guidelines on hand hygiene in health care (advanced draft). In: Hambraeus A 2006 Lowbury lecture 2005: infection control from a global perspective. Journal of Hospital Infection 64:217–223

Chapter 6

Mobility and moving

Jane Smallwood and David Lomas

KEY ISSUES

SUBJECT KNOWLEDGE
- The musculoskeletal system
- Physical effects of immobility
- Spinal anatomy
- Risk factors associated with back pain and injury
- Risks related to moving and handling
- Ergonomics
- Psychological and social aspects of mobility

CARE DELIVERY KNOWLEDGE
- Multidisciplinary assessment of mobility
- Principles of load handling
- Assessment of clients' mobility for moving and handling
- Planning to assist with mobility and movement
- Implementation and evaluation of assistance with mobility and movement

PROFESSIONAL AND ETHICAL KNOWLEDGE
- Facilities for mobility care
- Laws relating to disability
- Laws related to moving and handling
- Impact of Human Rights Act
- Professional guidelines
- Barriers to safe moving and handling

PERSONAL AND REFLECTIVE KNOWLEDGE
- Experiencing impaired mobility
- Caring for yourself
- Case studies

INTRODUCTION

Moving and handling and assisting patient mobility are often addressed separately, yet in practice an interdependent relationship exists. It is therefore useful to clarify our understanding of these terms from the outset. Dictionary definitions describe mobility as having the freedom or ability to move, whereas moving involves a change of place, situation or posture. Health professionals use 'mobility' to denote functional capacity, which means being able to get up, bend down, sit, stand, walk, run, dance, etc. and to perform such movements without assistance. 'Moving and handling' is reserved for interventions which assist moving or transferring people (or objects) from one situation to another. Essentially, 'mobility' and 'mobilizing' refer to patient or client activity while 'moving and handling' emphasize the carer's involvement. These two fundamental components of nursing are considered together in this chapter, as their related skills and knowledge are often combined to achieve goals of care.

Most people take mobility for granted, yet life's essential activities depend on it. In the first few weeks of life humans are incapable of independent movement but as small children learn to balance, they progress through sitting, standing, walking and more advanced moves. Beyond early childhood most individuals wake up each morning without restrictions or limitations, but for those whose mobility is impaired basic tasks such as getting out of bed or walking to the toilet require great effort or may be impossible without assistance. Impaired mobility may be experienced temporarily when health issues occur in life or as a progressive deterioration in response to disease or the ageing process. For some it is a routine and permanent way of life.

Definitions tend to depict mobility in purely physical terms, yet loss of function impacts on normal human development and quality of life. The concept of an optimum level of mobility changes throughout the lifespan and is not necessarily the same in all cultures. Where an environment caters primarily for those with optimum capacity, anything less tends to be regarded as a disability and may have consequences for a person's psychological and social health. As well as inherent physical, psychological or social issues, mobility may be compromised by therapeutic and diagnostic interventions. Caring for people with impaired mobility is therefore applicable to all branches of nursing and poses significant challenges.

As with mobility, handling situations are experienced in all aspects of life. Adults automatically lift babies and children, and processes of fetching, carrying, moving and rearranging are part of maintaining a functional environment. Back pain is associated with mechanical loading of the spine yet this chapter presents evidence of numerous factors affecting human performance. The nature of nursing work logically suggests that nurses are particularly at risk of back injury. The adult human form is an awkward load to move; it weighs several times more than a heavy bag of shopping, has no handles, lacks rigidity, may be uncooperative, and is liable to severe damage if mishandled or dropped. Add to this the confinements of clinical and community settings and the requirement to move people between beds, trolleys and toileting facilities, and nurses are faced with a situation that would be tolerated by few industrial workers. Injuries and accidents attributed to moving and handling constitute an enormous and costly problem in the health service (Department of Health 2004).

The overwhelming focus of literature relating to manual handling is staff health and safety, yet poor practice inevitably threatens the safety and potential recovery of patients. Legislation, supported by guidance from professional organizations, continues to be introduced, updated and amended to provide a framework for moving and handling practice. You will learn that this may pose conflicting demands in your day-to-day work. New methods rapidly evolve as knowledge in this field develops and innovative equipment continues to be manufactured. Moving and handling therefore represents a dynamic and rapidly developing area of health care that has implications for the safety and well-being of all involved.

The purpose of this chapter is to unravel some of the complexities surrounding moving and mobility and provide direction to your practice. It is important to recognize that practising patient handling in a skills laboratory or reading about recommended techniques is not enough to equip you with the skills required in clinical practice. This chapter does not describe specific manoeuvres but emphasizes principles of patient handling, incorporating an ergonomic approach, to promote safer practice.

OVERVIEW

Subject knowledge

For knowledge related to human mobility, the musculoskeletal system is examined. The effects of exercise and impaired mobility on the individual are explored, including perceptions and attitudes towards disability in society. Anatomy of the spine is described in relation to the causes of back injury and associated risks for moving and handling clients.

Care delivery knowledge

Explanation of practical aspects in assisting people to move and mobilize is covered, including information on assessment tools and procedures to select the most appropriate methods, equipment and human resources. Strategies for planning care, implementing and evaluating interventions are discussed.

Professional and ethical knowledge

Relevant legislation and professional guidelines are presented. Issues such as accountability and responsibilities in mobility care are addressed while recognizing and exploring barriers to safe and effective practice.

Personal and reflective knowledge

The exercises and case studies in this section will help you to understand some of the problems faced by people with mobility difficulties and to consider appropriate interventions. On pages 146–147 there are four case studies, each relating to one of the branch programmes. You may find it helpful to read one of them before you start the chapter and use it as a focus for your reflections.

SUBJECT KNOWLEDGE

BIOLOGICAL ASPECTS OF HUMAN MOBILITY

THE MUSCULOSKELETAL SYSTEM

Active movements of the body require coordination of connective, muscular and skeletal tissues (the musculoskeletal system) via the central and peripheral nervous systems (Palastanga et al 2004). Impairment of any one of these will interfere with or prevent normal mobility.

The skeleton has many functions, as listed in Box 6.1. It comprises two types of specially modified connective tissue, bone and cartilage. The human skeleton is made up of 206 bones which are categorized into five types (Tortora & Derrickson 2007):

- long bones
- short bones
- irregular bones
- flat bones
- sesamoid bones.

Each bone is enclosed in an outer layer of tissue called the periosteum, has an outer layer of compact bone and an internal network of cancellous bone (Palastanga et al 2004, Tortora & Derrickson 2007). Compact bone is also known

Box 6.1 Functions of the skeletal tissues (adapted with kind permission from Sarah Crowther 2008 The PH1 Handbook (functions of the skeleton), unpublished student handbook)

Support function

The skeleton is made up of two major bony components. The trunk or *axial* skeleton – comprising the spine, skull, ribs and sternum – and the limbs or *appendicular* skeleton. The axial skeleton is partly responsible for the upright posture of the body. It supports the appendicular skeleton, muscles, ligaments and tendons.

Movement function

The muscles that are attached to the bones move the skeleton. Bones also provide a system of levers (rigid rods that can be moved about a fixed point) on which a group of specialized tissues (muscles) act to produce motion. The fixed points around which the levers move are the joints.

Protection function

Bones protect internal organs from injury: the skull protects the brain, the rib cage protects the heart and lungs, the spine protects the spinal cord and the pelvis protects the lower bowel, bladder and the womb in females.

Blood–forming function

Through a process called haematopoiesis, the red marrow tissue contained within some bones produces red blood cells or erythrocytes; some white blood cells or leukocytes and platelets are also produced. The red blood cells transport oxygen around the body, leukocytes are vital to the immune system and platelets are vital to the clotting mechanism.

Storage functions

Bones store minerals (calcium, magnesium, sodium and potassium) and energy in the form of fat (yellow marrow). 97% of the body's calcium is stored in bone. Calcium may be removed from bone to maintain a normal blood calcium level, which is essentially for blood clotting and proper function of muscles and nerves. Yellow marrow is mostly fat and an important energy reserve. It can be converted to red marrow if necessary (e.g., after severe blood loss).

as Haversian bone because of the Haversian canals/tunnels running through it. These are surrounded by concentric rings of hard calcified lamellae. Nerves and blood vessels enter the bone through Volkmann's canals which connect to the Haversian canals. Spaces between the lamellae (lacunae) contain mature bone cells called osteocytes. Lacunae are interconnected by micro canals called canaliculi. The canal network facilitates nutrition and waste removal. The compact bone serves as attachments for muscles via tendons, thereby facilitating movement.

Cancellous bone is sponge-like in appearance. It has an internal network of mesh-like substance called trabeculae.

Red bone marrow lies between the mesh. This produces red blood cells. Two types of cells are associated with the trabeculae: the osteoclasts which reabsorb bone and the osteoblasts which lay down new bone. These cell types contribute to the formation of new bone after a fracture and the remodelling of bone in the later stages of healing.

Bone is very hard due to a matrix of fibrous connective tissue impregnated with calcium and phosphorus. Cartilage is supplementary to bone and is found wherever a combination of strength, rigidity and elasticity is required (Palastanga et al 2004).

Joints

The bones of the body come together to form articulations or joints. The articular surfaces at the end of bones are covered in cartilage which allows smooth movement. The type and extent of the movement depend upon the structure and function of the joint. Other functions of joints include providing stability during movement as well as maintaining body posture.

There are many types of joints in the body; not all are movable. To focus on mobility, only synovial joints will be considered. (For a full description of bones and joints see Tortora & Derrickson 2007: 7–16).

Synovial joints

Synovial joints are fundamental to full mobility and are termed 'freely movable'. They are enclosed within a fibrous capsule of connective tissue. Articular or hyaline cartilage lines the ends of the bones. Joint stability is enhanced by ligaments which connect one bone to another, and by surrounding muscles which are attached, via tendons, to bones. While providing stability, these same structures guide and limit movement. The nerve supply to joints comes from the surrounding muscles. The joint capsule is lined with synovial membrane containing microscopic villi, which secrete synovial fluid to lubricate and nourish the articular surfaces. All synovial joints have a similar structure to one another, but they vary in terms of their shape and range of movement (Drake et al 2005; Fig. 6.1).

There are basically seven types of synovial joints:

- ball and socket joint
- hinge joint
- pivot joint
- plane joint
- saddle joint
- ellipsoid joint
- condyloid joint (Drake et al 2005).

It is important to learn about synovial joints in order to identify normal movement and the range that exists. However, classification of joints is not always consistent. For example

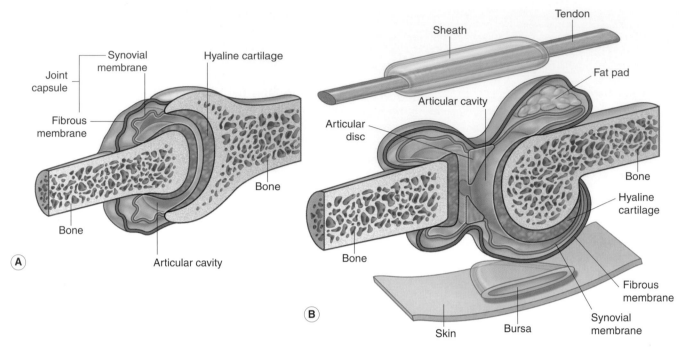

Figure 6.1 Synovial joints (from Drake et al 2005, with kind permission of Elsevier).

the knee is referred to as a hinge joint, but this is not an accurate description since it moves in rotational directions. In older varieties of artificial knee joints, this led to a problem of loosening since they were designed only to act as a hinge and did not take into account the rotational forces exerted on the knee.

Reflection and portfolio evidence

Gain access to a skeleton within your school or department and attempt the movements identified above on the skeleton.

- Attempt some of the common movements yourself.
- Make a note of the range that you may go through in a gym or exercise class when doing a 'warm up' or 'cool down' stretch.
- Sit on a chair and then flex and extend your knee; the movement created is that of a hinge. Now stand with your foot firmly fixed to the floor, try (within your limitations) to rotate at the knee joint. Notice how there is some rotational movement, but bear in mind that the ankle joint is also rotating.

Muscles

Skeletal muscles are attached to bones. Muscle is a unique connective tissue; it has specialized cells that allow contraction, which produces movement. Skeletal muscles are responsible for voluntary active movements which are coordinated by the nervous system. They are striated (striped) in appearance. For stability to be maintained and movement to occur, muscles need to work effectively. Muscle contractions not only allow movement but also maintain body posture. Another function of skeletal muscle is to produce heat, thus contributing to the body temperature (Drake et al 2005).

Active skeletal muscles require a great deal of energy. The nutritional aspects, especially sugar and carbohydrate intakes, are therefore of paramount importance. The full potential of mobility improvement or maintenance cannot be reached if there are nutritional deficits.

Blood and nerve supply of muscles

There is a rich blood and nerve supply to the skeletal muscles. Each muscle is supplied by at least one nerve that contains motor and sensory fibres. Impulses are transmitted to and from the muscles by chemical neurotransmitters. For further details see Evolve 6.1.

⊘volve

6.1 – MUSCLE ACTION

- Describe the terms 'origin' and 'insertion'.
- Identify how the blood and nerve supply contribute to movement.
- Define how neurotransmitters facilitate movement.

THE PHYSIOLOGY OF MOVEMENT

Body levers

In order for movement to take place a system of levers is used incorporating the structures of muscles, bones and joints. Muscles cross at least one joint between their attachments and movement is produced through a system of levers. These levers transmit energy through muscular contraction to move different parts of the body. All levers have a fulcrum, an effort arm and a resistance arm, and are classified according to the differing arrangement of these. By shortening the resistance arm, less effort is required to lift a weight. The relevance of this in assisting people to move is that holding the patient closer to your body reduces the muscular effort required to move them. (For a full description and explanation of the different body levers, see Palastanga et al 2004: 4–5).

Range of motion

The total amount of movement available at any joint is termed the range of motion. To be effective in care and protect our patients we need to know the extent of movement and the limitations that exist. Therefore it is important to know the normal ranges of motion, as given below and in Figure 6.2:

Single (plane) movements:

- flexion
- extension
- eversion
- pronation and supination
- abduction and adduction
- dorsiflexion and plantar flexion
- rotation.

Combined movements:

- protraction and retraction
- opposition
- circumduction (Palastanga et al 2004).

Movement at synovial joints is limited by the shape of the articulating bones and the structure of extracapsular (and sometimes intracapsular) ligaments. Other limiting factors are strength and tension of adjacent muscles or where two soft tissue surfaces come into contact with each other (Palastanga et al 2004).

PURPOSE AND BENEFITS OF MOBILITY AND EXERCISE

Joint range, muscle power, coordination and proprioception (awareness of the spatial position and movement of the body) are all vital to independent mobility. Exercise is fundamental in maintaining functional mobility because it improves or maintains these factors and contributes to general fitness, function, coordination, balance, relaxation, circulation and stability. Exercise also has psychological benefits with evidence suggesting improved self-concept and reduced anger, depression, anxiety and stress. Exercise is therefore necessary to maintain or improve our health. The level of an individual's physical fitness is determined mainly by their capacity for energy output, neuromuscular function, joint mobility, and psychological factors (e.g. motivation) (Bouchard et al 2007).

Evidence-based practice

National trends towards decreased physical activity have been identified, particularly in childhood, for over a decade (Wanless et al 2007). This has been matched by rising obesity levels and raises concerns about long-term effects such as high blood pressure, elevated blood cholesterol levels and coronary heart disease. Since government recommendations in 1996, improvements have been recognized; for example, 80% of pupils from schools participating in a national school sports initiative participated in at least 2 hours of physical education or sport each week in 2004. However, it was also recognized that a sustained effort up to and beyond 2011 was required to meet targets for adults (Wanless et al 2007). As a result of evidence of poor health, Scotland was one of the first countries in the world to develop a strategy for the development of physical activity (Scottish Executive 2003).

PHYSICAL EFFECTS OF IMMOBILITY

Reasons for impaired mobility are diverse. Physically, mobility is restricted when specific structures involved in facilitating movement (bones, joints, muscles and the nervous system) are affected by disease or injury. However, illnesses or degenerative conditions (such as cardiorespiratory disorders, Parkinson's disease or Huntington's chorea) and psychological and social problems can indirectly reduce functional mobility. Equally, impaired mobility, whether temporary or permanent, affects other systems of the body. This has important implications for nurses since many potential complications can be prevented or minimized by nursing interventions (Box 6.2).

Musculoskeletal changes

Muscular strength and endurance are essential for normal movement and performing everyday activities. However, deterioration of muscle mass and strength is influenced more by inactivity than other lifestyle factors (Brouwer & Olney 2004) and can occur in as little as 48 hours of disuse

Circumduction:
A combination of movements that makes the body part describe a circle.

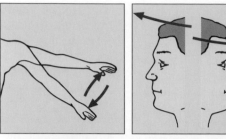

Rotation:
The pivoting of the body part around its axis, as in shaking the head. No rotation of any body part is complete (i.e. 360 degrees).

Protraction:
The protrusion of some body part, e.g. the lower jaw.

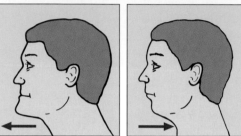

Retraction:
The opposite of protraction.

Abduction:
A movement of a bone or limb away from the median plane of the body. Abduction in the hands and feet is the movement of a digit away from the central axis of the limb. One abducts the fingers by spreading them apart.

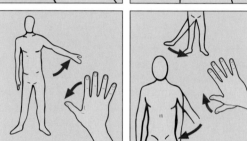

Adduction:
The opposite of abduction, involving approach to the median plane of the body or, in the case of the limbs, to the central axis of a limb.

Inversion:
An ankle movement that turns the sole of the foot medially. Applies only to the foot.

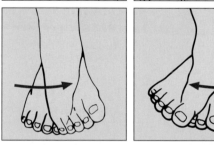

Eversion:
The opposite of inversion. It turns the sole of the foot laterally.

Supination:
The opposite of pronation. When the forearm is in the extended position, this movement brings the palm of the hand upward.

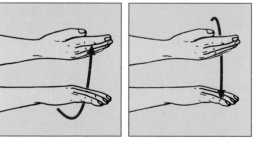

Pronation:
A movement of the forearm that in the extended position brings the palm of the hand to a downward position. Applies only to the forearm.

Extension:
The opposite of flexion, it increases the angle between two movably articulated bones, usually to a 180 degree maximum. If the angle of extension exceeds 180 degrees (as is possible when throwing back the head), this action is termed hyperextension.

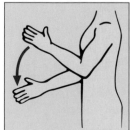
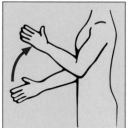

Flexion:
The bending of a joint; usually a movement that reduces the angle that two movably activated bones make with each other. When one crouches, the knees are flexed.

Figure 6.2 Types of movement of synovial joints (from Montague et al 2005, with kind permission of Elsevier).

Box 6.2 Potential problems of immobility	
Musculoskeletal	Muscle weakness and atrophy
	Contractures
Cardiovascular	Reduced venous return
	Venous stasis
	Deep vein thrombosis
	Pulmonary embolus
	Stroke
	Pressure ulcers
	Postural hypotension
	Oedema
Respiratory	Decreased lung expansion
	Bronchial pneumonia
Gastrointestinal	Decreased appetite
	Dehydration
	Constipation (and diarrhoea)
	Fluid and electrolyte imbalance
Metabolic and hormonal	Decreased metabolic rate
	Altered hormone secretion patterns
	Altered sleep patterns
	Bone reabsorption and osteoporosis
	Hypothermia
Neurological	Sensory–motor deprivation
	Diminished proprioception
	Reduced balance and posture control
	Disorientation
Other	Urinary stasis

(Prentice 2001a). A limb that has been immobilized in a cast is an excellent example. Muscle atrophy and weakness can be identified through girth measurements of the limbs, exercise tolerance and levels of fatigue. Where immobility is prolonged, connective tissue surrounding the joints, such as ligaments and the joint capsule, tend to lose elasticity and actually shorten (Prentice 2001b). This results in a reduced range of motion known as a contracture. Hips, knees, ankles, wrists, elbows and shoulders are at risk. Deformities such as joint fixed flexion or tendon shortening may result in pain, altered balance, diminished proprioception and postural impairment.

Cardiovascular changes

Since muscular activity promotes return of venous blood to the heart, reduced activity inevitably increases risk relating to poor venous return and venous stasis. In particular, thrombosis (formation of a clot on the interior wall of a blood vessel) often occurs in the lower extremities. Signs and symptoms of deep vein thrombosis (DVT) include mild fever and pain,

swelling and tenderness to the affected area. If portions of the clot detach, the mobile embolus can lodge in a distal blood vessel causing impaired circulation to major organs such as the lungs or brain.

Pressure sore development is exacerbated by numerous factors, but is essentially a result of two processes resulting in circulatory disruption; firstly, occlusion of blood vessels by external pressure and, secondly, damage to the microcirculation by friction and shearing forces. Where pressure is applied to the body, the resulting tissue ischaemia leads to discomfort. Individuals naturally respond by adjusting their position and posture to restore the blood supply. However, for those unable to move, ischaemia leads to tissue damage. Friction and shearing damage can be exacerbated by poor positioning and moving and handling techniques (see Ch. 15, 'Skin integrity').

When confined to bed, individuals may drop their blood pressure when assuming a standing posture (postural hypotension) leading to them feeling dizzy with potential to faint.

Respiratory changes

If, through immobility, recumbency (lying down) is increased, then the pressure of the abdominal contents pushing on the diaphragm reduces lung volume. Stress is placed on the muscles of inspiration, leading to inefficient respiratory muscular action. Reduced efficiency of the respiratory muscles can lead to an inability to cough effectively and subsequent accumulation of mucus. This creates a perfect medium for the growth and multiplication of bacteria. A chest infection is a major cause of sepsis which increases metabolic demand and systemic oxygen requirements. This affects oxygen supply to the skin making it more susceptible to pressure damage.

Gastrointestinal changes

Inactivity can affect gastrointestinal motility and appetite for food. Decreased food intake, also affected by a lowered metabolic rate, can result in constipation. 'Overflow' diarrhoea due to faecal impaction can, in turn, lead to dehydration and electrolyte imbalance.

Metabolic and hormonal changes

In periods of immobility, the basal metabolic rate decreases, since energy requirements are reduced, and protein is broken down due to muscle catabolism (demonstrated by increased urinary nitrogen). Both lead to increased body fat. Immobility is known to cause a range of other changes such as decreased bone density, calcium wastage, hypothermia and disruption of circadian rhythms (physiological patterns based on a 24 hour cycle such as sleeping, eating and secretion of hormones).

Neurological changes

Deprived of the ability to move, a person is also deprived of sensory–motor appreciation and control of posture and balance (Edwards 2001). An additional consequence is spasticity, a disorder of spinal reflexes that presents as increased muscle tone and overly brisk tendon reflexes (Edwards 2001).

Decision–making exercise

Reflecting on your practice placements, use the information provided in this section thus far, along with personal knowledge, to:

- Review reasons why some of your patients/clients had impaired mobility.
- Decide whether their altered mobility was temporary or permanent.
- Review the rationale for patterns of care and treatment you have seen to improve mobility or overcome the effects of immobility.

BIOLOGICAL BASIS FOR MOVING AND HANDLING

In dealing with the dual aspects covered in this chapter – that is, the 'mobility' of the patient/client and 'mobilizing', which deals with moving and handling patients – the following section focuses on the potential effects of moving and handling activities on the health and well-being of nurses or carers. In order to have a better understanding of the mechanisms involved, it is important to have some knowledge of the human spine.

THE SPINAL COLUMN

The spinal column comprises 33 bones (vertebrae) with discs between them. Its functions include distributing forces, providing attachments for ligaments, muscles and ribs, and as a protective cover for the spinal cord. For descriptive purposes it is divided into five sections (Fig. 6.3) but mechanically it functions as a single unit. Each vertebra is composed of a main body of bone at the front (vertebral body), the vertebral foramen (the vertebral arch) which surrounds the spinal cord, bony projections (spinous processes) situated at the back and at the sides (transverse processes). These provide the attachment for muscles and ligaments (Palastanga et al 2004).

The human spine, of which the spinal column and cord are component parts, forms a shallow 'S' shape when viewed from the side. These curves are a vital part of the

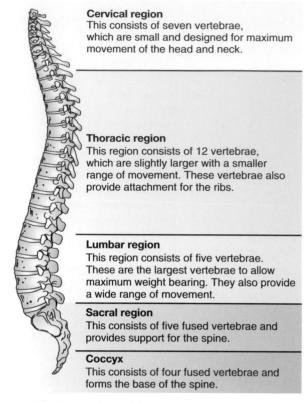

Cervical region
This consists of seven vertebrae, which are small and designed for maximum movement of the head and neck.

Thoracic region
This region consists of 12 vertebrae, which are slightly larger with a smaller range of movement. These vertebrae also provide attachment for the ribs.

Lumbar region
This region consists of five vertebrae. These are the largest vertebrae to allow maximum weight bearing. They also provide a wide range of movement.

Sacral region
This consists of five fused vertebrae and provides support for the spine.

Coccyx
This consists of four fused vertebrae and forms the base of the spine.

Figure 6.3 The five sections of the spinal column.

way the spine functions and give it strength and stability. The vertebrae are different shapes and sizes according to their type and function. For instance, the cervical vertebrae are smaller and their shape is designed to facilitate movement of the head and neck, whereas the lumbar vertebrae have larger bodies to carry more weight. Disc structure follows a similar pattern. The whole structure is designed to resist compressive forces and to facilitate a variety of movements (Fig. 6.4; Palastanga et al 2004). The spine is flexible but is strongest when maintained in its normal alignment ('S' shape). Persistent poor posture, such as forward bending, twisting and slumped seated positions, and excessive, repetitive or awkward manual handling tasks increase the risk of back disorders; however, a strong back that has adapted to mechanical loading is less likely to become injured (Adams & Dolan 2005).

Intervertebral discs

Between each vertebra is an intervertebral disc which consists of an outer fibrous cartilagenous ring and a soft jelly-like nucleus. They are designed to resist compression and rotational forces and have a small shock-absorbing effect. However, sustained pressure on the anterior wall of the disc (forward flexion of the spine, slumped sitting) forces the nucleus backwards, causing excessive pressure on the

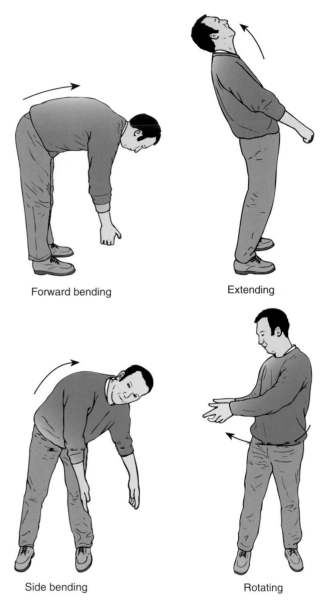

Forward bending

Extending

Side bending

Rotating

Figure 6.4 Movements of the spine.

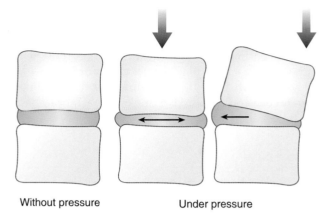

Without pressure

Under pressure

Figure 6.5 Under pressure, the disc is compressed and shapes itself to the angle and impact of pressure. When the pressure is released the disc returns to its original shape. Permanent one-sided pressure will cause wear and tear of the disc. Think of the disk as a jam doughnut – if you compress one side what happens to the jam? This can be likened to a herniation.

Precise data on the extent of back injury in our society are difficult to achieve since the pathology and associated risks are complex and diverse. For example, pain may be caused by disc herniation, muscle strain or bone degeneration; individuals may be at risk because of genetic and lifestyle factors as well as the nature of their work. However, evidence suggests that back pain is experienced by the majority of adults although most individuals cope without seeking treatment (May 2005). Episodes of back pain are often short-lived but they may be a precursor to more serious or prolonged disorders.

Certain predisposing factors help identify those who are at greatest risk of developing mechanical damage to spinal tissues (Adams & Dolan 2005) and these are listed in Box 6.3.

posterior disc wall (the weakest part of the disc). This can cause cracks to occur and further sustained pressure can cause the wall to break down completely and the nucleus material to herniate. This is commonly referred to as a 'slipped disc'. If the herniation compresses nearby nerves, acute pain and nerve damage can result. Figure 6.5 indicates how the disc modifies its position to take account of this pressure (Drake et al 2005).

BACK PAIN/INJURY

The relationship between back problems, poor posture and load handling techniques is explored along with the importance of an ergonomically friendly environment for moving and handling.

Box 6.3 Predisposing factors for damage to spinal tissues

Genetic inheritance
Advancing age
Repetitive loading
Excess weight
Smoking
Weak back or abdominal muscles due to absence of regular exercise
Extreme lordosis (increased degree of lumbar curvature in the back)
Loss of lordosis (normal lumbar curvature is decreased in flexed postures)

RISK FACTORS IN THE WORKPLACE

Risk factors refer to characteristics that make a person susceptible to a particular condition (May 2005). Although these are presented in a workplace context, they are equally relevant to other daily activities. In terms of low back pain, risk factors can be grouped into two major areas: biomechanical and psychosocial.

Biomechanical

Specific biomechanical risk factors have been identified from numerous studies. Key activities that result in back injury are described in Box 6.4. To summarize, during lifting or transferring, the weight of the load (and upper body if bending forward) generates compressive forces on the spine that can lead to damage. When these forces are combined with bending and twisting, the risks are increased. Individuals who have to work with their spine flexed forward (and rotated) for repeated or prolonged episodes are, therefore, more at risk.

Other work related physical stresses include moving heavy or uneven loads, generalized fatigue and environmental factors such as lighting, temperature and noise. Biomechanical factors have enormous implications for the way manual handling activities are performed (see Care Delivery section).

Psychosocial factors

Increasing evidence points to the significance of psychosocial factors (in particular, attitudes about work) in the onset or recovery from back pain and disability. Some perceptions of work that may act as barriers to recovery are listed in Box 6.5.

Taking measures to prevent back injury is important in nursing. Further information regarding taking care of yourself can be found in the Personal and Reflective Knowledge section.

RISKS ASSOCIATED WITH MOVING AND HANDLING

Risks to the client

Risks to those being assisted to move or transfer include the following:

Pain or discomfort

Most methods involve the person being held by handlers, equipment or both. Discomfort may be caused at the physical points of contact and careful attention should be paid to observing and preventing this. Research supports a relationship between nurses' skills in patient transfers and the safety and comfort of patients (Kjellburg et al 2004).

Box 6.4 Biomechanical risk factors associated with back pain

Stooping

Bending movements cause the spine to lose its natural curves and make it more vulnerable to injury. Normally, high levels of stress (external force) are only generated by bending forward to the maximum extent. However, when bending is repeated or continued, or after sustained spinal loading, bending stresses become high in more limited stooping positions

Twisting

Repeated activity that increases pressure on the intervertebral discs, particularly if the pressure is uneven, can ultimately lead to prolapsed discs. Adding torsion to bending and compression increases the risk of damage to discs and ligaments

Static or awkward postures

An environment that forces work to take place in non-neutral postures (see above) or at extremes of range of motion will increase stress to the tissues. Maintaining fixed postures is common in many healthcare settings and even if postures are neutral, fixed postures could lead to vulnerability

Cumulative strain

Most people think that trying to move an excessive weight, even if it be only once, is the situation most likely to result in injury. In fact this is rarely the case. Repeated movements of moderate weights have far greater potential for harm than a single maximal effort (Bridger 2002). This cumulative effect also relates to task duration since the longer tasks are performed the greater the applied loads. This concept is recognized as a contributing factor to injury among nurses. Poor practice, therefore, may not result in one identifiable injury but ongoing gradual wear and tear which may later cause pain and disability

---

Box 6.5 Psychosocial factors associated with back pain

Unable to make full use of skills
Low job satisfaction
Little control over nature and methods of work
Belief that work is harmful to the back
Insufficient rewards
Limited social interaction or support
Unhelpful management style
Repetitive or monotonous tasks where a pace is imposed

Injury

Falls are common and present significant risks to both patient and handlers (Patient Safety Observatory 2007). The risk of injury to patients through falls is therefore considerable, especially in the absence of a thorough assessment. Depending on severity, injuries could include soft tissue damage, joint dislocation, shearing and friction to the skin, bone fracture or severe head injury.

Resistance to future procedures

Perceptions of being moved vary considerably. The procedure may promote comfort and security for some and a loss of control for others. Negative experiences of being moved can lead to loss of confidence, self-esteem, dignity and, ultimately, reduced patient cooperation in rehabilitative and self-care processes.

Risks to nurses and other carers

Manual handling, in any context, is associated with back injury and other musculoskeletal disorders. Handling people poses additional problems particularly for nurses. Statistics are likely to underestimate the issue due to unreported incidents but additional studies clearly suggest that it is one of international significance (see Evidence-based Practice). The association between patient handling activities and musculoskeletal problems is evident, but the impact of value systems, such as stress, perceived lack of support and unpleasant work environments, needs to be recognized as well as the mechanical factors (Johnson 2005). What cannot be calculated from statistics is the personal suffering and social and financial impact on individuals who have been injured.

Evidence-based practice

The extent of work related back problems in UK

- A survey of self-reported work related illness (Health and Safety Executive 2007a) estimated that in 2005/6, 1% of people in Great Britain suffered from a back disorder that was caused or made worse by their work. This resulted in an estimated loss of 4.5 million working days.
- True costs to industry are difficult to ascertain, but at least 5 million adults consult their GP annually concerning back pain (Palmer et al 2000) and statistics from Back Care demonstrate that the financial burden of back pain is considerable (Back Care 2007).
- Health and social care is one of the occupations with above average prevalence rates of work related back disorders (Health and Safety Executive 2007b).

- In the health services, over 5000 manual handling injuries are reported each year which account for 40% of absence from work. Approximately half of these injuries occur during the handling of patients (Health and Safety Executive 2007b).
- The overall proportion of accidents related to moving and handling increased from 17% to 18% between 1996 and 2003, whereas a decrease of 6% was reported for slips, trips and falls (National Audit Office 2003).
- One in four nurses has taken time off work with a back injury sustained at work (Department of Health 2002).

ERGONOMICS

Since the publication of the Manual Handling Operations Regulations 1992, increasing emphasis has been given to ergonomic approaches to moving and handling (Nicholls 1997, National Back Exchange 2002). The word 'ergonomics' is Greek in origin and means natural laws ('nomo') of work ('ergo'). The guiding principle of this science is to optimize the match between the demands of a task, whether physical, social or psychological, and the capabilities of the individual performing it. This can be achieved by designing appliances, adapting the environment, introducing or reorganizing systems of work or changing the task.

Examples of ergonomic approaches to assisting people with mobility include:

- Provision of electric beds, hoists or other lifting/transferring devices to make the task easier and reduce risks.
- Designing hospital bed spaces and toilet areas to make the environment more appropriate to the task.
- Partnering practitioners in areas of high demand or storing 'single patient use' slide sheets at patients' bedsides to maximize efficiency and effectiveness in the activities undertaken.
- Interdisciplinary risk assessment tools to promote compatibility between the task and those performing it.

Ergonomics, therefore, aims to 'fit' the work situation to the people to improve performance, safety, health and well-being (Bridger 2002).

PSYCHOSOCIAL

PSYCHOLOGICAL AND SOCIAL EFFECTS OF IMMOBILITY

In order to understand some of the personal and social impact of immobility in our society, it is important to appreciate the significance of 'normality'. From birth, babies are assessed against criteria of normality. This continues as milestones are expected at specific points throughout the lifespan. Perceptions of normality vary according to cultural background but where criteria are delayed or not achieved people may be viewed as different or inferior. In societies that assume full mobility, reduced mobility can lead to stereotypical views and negative attitudes. Such stigmatization (acquiring an identity from the reactions of other people) can result in labelling (Walker et al 2007) which is often a false reflection of reality; for example, people with physical impairment can be perceived as having reduced learning capacity. Inappropriate interactions can lead to loss of self-esteem and subsequent withdrawal from society. (Further information on labelling and stigma can be found in Ch. 19, 'Rehabilitation and recovery'.)

Social exclusion manifests itself as the reluctance or inability to engage in everyday activities such as interacting with people, visiting friends and relatives, accessing services and undertaking domestic activities. It is arguable that, in many respects, society assists withdrawal by providing centres, homes and schools for those with special mobility requirements. In developed societies, older people tend to be associated with immobility and non-productivity which is usually related to the age of retirement. Clarke & Warren (2007) point out that although the notion of 'active ageing' permeates national and international policies, it tends to be interpreted in relation to physical activity and capacity to work rather than ability to realise individual potential in other ways.

Altered mobility may also affect close relationships and partnerships since the dynamics may be upset by one partner becoming physically dependent on the other. Where employability is affected, there may also be financial dependence and loss of self-esteem. Either partner's appetite for or enjoyment of sex can be affected by physical restrictions, fear of pain and doubts about attractiveness, and questions may be raised about the potential for pregnancy, childbirth or looking after young children (Arthritis Research Campaign 2004). Since most health professionals require full mobility to pursue their chosen career, it can be difficult to appreciate the practical and emotional challenges of reduced mobility. By examining psychological and social dimensions, insights into associated problems such as depression, isolation and loss of self-reliance and dignity can be gained.

PUBLIC PERCEPTIONS OF DISABILITY

In developed countries, full mobility is often viewed as the norm and impairment of this function as abnormal and undesirable. In other words, it is seen as a disability. This can create social, psychological and physical barriers in a society that is structured around 'able-bodied' people. Disability is a multi-faceted concept (LoBianco & Sheppard-Jones 2007) and it is important to examine this to appreciate how it might impact on everyday lives.

There are two major models of disability, the medical model and the social model. The first identifies a disabled person as someone with a physically limiting condition or impairment. For example, the Disability Discrimination Act (DDA) 2006 defines a disabled person as someone having a physical or mental impairment that has a substantial and long-term adverse effect on his or her ability to carry out normal day-to-day activities. (Further information on laws relating to disability can be found in the Professional Knowledge section.) The World Health Organization (WHO; 2008) defines impairment as any loss or abnormality of psychological, physiological or anatomical structure or function. These definitions would include, for example, people with learning difficulties, non-standard forms of communication, hearing or visual impairment or those requiring mobility aids. The impairment, therefore, is the physical or psychological deviation from 'normal' and the disability is what results from that change. A limitation of the medical model is that impairment and disability are not always directly related. It is possible to have a high degree of impairment (biomedical change) with a low degree of disability (loss of function) and vice versa. Consider an example where two individuals suffer from a prolapsed intervertebral disc. Scans may reveal the same degree of 'impairment', that is identical degrees of anatomical damage, but the disability or extent of function could vary greatly.

The social model of disability focuses on society's response to disability rather than the individual. It proposes that disability only exists because society refuses to remove environmental barriers that people with impairments encounter. As such it offers a very different meaning of disability. Public perceptions of disability do not distinguish between these concepts and the terms 'impairment' and 'disability' are used interchangeably. Goffman (1963) considers that the greatest problem faced by people with a disability is not their functional limitations but society's response to them (see Ch. 19 for further discussion).

From birth to adulthood, mobility related goals are perceived as part of normal development, not only by health professionals but also by the community. We need only to look at our own environment, where there are steps, narrow doorways and cramped workplaces, to see the boundaries created for a person with impaired mobility. Arguably, schools have been designed with the expectation that children are fully mobile and therefore 'disabled' children were expected to attend a special school. In the past, and to an extent today, institutions were designed to house those with disabilities for most of their lives which served to marginalize them from the rest of society. The introduction of the Special Education Needs and Disability Act 2001 makes it illegal for educational establishments, in particular in further and higher education, to discriminate against students with a disability. In general, progress has been made to ensure provision of access and facilities in schools and other public places. Recently, attempts have been made to integrate children with special needs into mainstream schools. This remains a controversial topic of debate since, although the notion of normality is promoted through socialization, it is argued that resources are insufficient to meet the children's particular needs.

Adolescence can be a challenging time for any individual and it brings the same bodily changes and sexual urges for those who are disabled as for anyone else. This is easily overlooked and a young person with mobility impairment may feel frustrated and inadequate because of their physical limitations.

People tend to experience more problems with mobility as they get older. Musculoskeletal system changes tend to cause people to walk slower, take shorter steps and become more unsteady. Consequently, older people become associated with disability. It is interesting to speculate how, with an increasingly ageing population, our concept of normality may change.

Reflection and portfolio evidence

Next time you have an opportunity to observe a carer assisting a disabled person or pushing a person in a wheelchair in a public setting:

- Notice interactions between the disabled person, carer and others.
- Do others concentrate upon the carer or the disabled person?
- Is there any lack of interaction?
- Is there any inappropriate interaction such as staring?
- Recall, honestly, how you feel and react when you meet a disabled person, particularly of your own age, in a social setting.
- How could knowledge gained from this chapter affect your attitude and feelings in future?

CARE DELIVERY KNOWLEDGE

This section addresses multidisciplinary assessment of mobility and explores the principles of mobility care. It focuses in more detail on the assessment and safe management of moving and handling people.

MULTIDISCIPLINARY ASSESSMENT OF MOBILITY

Caring for people in hospital and community environments involves not just nurses but healthcare professionals from a range of disciplines. The terms 'interprofessional working', 'integrated care', 'interagency working' and 'collaboration' are all terms currently used to describe integrated approaches to health care (Atwal & Caldwell 2002). Integrated care pathways (ICPs) are structured, multidisciplinary care plans which outline essential steps in the care of a patient with a specific clinical problem (Campbell et al 1998). A single document may therefore be used to facilitate the management of patients or clients with mobility problems where several disciplines are involved. Where appropriate, individual care plans may be written by occupational therapists, physiotherapists or nurses. This is usually determined by whichever profession makes first contact. The 'single assessment process' is a key target in the National Service Framework for Older People (Department of Health 2001) that involves *one* person-centred assessment to which different disciplines contribute. This aims to facilitate integrated provision of services and effective management of care. Nurses play an important part in this coordinated approach because of their close, regular contact with patients.

Decision-making exercise

Make a list of those professionals and non-professionals who may directly or indirectly contribute towards the care of people with limited mobility. From this list identify their different priorities in caring for:

- an adult
- a child
- a person with a mental health problem
- a person with a learning disability.

How could a nurse contribute to the decision-making process of this team?

Using tools and scales has become increasingly important in helping nurses to manage individual care more effectively. They assist in producing a more objective assessment of an aspect of care or provide a numerical measure of risk. In addition, they provide evidence that these processes have been undertaken. For example pain may impede a person's mobility which may in turn place them at risk of developing pressure ulcers. In these instances tools such as pain scales and risk assessment tools for pressure ulcers would be useful in the overall management of this type of patient (see Ch. 11, 'Pain', and Ch. 15, 'Skin integrity', for full descriptions). Various tools exist to assess mobility. One example is the Barthel Activities of Daily Living (ADL) scale (Mahoney & Barthel 1965) which measures dependency on a 0 to 20 point scale. Another is the Assessment of Motor and Process Skills (AMPS) which is considered to be more sensitive in community settings (http://www.ampsintl.com/).

To provide a holistic approach to mobility assessment it is important to remember that factors such as the person's beliefs, motivation and their perceptions of mobilizing need to be taken into consideration. Similarly, when assessing children or individuals with learning disabilities or mental illness their levels of understanding need to be taken into account. When preparing for discharge it is useful to undertake assessment in the patient's own home or in very similar conditions. For more information please access Evolve 6.2.

6.2 – FUNCTIONAL ASSESSMENT OF MOBILITY

- Outline the use of integrated care pathways.
- List the mobility assessment tools available.
- Describe common features of the different tools.
- Gain an understanding of their application.

MANAGEMENT OF MOBILITY CARE

Management of mobility care and rehabilitation requires knowledge and understanding of specific factors relating to functional capacity. These include:

- range of movement
- gait and body alignment
- balance
- tolerance to exercise and activity.

Range of movement

If a person's joints are stiff from limited movement, muscles are not able to function to their maximum capacity or control movement of the joint through full range of motion. There is little benefit in strengthening muscles around a stiff joint as this merely gives a person control over a restricted range and function remains limited. In certain instances, such as joint replacement or ligament repair, flexion or extension may need to be temporarily limited but generally joint movement should be encouraged. This not only maintains and increases range of movement but also helps to maintain muscle strength and joint stability which are essential for mobility. As a rule, joint range should be maximized before muscle strengthening.

When joints are not moved, a fixed flexion deformity can occur. This is abnormal shortening of muscle tissue that becomes resistant to stretching and can lead to fibrosis of the muscle or joint. The aim therefore is to prevent such an occurrence as this will severely hamper rehabilitation and can lead to permanent disability. Patients may simply need to be reminded to move their knees, ankles or hips or, if assistance is required, their limbs may need support to achieve a full range of movement.

Gait and body alignment

Gait is the style and manner of walking and an observation of the patient's gait can be made at any time while he or she is walking. Normal walking consists of three basic movements:

- the swing, in which the foot does not touch the ground and the weight is taken on the opposite side.
- the heel strike, in which the heel of the swinging foot touches the ground immediately prior to the weight being taken over the foot.
- the stance, in which one leg bears most of the body weight at one point in the movement.

A detailed analysis of gait further subdivides these stages (Magee 2002).

There can be many styles of gait, most of which present no problem. However, problems may occur when gait and alignment of body segments give rise to, or arise from, instability and these should be corrected. Where this is not possible, for example where a person has spina bifida or cerebral palsy, care should focus on preventing further damage and maintaining maximum function. A person's age is significant since, for example, a child's gait is not the same as that of an adult although abnormal gaits can be similar in both children and adults.

Along with many types of gait are different strategies to control balance – some people use their ankles, others use their hips. Causes of instability can be multifactorial and programmes of correction may involve, for example, reduction of pain through analgesia or local application of heat or cold.

Balance

Balance, or the state in which the body is in equilibrium, is important for mobility (Umphred 2007). The ability to balance depends on complex mechanisms and the integrity of the central and peripheral nervous system and the musculoskeletal system. It also relies upon adequate functioning and coordination of:

- vision
- the vestibule (the cavity in the middle of the bony labyrinth or inner ear)
- proprioception
- sensory input, especially to the feet and hands
- the central nervous system to integrate all stimuli
- visuospatial perception
- muscles and joints.

Disruption to any of these factors needs be considered before, during and after assisting with mobility. For example, the ear is important for balance and deterioration in function can lead to increased risk of falls. In such circumstances hearing tests and appropriate aids can improve and maintain a person's balance. Eyesight is especially relevant as deterioration often occurs with ageing. Longsightedness (presbyopia) may begin to develop around the age of 40, so it is important to initiate checks if there is any doubt. Rooms that may seem adequately lit to a person with normal eyesight may be inadequate for those with visual impairment.

Tolerance to exercise and activity

Exercise is the undertaking of physical exertion with the aim of improving fitness and health. Along with activity, it is fundamental to mobility.

Types of therapeutic exercise include:

- Passive – exercises carried out by the therapist or nurse without assistance from the patient.
- Active assisted – exercises performed by the patient with assistance from the therapist or nurse.
- Active – exercises undertaken by the patient without assistance.
- Resisted – exercises performed by the patient working against manual or physical resistance.
- Isometric or static – exercises performed by the patient where muscles are alternately contracted and relaxed while that body part remains in a fixed position (Gormley & Hussey 2005). See Evolve 6.3 for information on exercise programmes.

---

evolve

6.3 – EXERCISE PROGRAMMES

- Demonstrate an understanding of the role of exercise.
- Explain the effects and application of exercise concepts to influence rehabilitation.
- Understand safe and appropriate application of exercise.

Individuals cope with mobility problems or disability in different ways. This may depend on whether the onset is sudden (injury) or insidious (a chronic condition). The former is more likely to cause denial or anger whereas a person who has been gradually experiencing difficulties may have come to terms with some functional incapacity. Coping mechanisms and readjustment will depend on the individual's degree of acceptance of their physical limitations.

The main purpose of any management strategy is to maximize independence and quality of life. This requires a coordinated and holistic approach that involves the multidisciplinary team and, as far as possible, the client/patient and their family or significant others. Information collected and recorded during assessment is used to identify general and specific problems or needs. Depending on the cause, extent and nature of immobility, goals may be short or long term but must be realistic and achievable. Planning and implementing a care programme requires consideration of a range factors. These can be classified into three areas – *personal, environmental* and *disability* – and are listed in Box 6.6. Decision making should be based on ongoing assessment and evaluation of the progress to ensure that the person's psychological, emotional, social and cultural needs are met.

Box 6.6 Factors involved in mobility care management

Personal factors
Age and gender
Social and cultural background
Personal values, attitudes and beliefs
Denial or acceptance of mobility problem
Ability to cope, self-efficacy and personal coping mechanism
Willingness to participate in care management and motivation
Health status and level of dependency
Personal care deficits
Anger, fear and anxiety
Level of knowledge and understanding of condition
Confidence, self-esteem, helplessness or despair

Environmental factors
Hospital and primary care settings
Services in community
Social security and welfare
Family and support networks
Self-help groups
Users' and carers' associations
Statutory and voluntary groups
Policies – local, national and international
Public and work places, leisure facilities – amenities and access
Equipment, aids and assistive technology
Health professionals and significant others
Transport facilities – personal and public
Accommodation and housing
Public attitudes

Disability factors
Causes – primary or secondary
Nature of immobility – sudden or insidious onset
Degree of immobility – partial or full
Types of immobility – temporary or permanent
Functional capacity – range of movement, gait/body alignment, balance and exercise/activity tolerance

Decision-making exercise

With fellow students or workplace colleagues from other branches of nursing, consider the following clients:

- A 50-year-old man suffering from chronic bronchitis.
- A 5-year-old child who has been diagnosed as having cystic fibrosis.
- A 20-year-old woman with learning disability.
- A 60-year-old man who is depressed.

What factors, excluding musculoskeletal problems, may lead to mobility difficulties for each client?

Reflecting on specific clients, what would you do to encourage, maintain or improve function and mobility?

Compare approaches that will be needed for different client groups in differing contexts of care.

PRINCIPLES OF LOAD HANDLING

This section outlines the principles that currently underpin assessment, planning, implementation and evaluation of moving and handling in health and social care. You will see that many are based on biomechanics and causes of back injury that are discussed in the Subject Knowledge section. Although principles are described in the context of patient care, they equally apply when moving inanimate objects and are relevant to all aspects of your work and personal life. Box 6.7 outlines the key principles when carrying out a moving and handling task and additional considerations are described below.

Avoid the task

You should first consider whether the task is essential, or whether the patient or client could perform it without manual assistance. For example, provision of a transfer board might enable an individual to transfer from bed to chair independently; explanations and encouragement may be all that a surgical patient requires to move from a bed to a theatre trolley.

Avoid lifting

The risks of manual lifting are well documented. Numerical guidelines (Health and Safety Executive 2004) help to make a quick and easy assessment for lifting and lowering loads but the normal weight range of most people falls widely outside of these figures (see Evolve 6.4). In the main, techniques that involve lifting people are regarded as unsafe and equipment-based methods should be employed. However, assessment may determine that, in

Box 6.7 Key principles when carrying out a moving and handling task

1. **Adopt a stable position**

   A stable base is required for balance. This can be achieved by placing your feet approximately shoulder width apart with one foot forward, pointing in the direction of movement. Sometimes a knee or hand may form part of this base. During a manoeuvre, transfer of weight or movement of feet maintains stability. In tasks such as 'sit to stand', the person being assisted will also require a stable base

2. **Achieve a good hold**

   A good grip is essential when moving inanimate objects, although hugging the load close to the body is better than gripping tightly with only your hands. When assisting people to move, you need to consider their skin integrity, comfort and dignity as well as physical support and safety. Using the flat palms of hands reduces the risk of pain or soft tissue damage to the patient and prevents lifting forces being exerted by the handler. As manual handling can often be quite intrusive it is important to ask permission before touching a person. You may wish to consider asking patients or clients to place their own hand on the appropriate part of their body before you make contact with your own hand

3. **Keep your spine in 'normal' alignment**

   As previously discussed, a key principle is to avoid stooping and twisting during manual handling procedures. Other principles such as keeping your knees slightly bent and your head up, rather than looking at the person or load, also help to achieve correct spinal alignment. Before performing a manoeuvre, it is useful to check if your shoulders are level, above your hips and facing the same direction as your hips

4. **Keep the load close to your body**

   By the principles of levers, the further away a load is from your centre of gravity, the greater the force needed to counterbalance it. In other words, a greater strain is placed on the ligaments and muscles in your back. Manoeuvres should take place within your base of support and involve the load being moved towards you or being held as close to your body as possible. (See Evolve 6.5 for an exercise you can do to demonstrate this principle.)

5. **Use easy, flowing movements**

   The force required to move a given load depends on its mass and the acceleration of movement. Loads should therefore be moved using slow, controlled movements where little effort is required. Fast, jerky movements or snatching not only increase risk of injury but also make the load harder to control very limited and defined situations, manual lifting may be necessary (further information in Evolve 6.4).

6.4 – LIFTING AND LOWERING LOADS

- Assess a load handling task using Manual Handling Operations Regulations (MHOR) guidelines.
- Describe and experience how the weight of a load differs according to its position relative to your body.
- Utilize Statutory and Professional Guidelines in decisions about lifting loads and people.

Use handling aids and equipment

Guidelines emphasize the use of equipment to reduce risks and an enormous range of such devices exist. However, equipment may also introduce disadvantages to moving and handling situations, such as the time involved for handlers and the risk of infection or loss of dignity for the person being assisted. Comprehensive assessment and an intimate knowledge of the equipment are therefore essential in ensuring that aids are suitable for each individual.

Reduce friction

Many aids, for example slide sheets and transfer boards, lessen the effort of manual handling by reducing friction between the load and the resting surface(s). Horizontal movements such as assisting a person up the bed or to sit back in a chair subsequently require less effort.

Prepare the environment and plan the manoeuvre

Both clinical and community environments may present limited space. Moving furniture and other obstacles before proceeding with a manoeuvre can prevent awkward or prolonged positions that increase the risks of the task.

Communicate clearly

Effective communication includes documentation as well as the spoken word. A manoeuvre is more likely to be successful if all involved, including those being assisted, are clear about what will happen and about their specific contribution to the task. Commands are necessary for correct timing of movements to avoid some people exerting greater effort than others. Participants need to know what the command will be as well as on which part they should instigate the move. Commands involving a verb such as

'Ready, steady go/push/stand' are more likely to result in synchronized actions rather than, for example 'One, two, three'. Planning and clear communication is predictably facilitated by identifying a leader for the task.

Use major muscle groups

In the human body, the largest and most powerful muscles and ligaments surround the hip joints. The effort in manual handling should be exerted through these rather than those in the back or upper limbs.

Avoid prolonged effort and repetitive movements

The impact of fixed, awkward postures and sustained effort has previously been discussed. This has clear implications for routine nursing procedures, such as taking a series of blood pressure readings, in a stooped position. The nature of health care often demands 24 hour a day nursing provision but it is important that sufficient rest and recovery time is taken. Therefore, staff breaks and days off require careful planning.

Avoid large vertical distances

Greater effort is required where moving objects/people involves starting or finishing near the floor or overhead. The need to bend or reach to access clinical equipment such as operating theatre trays could be avoided with a review of storage facilities. Attempting to manually move a person from the floor poses obvious risks and suitable equipment should be used wherever possible.

Wear suitable clothing

Clothing should be loose enough to allow free range of movement. In most healthcare organizations nurses are provided with a uniform but this may need renewing if your size alters. Shoes should fully enclose the foot to provide support and protection and have a sole that provides sufficient grip during procedures. Before proceeding, risks presented by jewellery and personal accessories should be considered, along with the need for protective clothing (for example, gloves and aprons). In cases of back injury, the wrong footwear or clothing could nullify or reduce a claim for compensation.

Literature relating to back pain emphasizes two factors that are significant in affecting back injury; these are posture and level of activity. Many of the principles outlined above are based on mechanical forces but the relevance of psychosocial, physiological and organizational dimensions of movement is also recognized.

Reflection and portfolio evidence

Reflect on a particular experience you have had in handling and moving a patient/client in your clinical placement area:

- Write a short description of the situation - what decisions were made and by whom?
- Using knowledge you have gained from this chapter and guidelines/protocols in your practice setting, analyse whether these decisions were the most appropriate for safe and effective practice.
- Add your analysis to your personal portfolio.

Evidence-based practice

An exploratory study was undertaken by Karahan & Bayraktar (2004) to identify the occurrence of low back pain among nurses and their use of body mechanics in clinical settings. Data were collected by observation and interviews from a sample of nurses working in acute settings in a state hospital in Turkey. Results from this research demonstrated that the majority of nurses experienced back pain and that some nurses do not use correct body mechanics either through lack of thought or care or through trying to do the task quickly. The study indicated a relationship between back pain and wearing high heels and lifting.

ASSESSMENT OF CLIENT MOBILITY FOR MOVING AND HANDLING

Risk assessment

Responsibilities of healthcare professionals are determined by numerous regulations relating to manual handling (see Professional and Ethical Knowledge). The Manual Handling Operations Regulations (MHOR) (Health and Safety Executive 1992) placed particular emphasis on risk assessment prior to carrying out any manual handling procedure. This includes risks to the handler and to the person being moved. Before discussing requirements of risk assessment, it is necessary to define some basic terms:

- Load – any discrete movable object.
- Manual handling operation – involves the movement of loads by direct human effort or indirectly via the use of equipment; includes lifting, putting down, pulling, pushing or carrying.

Risk factors related to moving and handling can be categorized as those relating to:

- the Task itself
- the handler's Individual capacity

- the Load to be moved
- the Environment.

Each needs to be considered during the assessment process and is easily remembered by the acronym TILE or LITE.

The Task (T)

Important considerations related to the task include whether it involves unsatisfactory postures (such as twisting, stooping, reaching overhead, holding or manipulating the load at a distance from the trunk) or body movements (such as moving the load through a large range), especially when raising or lowering or carrying long distances. Does the task require excessive pulling or pushing and is there risk of sudden movement of the load? Some situations require frequent or prolonged physical effort and the potential for insufficient rest or recovery periods, especially if the rate of work is imposed by processes or regimes. An example would be assisting people in care settings out of into bed within stipulated time periods.

Individual capacity (I)

Risk assessment should consider the abilities of those carrying out the task. This will include whether handlers have the skills and capacity to move the load, have undertaken recent training or have disabilities or impairments that could affect safety. Does the task require unusual strength or pose a hazard for those who are pregnant or have health problems?

The load (L)

Considerations should include whether the load is heavy, bulky, unwieldy, difficult to grasp or potentially unstable; the exterior may be sharp, hot, cold or otherwise potentially harmful. Where the load is a person, it is not only their physical abilities (joint movement range, muscle strength) but their age, gender and cultural and religious beliefs that are relevant. If mobility is restricted, what are the reasons for these limitations? Patients' diagnoses or symptoms need to be taken into account, for example areas of pain or discomfort, pressure sores or surgical wounds, heart or breathing problems or orthopaedic interventions such as joint replacement. Attachments (urinary catheter, intravenous infusion) or clothing may hinder the manoeuvre or affect cooperation. It is essential to assess communication and whether the person can understand instructions. A person's attitudes, feelings, expectations and goals will influence the success of moving and handling. Previous experiences of being assisted may lead to ongoing problems. A person's views and personal values should be taken into consideration and whether the planned move infringes on duty of care or human rights.

The Environment (E)

This can affect the safety of all involved. Space should be adequate for the task and free from constraints or obstacles. The floor should be observed for spillages, tripping hazards, variations in level and type of surface (slippery, carpeted). Extremes of temperature, humidity, lighting conditions and possible distractions, for example noise, can affect people's ability to function effectively. Equipment should be safe, in good order, clean and regularly checked or serviced. Handlers wearing inappropriate clothing, jewellery or shoes could be hazardous.

Reflection and portfolio evidence

Look at the documentation for manual handling risk assessment and care planning in your clinical area.

- Talk to your mentor or moving and handling advisor about the assessment process.
- Undertake an assessment of a patient using the TILE or LITE format.
- How long did it take you? Did this surprise you?
- Talk to the patient about your plan and note the responses for your reflection.
- Write up and add to your personal portfolio.

PLANNING TO ASSIST WITH MOBILITY AND MOVEMENT

Once assessment has been undertaken the information is used to plan moving and handling procedures for an individual patient or client. Risks can never be fully eliminated when assisting people to move but a documented plan promotes development and dissemination of strategies for reducing these risks. A plan may be relatively simple (for example, where a person only requires assistance with standing) or more comprehensive, for someone who has difficulty with many aspects of mobility. It should specify the tasks that require intervention, key risks associated with those tasks and methods to be used. A plan should also include a review date and, as with all patient documents, be signed and dated. Detailed information such as the number of handlers required, the size of sling to use, or the client's wish to give the command is crucial to the success of the procedure and it is worth considering if pictures may be more effective in communicating some of this detail. Reasons for using or not using particular methods or equipment, such as environmental restrictions or patient comfort, should also be clearly documented. A plan should take into account the goals and perspectives of members of the multidisciplinary team and the personal preferences of the person being handled. It should be kept in a place that is easily accessed by all staff, such as at the patient's bedside or with their notes. Fig. 6.6 shows an example of such a plan.

A major factor to consider in the planning process is availability of equipment and human resources. A range of handling equipment is now available, some of which is sophisticated and expensive while others items are simple and relatively inexpensive. The main examples are described below.

Sliding equipment

Devices such as sliding sheets, transfer boards and inflatable transfer mattresses allow repositioning or transferring (for example, from bed to trolley) to be achieved by sliding rather than lifting. Although they are not taking the full weight of the load, effort is still required by handlers to complete the manoeuvre and therefore the task should be planned carefully and carried out in manageable stages. Extra caution should be taken to protect the patient, particularly when a combination of sliding equipment is used, as the effort required to move them becomes considerably less than conventional means. This could result in the patient being moved much further than intended with potentially detrimental results.

Other simple transfer aids

Choice of transfer aid will be influenced by the weight, capability and cooperation of the person being transferred. As with selection of any equipment, risk assessment is required. Small, rigid transfer boards are used to bridge the gap between one surface and another (for example, bed, commode, wheelchair or chair) to aid transfers in a seated position. They promote independence in people with limited weight-bearing capacity but upper body strength such as those with lower limb amputations or lumbar spinal cord injury. Turntable devices are circular discs used on the floor to rotate a standing person; many have elaborate frames and support features to promote stability and are useful for people with impaired leg movement. Turning discs can be used on beds, chairs and inside cars to turn a seated person into position.

Beds and mattresses

For highly dependent patients, special beds and mattresses can assist with repositioning. Electrically powered profiling beds enable the patient or nurse to alter a flat surface to different positions for sitting. Adjustable leg sections prevent the patient from slipping down. These beds are essential for those who lack the strength to sit forward with simple aids and where manual handling has been assessed as

Patient's name		District nurse		
Body build Obese ☐ Above average ☐ Average ☐		Below average ☐ Tall ☐ Medium ☐ Short ☐		
Weight (if known)		**Risk of falls** High ☐ Low ☐		

Problems with comprehension, behaviour, cooperation (identify)

Handling constraints, e.g. disability, weakness, pain, skin lesions, infusions (identify)

Tasks (see examples)	**Methods to be used** (see examples)	**Describe any remaining problems, list any other measures needed** (see examples)

Date(s) assessed:				
Assessor's signature:				
Proposed review dates:				

Finishing date:

Examples of tasks:
✓ sitting/standing
✓ toiletting
✓ bathing
✓ transfer to/from bed
✓ movement in bed
✓ sustained postures
✓ walking
✓ in/out of car

Examples of methods/ control measures
Organization
✓ Number of staff needed?
✓ Patient stays in bed
Equipment
✓ Variable height bed
✓ Hoists
✓ Slings/belt
✓ Bath aids
✓ Wheeled sani-chair
✓ Monkey poles
✓ Patient hand blocks
✓ Rope ladders
✓ Turntable
✓ Sliding aids
✓ Stair lift
Furniture
✓ Reposition/remove

Examples of problems/ risk factors
Task
✓ Is it necessary? Can it be avoided?
✓ Involves stretching, stooping, twisting, sustained load?
✓ Rest/recovery time?
Patient
✓ Weight, disability, ailments, etc.
Environment
✓ Space to manoeuvre, to use hoist?
✓ Access to bed, bath, WC, passageways?
✓ Steps, stairs?
✓ Flooring uneven? OK for hoist?
✓ Furniture: movable? height? condition?
✓ Bed: double? low?
Carers
✓ Fitness for the task, freshness or fatigue?
✓ Experience with patient and with handling team?
✓ Skill: handling, using equipment?
Furniture
✓ Reposition/remove

Figure 6.6 Royal College of Nursing community care plan (reproduced by kind permission of Royal College of Nursing 2003).

inappropriate. Inflatable mattress inclinators can be placed under an ordinary mattress or pillow to help a person sit up or turn over. Turning beds remove the need for manual handling where patients are at risk of pressure ulcers and cannot turn themselves.

Lifting equipment

Hoists are the most common type of lifting equipment and are designed to take the full weight of a person. Box 6.8 lists the main types of hoists and more details can be found

Box 6.8 Types of hoist	
Type	**Function**
Mobile hoists	Portable devices mostly used for lifting and transferring a person who is unable to take their own weight (or where assessment deems this to be the most appropriate method). They are not a means of transportation and should only be used over short distances
Standing hoists	A type of mobile hoist that lifts a seated person to standing position. Once standing, transfer to another seat is easily achieved
Overhead track hoists	Usually attached to the ceiling but also available as a freestanding gantry to span over a patient's bed and chair. Elimininates problems of limited space and can be adapted for home use. The person requiring assistance may use it independently
Fixed hoists	These are fixed to a wall or floor or set inside a bath. Useful in small spaces where overhead tracks cannot be fitted
Walking hoists	A harness or sling takes some of the person's weight during walking. Can be used for clients who have problems with balance or cannot fully take their weight

in Evolve 6.5 (see also http://www.arjohuntleigh.com/int/ for photographs and descriptions of examples of equipment).

6.5 – HOISTS AND THEIR USES

- State the four main types of hoists.
- Explain the principal uses of each type of hoist.
- Describe the preliminary checks before using a mobile hoist.

Lifting cushions or seats are inflatable devices used to lift fallen patients from the floor. They consist of a compressor unit and an inflatable cushion which is fitted under a sitting person (an inflatable seat with an integral back rest is used for a lying person who cannot sit forward). The cushion is inflated to a height that enables the patient to stand easily or transfer to another surface. Prior to using this device, it is essential to assess the person for injuries and their capacity to balance and cooperate. Findings should be documented in their notes. Inflatable devices may be used for other purposes such as lifting heavy or immobile limbs.

Riser chairs are electrically powered or spring loaded to lift or assist a person upwards and forwards into a standing position.

Other moving and handling equipment

A range of equipment, from hand blocks to walking frames, is available to provide support for people with difficulty moving and to promote independence. Attachments such as grab handles, monkey poles and rope ladders can assist with movement in bed while chair and bed raisers simply adjust the height to make it easier to get in and out. Handling equipment usually takes the form of slide sheets, belts and slings which can be purchased in different sizes. Careful assessment, however, of the type of task and the condition and understanding of the patient is required to prevent manual lifting during use.

Equipment has the potential to reduce risks associated with moving and handling but, without assessment and planning, injuries may be caused. Selecting suitable methods requires knowledge of the negative aspects of equipment as well as the benefits. For example, a hoist removes the need for manual lifting but impedes rehabilitation; a sliding board, intended for transfers from one seated position to another, is hazardous if the person lacks upper body strength and sitting balance. It is therefore important to be aware of a range of options, available equipment and further resources. Equipment not available in a given clinical area can often be loaned from other sources. Information and advice is available from back care advisors, local groups and specialist forums. Remember that ordering special equipment may also require organization of specialist training for those that will be involved in its use.

Often, a forgotten resource is the patients themselves. Involving patients in the planning process will identify their particular needs and preferences, gain cooperation and clarify their contribution to the procedure, for example physical assistance or how they prefer to give the command. If consulted, patients can often move themselves with small adjustments such as hand blocks (although rarely used these days), a monkey pole or transfer board.

Procedures cannot be planned without considering the environment. For example, a hoist is of little use if the legs do not fit under or around the furniture; a walking frame with wheels is likely to cause greater risks if it cannot be pushed along the carpet; installation of a special bed may be resented if it prevents a person from sleeping with their partner. Achieving the task may require rearranging furniture in a hospital environment or making more permanent adjustments in someone's home. Ergonomic principles should be applied to address space constraints, staffing levels, equipment provision and ways of working.

To conclude, key principles of planning are to avoid manual lifting and handling wherever possible, optimize safety and achieve goals of care. Methods need to be chosen using professional judgement, based on comprehensive and holistic assessment. Negotiation with patients should be incorporated whenever possible so that they know what to expect and are in agreement with the plans.

Decision-making exercise

Martin Richards is a 15 year old boy with learning disabilities. He weighs 8 stone (50 kg), lives at home with his parents and attends a day centre during school periods. His mobility needs are met by transporting him in a wheelchair but he requires assistance to transfer from wheelchair to toilet and vice versa on a regular basis. He is subject to bouts of anger that make him uncooperative at times.

In relation to assisting Martin with his toileting requirements at the day centre:

1. Identify pertinent factors that need to be taken into account and potential hazards relating to this task (use TILE or LITE to guide you in this process).
2. Make notes of what you might include in a moving and handling plan for this particular task with regard to:
   – equipment
   – people
   – adaptations to the environment.

Compare your ideas with the thoughts of the authors in Evolve 6.8.

IMPLEMENTING ASSISTANCE WITH MOBILITY AND MOVEMENT

General principles

Documentation is essential to provide a consistent approach to care. However, as no two moving and handling situations are the same, 'on-the-spot' assessment and planning is required each time the task is performed. The condition of the person is often critical, since they may be unable to cooperate or contribute as expected if tired, upset, unmotivated or in pain. Their clothing may compromise the manoeuvre if it is likely to result in them being exposed or if slippery material prevents a suitable hold. Equipment needs to be available and in good working order and handlers should be familiar with its function and safe operation.

There should be time to access necessary staff for the procedure and assess the risks of using handlers of different heights. Where several handlers are required a leader is required to avoid confusion. Those assisting need to agree to the manoeuvre and have the expertise and personal capacity to undertake the task. Inexperienced handlers must take care not to act beyond their level of competence. Commands need to be agreed in advance to ensure that handling is coordinated and weight is evenly distributed between

handlers. The patient, too, needs to know the commands and what they are to expect or is expected of them at the specified time. Preparation of the environment, beyond positioning furniture for transfers, is often overlooked but creating sufficient space may prevent hazardous postures and interruptions during handling. Moving bedside tables and lockers and the assortment of objects usually placed on them is a worthwhile investment of time. Similarly, other hazards such as patient attachments need to be dealt with before proceeding. An ergonomic approach needs to be adopted by using equipment and systems, such as adjustable height beds, to full advantage.

It should be apparent that moving and handling people does not consist of set of techniques that are employed for given tasks, rather, the application of principles and professional judgment based on assessment of the situation. Nonetheless, knowledge of potentially suitable methods is required and these are examined, through all ranges of dependency, in *The Guide to the Handling of People* (Smith 2005).

The following sections offer a brief overview of key tasks associated with moving people and some key points for consideration.

Helping a person move in bed

Dependent patients who are confined to bed require assistance with mobility to achieve many activities of living. Handlers should adjust the height of the bed, where possible, so that these activities can be performed without bending. Where fixed-height beds, special beds and cots are used, hazards should be minimized by choosing appropriate aids and adapting methods. Many movements in bed can be achieved more safely with the use of slide sheets, which should be inserted under all areas of the body to prevent friction damage to skin and hindrance to the manoeuvre. If the sheets are tubular, the closed ends should be in the direction of movement. Less dependent patients should be encouraged to assist, for example, by lifting their pelvis to insert a slide sheet or grabbing a hand rail to assist with turning.

Generally, handlers should move a person towards them by transferring their weight backwards from their front foot to the other. When moving a supine person up the bed, this will necessitate handlers standing behind the head of the bed. If there are space constraints, handlers can pull by standing either side of the bed but extra vigilance is necessary to avoid twisting or lateral flexion. Moving a dependent person from a bed to a trolley or another bed must be carried out by at least two people using a transfer device such as a full length sliding board or inflatable transfer mattress. The surfaces must be the same level and high enough to prevent stooping. A person who has capacity to assist may simply require verbal instructions. Bed or trolley rails should be used as appropriate and brakes applied to prevent falling.

Assisting a person from lying to sitting in bed, without equipment, requires the person to have the cognitive ability and physical strength to move themselves. Prior to undertaking this task, it is essential to assess a person's capacity to support themselves once sitting and plan to provide support as required. Techniques involve the person rolling onto their side before pushing up as this is less demanding on their abdominal muscles. This may be achieved with verbal instructions or may require some manual assistance. Aids such as rope ladders, grab rails or bed levers may assist a person to sit independently. For people with limited function and ability, particularly if they cannot support their head, profiling equipment should be considered a priority. Manually lifting a person from lying to sitting without equipment should only be used as an interim measure as this carries numerous risks unless performed in clearly defined circumstances by handlers who are practised in the techniques. Consideration should therefore be given to using a hoist for sitting a person up and repositioning them in bed.

Helping a seated person to stand and a standing person to sit down

Moving from a seated to standing position is a regular and essential activity in the lives of most people. Difficulty in achieving this task may reduce a person's ability to mobilize and, hence, participate in vital and meaningful activities. Assistance involves preparation and promoting patterns of normal movement. A person needs to be in an appropriate sitting position before standing can be achieved, that is with their hips or bottom close to the edge of the chair and their feet behind their knees, with one foot slightly apart and in front of the other. This position allows them to push to a standing position with a stable base (Fig. 6.7). Their hands can be placed on the arms of the chair, the edge of the bed, or, if necessary, on their thighs. The transition to standing is initiated by the person leaning forward and lifting their head. Their weight is lifted by pushing with their arms and legs. Clients should not be encouraged to hold the carer's hand. It is always better to encourage the client to push themselves up into standing by pushing on the arms of the chair. If following assessment, it is agreed to be necessary, some options are illustrated in Figure 6.8. In order for this procedure to be successful, the person needs the strength to push, the capacity to take their full weight on their feet and the ability to balance through all stages of the manoeuvre. Equally, success depends on the suitability of the seat, that is height, position and form of the arms, angle between seat and chair back and the space in front of it. Sitting down from a standing position involves the same muscles and joints as standing up and, while it requires less physical effort, weak muscles or painful joints can make this manoeuvre difficult to control.

Since assistance often involves detailed verbal instructions, the person's cognitive as well as physical ability must be assessed. Where manual assistance is required, handlers need to ensure that they support normal movements and avoid lifting or holding the person if they cannot take their

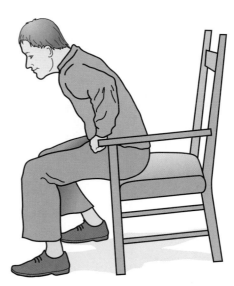

Figure 6.7 Preparation for standing (courtesy of LPS Training and Consultancy Ltd.).

full weight. Provision of aids such as ejector seats, toilet frames and standing devices enable people to stand independently or with minimal assistance or supervision. If a person does not fulfil the assessment criteria described, a standing hoist will be necessary.

Helping a seated person to transfer

Transferring a seated person can be facilitated through standing or by direct horizontal transfer from one surface to another. The success of the procedure depends on numerous factors because more than one manoeuvre is likely to be involved. In particular, the dimensions and positions of the seated surfaces (for example, bed, wheelchair, toilet), the presence of chair arms or attachments and the space around them all need to be considered as well as the capacity of the patient and handlers to perform each component of the task. Once in a standing position a person can step around to another seating surface with verbal instructions or minimal assistance. Turning devices, some of which incorporate a standing frame, can facilitate those with more limited capacity. A standing hoist can be used for someone who has difficulty standing from a seated position but has some weight-bearing ability. For a person who cannot take weight through their legs, but has upper body strength and balance, transfer boards allow movement from one seating surface to another. However, a dependent person, unable to assist with transfer, will require a traditional mobile hoist.

Helping a person to walk

Factors affecting a person's ability to walk extend beyond muscle and joint function. Balance, coordination, proprioception, sensory awareness and confidence are also required. Walking can be affected by normal aging processes as well as by many disabling conditions.

Clients should not be encouraged to hold the carer's hand. It is always better to encourage the client to push themselves up into standing by pushing on the arms of the chair. If, following assessment, it is agreed to be necessary, there are some alternatives:

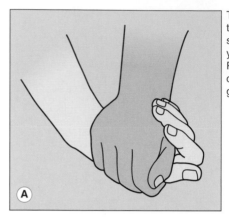

The palm to palm. Has the advantage of good support whilst leaving your thumb out of grip. Particularly useful if the client has a tendency to grip your thumb too hard.

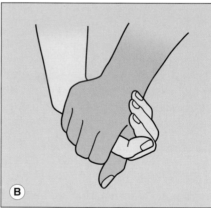

The thumb to thumb. This is a very strong and supportive hold but might not be appropriate as the client could grip, and the carer may not be able to release their hand.

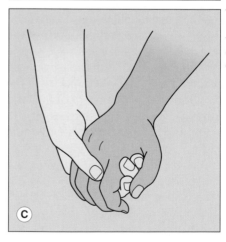

The finger to finger. Can be useful for a client if there is a risk of them gripping too hard, nipping or scratching.

Remember
- Handholds should be included in the client's handling care plan.
- When holding the client's hands, ensure their hands are below their elbows.
- Ensure the client does not put too much weight through their hands (and then yours).

Figure 6.8 Hand holds. (A) The palm to palm (B) The thumb to thumb (C) The finger to finger. (Courtesy of LPS Training and Consultancy Ltd.)

Assisting with walking is hazardous since it is a task where falls commonly occur (others are moving from bed to chair or using a toilet or commode; Patient Safety Observatory 2007). One of the most important aspects of assessment, therefore, is identifying a person's risk of falling as this will impact on decisions about equipment, holds and number of handlers involved.

Many aspects of 'on-the-spot' assessment and preparation are required before undertaking this task. The person requires appropriate footwear and clothes that will not compromise their dignity. Attachments such as urinary catheters and intravenous infusions need to be transported without hindering the process. The route should be checked for obstructions, steps or slippery surfaces and, in a hospital environment, anything that is likely to upset the patient. Doors need to be open before you reach them and wide enough to pass through. The person needs to be alert enough to follow instructions and have the stamina and motivation to walk; previous activity, lack of sleep or rest, pain and the presence of other people may influence their performance.

Provision of walking aids promotes independence but, during periods of rehabilitation or altered health, manual assistance may be required. This may involve staying close to the person's side and providing support by holding their nearside hand. A number of holds can be used but decisions should take into account patient comfort (they may have painful joints) and the ability of the handler to release the grip if the person panics or falls (Fig. 6.8).

A handling belt may be useful to gain a secure hold or avoid direct body contact but this is controversial as evidence suggests they make it more likely that a nurse will 'grab' the person if they fall (Fray, conference presentation, 2006). Communication is essential throughout the procedure to provide instructions, guidance and encouragement. Where a risk of falling is identified, strategies such as having a carer follow with a wheelchair may be considered or if the person urgently needs the toilet, a wheelchair is used to take them but walking is assisted on return. If a person loses their balance or begins to collapse when walking the situation needs to be managed appropriately. Training can be sought from your manager or manual handling advisor and you should be aware of your organization's policies or guidelines. Further information on the consequences and management of falls can be found from the Patient Safety Observatory report (see National Patient Safety Agency in Annotated Further Reading).

Most types of walking aids reduce the need for manual assistance by transferring some of the weight from the lower limbs to the upper limbs. These include sticks, crutches, frames and wheeled 'walkers' (Fig. 6.9). Most mobility aids are initially ordered by physiotherapists but community nurses frequently evaluate patients discharged with these aids. Points to consider in the home environment include whether there is sufficient space, whether steps need to be

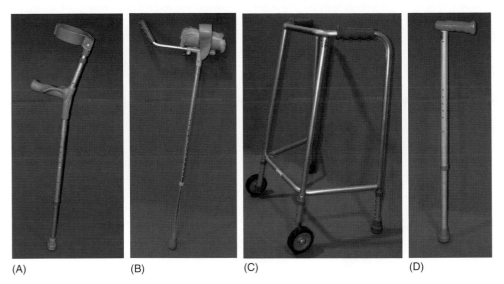

(A) (B) (C) (D)

Figure 6.9 Walking aids. (A) Elbow crutch. (B) Gutter crutch. (C) Roller frame. (D) Stick. (Courtesy of Sheffield Hallam University.)

negotiated, whether the device is to be used for indoor or outdoor use, and whether it needs to be accommodated in public or private transport.

In the absence of physiotherapists, nurses who prescribe, administer and assist people to use walking aids need a working knowledge of the equipment, the ability to ascertain the correct size and understanding of some of the basic principles involved. For example, the higher a person takes their weight and the wider the weight-bearing area of the aid, the greater the stability. Therefore, patients using gutter frames are more stable than those using the more common waist high frames, and those using axilla crutches are more stable than those using elbow crutches. It is important to note that axilla crutches are designed to rest two or three fingerwidths below the axilla to stabilize the body while the weight is taken through the hands, wrists and arms. Taking body weight through the axilla causes pressure on the brachial plexus which could result in a crutch palsy. Appropriate assessment and evaluation also requires an awareness of gait patterns associated with different aids. Fig. 6.10 illustrates the weight-bearing areas when walking with a frame or crutches while Fig. 6.11 shows the correct technique for ascending and descending stairs with crutches. Walking aids need to be in good working order and, if able, patients or carers can be taught how to make regular safety checks and necessary adjustments. Although nurses may not have the relevant expertise to make necessary adjustments or changes to equipment, a referral can be made to appropriate personnel or departments. (For information on the use of walking hoists see Evolve 6.5).

Reflection and portfolio evidence

During your practice placements, observe how clients with impaired mobility are assisted or instructed to move from lying to sitting and standing.

- Note the rationale for the specific methods used and relate these to the knowledge gained from this chapter.
- Monitor your own technique or get a member of the multidisciplinary team to assess your ability in this area.

For additional information on promoting and helping certain clients in various circumstances to improve their mobility see Evolve 6.6.

evolve

6.6 – PLANNING AND IMPLEMENTING CARE IN SPECIFIC CIRCUMSTANCES OR WITH SPECIFIC GROUPS OF PEOPLE

Identify the main hazards and ways of avoiding these when:
- Handling in confined spaces.
- Handling inanimate objects.
- Handling children.
- Handling heavier patients.
- Handling people who may be unpredictable or uncooperative.

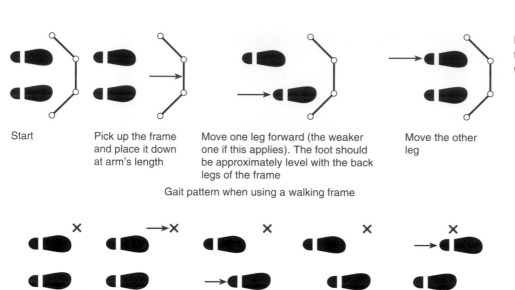

Start

Pick up the frame and place it down at arm's length

Move one leg forward (the weaker one if this applies). The foot should be approximately level with the back legs of the frame

Move the other leg

Gait pattern when using a walking frame

Start   Move one aid   Move opposite leg   Move second aid   Move second leg

Example of four-point gait. ✗ represents an axillary or elbow crutch in the early stages of recovery, or a stick in the later stages

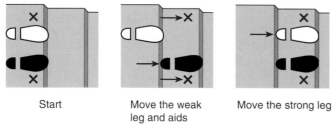

Start

Move the weak leg and aids

Move the strong leg

Descending stairs using crutches. The black area represents either the weak or non-weightbearing leg

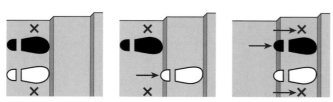

Ascending stairs using crutches. The black area represents either the weak or non-weightbearing leg

Figure 6.11 Ascending and descending stairs with crutches (from Judd 1989, with kind permission).

EVALUATION

Evaluation is an integral part of the systematic approach to nursing and is necessary to identify the level of success of care delivered. The outcomes of assisting a person to move or mobilize should be documented, along with any problems and the actions taken to resolve them. Evaluation thus provides the basis for ongoing assessment and further

planning. The importance of good record keeping cannot be overemphasized. Records should provide clear, accurate, current and comprehensive information about a patient and are vital in multidisciplinary risk management of moving and handling situations (Nursing and Midwifery Council 2008). Records may be used as evidence in legal proceedings and panel hearings.

Evidence-based practice

Many techniques and recommendations relating to moving and handling people have evolved through expert opinion rather than empirical research. Hignett (2003) carried out a systematic review with the aim of providing an evidence base for future professional guidelines in this area. Evidence supported the use of hoists (for non-weight-bearing patients), standing aids, slide sheets, lateral transfer boards, handling belts and adjustable-height beds and baths. It is suggested that these items are a minimum requirement in any clinical environment where patient handling regularly occurs and, until more research is available, practitioners should follow professional guidelines and continuously review and reflect on their practice.

A later study by Hignett & Evans (2006), to determine spatial requirements in hospital shower and toilet rooms, demonstrated that a mobile hoist needed significantly more space, took significantly longer and exposed the handlers to higher postural risk than an overhead hoist.

PROFESSIONAL AND ETHICAL KNOWLEDGE

This section highlights the interface between laws and professional guidelines relevant to mobility and moving and some of the ethical issues that are presented to nurses.

FACILITIES FOR MOBILITY CARE

As health promoters, nurses need to be aware of facilities available in the community and where they and their patients/clients can obtain expert advice. Disabled Living Centres give unbiased physiotherapy and occupational therapy advice on a wide range of disability equipment and can be accessed by anyone, for example patients, relatives, voluntary carers, voluntary organizations and health professionals. They are located throughout England, Wales and Scotland and financed by various means such as charities, health authorities, social services and personal donations. Staff in these centres are an excellent source of information about many aspects of mobility. They assess the suitability of mobility aids for individual clients and advise on where equipment can be obtained. Equipment is sometimes available for trial. Staff also facilitate negotiations between clients and relevant mobility or disability departments and offer contact details for financial aid or physical and psychological care. These centres also assess new equipment and provide training and advice for professional and non-professional carers (see Annotated Websites for contact details).

LAWS RELATING TO DISABILITY

The main legislation addressing rights of disabled people is the Disability Discrimination Act 2006. The Act was first passed in 1995 to end discrimination in terms of employment, access to goods, facilities and services, and the management, buying or renting of land and property. In 1999 the Disabled People (Duties of Public Authorities) Bill placed a responsibility on employers and service providers to make 'reasonable adjustments' to meet the needs of disabled individuals. Also in 1999, the Disability Rights Commission Act led to the establishment of the Disability Rights Commission (DRC). This is an independent body whose duties are to secure civil rights and promote equal opportunities for disabled people while eliminating discrimination and encouraging good practice. It also advises the government on the working of disability legislation.

LAWS RELATING TO MOVING AND HANDLING

The law relating to moving and handling operations is derived from various sources. It includes a number of different statutes and regulations based on Acts of Parliament, European Community Directives and common law (law based on the outcomes of previous court cases). As such, the impact on practice can appear complex and confusing. One of the key statutes relevant to moving and handling is the Health and Safety at Work Act 1974 (see Ch. 3, 'Safety and risk', for more details on regulations within this act), which addresses health and safety issues in all aspects of work. Tensions can arise when employers do not provide adequate resources to fulfil the requirements of the Act or employees do not ensure they access and comply with appropriate training provided by employers.

More recently, UK law specifically relating to manual handling has arisen from European Directives. The Manual Handling Operations Regulations (MHOR) 1992 emphasize the importance of risk assessment and clearly state employers' responsibilities as:

- Avoiding hazardous manual handling so far as is reasonably practicable.
- Making suitable and sufficient assessment of any hazardous manual handling operations that cannot be avoided.
- Reducing the risk of injury from those operations as far as is reasonably practicable.
- Reviewing the assessment when it is no longer valid or when injury has occurred.

Certain regulations relate exclusively to equipment, for example, the Lifting Operations and Lifting Equipment Regulations (LOLER) 1998 stipulate employers' responsibilities in relation to equipment used for lifting and lowering loads. These include consideration and assessment of ergonomic risk factors and whether the equipment is strong, stable and positioned and installed in a way that minimizes risks to the operator.

Another aspect related to safety in moving and handling is the reporting and monitoring of accidents and incidents. This is governed by the Reporting of Injuries, Diseases and Dangerous Occurrences Regulations (RIDDOR) (Health and Safety Executive 1995) and requires employers to keep records of specific events. Incidents such as back pain, whether it requires follow-up advice or treatment or simply prevents you from functioning normally, should be recorded in detail according to the workplace protocol. This information enables occupational health personnel to identify areas where practices should be investigated and appropriate support can be implemented. In certain situations it may be appropriate for the Health and Safety Executive to investigate working practices. This information may also be of use should an injured party seek legal compensation.

Many additional regulations exist to provide a framework for practice to reduce or, wherever possible, eliminate the risks of injury to workers. In the clinical workplace this also means reducing or eliminating the risk of injury to patients/clients that might be caused by controversial or inappropriate methods of moving or lifting.

THE IMPACT OF THE HUMAN RIGHTS ACT

Since the introduction of the Human Rights Act 1998 the High Court has revisited the interpretation of 'reasonably practicable' that is frequently stated in other regulations (Griffith & Stevens 2004). In cases relating to manual handling, emphasis is now placed on the needs and wishes of clients as well as the balance between risk to staff and cost. The articles most relevant to assisting mobility are:

- Right to life – there would be a duty to manually lift a person from a life-threatening situation (e.g. fire or a collapsing building) if this was the only means of moving them.
- Prohibition of torture, inhuman or degrading treatment or punishment – this would be relevant to patients who, for example, are unable to attend to their own hygiene or toileting needs or may be at risk of pressure sores, and there is no suitable alternative to manual lifting.
- Right to and respect for private and family life – examples where this might be relevant include patients who find the use of a hoist undignified and distressing or those who have fallen and can't be moved without manual assistance.

Mandelstam (2004) emphasized the need to consider the overall legal framework and not just what is 'reasonably practicable' to assess and reduce risks as stated in MHOR 1992. In other words, human rights legislation and the duty of care that is owed to patients in both statute and common law should redress the balance in decision-making processes. Because of changing perspectives, confusion often arises regarding manual handling procedures and whether or not patients should be lifted (see Evolve 6.4 for more detailed information to aid your decision-making processes).

PROFESSIONAL GUIDELINES

Registered nurses are responsible professionals and are accountable to patients/clients. To protect the public, practice is governed by *The Code: Standards of Conduct, Performance and Ethics for Nurses and Midwives* (Nursing and Midwifery Council 2008). One clause states that nurses must act without delay to prevent someone being put at risk. This reinforces the importance of assessment and decision making when assisting to mobilize. Nurses also have a duty to maintain and update their knowledge and skills and comply with local and national policies. If you are unsure of your responsibilities when assisting mobility, they need to be ascertained. If responsibility lies with others, such as a community physiotherapist, you must ensure referral to the appropriate person or department. The Code also highlights cooperating with other team members and respecting the patient or client as an individual.

Guidance by the Royal College of Nursing (RCN) and other professional organizations is also applicable to your practice. The RCN produces numerous publications relevant to this field and their *Code of Practice for Patient Handling* (Royal College of Nursing 2002) offers a framework for implementing national regulations and recommendations. The latest edition states the aim is to eliminate hazardous manual handling in all but exceptional or life-threatening situations. Inevitably, patients often require manual handling but this should only be considered if it does not involve lifting all or most of the their weight. In light of the legislation described above, it is possible to identify situations where conflict may arise but, as far as possible, the RCN advocates using aids to reduce risks and encouraging clients to assist wherever possible.

Potential conflict between safer handling policies and people's rehabilitation or maintenance needs is recognized by other allied health professional bodies. The Chartered Society of Physiotherapists (2005) recognizes that manual handling may be a key requirement of rehabilitation and its avoidance may be detrimental to service users. The College of Occupational Therapists (2006) holds a similar view on blanket bans on manual lifting and emphasizes the importance of professional judgement in balancing the safety of handlers with the needs and wishes of service users and carers.

In emergency situations, recommended handling techniques are often forgotten. The Resuscitation Council (UK) (2001) offers guidance for safer handling during cardiopulmonary resuscitation in hospital. Rapid assessment skills, effective communication to coordinate team working and knowledge of techniques applicable to such circumstances will help to reduce risks to rescuers (see Ch. 4, 'Resuscitation and emergency care').

BARRIERS TO SAFER MOVING AND HANDLING

Risks associated with moving and handling people are well established although evidence largely relates to musculoskeletal disorders among practitioners (Retsas 2000, Department of Health 2002) rather than patient-related outcomes. Despite legislation, guidance, trust policies and other strategies (for example, employment of back care advisors), evidence indicates a sustained prevalence of back disorders among healthcare workers (Crumpton & Bannister 2002, Department of Health 2002). As a consequence, the effectiveness of traditional, techniques-based training has been questioned (Hignett 2003). Changes in workload, staffing provision and the nature of healthcare delivery mean that the effectiveness of such strategies is difficult to establish but it is clear from numerous studies that, despite knowledge and training, nurses do not always comply with taught techniques (Smallwood 2006).

Listed below are some reasons, other than knowledge and training deficits, why practice may fall short of the ideal. Often, there is no easy or immediate solution but it is anticipated that raising your awareness of these constraints will prompt reflection on your practice and help you to evaluate assisting with mobility from a wider perspective.

Lack of time

'Not enough time' is often quoted by nurses as a reason for not complying with regulations; yet this is a symptom of other issues such as workload, staff shortages and the competing demands of nursing practice. If recommended moving and handling methods are perceived as time consuming, nurses may adopt less safe alternatives or take shortcuts. Provision of additional staff may be the only way to resolve these difficulties, but consideration also needs to be given to the way work is allocated and organized. For example, staff working in partnership may be more efficient than dividing a caseload between two.

Lack of space

Assisting people to move requires space. In a hospital environment, allocation of a patient to a bed space should take into account the assistance required with moving or repositioning. For example, a single room may not allow sufficient space for handlers to reposition a patient in a large, special bed. Preparing the environment by rearranging furniture and removing clutter can reduce risks of imbalance and hazardous postures but safe principles equally apply to these tasks.

Unavailable or inaccessible equipment

Given pressures of time and workload, nurses may be reluctant to use equipment if they have to rummage through store cupboards or walk to the other end of a ward to obtain it. Equipment needs to be accessible. In a hospital environment, smaller aids for single patient use can often be kept at the bedside. In the home, patients can apply for funding to purchase personal aids or borrow them for long or short term use. Where equipment is lacking (for example, you feel a standing aid will reduce risks on a rehabilitation ward), a comprehensive risk assessment, which includes a cost-benefit analysis, is an effective means of persuading managers that money will be well spent.

Social and cultural barriers

The significance of social and cultural influences in patient moving and handling is increasingly being recognized. Kneafsey (2000) explored the concept of occupational socialization in this aspect of care: that is, the influence of established norms of behaviour in a given place of work which serve to perpetuate poor practice. Her argument that compliance with recommended techniques is influenced by peer pressure has since been reinforced by several studies (Crumpton & Bannister 2002), particularly where student nurses are concerned (Swain et al 2003, Smallwood 2006). The Royal College of Nursing (2003) states that attitudes, behaviours and cultures that prioritize safe practice are essential to achieving successful patient handling. A culture of best practice can be fostered through leadership, change management and supportive policies but there is also a need for individuals to develop the requisite interpersonal and problem-solving skills to tackle these barriers. Declining to participate in a manoeuvre that carries unnecessary risks can be difficult, particularly when those expecting you to assist are of a higher ranking. This situation is compounded by pressures of time, the need to fetch equipment or urgency of patient care needs. Suggesting a safer technique is an obvious strategy but where alternatives are not immediately apparent, it can be difficult to resolve such dilemmas. Clear and accessible records of risk assessment and care planning will promote a coordinated approach but, as professionals, each of us is accountable for our actions and decisions in any given circumstances.

Diversity of knowledge and understanding

Patient handling techniques have evolved rapidly over recent years. Knowledge development and creative thinking means that new ways of moving people are continually introduced and techniques once regarded as suitable are now controversial. (You are advised to access information about these controversial techniques in Evolve 6.7 as you may witness them in practice and need to understand the associated risks.) Additionally, goals relating to moving and mobility are not achieved by following a formula and the complexity of decision making is likely to result in differences of opinion. Assistants may feel unable to cooperate with a task because they are unfamiliar or disagree with suggested techniques. Others may be unwilling because they underestimate the risks. Again, disputes may be avoided by careful planning and documentation of selected methods which take into account the skills of those likely to be involved.

6.7 – CONTROVERSIAL TECHNIQUES

- Define what is meant by a controversial technique.
- Identify at least three types of manoeuvres that are regarded as controversial.
- Identify risks to handlers and patients/clients for a specified technique.

Client expectations and preferences

Everyday demands of nursing work can leave you feeling in a 'no win' situation. For example, lifting a person onto a commode presents numerous risks but using a standing hoist may be undignified and distressing to the patient. In addition, traditions of nursing appear to have cultivated an expectation among patients that nurses should lift them and an acceptance among nurses that a 'bad back' is just part of the job. Many authors comment on the role of altruism (the inclination to prioritize patients' needs and wishes over personal safety) in nurses' decision making (Kneafsey 2000, Crumpton & Bannister 2002, Swain et al 2003), yet Mandelstam (2003) points out that a balanced approach is laid down in existing laws and good professional practice. Decisions are not always easy and service users are likely to have different priorities from the professionals. Individual assessment provides the opportunity to develop constructive relationships with patients and carers and an understanding of their personal perspectives. Patients might presuppose the use of equipment to be uncomfortable or frightening but this should not be assumed, as evidence indicates that nurses' reluctance to use equipment for this reason can be

misplaced (McGuire et al 1996). Equally, care needs to be taken that manual handling is not intrusive. Explanations and negotiation can resolve many dilemmas and strategies based on safe principles are often those that promote patient comfort and independence.

Evidence-based practice

To examine factors that influence patient handling practices from the perspectives of student nurses, Smallwood (2006) conducted a study that focused on their placement experiences. Using a purposive sample, data collection consisted of a self-report questionnaire to ascertain the extent to which factors described in the literature influenced their practice. Responses ($n=51$) were analysed using descriptive statistics and presented for discussion to the same sample to clarify understanding and gain further insights.

The effects of peer pressure and socialization, conflict between personal and patient well-being and difficulties transferring classroom skills into practice were acknowledged as barriers to recommended practice. However, disparity was demonstrated in the responses suggesting that some students were able to resist these pressures better than others. The significance of clinical placement areas in influencing students' patient handling behaviour emerged from the questionnaire and discussion group data.

The study contributes to evidence of poor compliance with patient handling directives and suggests a need to address potential barriers through educational strategies.

In summary, successful moving and handling requires consideration of 'the human factor'. Compliance with recommended practice relies on personal disposition and interpersonal skills yet many barriers can be lessened by strategies relevant to specific clinical areas; for example, suitable equipment that is easily accessible, communication structures that encourage reporting of problems and staff training that acknowledges the value of teamwork.

PERSONAL AND REFLECTIVE KNOWLEDGE

As a professional practitioner, you are required to be knowledgeable in your area of practice and proficient in skills relevant to your particular client population. This requires ongoing revision and review of theory, legislation, guidelines and practices. This section focuses on gaining awareness of difficulties experienced by those with impaired mobility and reflecting on your personal capacity to assist with moving and handling. In addition to further information and theoretical exercises, we have provided a variety of practical exercises that are designed to be undertaken within care settings or a formal educational environment.

USING MOBILITY AIDS AND APPLIANCES

The exercises suggested are for groups of learners. A facilitator who is fully trained in the use of the appliances is required for advice and supervision regarding appropriate techniques. The facilitator should stress the importance of safety which should not be compromised during these exercises.

Learners should maximize their experiences by including the following:

- asking for directions
- obtaining money from a bank or cashpoint
- making a purchase at a shop
- having refreshments in a cafe
- sitting in a public area.

Elbow or axillary crutches

After instruction and assessment, learners go into the care setting and/or local area to:

- experience what practical difficulties exist
- identify whether planners and architects have made adequate provision for anyone using crutches
- experience how users of crutches are perceived and treated by the general public.

Two learners need to work together. One will use the crutches and one will identify (in writing) the findings. Both should have equal opportunity to participate in each task. To fully appreciate the experience, it should ideally be conducted over one day with group discussion the following day.

Wheelchairs

This exercise is similar to the previous one, with the same three questions to be answered. There are two methods:

- Three learners – one learner sits in the wheelchair, one assists and the other records their observations.

- Two learners – one learner uses the wheelchair independently and the other observes and records.

Each team should discuss their experiences so that additional points can be made before feeding back to the whole group.

Obstacle audit

This exercise is helpful where use of mobility aids is not feasible. Initially, learners are given guidance about potential obstacles for people with impaired mobility. Working in pairs, they venture into the community or hospital to identify the obstacles they observe. A video camera is useful for this exercise.

When back in the classroom setting, discussion should include:

- items identified
- difficulties that may be encountered
- suggested reasons why changes or adaptations have not been made.

One might expect that the hospital planners and managers would have looked closely at such difficulties but this is not always the case. Again, why is this and what can be done?

CARING FOR YOURSELF

The importance of exercise and activity has been highlighted in the Subject Knowledge section. As a nurse, you need to keep fit and care for your back both at work and in daily life. Gentle exercise programmes such as regular walking, yoga, pilates and swimming are recommended. Keeping to your desirable weight will also help to prevent back problems. Further reading on this subject can be found in publications and websites (see Annotated Websites).

REFLECTION ON PERSONAL PRACTICE

There are likely to be occasions in practice when you feel you have breached recommended principles when assisting patients. The 'theory–practice' gap, a concept in nursing that refers to the differences between theory and the reality of practice, is particularly manifest in moving and handling due to the challenges it presents and pace of developments. Achieving the 'ideal' depends on the particular complexities of the task, including psychosocial factors as well as knowledge and skills of handlers. A sense of failing to perform to the highest standards or being in a 'no win' situation can be experienced equally by student nurses and senior practitioners. It is important not to feel disheartened and remember that no moving and handling task is completely safe. The aim is to reduce risks as far as reasonably practicable while considering the best interests of the patient or client. Reflection on personal experiences can help to improve your practice.

CASE STUDIES

The following case studies are designed to consolidate the knowledge you have gained from this chapter and your practice experiences. After completion, compare your ideas with the thoughts of the authors in Evolve 6.8.

℮volve
learning system

6.8 – CASE STUDIES FEEDBACK

- Identify mobility and moving and handling needs in patient/client scenarios.
- Identify factors that present a hazard to carers and patients/clients.
- Plan care to meet the needs of patients/clients and their family or carers.
- Identify facilities and other personnel that may be involved in this care.

Case study: Adult

Mary Reed is a 67-year-old widow, lives alone and claims to be independent. She has always had problems with her weight and this has caused degeneration in her joints. She currently weighs 15 stone (95 kg). She walks slowly with a shuffling gait and is able to visit the local shops to meet her daily needs. However, she is finding it increasingly difficult to climb stairs and to sit down and stand up from her chair. She loves to have a bath but has not been able to do so for over 6 months. Her daughter is concerned that she will sustain a fall and has tried to persuade Mary, without success, to move into a rest home. She has contacted her mother's general practitioner for help and the district nurse is asked to assess the situation.

- What facilities and personnel are available to help in this situation?
- List the tasks that will require a moving and handling assessment.
- Using a holistic approach, note the factors relating to Mary that need to be taken into account. What factors in particular have implications for handlers that might be involved? What environmental factors may affect the situation?
- How would you deal with the conflict of interests between mother and daughter?
- Devise a care plan for Mary to address her mobility and moving and handling needs by considering suitable options for her situation. What resources, equipment or adaptations to the environment are needed? State why you have chosen particular

strategies or methods to assist with the required tasks. What factors relating to individual handlers need to be taken into account?
- Multidisciplinary assessment advocates instalment of a bath hoist and a care assistant to assist with bathing once a week. Although Mary is happy for someone to assist, she does not want to be hoisted as she feels this would be undignified. Considering the best interests of the patient/client and safety risks to handlers, how would you handle this situation? Would a compromise be in order and, if so, what would it be?

Case study: Mental health

Doreen Jones is a 66-year-old lady who lives in a care home. She has advanced dementia and her communication is limited to only expressing pain by screaming at the nurses. Doreen weighs 11 stone (70 kg) and requires assistance with activities of living as her body is permanently rigid with her arms and legs flexed. She frequently slips down the bed but is unable to sit in a chair because she arches her back, which puts her at risk of falling out. Much of her surrounding space is taken up by bedside tables, chairs and residents' personal belongings to make it more homely. She has two daughters who visit regularly but feel helpless and distressed about their mother's condition.

- How do Doreen's mental health problems impact on her mobility?
- List the tasks that require a moving and handling assessment.
- Using a holistic approach, note key factors relating to Doreen that need to be taken into account. What factors in particular have implications for handlers that might be involved? What environmental factors may affect the situation?
- Devise a care plan for Doreen to address her mobility and moving and handling needs by considering suitable options for her situation. What resources, equipment or adaptations to the environment are needed? State why you have chosen particular strategies or methods to assist with the required mobility tasks. What factors relating to individual handlers need to be taken into account?
- How could you involve the family in addressing Doreen's needs and what might be the benefits of this?

Case study: Child

Mandy Roberts is a 7-year-old girl who fell and fractured her right tibia when performing gymnastics in a regional competition. She had an external fixator placed in situ (a large, heavy metal frame attached to her leg) 2 days ago and is being cared for in a children's hospital ward. Mandy is small for her age and slightly built. So far, she has spent most of her time in bed with her fractured leg supported on a pillow. However, she was assisted into a chair yesterday where she sat for a couple of hours. She has been instructed not to bear weight on her right leg. Mandy is a motivated child who is quite frustrated by her limited mobility. She wants to get back to school and is concerned about how the injury will affect her gymnastics. Mandy's parents are with her whenever possible and want to support her recovery. They are also concerned about how this injury will affect their daughter's general progress.

- List the tasks that will require a moving and handling assessment.
- Using a holistic approach, note key factors relating to Mandy that need to be taken into account. What factors in particular have implications for handlers that might be involved? What environmental factors may affect the situation?
- Devise a care plan for Mandy to address her mobility and moving and handling needs by considering suitable options for her situation. What resources, equipment or adaptations to the environment are needed? State why you have chosen particular strategies or methods to assist with the required mobility tasks. What factors relating to individual handlers need to be taken into account?
- How would you deal with Mandy's frustration and assist her in complying with keeping weight off her right leg?
- How might you involve Mandy's parents?
- What other facilities and personnel would help Mandy's recovery?

Case study: Learning disabilities

Stephen White is an 11-year-old boy who suffers from severe brain damage following a road traffic accident 2 years ago. He lives with his parents and 15-year-old sister. Steven is unable to walk although he has some weight-bearing capacity. He is transported in a wheelchair and assisted with other mobility tasks (for example, transferring between his wheelchair and toilet, his bed and the family car) by one or two family members manually transferring him; in doing so, they often take all or most of his body weight. His arms and legs have developed flexion contractures and he can no longer talk coherently. He attends the local physiotherapy department twice a week. Stephen's mother, Margaret, is the main carer in the family and worries that Stephen is about to lose the little mobility he has. She does not want Stephen to be placed in a permanent care facility.

- How does Stephen's learning disability impact on his mobility?
- Using a holistic approach, note key factors relating to Stephen that need to be taken into account when assessing his moving and handling needs. What factors in particular have implications for handlers that might be involved? What environmental factors may affect the situation?
- Devise a care plan to address Stephen's moving and handling needs by considering suitable options for his situation. What resources, equipment or adaptations to the environment are needed? State why you have chosen particular strategies or methods to assist with the required mobility tasks. What factors relating to individual handlers need to be taken into account?
- What strategies would you consider to deal with Stephen's mobility problems? What facilities and personnel are available to help and how would you involve his family?
- How would you deal with the potential discrepancy between meeting Stephen's needs and the wishes of his mother?

SUMMARY

This chapter has introduced you to the knowledge required to promote and support mobility and to undertake safe and effective nursing decisions in moving and handling situations. It has included:

1. An outline of the musculoskeletal system and the applied anatomy of the spine to include risk factors in relation to back pain and injury, especially in the work place.
2. A consideration of mobility and its meaning to individuals and to society in terms of good health; the long and short-term impact of immobility; and attitudes to disability.
3. A critical review of multidisciplinary assessment tools in planning and implementing care for those with mobility deficits.
4. An outline of mobility care management to include relevant exercise programmes.
5. A description of the principles of load handling and an outline of elements in a risk assessment tool and a handling and moving plan.
6. A review of handling equipment and its use and an overview of how to move people in various situations at home or in hospital.
7. The professional role of the nurse in providing mobility care; the implications of disability legislation; and the importance of legislation on moving and handling.
8. A review of potential legal and ethical problems arising in handling situations and mobility care.
9. An emphasis on following professional guidelines and the need to care for your own back.

Annotated further reading and websites

Health and Safety Executive 2002 Handling home care: achieving safe, efficient and positive outcomes for care workers and clients. Health and Safety Executive, Sudbury

This book is aimed at organizations that provide home care services. It contains practical advice on minimizing risks from manual handling and contains case studies of real situations.

Health and Safety Executive 2004 Getting to grips with manual handling: a short guide. Health and Safety Executive, Sudbury

This booklet outlines the problems of manual handling and best practice in dealing with them. It provides a clear summary of basic principles.

Royal College of Nursing 2002 RCN Code of practice for patient handling. Royal College of Nursing, London (Reorder code 000 604)

This publication provides a framework for implementing manual handling regulations. It includes a summary of employer and employee responsibilities.

Royal College of Nursing 2003 Manual handling assessments in hospitals and the community. Royal College of Nursing, London (Reorder code 000 605)

A useful and practical guide on assessment for patient handling.

Smith J 2005 The guide to the handling of people, 5th edn. BackCare, Middlesex

A definitive book for health professionals involved with moving and handling people. Each chapter is written by experts in their field and provides recent evidence for the safer handling of people. The detailed text is aimed at advanced and specialist practitioners but the practical chapters, providing illustrations and reviews of evidence for a range of tasks, are a useful reference for students and qualified practitioners of all levels.

www.arc.org.uk

The Arthritis Research Campaign (arc) produces a range of free information booklets and leaflets.

www.backcare.org.uk

BackCare is a charity promoting prevention of back pain and supporting back pain sufferers through education and information. It produces a range of publications.

www.disabilitynet.co.uk

This site provides a route out to other websites regarding information on various subjects, including policies.

www.iea.cc

This is the site of the International Ergonomics Association.

www.independentliving.org

Website containing views, experiences and articles dealing with disability issues.

www.Motability.co.uk

Motability is an organization that helps people with disabilities and their families with mobility issues.

http://www.nationalbackexchange.org/

The National Back Exchange (NBE) provides a multidisciplinary forum to support health professionals and promote exchange of information on back care.

www.nhs.uk/Livewell/Backpain/Pages/Backpainatwork.aspx

This is a useful website aimed at everyone working in the NHS. It contains articles, videos and useful tips on looking after your back. It also provides links to other useful information. Well worth a look.

References

Adams MA, Dolan P 2005 Biomechanics of low back pain. In: Smith J (ed) The guide to the handling of people, 5th edn. Backcare, Middlesex

AMPS Project International 2007 Assessment of motor and process skills. Available online: http://www.ampsintl.com/ (accessed February 2008)

ArjoHuntleigh website. Available online: http://www.arjohuntleigh.com/int/ – ArjoHuntleigh company website for moving and handling equipment (accessed February 2008)

Arthritis Research Campaign 2004 Sexuality and arthritis. ARC, York. Available online: http://www.arc.org.uk/arthinfo/patpubs/6037/6037.asp (accessed 10 August 2008)

Atwal A, Caldwell K 2002 Do multidisciplinary integrated care pathways improve interprofessional collaboration? Scandinavian Journal of Caring Sciences 16(4):360–367

Back Care 2007 Back facts. Available online: http://www.backpain.org/pages/b_pages/backfacts-2007.php (accessed 9 March 2007)

Bouchard C, Blair SN, Haskell W (eds) 2007 Physical activity and health. Human Kinetics, Leeds

Bridger RS 2002 Introduction to ergonomics, 2nd edn. Taylor & Francis, London

Brouwer B, Olney S 2004 Aging skeletal muscle and the impact of resistance exercise. Physiotherapy 56(2):80–87

Campbell H, Hotchkiss R, Bradshaw N, Porteus M 1998 Integrated care pathways. British Medical Journal 316:133–137

Chartered Society of Physiotherapists 2005 Core standards of physiotherapy practice (2005). Chartered Society of Physiotherapists, London

Clarke A, Warren L 2007 Hopes, fears and expectations about the future: what older people's stories tell about active ageing. Ageing and Society 27:465–488

College of Occupational Therapists 2006 Manual handling. College of Occupational Therapists, London

Crumpton E, Bannister C 2002 Survey to investigate NHS trusts compliance with the RCN safer patient handling policy 1996. Royal College of Nursing, London

Department of Health 2001 National service framework for older people. Department of Health, London

Department of Health 2002 Back in Work back pack: everything you need to know about the national Back in Work campaign. Department of Health, London

Department of Health 2004 Back in Work. Stationery Office, London

Disability Discrimination Act 2006 HMSO, London

Disability Rights Commission Act 1999 HSMO, London

Disabled Persons (Independent Living) Bill 1999 HMSO, London

Drake RL, Vogel W, Mitchell AWM (eds) 2005 Gray's anatomy for students. Elsevier, Edinburgh

Edwards S 2001 Neurological physiotherapy: a problem solving approach. Churchill Livingstone, Edinburgh

Goffman E 1963. Stigma: notes on the management of spoiled identity. Prentice Hall, Englewood Cliffs

Gormley J, Hussey J 2005 Exercise therapy: prevention and treatment of disease. Blackwell, Oxford, ch 10

Griffith R, Stevens M 2004 Manual handling and the lawfulness of no-lift policies. Nursing Standard 18(21):39–43

Health and Safety at Work, Etc. Act 1974 HMSO, London

Health and Safety Executive 1992 Manual Handling Operations Regulations. HMSO, London

Health and Safety Executive 1995 Reporting of Injuries, Diseases and Dangerous Occurrences Regulations 1995. HMSO, London

Health and Safety Executive 2004 Getting to grips with manual handling: a short guide. Health and Safety Executive, Sudbury

Health and Safety Executive 2007a Self reported work related illness and workplace injuries 2005/06: results from the labour force survey. Health and Safety Executive, Caerphilly. Available online: http://www.hse.gov.uk/statistics/lfs/lfs0506.pdf (accessed 11 August 2008)

Health and Safety Executive 2007b Musculoskeletal disorders. Worried about aches and pains. OPSI, Norwich. Available online:

http://www.hse.gov.uk/healthservices/msd.htm (accessed 25 September 2007)

Hignett S 2003 Evidence-based patient handling: systematic review. Nursing Standard 17(33):33–36

Hignett S, Evans D 2006 Spatial requirements in hospital shower and toilet rooms. Nursing Standard 21(3):43–48

Human Rights Act 1998 HMSO, London

Johnson C 2005 Manual handling risk assessment: theory and practice. In: Smith J The guide to the handling of people, 5th edn. BackCare, Middlesex, p 108

Judd M 1989 Mobility: patient problems and nursing care. Heinemann Nursing, Oxford

Karahan A, Bayraktar N 2004 Determination of the usage of body mechanics in clinical settings and the occurrence of low back pain in nurses. International Journal of Nursing Studies 41(1):67–75

Kjellburg K, Lagerstrom M, Hagberg M 2004 Patient safety and comfort during transfers in relation to nurses' work technique. Journal of Advanced Nursing 47(3):251–259

Kneafsey R 2000 The effect of occupational socialisation on nurses' patient handling practices. Journal of Clinical Nursing 9:585–593

Lifting Operations and Lifting Equipment Regulations 1998 No. 2307. HMSO, London

LoBianco AF, Shepppard-Jones K 2007 Perceptions of disability as related to medical and social factors. Applied Social Psychology 37(1):1–13

McGuire T, Moody J, Hanson M et al 1996 A study into clients' attitudes towards mechanical aids. Nursing Standard 11(5):35–38

Magee DJ 2002 Orthopaedic physical assessment, 4th edn. Saunders, Toronto, ch 14

Mahoney FI, Barthel DW 1965 Functional evaluation: the Barthel index. Maryland State Medical Journal 14:61–65

Mandelstam M 2003 Disabled people, manual handling and human rights. British Journal of Occupational Therapy 66(11):528–530

Mandelstam M 2004 Balanced decision-taking, legal principle, practical implications. The Column 16, 1 February 2004

May S 2005 The prevention and management of simple low back pain. In: Smith J The guide to the handling of people, 5th edn. Back Care, Middlesex, p 79

Montague SE, Watson R, Herbert R 2005 Physiology for nursing practice, 3rd edn. Elsevier, Edinburgh

National Audit Office 2003 A safer place to work: improving the management of health and safety risks to staff in NHS trusts. The Stationery Office, London

National Back Exchange 2002 Essential back-up revised 2002. An employer's guide for setting up and maintaining an effective back care advisory service. National Back Exchange, Towcester

Nicholls JA 1997 Patient handling training and work-related back pain. British Journal of Therapy and Rehabilitation 4(8):429–434

Nursing and Midwifery Council 2008 The Code: standards of conduct, performance and ethics for nurses and midwives. Nursing and Midwifery Council, London

Palastanga N, Field, D, Soames R 2004 Anatomy and human movement: structure and function, 4th edn. Butterworth Heinemann, Edinburgh

Palmer KT, Walsh K, Bendall H, Cooper C, Coggon D 2000 Back pain in Britain: comparison of two prevalence surveys at an interval of 10 years. British Medical Journal 320:1577–1578

Patient Safety Observatory 2007 Slips, trips and falls in hospital: the third report from the Patient Safety Observatory. National Patient Safety Agency, London

Prentice WE 2001a Impaired mobility: restoring range of motion and improving flexibility. In: Prentice WE, Voight MI (eds) Techniques in musculoskeletal rehabilitation. McGraw-Hill, London, p 62

Prentice WE 2001b Impaired mobility: restoring range of motion and improving flexibility. In: Prentice WE, Voight MI (eds) Techniques in musculoskeletal rehabilitation. McGraw-Hill, London, p 84

Resuscitation Council (UK) 2001 Guidance for safer handling during resuscitation in hospitals. Resuscitation Council, London

Retsas A 2000 Manual handling activities and injuries among nurses: an Australian hospital study. Journal of Advanced Nursing 31(4):875–883

Royal College of Nursing 2002 RCN Code of Practice for patient handling. Royal College of Nursing, London

Royal College of Nursing 2003 Safer staff, better care: RCN manual handling training guidance. Royal College of Nursing, London

Scottish Executive 2003 Lets make Scotland more active: a strategy for physical activity. Stationery Office, Edinburgh. Available online: http://www.scotland.gov.uk/Publications (accessed 3 October 2007)

Smallwood JA 2006 Patient handling: student nurses' views. Learning in Health and Social Care 5(4): 208–219

Smith J 2005 The guide to the handling of people. BackCare, Middlesex

Special Education Needs and Disability Act 2001 OPSI, Norwich

Swain J, Pufahl E, Williamson GR 2003 Do they practice what we teach? A survey of manual handling practice amongst student nurses. Journal of Clinical Nursing 12(2):297–306

Tortora GJ, Derrickson B 2007 Introduction to the human body, the essentials of anatomy and physiology, 7th edn. Wiley, New York

Umphred DA 2007 Neurological rehabilitation, 5th edn. Mosby Elsevier, St Louis, ch 23

Walker J, Payne S, Smith P et al 2007 Psychology for nurses and the caring professions, 3rd edn. Open University Press, Edinburgh

Wanless D, Appleby A, Harrison A, Patel D 2007 Our future health secured? A review of NHS funding and performance. King's Fund, London

World Health Organization 2008 Health topics: disabilities. World Health Organization, Geneva. Available online: http://www.who.int/topics/disabilities/en/

Chapter 7

Homeostasis

Jeff Evans

KEY ISSUES

SUBJECT KNOWLEDGE
- Behavioural, cultural and environmental factors that affect health
- Mechanism of feedback loops in maintaining homeostasis
- Biological basis of thermoregulation, blood pressure maintenance, pulse and respiratory homeostasis

CARE DELIVERY KNOWLEDGE
- Measurement and assessment of body temperature
- Measurement and assessment of blood pressure
- Measurement and assessment of respiration

PROFESSIONAL AND ETHICAL KNOWLEDGE
- Accountability
- Consent
- Health promotion

PERSONAL AND REFLECTIVE KNOWLEDGE
- Ideas for portfolio and skills laboratory learning
- Case study consolidation

INTRODUCTION

La fixité du milieu intérieur est la condition d'une vie libre et indépendante.

Claude Bernard (1878–9)

('To have a free life, independent of the external environment, requires a constant internal environment')

Claude Bernard was a pioneering physiologist working in the early 19th century. Through his various experiments and investigations he noticed that certain physiological values stayed within a very narrow range. He proposed that the body works hard through compensatory mechanisms to maintain certain key parameters such as oxygen and carbon dioxide levels, water and electrolyte balance, blood glucose, body temperature and blood pressure within an optimal range. This idea of a fixed internal environment is termed *homeostasis*. By maintaining homeostasis, the body can provide the best conditions possible for cells and organs to function. Illness can be seen to arise when there is a deviation away from the normal, one that the body cannot cope with or adapt to.

A change in internal environment creates an automatic response by the body which enables mechanisms to redress deviation from normal. Our biology returns to a point of homeostasis. In the same way, in everyday life we adapt to, and cope with, all of the problems and opportunities thrown at us by an ever changing world. Nursing theorists such as Betty Neuman and Sister Callista Roy see nursing as working with people to help them cope with or adapt to problems they encounter (Marriner-Tomey & Alligood 1998). These problems may be biological in nature, involved with thinking, emotions and beliefs, or may be social in nature. More often than not, however, problems span all three domains. There is thus a holistic view of health and nursing in which the nurse and client work together to achieve a sense of control and balance in the everyday life, and also optimal biological functioning.

As an example of homeostasis, this chapter will examine the ways in which the body responds in an attempt to meet the specific demands placed upon it by changing blood pressure, body temperature and respiration. The role of the nurse in monitoring temperature, blood pressure and respiration will be explored and related professional and ethical issues considered. As the content of this chapter focuses on these three specific areas of homeostasis, it is expected that you will cross-reference with many other chapters for other complementary aspects of homeostasis (e.g. Ch. 4, 'Resuscitation and emergency care', Ch. 15, 'Skin integrity', Ch. 8, 'Nutrition' and Ch. 9, 'Stress, relaxation and rest').

OVERVIEW

Subject knowledge

The mechanisms of feedback loops are explored. These are essential to maintaining homeostasis. The chapter will concentrate on how normal temperature, blood pressure and respiration are maintained and controlled by the body.

Individual behavioural, environmental, social and emotional factors also have an effect on how the internal body balance is maintained. These factors are explored under psychosocial and environmental subject knowledge.

Care delivery knowledge

The knowledge needed by the nurse for making a comprehensive assessment of temperature, blood pressure and respirations is explored. The nursing management of some common problems that threaten homeostasis are also included in this section.

Professional and ethical knowledge

Professional issues that influence the role of the nurse in the assessment of homeostasis are identified. The discussion includes an exploration of how the issues of consent, professional accountability and health promotion apply to the nurse's role when undertaking observations and measurements.

Personal and reflective knowledge

Suggestions are made for portfolio development and experiential exercises in which assessment of homeostasis can be practised in a safe environment. Consolidation of knowledge gained from the chapter and through your practice experience is facilitated through case study work.

On pages 172–173 there are four case studies, each one relating to one of the branches of nursing. You may find it helpful to read one of them before you start the chapter and use it as a focus for your reflections while reading.

SUBJECT KNOWLEDGE

MECHANISMS IN HOMEOSTASIS

Before outlining specific knowledge needed for clinical decision making regarding body temperature, blood pressure and respiration, it is important to understand the internal mechanisms involved in maintaining balance in all body systems and also to consider potential external influences.

Before discussing control loops, it is useful to consider an everyday occurrence. Sian is running a bath for her toddler, Tom. She runs in hot and cold water and tests the temperature with her hand. If it is too cold she turns off the cold tap and runs in more hot, if it gets too hot she runs in more cold. Eventually she ends up with a bath full of water at the right temperature. What Sian has just done is an illustration of how the body controls all of our physiology through *feedback loops*. The elements of a feedback loop are:

1. Detector (Sian's hand).
2. Sensory pathways (nerves in Sian's arm and spinal cord).
3. An integrator to bring all the information together and make a response (Sian's perception of whether or not the bath is too hot or too cold).
4. Pathways carrying the decision out (motor nerves in Sian's spinal cord and arm).
5. An effector to put into effect the decisions of the integrator (Sian's hands that turn on and off the taps).

This situation described is an example of negative feedback. In negative feedback, the response that is triggered by the detector negates the deviation from the desired point. Negative feedback loops are the most common mechanism for controlling body functions. Positive feedbacks tend to amplify the trigger rather than reduce it, thus moving the body further away from homeostasis. They are rarely found in healthy individuals (Seeley et al 2008). However, many diseases are characterized by positive feedback, including rheumatoid arthritis, asthma and heart failure. Positive feedback also has a role to play in mental health settings; panic attacks and phobias have elements of positive feedback, where, for example, awareness of sweating and a pounding heart increase anxiety levels even further.

The hypothalamus is a key control and integration centre in the brain and is part of the limbic system, which helps to maintain homeostasis. The hypothalamus regulates eating and drinking, sleeping and waking, body temperature, hormone balances, heart rate, sex drive and emotions (Seeley et al 2008). It also directs the master gland of the brain – the adenohypophysis (pituitary gland) – which is responsible for regulating hormonal balance within the body. The brain is therefore a major organ of adaptation and can respond to changes in the external and internal environment quickly and flexibly to maintain health (Shmaefsky 2007). How homeostasis is specifically maintained is the major focus of this chapter, but although homeostasis is concerned with the stability and maintenance of internal physiological systems, it is also important to consider such balance as being within a context of some external influence.

---

evolve *learning system*

7.1 – SYSTEMS, ADAPTATION, HOMEOSTASIS AND NURSING

- Learn about different systems and the human being as a complex open system.
- Consider how nursing can help people to adapt to maintain homeostasis.

EXTERNAL INFLUENCES ON HOMEOSTASIS

Psychosocial, cultural, economic and environmental factors can affect homeostasis and need to be considered. Influences on behaviour are individual to each person, but are usually associated with the family and school in childhood, peers in early adolescence, and social groupings, religious beliefs, the media and multiple other sources in adult life. The beliefs of society are influential and how individuals become ill or remain healthy is affected by cultural beliefs on what is good and bad 'healthy' behaviour. In the past, many sociologists have commented on the 'lay' perceptions of health as opposed to how professionals describe, label and classify 'ill-health' (Kleinman 1980, Mishler 1981, Helman 1994).

Understanding differences in perception can be important in deciding how to approach individuals and groups when involved in health promotion activities. Cultural beliefs can also lead to misunderstandings and may even be a threat to health. An example would be using a hot water bottle during the shivering phase of a fever for a young child aged between 6 months and 3 years. Besides the danger of burning the skin, the child's temperature may rise rapidly, leading to an increased risk of febrile convulsion.

Health can also be detrimentally affected by environmental factors, which include political and economic factors over which individuals have limited control. Correspondingly, government legislation and policy can be influential in controlling situations where detriment to health is likely (see Ch. 3, 'Safety and risk').

In order to cope and adapt to illness and life problems, people need resources. This is another way the government can influence a person's level of wellness, through controlling what services and resources are available to people to help them overcome or live with their health problems. So, for example, the Scottish Executive introduced free personal and nursing care in 2002, and the Welsh Assembly Government introduced free prescriptions for all in 2007. Both of these policies are likely to have dramatic effects upon people's abilities to maintain their own health and well-being.

Government economic policy has also had a direct impact on individuals in society. It could be argued that imposing a tax on fuel and limiting extra payments to the elderly and disabled until certain low temperatures have been reached over consecutive days has little impact overall on reducing morbidity and mortality due to hypothermia during the winter months. Research in this area is fraught with difficulties as hypothermia is often not the main recorded cause of death (Watson 1996, Age Concern 2008); however, the Department of Health (2001a) suggest that there are about 80 000 cold-related deaths each year in the UK. Although health promotion may be addressed at the levels of behaviour and lifestyle, it may still be the cost factor that predominates in an individual's ability to keep warm in winter.

A more recent concern is that of the health effects of climate change in the UK (Department of Health 2001a). It is anticipated that there will be a gradual fall in cold-related deaths and an increase in heat-related deaths due to global warming over the next few decades.

Evidence-based practice

During a nine day heat-wave from 4–13 August 2003, there were 2091 more deaths than expected in England; likewise there were 1311 more emergency hospital admissions than expected, with the over 75 age group suffering particularly badly (Office of National Statistics 2006). This kind of statistic has clear implications for nursing and the management of resources in the future.

Whether a person's health status is considered as an individual matter, a disturbed internal biology or a mental health problem is continuously debated. In some respects it is simpler to take this view as the individual's health status is focused clearly as their own personal concern and can be identified as their problem when health is poor. However, by considering people as interacting with the world they live in, we can see that local, national and even international factors often have a role to play in determining a person's health status. Nurses must be cognizant of these debates, for they can respond in a number of ways. On an individual basis, nurses may need to help a person cope with, or adapt to the challenges these factors present in their lives, while on a wider scale the role of the nurse in advocating for patient communities is relevant.

Optimum health is a fundamental building block of wider well-being and the body strives to maintain balance and adapt to changes to ensure optimum health through homeostasis. The rest of this chapter will focus upon the maintenance of homeostasis within the three key areas already identified: control of body temperature, blood pressure maintenance and respiratory regulation.

THE BALANCE OF BODY TEMPERATURE

The main organ for maintaining normal body temperature (thermoregulation) is the skin. The skin has many vital functions. However, in this particular section, thermoregulation and its homeostatic control will be the main focus (see Chapter 15 for other functions of the skin).

Humans are homeothermic and strive to maintain a core temperature within a narrow range of 36–38 °C despite the day-to-day fluctuations encountered as a consequence of environmental temperatures and our own metabolic activities. Homeothermy is dependent upon continual thermoregulation with the scales finely balanced between heat production and heat loss. We need to maintain a body temperature of around 37°C because this is the optimal temperature for our metabolism and enzyme systems to function at. Deviation above or below the normal range of body temperature will have increasingly severe consequences for our health and will eventually lead to death (Montague et al 2005).

Heat production occurs in two ways. Firstly, muscle contraction generates large amounts of heat as a waste product. This excess heat is removed from active muscles and distributed around the body by the circulatory system, using blood as a heat transfer medium. If we begin to feel cold we naturally increase our level of activity, almost unconsciously, and might even start to shiver to increase heat production. If we are not exercising – resting on the sofa watching television, for example, or asleep – heat is generated through metabolism. The liver is highly active metabolically and generates a large amount of heat that can be distributed around the body via the bloodstream.

The general level of metabolic activity in the body is chiefly governed by the hormone thyroxine, and levels of this hormone increase when we are cold to increase heat production (Martini 2006). This mechanism is particularly important in young babies who may not have developed the ability to shiver.

Four major physical processes are involved in the loss of heat from the skin to the environment:

- evaporation
- conduction
- radiation
- convection.

Each of these processes is important to understand when managing the care of patients and clients.

Evaporation (22% of heat loss)

Large amounts of heat energy are needed to convert liquid water into water vapour, a process known as evaporation. If you wet your hands the liquid water strips heat out of the tissues of your hand and uses this heat energy to turn from liquid to vapour. We experience two things: firstly, our hands chill and secondly, they dry. Sweat is composed mainly of water and as it evaporates the energy used in the process of evaporation cools the body. Water is constantly being lost from the body; insensible water loss (i.e. too small or gradual to be perceived) is approximately 500 mL/day as a result of evaporative loss from the skin and the respiratory passages. This loss can be increased as a result of exercise or sweating. This is why on a hot day the cooling of the body through cool sponges may be soothing. In nursing the use of cooling liquids to reduce temperature is recognized with some caution. In children, whose surface areas are large, there is a risk of too rapid cooling leading to discomfort and in most patients there is a risk of shivering, which is counterproductive as it is a mechanism which generates heat.

Conduction (3% of heat loss)

In conduction, heat loss or gain is brought about by contact between the surface of the skin and some other object that is either warmer or cooler, for example jumping into a hot bath after being outdoors in the winter for 2 hours in the freezing cold, or having a lovely chilled drink on a hot day. Heat loss to cold objects can be decreased by insulation and clothing, for example wearing thick socks and boots when walking in snow.

Radiation (60% of heat loss)

Radiation is a process whereby heat is transferred from one heat source to another via infrared radiation without direct contact. For example, when you are cold it is possible to gain heat by standing in the sunshine. The human body also loses heat via radiation. The amount of heat lost through radiation is directly proportional to the amount of skin exposed. Babies and small children have a relatively large skin surface area when compared to their size so they tend to lose heat rapidly via radiation. Conversely, they can also be re-warmed by radiation too, and baby resuscitation equipment often includes overhead infrared warming lamps.

Convection (15% of heat loss)

As air moves over the skin heat is lost through convection. When there is little movement of air, the still air forms an insulating barrier and reduces the amount of heat lost;

when air movement increases heat loss also increases. Fleecy clothing works by trapping a warm layer of air against the skin, thus reducing the heat lost by convection. The use of electric fans to cool clients with fevers is an example of this principle.

Reflection and portfolio evidence

- Compare and contrast the ways a child under the age of 8 years and an adult can be safely cooled if they have a fever of 39°C.

Homeostatic control of body temperature

Body temperature is regulated by a feedback loop. As discussed above, heat is constantly being produced by metabolic activity. In order for this heat production to become and remain homeostatically balanced, there has to be a heat loss of the same proportion. This is obtained by balancing the scales between heat input and heat output (Fig. 7.1).

Physiological response to low temperatures

Thermoreceptors located in the periphery and central nervous system respond to a lowering of temperature and transmit impulses to the preoptic area of the brain, located in the hypothalamus, stimulating the heat promoting centre. As a consequence there is sympathetic nervous system stimulation resulting in vasoconstriction of the blood vessels in the skin, and shivering is increased (Fig. 7.2). The sympathetic nervous system response also triggers the release of epinephrine and thyroxine, both of which increase metabolic activity throughout the body, thus increasing heat production.

Sympathetic stimulation resulting in the release of epinephrine and thyroxine increases the basal metabolic rate by mobilizing the fat stores from adipose tissue and as a consequence generating heat. This process is known as chemical thermogenesis or non-shivering thermogenesis, and its function is vital in the newborn because their heat loss is large due to their large surface area, and in the early years the shivering response is poorly developed. This adipose tissue is called 'brown fat' and humans have only a

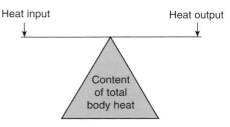

Figure 7.1 Balancing the scales of body heat.

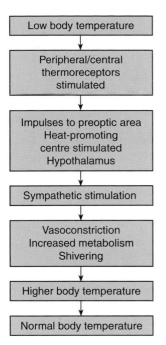

Figure 7.2 Thermoregulatory mechanism when the body temperature is low.

small quantity and can therefore only raise their body heat production by 10–15%.

We also see goose bumps developing. In mammals and birds this response results in raising the fur or feathers to trap a layer of warm air against the body. As humans are largely hairless this mechanism has little effect in heat conservation and is largely redundant.

The other important set of responses to low temperatures are the non-physiological behavioural responses such as finding shelter, dressing in warm clothing, turning up the heating in a house. These factors are important to consider as it is often a failure of behaviour rather than a failure of physiology that results in unplanned and life-threatening heat loss.

Physiological response to high temperatures

A rise in temperature is recognized by peripheral and central thermoreceptors; they relay this information to the preoptic area of the hypothalamus and the heat losing centre is stimulated. As a result, there is parasympathetic stimulation; cutaneous vasodilatation, diaphoresis (sweating) and decreased metabolism ensue and heat loss is increased. Shivering is inhibited.

In addition to the physiological mechanisms, nurses must remember the important role played by a person's behaviour. Cooling behaviours include taking off clothes, seeking shade and a cool environment, drinking fluids, and active cooling, for example jumping in a swimming pool.

Physical factors that affect thermoregulation

These include:

- exercise
- hormones
- drugs
- food intake
- circadian rhythms
- age.

Reflection and portfolio evidence

- Review the relative effects of circadian rhythms on temperature.
- In your practice placements, note the times of day when temperature is recorded.
- Discuss with your practice supervisor how you would differentiate the effects of time of day on temperature from possible upsets in thermoregulation.

Thermoregulation failure

Under certain conditions the normal thermoregulatory mechanisms can be compromised. These include:

- fever (pyrexia)
- hyperthermia
- hypothermia.

Fever

Fever (pyrexia) is an elevation in body temperature up to 41°C. It can be caused by inflammation as a result of pyrogen/interleukin-1 released in response to the invasion of the body by microorganisms or other foreign substances (Seeley et al 2008). This initiates an upward displacement of the hypothalamic 'set point' for temperature control. As the set point has been raised the body responds by increasing temperature to this new level. We usually associate fever with infection and it cannot be denied that a fever is one of the signs of infection. However, any large scale tissue damage within the body will result in an inflammatory reaction and hence a rise in body temperature. You might see this in clients following major surgery, or following a myocardial infarction, where a spike in temperature might be seen in the first 24–36 hours after the event. A rise in temperature is said to help the body's immune responses eliminate the pathogens. In addition, metabolism in all cells is increased as their temperature rises; thus healing and repair processes are accelerated.

Hyperthermia

This is caused by a failure of the thermoregulatory system. The body becomes dangerously overheated when there has been prolonged exposure to heat (often as a result of high ambient air temperatures); exercise in the heat is usually a contributory factor, as is high humidity and a failure to maintain fluid intake.

In the early stages loss of energy, cramps in the legs, arms or back with associated fatigue, dizziness and irritability emerge. As the body temperature rises further, more serious neurological and mental disturbances occur such as fitting or periods of unconsciousness. Due to the loss of large volumes of fluid as sweat there may be circulatory collapse with the client showing signs of hypovolaemic shock. As the temperature rises even higher there is a large reduction in sweating and coma usually occurs as the core body temperature approaches 42 °C (Montague et al 2005).

Heat exhaustion and heat stroke are sometimes defined as different stages of hyperthermia. However, such a distinction is usually arbitrary and difficult to define, and the treatment for both conditions follows the same principles (controlled cooling, rehydration, protection from the environment). There is also a risk that some people's condition may be seen as not that serious – 'it's only heat cramps'. All clients with hyperthermia require expert care and attention.

Hypothermia

The effects of hypothermia vary with the speed of onset and how far the temperature falls. At 35°C there may be shivering, cold, pale, dry skin and apathy. A fall of body temperature to below 34°C causes mental confusion and sluggishness and further reductions result in dysfunction of the thermoregulatory system. Shivering in an attempt to gain heat ceases and loss of consciousness results. Muscle rigidity follows with associated cardiac dysrhythmias and eventual death (Holtzclaw 1993, cited by Montague et al 2005). The elderly, the very young and homeless people are particularly vulnerable during the winter months in the UK.

Alcohol and drugs can exacerbate hypothermia. The role of drugs and alcohol in causing hypothermia cannot be underestimated; it is quite possible to develop profound hypothermia in mid-summer by ingesting a cocktail of alcohol, street drugs and prescription medications either for pleasure or with the intention of suicide.

Children have a protective mechanism that is triggered if they fall into cold water. This response is referred to as the dive reflex, and results in a decreased heart rate and an increased cerebral and cardiac blood flow. As children are small in size they have a relatively smaller circulating blood volume, which means that the cold water in the lungs rapidly chills the blood in the pulmonary circulation which then results in brain cooling and a reduction in the brain's oxygen (O_2) requirements. Consequently, a child may survive immersion in cold water for longer periods of time than an adult.

THE CONTROL OF BLOOD PRESSURE

Blood pressure is the pressure that is exerted on the walls of the blood vessels in which blood is contained. Its level is dependent upon the interaction of three components:

- the volume of blood in the circulatory system
- the heart rate (velocity)
- the resistance offered by constricted blood vessels (peripheral resistance).

Blood pressure is usually recorded as a pair of figures, one higher than the other. Systolic blood pressure (the upper value) reflects the maximum pressure produced by the left ventricle during contraction, or systole. Diastolic blood pressure (lower value) represents the pressure in the artery at the end of relaxation of the left ventricle, known as diastole. The range of normal blood pressure (normotension) varies according to age (Table 7.1).

Factors contributing to a change in blood pressure

Blood pressure is needed to drive blood around the circulatory system, ensuring delivery of oxygen and nutrients and the removal of wastes. This is known as perfusion. Blood flow varies in different regions of the body and in different organs; thus we might talk of renal perfusion or cerebral perfusion. The body uses a range of compensatory mechanisms to maintain adequate blood pressure and hence perfusion. If the needs of an organ or region of the body increase then the delivery of blood to that area will also have to increase to meet the needs.

The pumping action of the heart is one of the main factors that generates blood pressure. The speed with which the heart contracts each minute (heart rate) multiplied by the amount of blood it expels per contraction (stroke volume) is referred to as the cardiac output (i.e. cardiac output = heart rate × stroke volume), and should this increase, a corresponding increase in blood pressure will be observed (Seeley et al 2008).

Another factor that must be borne in mind is the degree of friction created when blood travels rapidly through the blood vessels. This is referred to as peripheral resistance.

Table 7.1 Average blood pressure values, taken from 250 000 healthy individuals (from Durkin 1979)

Age (years)	(mmHg) Systolic	Diastolic
Newborn	80	46
10	103	70
20	120	80
40	126	84
60	135	89

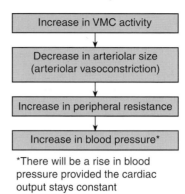

*There will be a rise in blood pressure provided the cardiac output stays constant

Figure 7.3 Increase in vasomotor centre (VMC) activity.

The widening (vasodilatation) or narrowing (vasoconstriction) of a blood vessel will result in either a reduction or increase in this friction of blood against the walls of the blood vessels and, as a consequence, a decrease or increase in the blood pressure. A division of the autonomic nervous system called the sympathetic nervous system regulates the size of blood vessels. The middle layer in the arteriolar wall, called the tunica media, is in a state of partial contraction as a result of continual activity by the sympathetic division of the autonomic nervous system. This is referred to as sympathetic tone and the tone derives from a group of cells in the vasomotor centre within the medulla oblongata in the brain. An increase or decrease in vasomotor centre (VMC) activity will lead to a corresponding increase or decrease in blood pressure (Fig. 7.3).

Reflection and portfolio evidence

Using your biological sciences textbook, review the effects on the homeostatic control of blood pressure of:

- The baroreceptor control system.
- A drop in blood flow through the kidney (renal perfusion).

Review the relative effects of each of these mechanisms when:

- You get patients up suddenly from a lying position to a standing position and they complain of feeling dizzy and faint.
- A victim of a stabbing loses a large amount of blood.

THE PULSE

Contraction of the left ventricle forces blood into the aorta and as a result creates distension and elongation in the arterial wall. As a consequence of this distension, the wave passing along an artery can be felt whenever it is pressed carefully against a bone in places such as the wrist (radial and ulnar pulses), ankle (posterior tibial pulse), neck (carotid pulse) and groin (femoral pulse) areas (Fig. 7.4).

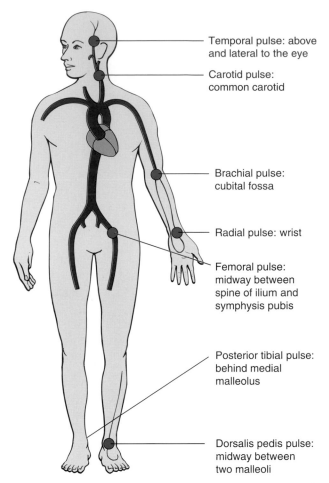

Temporal pulse: above
and lateral to the eye

Carotid pulse:
common carotid

Brachial pulse:
cubital fossa

Radial pulse: wrist

Femoral pulse:
midway between
spine of ilium and
symphysis pubis

Posterior tibial pulse:
behind medial
malleolus

Dorsalis pedis pulse:
midway between
two malleoli

Figure 7.4 Common sites in the body where pulses can be felt (from Montague et al 2005, with kind permission of Elsevier).

In babies less than 1 year of age heart rate is measured by listening with a stethoscope to the apex beat. This is defined as the heart beat which is heard at the apex or lower tip of the heart. The nurse listens for the characteristic 'lub-dub' sounds and counts each full cardiac cycle for 1 minute to determine the apical rate (Lewis & Timby 1993). In young children the brachial pulse is the most common site for measurement of pulse.

When trying to establish information about a patient's pulse, it is important to consider three factors:

- rate
- rhythm
- strength of the pulse wave.

Pulse rate

Pulse rate (Table 7.2) indicates the speed with which the heart is beating, and it varies with age. A rapid pulse is called a tachycardia and may be triggered by excitement, anxiety or exertion; however, it is also indicative of

Table 7.2 Normal pulse rates per minute at various ages

Age	Approximate range	Approximate average
Newborn	120–160	140
1 month to 12 months	80–140	120
2 years	80–130	110
2 years to 6 years	75–120	100
6 years to 12 years	75–110	95
Adolescence	60–100	80
Adulthood	60–100	80

problems such as haemorrhage or fever. Conversely, a slow pulse is referred to as bradycardia. In health, a well-trained athlete may exhibit bradycardia because their heart muscle is very efficient. Bradycardia can be indicative of heart and neurological disease and is also caused by stimulation of the parasympathetic nervous system.

Pulse rhythm

The normal pulse is regular and the time between each beat is constant. If the normal rhythm of ventricular contraction alters, the interval between beats is interrupted. This can be due to a heart beat occurring earlier (premature) or later or a missed beat. An irregular pulse pattern is called an arrhythmia or dysrhythmia. Some dysrhythmias are there all the time and are continuous; others come and go and are intermittent, and may be triggered by certain events, or even something as simple as a cup of coffee! Sinus arryhthmia is a change in rhythm more commonly found in children and is associated with an increase in heart rate on inspiration and a decrease on expiration (Montague et al 2005). Other changes are often associated with cardiovascular disease and can be life-threatening if cardiac output is seriously affected (see Ch. 4, 'Resuscitation and emergency care').

Pulse strength

Pulse strength can be separated into two important factors:

- volume
- tension.

Pulse *volume* is the degree of distension felt in the arterial wall in response to the pressure wave exerted on ventricular contraction. It usually relates to the amount of blood pumped out with each contraction.

An altered pulse volume is often described as being:

- Weak and thready – here the pulse is difficult to feel and disappears if slight pressure is exerted.
- Bounding and full – here the pulse is easy to feel; it is pronounced and strong and does not disappear with moderate pressure (Torrance & Elley 1997).

Tension is specifically related to blood pressure. More force is needed when compressing the artery to feel for a pulse when the blood pressure is high. Conversely, less force is required when the blood pressure is low. When automated equipment is used to measure the pulse rate, such as a pulse oximeter, it is important to manually check rhythm and strength as the equipment will not detect this.

Reflection and portfolio evidence

In the practice laboratory:

- Measure and comment on the rate, rhythm and strength of the pulse rate of your peer group.
- Note any differences related to age and other factors such as recent exercise.

In your practice placements:

- Observe the different sites for taking the pulse in different client groups.
- Under supervision, practise taking the pulse of individual clients and note any changes and the reason for those changes in rate, rhythm and strength.

RESPIRATORY HOMEOSTASIS

This section is concerned with the physiology of breathing and gaseous exchange, and the way that respiratory and cardiovascular systems work together to maintain homeostasis.

The balance of respiration

The primary purpose of respiration is to supply the cells of the body with oxygen (O_2) and remove carbon dioxide (CO_2). The three basic processes involved are:

- Pulmonary ventilation (otherwise known as breathing), which is concerned with air passing into (inspiration) and out of (expiration) the respiratory passageways in an exchange with the atmosphere.
- External respiration, which refers to the exchange of respiratory gases between the lungs and the blood.
- Internal respiration, which is the exchange of respiratory gases between the blood and the cells of the body.

The process of pulmonary ventilation relies upon two characteristics of gases such as air. Firstly, gases move from areas of high pressure to areas of lower pressure along pressure gradients. Secondly, there is an inverse relationship between volume and pressure – i.e. if you increase the volume the pressure goes down and if you decrease the volume of a fixed amount of gas the pressure rises. This universal property of gases is termed Boyle's law (Cree & Rischmiller 2001). In the respiratory system there is a continuous movement of air into and out of the lungs along pressure gradients. Upon inspiration, contraction of the diaphragm and the intercostal muscles cause the volume of the chest cavity, and hence the lungs, to increase. This causes the pressure inside the lungs to drop below atmospheric pressure. This leads to a movement of air from the atmosphere to the lungs during inspiration. However, on expiration, when the diaphragm and the intercostal muscles return to their normal position, the pressure gradient is reversed and air moves out of the lungs.

Once the tissues of the body have used the O_2 it is essential not only that the waste product CO_2 is removed, but also that O_2 concentrations are replenished. Gas exchange in the lungs is the process whereby there is a movement of O_2 into the blood in the pulmonary blood capillaries, while CO_2 moves outwards into the lung alveoli. This movement of gases is brought about by their movement along concentration gradients; this is where gases move by diffusion from areas of higher concentration to areas of lower concentration (Cree & Rischmiller 2001). In mixtures of gases, concentration is often measured as partial pressure in mmHg or kPa rather than in grams or litres. Figure 7.5 refers to the partial pressures of O_2 (pO_2) and CO_2 (pCO_2). Because the pO_2 in the alveoli is greater than in the pulmonary blood vessels, O_2 moves down the concentration gradient. The diffusion of O_2 from alveoli to blood capillaries allows deoxygenated blood to be converted to oxygenated blood. The diffusion of CO_2 from the blood capillary to the alveoli works on exactly the same principle as O_2 diffusion. Due to the relatively high partial pressure of CO_2 (pCO_2) in the pulmonary blood capillary and the low pCO_2 in the alveoli, CO_2 diffuses down its concentration gradient (see Fig. 7.5).

On completion of gas exchange in the lungs, oxygenated blood is transported back to the left atrium via the pulmonary veins, and thence to the circulation and tissue cells via the aorta. Exchange of gases between the blood capillaries of the tissues and the tissue cells themselves is referred to as internal respiration and works on the same principles as the exchange of gases seen in the lungs (see Fig. 7.5).

Oxygen transport

Blood plasma, i.e. blood without red blood cells, can only carry 0.3 mL of oxygen per 100 mL, far too little to meet the oxygen demands of the body. The addition of red blood cells (erythrocytes) increases the oxygen carrying capacity of the blood to 20 mL per 100 mL. The reason that red blood cells are so efficient at carrying oxygen is due to the presence of large amounts of haemoglobin (Hb) in each erythrocyte. Haemoglobin is a protein in which the haem portion contains

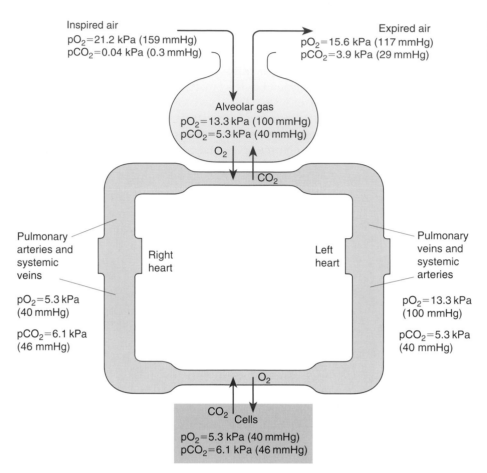

Inspired air
pO_2=21.2 kPa (159 mmHg)
pCO_2=0.04 kPa (0.3 mmHg)

Expired air
pO_2=15.6 kPa (117 mmHg)
pCO_2=3.9 kPa (29 mmHg)

Alveolar gas
pO_2=13.3 kPa (100 mmHg)
pCO_2=5.3 kPa (40 mmHg)
O_2
CO_2

Pulmonary arteries and systemic veins

Right heart

Left heart

Pulmonary veins and systemic arteries

pO_2=5.3 kPa (40 mmHg)
pCO_2=6.1 kPa (46 mmHg)

pO_2=13.3 kPa (100 mmHg)
pCO_2=5.3 kPa (40 mmHg)

O_2
CO_2 Cells
pO_2=5.3 kPa (40 mmHg)
pCO_2=6.1 kPa (46 mmHg)

Figure 7.5 The process of respiration (from Montague et al 2005, with kind permission of Elsevier).

four atoms of iron, each of which is capable of attaching itself to a molecule of O_2. Therefore, four molecules of O_2 can combine with one molecule of Hb (Fig. 7.6). When the Hb is fully saturated with O_2 (oxyhaemoglobin) it is bright red, while a gradual diminution in the O_2 content results in a dark red coloration (deoxyhaemoglobin).

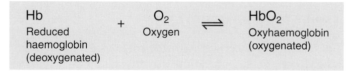

Hb
Reduced haemoglobin (deoxygenated)

$+$

O_2
Oxygen

$\rightleftharpoons$

HbO_2
Oxyhaemoglobin (oxygenated)

Figure 7.6 The association of oxygen with haemoglobin. This is a reversible reaction as denoted by the two-way arrow.

Control of the respiratory system

The control of the respiratory system is an interrelated one between neural and chemical stimuli, which regulate the underlying rhythm of breathing in order to meet the metabolic requirements of the body. Many factors affect respiratory rate and they are summarised in Figure 7.7.

Chemical control is related specifically to levels of acidity (pH). The biggest factor influencing blood pH is CO_2 in the blood, hence the control of breathing is usually seen as being a response to CO_2 levels; however, you need to remember that anything altering levels of blood acidity will alter the breathing pattern. Changes in pH or CO_2 are quickly reflected in similar changes in the cerebrospinal fluid (CSF)

Reflection and portfolio evidence

Haemoglobin (Hb) is so important in the carriage of O_2 that a reduction in Hb concentration from whatever cause will be a threat to the patient or client. In maintaining or restoring homeostasis the patient or client may need to have a blood transfusion. During your practice placements:

- Find out where, how and from whom blood is obtained for transfusion.
- How soon after obtaining blood from a donor should it be transfused into the recipient and what changes can occur to donor blood during storage?
- Are there any other intravenous fluids that can be given as a replacement for blood? What are the problems with these fluids in relation to restoring O_2 homeostasis?

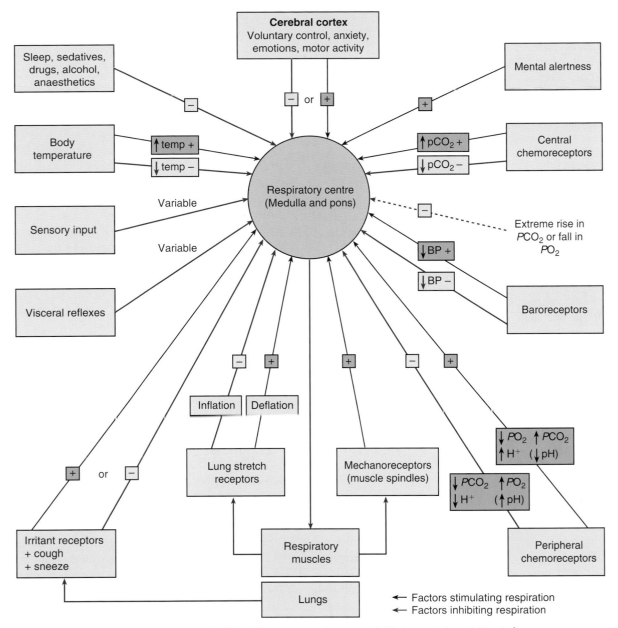

Figure 7.7 Factors that affect respiratory homeostasis (from Montague et al 2005, with kind permission of Elsevier).

found within the ventricles of the brain. Chemoreceptors in the brain detect any increase in CO_2 concentration in the CSF, likewise peripheral chemoreceptors in the arch of the aorta monitor pH/CO_2 concentrations of arterial blood. High levels of CO_2 stimulate a feedback loop through the respiratory centre that will result in an increase in the rate and depth of breathing in order to return the blood CO_2 concentration to normal and therefore maintain homeostasis. Low blood oxygen levels (hypoxia) can act as a respiratory stimulant but the body is relatively insensitive to hypoxia as a respiratory drive. If someone's breathing increases it is usually a response to expel more CO_2 rather than a lack of oxygen.

Neural control is via areas within the respiratory centre, which have the ability to stimulate and inhibit respiration. These areas include the following:

- The medullary rhythmicity area controls the rhythm of respiration.
- The pneumotaxic area controls the smooth transition between inspiration and expiration and inhibits inspiration to prevent over-inflation of the lungs.
- The apneustic area controls the smooth transition between inspiration and expiration and inhibits expiration.

An understanding of the neural and chemical control of respiration is helpful when assessing respiration.

The voluntary control of breathing is achieved through descending pathways from the cerebral cortex to the medullary respiratory centre. Voluntary control is limited in duration, it is demonstrated during hyperventilation, breath holding, singing, speech and deep breathing for relaxation. Enhancing voluntary control through teaching patients how to adapt their breathing can be useful in managing respiratory problems.

CARE DELIVERY KNOWLEDGE

A fundamental component of a nurse's role is the thorough and accurate physiological assessment of children and adults in whatever healthcare setting. The information gained provides the foundation for nursing decisions and contributes towards the decisions of other health professionals. It is vital that changes in homeostasis are detected promptly and monitored as they can indicate serious alterations in health due to disease, injury, treatments, surgery and medications. Screening for changes that occur more slowly is also important within the context of health promotion and the prevention of disease.

Physiological assessment involves the collection of both measurable and subjective information, the most common of which are:

- blood pressure
- pulse
- temperature
- respiration
- fluid balance
- skin condition and pallor.

These measurements and observations are often referred to as vital signs.

It is important to recognize that vital signs can remain within the normal range despite serious illness or injury. Compensatory mechanisms can mask an underlying problem as the body strives to maintain homeostasis. It is therefore crucial always to assess the whole patient for any change, using a range of measurements and observations, and listen to how the patient reports feeling. The converse situation can also arise; you may detect a low blood pressure in a patient who appears perfectly healthy.

Single measurements are not generally acted upon in isolation as temporary changes can occur in response to emotional, physical and environmental factors such as pain and anxiety, or the measurement could be inaccurate. Monitoring for any pattern or trends emerging in the observations is a more reliable indication of a change (Oakey & Slade 2006).

GENERAL PRINCIPLES

When carrying out observations the nurse must ensure that the person's privacy, dignity, safety and comfort are maintained and that, when possible, verbal consent is sought before commencing a procedure (this is discussed later). The results of observations should be explained to the patient. The nurse must also ensure that:

- Correct equipment is used and maintained in good working order.
- Correct techniques are followed and reflect local/national guidelines.
- Measurements taken are accurate, clearly documented and communicated to the patient's doctor and nurse if they fall outside the normal range for that person.
- Measurements are performed when there is a rational patient-centred reason to do so.
- Any problems identified and subsequent nursing interventions are recorded in the patient's nursing records.
- Measurements are performed by competent healthcare staff.

MEASUREMENT OF TEMPERATURE

A thorough knowledge of thermoregulation and the factors that influence it provides a valuable contribution to decision making in many aspects of nursing practice. This knowledge can be applied to health education, for example when advising an elderly person on how to prevent hypothermia. It influences decisions about the environment of care, such as minimizing an infant's heat loss during bathing by ensuring a warm, draught-free environment. Importantly, this knowledge also forms the basis for the assessment, planning, implementation and evaluation of care of those individuals who have the potential for or an actual altered body temperature. Those most at risk of thermoregulatory disturbance are the very young, the elderly and people with chronic or acute illness. People with mental health problems and people with learning disabilities are also at risk as they may not perceive danger or be able to alter their behaviour accordingly. The effects of limited mobility and an inadequate nutritional intake are particularly important as they limit heat-gaining mechanisms. Alterations in body temperature may indicate a physical problem, as occurs when temperature is raised due to an infection, or a behavioural problem such as dressing inappropriately for the weather conditions.

Assessment of temperature

The assessment of temperature involves observing and touching the skin, noting any change in behaviour, and listening to how the patient reports feeling (Woollons 1996). Specific aspects to consider are:

- Is the skin excessively warm or cool, dry or moist? (Use the back of your fingers as they are more sensitive to temperature.)

- Are the extremities pale, mottled or flushed?
- Is the patient shivering? Shivering can occur when a person is cold or during the heat-gaining phase of pyrexia. It causes discomfort in the short term; however, prolonged uncontrolled shivering can lead to exhaustion, pain and helplessness (Montague et al 2005). It is also important to remember when caring for young infants (under 1 year of age) that they cannot shiver.
- Has the patient's behaviour changed (e.g. restlessness, lethargy, delirium)?
- Does the client's behaviour indicate that they are feeling hot or cold?
- You may also need to take a history, such as are there any signs of infections, e.g. chest infections, wound infections or urinary tract infections; how much have they been eating and drinking recently; are they on any medications?

It is important both in the home and in institutional settings to assess the environment, particularly air temperature, heating and ventilation, dampness and draughts, and if appropriate to ensure that clothing and bedding are available. Nurses are responsible for providing a safe and comfortable environment of care and must report promptly any problems that arise.

Reflection and portfolio evidence

Consider what sort of actions or behaviour an adult, an infant and a child might demonstrate with decreased body temperature and raised body temperature.

- During your practice placements, note any differences between expected behaviour and what you witness.
- Discuss the possible reasons for these differences with practice staff and your tutor.

Accurate measurements of temperature

The aim of temperature measurement is to provide an objective approximation of core body temperature. Measurements must be accurate and the method used safe and acceptable to the patient.

Safety is particularly relevant when considering the risks of broken glass and mercury toxicity associated with the use of a glass and mercury thermometer. Although used less frequently these are still available in some healthcare settings. Mercury is a highly toxic substance and is extremely hazardous. If a thermometer breaks, mercury vapour is emitted into the atmosphere and may be inhaled or absorbed through the skin, and if not correctly disposed of, mercury remains in the environment for years (Cutter 1994). The handling and disposal of mercury is controlled by the 1989 Control of Substances Hazardous to Health (COSHH) regulations (Health and Safety Commission 1988). The Medicines and Healthcare products Regulatory Agency (MHRA) (2008) gives information on the use of safer alternatives. The clinical thermometer has been largely replaced by the use of electronic/digital probes and disposable and infrared tympanic thermometers. These devices are quicker and safer to use and generally considered to be accurate (Carroll 2000).

The nurse needs to consider the three main variables that influence the accuracy of temperature measurement (Woollons 1996). These are:

- the site
- the measuring device
- the technique.

Choosing a site

The best sites for core temperature measurement are those that are in close proximity to major arteries and organs in the central core of the body and are well insulated from external factors. The pulmonary artery is considered the optimal core site, but this measurement requires the insertion of a pulmonary artery catheter and thermistor, which are only suitable for use in high-dependency or critical care areas. Key factors to consider when choosing a site are:

- the individual's age and health status
- the degree of accuracy required
- accessibility and acceptability
- the degree of cooperation.

The most commonly used sites are the mouth, tympanic membrane, axilla and less frequently the rectum. All have relative advantages and disadvantages that require consideration. Table 7.3 lists these and the devices suggested to take the measurement.

Evidence-based practice

Research available that compares the accuracy of different sites includes the following:

- Moran et al (2007) examined the use of tympanic temperature measurement in critically ill adults. They compared the performance of tympanic thermometers against the gold standards of pulmonary artery temperature measurement and urinary bladder temperatures. They found that tympanic thermometers performed poorly in this sub-group of patients
- Gilbert et al (2002) examined the use of tympanic and oral temperatures in adult surgical patients. They found no significant difference between the average tympanic and oral temperatures. They support the use of tympanic temperature measurements.

Table 7.3 Advantages and disadvantages of different thermometry sites

Site	Advantage	Disadvantages	Thermometer
Oral	• Good correlation with core temperature due to close proximity of the lingual and sublingual arteries and thermoreceptors • Suitable for most older children and adults • Easily accessible and usually acceptable to patients	• Needs accurate positioning of the thermometer in the sublingual pocket • Prior eating, drinking and smoking or mouth breathing, poor lip seal and talking during the measurement can influence accuracy • Not suitable for infants, young children and confused or restless adults • Cross-infection is a potential risk with any shared thermometer	• Glass and mercury • Electronic/digital • Tempadot
Tympanic	• Good correlation with core temperature due to close proximity of the eardrum to the carotid artery and hypothalamus • Suitable for most children and adults • Ease of access and very rapid reading time	• Poor positioning, use of incorrect probe size and poor operating technique can influence accuracy	• Tympanic infrared
Axilla	• Useful for patients when you can't use the oral or tympanic site, e.g. following surgery or trauma • Provides a good approximation of temperature, as long as site is documented	• Peripheral measurement, therefore not to be used in hypothermia or shock • Site not well insulated from the environment; position difficult to maintain • Need to disrupt bedding and clothing	• Glass and mercury • Electronic/digital • Tempadot
Rectal	• Good correlation with core temperature • Useful for patients with hypothermia or who are unconscious. Although very accurate in young children, its use is in decline and questioned	• Potential discomfort, trauma/rectal perforation and embarrassment • Site not easily accessible • Unsuitable for a restless child or adult • Accuracy affected by presence of stool	• Glass and mercury • Electronic/digital

Choice of thermometer

The devices available are:

- glass and mercury thermometer
- electronic (probe and digital display) thermometers (Fig. 7.8)
- liquid crystal thermometer (disposable forehead strip)

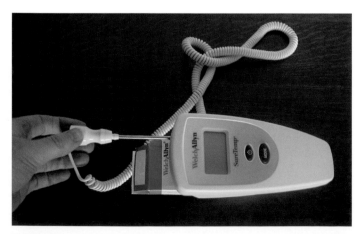

Figure 7.8 An electronic thermometer (courtesy of Welch Allyn UK Ltd).

- TempaDOT™ (a disposable strip impregnated with heat-sensitive chemicals, which change colour as temperature alters)
- tympanic membrane thermometers (Fig. 7.9).

The criteria for choosing a device include accuracy, reliability, adaptability across age groups and sites, safety, ease of use, low risk of cross-infection, cost-effectiveness, full range of temperature measurements, durability, maintainability and anti-theft properties. Careful consideration needs to be taken in choosing an appropriate site and device for children; a recent study identified that children preferred the tympanic thermometer because it was fast and comfortable (Pickersgill 2003).

Technique

Using the correct technique should ensure a safe and accurate temperature measurement. This involves having knowledge of both the site and the device being used and minimizing extraneous variables such as drinking before an oral measurement. Manufacturer's guidelines must be followed and electronic equipment will need regular servicing to ensure accuracy. Minimizing the risk of cross-infection with any device is paramount and disposable covers must be used with all probes.

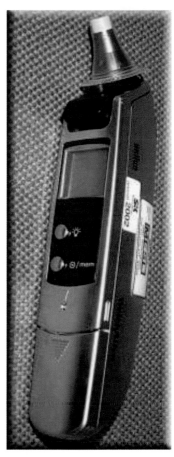

Figure 7.9 A tympanic thermometer (courtesy of Welch Allyn UK Ltd).

Pyrexia

Pyrexia is defined as a core temperature above 37.2 °C (Martini 2006); this commonly occurs in response to an infection or tissue damage. Decisions about nursing care are determined by the stage of the pyrexia (Table 7.4). If the rise in temperature is slight, symptoms may not be observable.

If the temperature rises above 40 °C it can affect cerebral function and cause restlessness and delirium due to nerve cell irritability. Febrile convulsions are a particular risk in infants and young children because their thermoregulation mechanisms are immature.

Decision–making exercise

Oliver is 3 years old and has been generally unwell for the past 2 days with a temperature fluctuating between 38°C and 39°C. The general practitioner diagnoses an ear infection and prescribes antibiotics. Oliver's parents ask you for advice on using paracetamol to reduce his temperature.

- Decide on what advice you would give Oliver's parents on how to manage the pyrexia.
- What is the likely cause of the pyrexia?
- What are the latest National Institute for Health and Clinical Excellence guidelines on the use of paracetamol in fever in children (National Institute for Health and Clinical Excellence 2007)?
- Find out how paracetamol reduces temperature and review the advice you would give Oliver's parents about its use in this case.

Table 7.4 Stages in pyrexia with nursing management

Stage	Features	Nursing management
Stage 1: heat gaining	• Patient complains of feeling cold and shivery • If a child, looks pale and feels cold to the touch peripherally	• Promote rest and comfort in a warm draught-free environment and adjust bedding to maintain comfort • Administer prescribed antipyretics
Stage 2: heat dissipation	• Patient looks flushed and complains of feeling hot • Diaphoresis (sweating) • Thirst and dry mouth • Headache • Reduced appetite • Disorientation • Lethargy • Aching • Weakness • Pulse and respiratory rate increase	• Promote rest • Adjust environment and bedding to increase the circulation of cool air – use a fan, but do not direct at the patient as this causes vasoconstriction • Encourage fluids • Reassure and explain what is happening • Administer prescribed antipyretics
Stage 3	• Return to normal	

Hypothermia

Hypothermia is defined as a core temperature below 35°C (Montague et al 2005). It can develop gradually over a period of time or have a sudden acute onset. The main aims of care are to reduce further loss of heat and to promote the return of a normal body temperature with the minimum of complications, if possible by natural warming. The temperature should return to normal at a rate of no more than 0.5°C/hour. Rapid uncontrolled rewarming will lead to peripheral vasodilatation; this causes a fall in blood pressure and the return of cold acidotic peripheral blood to the heart. This may precipitate a cardiac arrest.

Early signs of hypothermia (i.e. when the core temperature is between 35°C and 33°C) are:

- patient looks and feels cold
- puffy face and husky voice
- pale, cool and waxy skin
- shivering (the ability to shiver decreases as temperature falls below 34°C)
- fatigue and impaired cognitive function
- drowsiness.

Later signs of hypothermia (i.e. when the core temperature is lower than 32°C) are:

- reduced heart and respiratory rate and blood pressure
- cyanosis and mottled peripheries
- cardiac arrhythmias
- reduced responsiveness leading to loss of consciousness.

Prevention is central to caring for individuals who are at risk of hypothermia and this is best achieved by educating such individuals and their family and friends about their personal vulnerability and how to minimize their risk (Webster 1995).

Slow, natural rewarming can be achieved by caring for the patient in bed, with lightweight blankets and maintaining a warm environment (26–29 °C). Warm drinks and food can commence as the patient's condition improves. Active strategies are usually decided upon by the medical staff and may include the use of a warming mattress and administering warm intravenous (IV) fluids.

MEASUREMENT OF BLOOD PRESSURE

Blood pressure is a frequently undertaken assessment procedure in adults. It is completed less frequently in children, in whom abnormal blood pressure is usually secondary to an underlying disease (Goonasekera & Dillon 2000).

Assessment

Blood pressure can only be recorded by a physical procedure, unlike some other observations. However, common physical symptoms are associated with abnormal blood pressures. These are listed in Table 7.5. An absence of symptoms does not exclude a problem. People can adapt to an abnormal blood pressure and have no symptoms at all.

There are several ways in which blood pressure can be measured.

> **Reflection and portfolio evidence**
>
> During your practice placements:
>
> - Observe any differences in the way the blood pressure is measured and recorded for different client groups, especially infants and children.
> - Find out if there are local standards for accurately measuring the blood pressure and note how often these standards are audited.

Direct/invasive

This method is infrequently used as it requires insertion of a catheter into an artery, which can be attached to a monitoring system via a pressure transducer. It is a technique used frequently in high dependency and intensive care settings and provides a continuous reading which is very accurate. However, it is impractical and invasive, and therefore unsuitable for most practice situations.

Indirect/non-invasive

Non-invasive methods are the most frequently used. This can be done using automated machines or manual equipment.

- Automated machines

Automated blood pressure equipment is now the most common method of measuring blood pressure in most clinical settings. It is often the preferred method in children, who can become distressed or impatient with manual measurement and as such can make detecting the sounds required (see below) very difficult.

Table 7.5 Symptoms associated with abnormal blood pressure

Hypertension	Hypotension
Pounding headache	Dizziness
Nose bleeds	Fainting
Visual disturbances	Confusion
Chest pain	Palpitations

These machines usually use the oscillometric method (detect vibrations). A compressive cuff is attached to a machine and is inflated either on a timed setting or by the user. The machine then detects oscillations in pressure due to arterial wall movement beneath the cuff. Most-machines detect the mean blood pressure reading; the machine then uses empirically derived algorithms to determine the systolic and diastolic values.

Research is being undertaken to determine the accuracy of these machines, and the British Hypertension Society has made equipment recommendations as a result (O'Brien et al 2001).

It is still important, despite the accuracy of the recommended machines, that healthcare workers have the skill to perform manual blood pressure measurements. Mechanical errors/failures can occur and readings may need verification before treatment is commenced.

- Manual

This technique requires a measuring device with means of manually inflating the compressive cuff. It also requires some means of detecting the reading, usually by auscultation (listening).

The measuring device used is called a sphygmomanometer, of which the most common is the mercury device. As identified in temperature measurement, mercury use is controversial. The Medicines and Healthcare Products Regulatory Agency (MHRA) (2008) gives information on using alternatives.

Aneroid sphygmomanometers can be used, and are safer. However, they need regular calibration as they lose accuracy over time. It is for this reason that mercury sphygmomanometers are often still used (O'Brien et al 2001).

A stethoscope is the most common means of listening to the Korotkoff sounds that enable the pressures to be identified (Fig. 7.10). However, in small children it can be difficult to hear, and therefore a Doppler flow detector may be used. This device uses ultrasound technology to amplify the sound. Only systolic recordings can be detected with the Doppler.

It is important to note that in some patients there is an auscultatory gap in the Korotkoff sounds. After the systolic pressure appears it can briefly disappear again and this can be mistaken for the systolic pressure reading.

Palpation is a means of estimating the location of the systolic pressure. This is done by feeling for the pulse disappearing when inflating the cuff. The cuff can then be inflated to 30 mmHg above this value for auscultation to increase accuracy.

Some very skilled health professionals can accurately palpate the systolic pressure and do not use an auscultatory method at all.

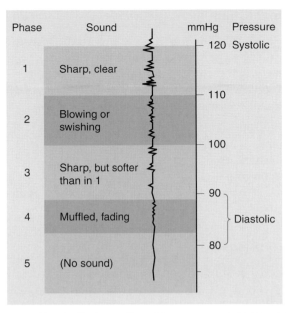

Figure 7.10 Korotkoff phases (from Montague et al 2005, with kind permission of Elsevier).

Procedure

Blood pressure measurement is a skilled procedure that requires practice and consistency. The British Hypertension Society has made recommendations that enable uniform practice when adhered to (O'Brien et al 1997):

- Patients should sit for 3 minutes before measurement takes place.
- Full explanations are needed regardless of age to gain consent and reduce anxiety.
- Equipment should be checked for condition and maintenance before use.
- Cuff selection is very important. Guidelines state that the bladder in the cuff should circle at least 80% of the limb. A selection of cuffs should always be available, particularly in areas attended by children.
- The cuff should be inflated to 30 mmHg above estimated systolic pressure and deflated by 2–3 mmHg/per second. This ensures accurate visualization of reading.
- The limb should be at heart level during measurement.
- Pressure should be recorded to the nearest 2 mmHg. Rounding off to the nearest 5–10 mmHg creates inaccuracies.
- The diastolic reading should be recorded as phase 5 during auscultation (this is when the sounds disappear). In some patient groups the sound may still be present at 0 on the device. If this occurs phase 4, when muffling occurs, should be used. This should be clearly recorded.
- Clinical decisions should never be made on a single reading; the reading should be repeated and other factors disregarded first. For example, patients with coarctation of the aorta will have a high reading on one arm but not the other.

(See also the British Hypertension Society website.)

Documentation

Accurate documentation is very important. Measurement of blood pressure is most useful when considering trends. Therefore each recording needs to be comparable.

The following information should be recorded, and subsequent readings performed in the same way:

- the limb used
- the size of cuff
- equipment used
- position of patient
- status of patient (any other important observations such as anxiety).

Hypertension

Hypertension (high blood pressure) is the chronic elevation of blood pressure above a normal value which is acceptable for the patient's age. This is usually accepted as 100 plus the chronological age of the patient for systolic pressure, and for the diastolic pressure it is usually above 90 mmHg. Hypertension may be mainly systolic, or a combination of systolic and diastolic (Thomas et al 1992). Hypertension can be separated into two categories:

- primary hypertension
- secondary hypertension.

One of the problems with hypertension is that it can be present without symptoms. Longstanding undetected and un-treated hypertension can result in heart failure, stroke and even myocardial infarction.

Primary hypertension

This is commonly referred to as essential hypertension and usually occurs in people who are 35–45 years of age. It is not caused by any specific disease but is associated with a combination of factors. The effects are insidious and develop over many years. Hypertension is frequently discovered by chance at routine health checks. Factors known to predispose individuals to primary hypertension include:

- genetic factors
- racial factors
- age and sex
- diet
- smoking
- environmental factors
- stress.

Secondary hypertension

This develops as a consequence of an underlying disease, and occurs in approximately 5–10% of patients with hypertension and is more common in young patients. The primary causes for secondary hypertension are:

- renal in origin
- stenosis of the aorta, commonly called coarctation
- arteriosclerosis, which causes a narrowing of the lumen of blood vessels leading to increased peripheral resistance.

White coat hypertension

Patients, particularly children, can become very anxious during procedures involving health professionals. This can cause a rise blood pressure, which could be misdiagnosed as hypertension (Sorof & Portman 2000). Ambulatory blood pressure measurement (ABPM) is used to detect this group of patients, for whom treatment is not necessary. A compact automated device is worn at home continuously for 24 hours, and is preset to take regular readings. The data are then downloaded once the equipment is collected, when a trace can be analysed. Other individual/biological factors that should be considered when assessing blood pressure are listed in Table 7.6.

National Service Framework for coronary heart disease

Hypertension is just one risk factor in heart disease, and is closely linked to myocardial infarction and stroke (Beevers et al 2001). Over 110 000 people die from heart problems each year and 300 000 have heart attacks.

This is a serious issue, which has become the target for one of the National Service Frameworks. Prevention is a major focus, identifying people who are at high risk. Monitoring of people with hypertension is an area that is identified, and national strategies are being developed as a result. If myocardial infarction does occur many factors need to be taken into account (this is developed in Evolve 7.2).

Table 7.6 Factors that may alter blood pressure

Increased blood pressure	Decreased blood pressure
Environmental/physiological factors which alter blood pressure	
Exercise	Sleep
Environmental factors Full bladder Alcohol Smoking	
Procedural errors which alter blood pressure	
Limb below heart level Cuff too small Limb unsupported during measurement	Limb above heart level Cuff too large

7.2 – HELPING PEOPLE ADAPT TO CHANGE AND MAINTAIN A SENSE OF BALANCE

• Consider how nursing based on adaptation and maintenance of homeostasis may help your patients.
• Learn about how nursing can help a patient adapt to living following myocardial infarction.

Hypotension

Hypotension is usually a condition in which the systolic blood pressure falls below 100 mmHg in the adult. Remember that a child's normal blood pressure is age related (see Table 7.1). A hypotensive state can be precipitated by either a loss of blood or a fluid shift from one physiological fluid compartment to another. Children are particularly vulnerable as they have a relatively low circulating blood volume and can develop hypovolaemic shock very rapidly. A fall in blood pressure initiates a cyclical chain of events, which initially brings about hypoxia (i.e. a reduction of O_2 to the tissues). Hypoxia leads to cell and tissue damage, resulting in the release of vasodilator substances and a further fall in blood pressure.

MEASUREMENT OF RESPIRATION

Nurses require a sound knowledge of normal respiration together with an understanding of how and why respiratory homeostasis can be disrupted. The factors that influence respiration are complex, often interrelate and can be broadly described as being physical, psychological, social and environmental. In fact very few health problems do not affect respiration in some way.

Knowledge of factors affecting respiration can be effectively used by nurses to:

• promote health and provide health education
• detect respiratory problems through screening
• assess and monitor respiratory status
• provide competent care for individuals with respiratory problems.

Many of the frequently encountered respiratory diseases such as asthma, chronic obstructive pulmonary disease and lung cancer have been closely linked to environmental factors and individual lifestyle and are considered by health professionals to be largely preventable.

Reflection and portfolio evidence

With reference to *The Health of the Nation* (Department of Health 1997):

• Review the targets the government has set that relate to respiratory disease.

• Make a list of the possible opportunities nurses have to promote healthier living that could reduce the incidence and symptoms of respiratory disease.

Assessing respirations

It is relatively simple for a nurse to assess breathing directly by observing the rate, depth and rhythm of respiration (Table 7.7). It is also important to remember that breathing should be quiet and effortless. First level assessment of respiratory function may involve nothing more than listening and watching respiratory effort. These observations provide a good basic indicator of respiratory function. Impaired gas exchange during external and internal respiration is more difficult to assess. If more detailed information is required additional assessment methods can be used, such as:

• an oximeter, which measures the O_2 saturation level in the blood
• laboratory equipment to measure arterial blood gases
• apnoea monitors, which alarm if an infant has an episode of apnoea.

The use of technology supplements the information gained through observation and measurement and allows the nurse to note both subtle and rapid change in a patient's condition. In children there can be a rapid deterioration in condition with diseases such as asthma and bronchiolitis. The oximeter and apnoea monitors are essential.

Table 7.7 Respiratory rates and volumes for infant, child and adult (from Wong 1993)

Age	Rate (breaths/min)
Newborn	35
1 to 11 months	30
2 years	25
4 years	23
6 years	21
8 years	20
10 years	19
12 years	19
14 years	18
16 years	17
18 years	16–18

Observation of breathing

At rest, normal respiration is passive and quiet, and the chest wall and abdomen gently rise and fall with each breath. In more active breathing (e.g. following exercise) there is an increase in the use of the intercostal and accessory muscles, which allows greater lung expansion. This increase in depth of respirations can be observed by the rise and fall of the shoulders, increased movement of the ribcage and the contraction of the accessory muscles in the neck during inspiration. It is important to assess the symmetry of chest movement and the type of breath, while noting the amount of effort required to breathe at rest and during activity. Prolonged laboured breathing at rest and use of the accessory muscles is a cause for concern and indicates serious respiratory dysfunction. Nasal flaring, rib recession and head bobbing in the infant and young child indicate problems that lead to a rapid deterioration in the child's condition (see Ch. 4, 'Resuscitation and emergency care').

It can be difficult to assess breathing during sleep, especially with children; placing a hand gently on the upper abdominal area allows respiratory movement to be felt.

Respiratory rate

The respiratory rate is simply assessed by counting each full breath over 1 minute. Extraneous variables such as talking and the effects of activity need to be considered. An awareness of being observed may alter respiratory rate and depth; counting respirations while appearing to take the patient's pulse can minimize this. The rate of pulse and breathing tends to maintain a ratio of approximately 5:1 (Faulkner 1985). Table 7.7 indicates normal respiratory rates.

Tachypnoea is a respiratory rate above age-adjusted normal values. Tachypnoea is a normal response to increased activity, but can also be an indication of hypoxia (low O_2), hypercarbia (high CO_2), acidosis, raised temperature, pain, stress and anxiety. These latter observations are important in dealing with clients with phobias and anxiety related conditions.

Bradypnoea is a respiratory rate lower than the normal age-adjusted values. It is less commonly seen than tachypnoea and can be an indication of severe hypothermia, opiate drug overdose, acid–base imbalance and neurological dysfunction.

Apnoea is the absence of breathing for at least 10 seconds. It can be transitory, as in 'sleep apnoea', which is associated with a brief obstruction of the upper airway and causes snoring, or it may be life-threatening, as in sudden infant death syndrome.

Respiratory rate is a key indicator of the general level of wellness or illness of clients. It is a sensitive and early indicator of deterioration and is now a cornerstone of early warning scores (Oakey & Slade 2006).

Respiratory depth

The depth of respiration is dependent upon the amount of air inhaled, which is known as the tidal volume. For an average adult at rest it is about 500 mL of expired air. Depth is assessed by observing the degree of movement of the chest wall during inspiration. A more objective way is to measure the amount of air exhaled with a spirometer or peak flow meter (Fig. 7.11). This method is particularly beneficial when caring for individuals with respiratory problems such as asthma and chronic obstructive pulmonary disease.

Posture can affect the depth of respiration; supine, lateral and slumped positions can limit chest expansion. *Orthopnoea* is the term used to describe difficulty in breathing when lying down. Depth is also reduced when the movement of the diaphragm is restricted by obesity, pregnancy or ascites. Patients with respiratory disease tend to feel more comfortable sitting well up and leaning slightly forward or standing as gravity enhances lung expansion. Before making decisions it may be valuable to assess which position if any provides relief from symptoms.

Respiratory rhythm

Normal breathing in adults is regular and uninterrupted except for the occasional sigh, but infants and young children can have a less regular pattern. The rhythm is maintained by the carefully controlled timing of the respiratory cycle. Many of the abnormal patterns in breathing occur as the result of brain injury or disease that affects the respiratory centres in the brain such as the apneustic or pneumotaxic centres mentioned above.

'Cheyne–Stokes respiration' may occur and is characterized by a gradual increase in the rate and depth of respiration followed by a gradual decrease over 30–45 seconds in the depth and rate of respiration. This cycle may be followed by a period of apnoea for up to 20 seconds (Montague et al

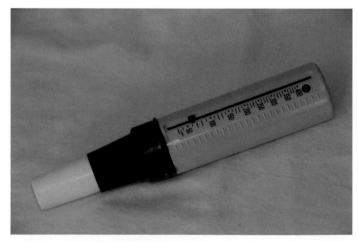

Figure 7.11 Peak flow monitor.

2005). It can be distressing to observe and families need an explanation and reassurance.

Breath sounds

Further information can be gained by assessing the sounds of breathing. Normal respiration is almost silent, therefore any respiratory sound requires investigation. Noisy respiration is referred to as stertorous breathing and can be caused by:

- secretions in the trachea and bronchi, which make a gurgling type of noise
- obstruction to air flow, which sounds like a wheeze or a harsh crowing sound (e.g. stridor in children).

Reflection and portfolio evidence

Learning to use a stethoscope to listen to particular breath sounds is a skill you may have an opportunity to observe if you are involved in specialist nursing of patients with respiratory difficulties or if you work with a specialist nurse practitioner, in a general practitioner practice or alongside a physiotherapist who is also caring for clients with respiratory problems.

- In appropriate practice placements listen to breath sounds that are normal and abnormal under the guidance of the experienced health professional.
- Note and record in your reflective diary your experiences and continue to develop your skills as you gain further experience.

Observation of skin colour

Cyanosis occurs when the blood is not carrying sufficient O_2 to the tissues and deoxygenated haemoglobin accumulates in the tissues. A grey, blue or mauve discoloration of the skin occurs. Peripheral cyanosis is usually seen in the hands and feet and occurs when the circulation is restricted. Central cyanosis is more serious and indicates a lack of arterial blood from the lungs. It is most clearly seen in the tissues of the face and trunk. It can be difficult to assess in dark-skinned people but may be seen on the inside of the lips of inside of the eyelids. Cyanosis is an unreliable and late sign of hypoxia so you should be alert to alterations in the rate and depth of breathing and any behavioural changes in the individual. The use of an oximeter to monitor oxygen saturation levels is strongly indicated in the assessment and monitoring of patients who are at risk of hypoxia.

Behavioural changes

Common responses to inadequate respiratory function include restlessness, confusion, anxiety, fatigue, agitation and loss of concentration. There can be an altered level of consciousness, which will depend upon the degree of cerebral hypoxia and acidosis.

Cough, sneeze and sputum

Coughing and sneezing are the respiratory system's protective mechanism against irritants and obstructions. However, if the nature and frequency of a cough change there may be a respiratory problem. Sputum coughed up from the lungs provides valuable information, and the amount, consistency, colour and odour need to be assessed. Blood-stained sputum is referred to as haemoptysis.

Pain and dyspnoea

Pain on breathing needs to be assessed to determine its cause and can indicate infection, inflammation or trauma. Dyspnoea describes the feelings experienced by a patient of difficult and laboured breathing. Gift (1990) describes dyspnoea as a subjective sensation that is often associated with chronic lung disease and stresses that the intensity of the dyspnoea is not always reflected in the findings when respiratory function is assessed. Gift also provides a useful model based upon three dimensions of dyspnoea: physical, psychological and social. This model is very important for nurses to consider as it reminds us of the holistic needs of our patients and focuses our attention on the effects of living with dyspnoea.

PROFESSIONAL AND ETHICAL KNOWLEDGE

ACCOUNTABILITY

Clinical decision making is an area that is reliant upon professional judgement and knowledge. This is especially important in an age where the use of technology is increasing, and it can be very easy to become dependent upon its use. As identified earlier in this chapter, there are other means of assessing homeostasis which should also be used, such as visual observation. Equipment can produce inaccuracies, and means of verifying abnormal results are needed.

Equally nurses need to be aware of their own limitations in practice. If they are not confident in the results they are obtaining they should seek clarification and guidance. This can be difficult to acknowledge; however, ritualistic practices and inaccurate documentation of observations are not acceptable (Nursing and Midwifery Council 2008). Registered nurses also need to be aware of their responsibilities and accountability when delegating activities to other members of staff, for example students or healthcare assistants, or even to family members (Nursing and Midwifery Council 2008).

CONSENT

Consent is also addressed in the Nursing and Midwifery Council's publication *The Code: Standards of Conduct, Performance and Ethics for Nurses and Midwives* (2008).

In 2001 the Department of Health published revised good practice guidelines for consent. Within this it states that: 'Patients have a fundamental ethical and legal right to determine what happens to their own bodies' (Department of Health 2001b: 9). Observations such as measuring blood pressure, pulse and temperature that involve physically touching patients need to be considered within these guidelines.

Informed consent is fundamental to this, but can become very complex in situations where a patient's health status (physical or mental) is compromised. Although in most situations it is unnecessary to document consent for observation, it may be important to do so in these circumstances.

HEALTH PROMOTION

An important aspect of the nurse's role in health promotion is to empower the patient through sharing information so that they can take an active role in their care and contribute to their own well-being. Explaining why observations are made and the results will often provide the opportunity to answer the patient's questions and discuss related health issues. This may lead to increased insight into their health and promote healthier choices.

PERSONAL AND REFLECTIVE KNOWLEDGE

IDEAS FOR PORTFOLIO AND SKILLS LABORATORY LEARNING

Undertaking the assessment of patients involves understanding a considerable amount of theoretical knowledge as well as mastering a wide range of skills and being able to use your professional judgement. This chapter has alerted you to the scope of knowledge and skills needed, but this should be supplemented by other more specialized texts and consolidated through reflection and discussion of learning in your practice placements. Many of the exercises throughout the chapter will have encouraged you to reflect on your practice experiences. Keeping a record and reviewing these experiences will help you to develop your portfolio.

It is recommended that you take the opportunity to practise your skills in a learning laboratory before commencing your placements. This will help develop your confidence and is important in terms of the quality of care being delivered to clients. When learning how to assess temperature, pulse, respirations and blood pressure on your peers take note of any differences you observe. Experiential exercises could include testing the effects of factors such as exercise, rest, noise, time of day on 'vital signs'.

CASE STUDIES RELATING TO HOMEOSTASIS

The following case studies are included so that you can consolidate knowledge gained from this chapter and your practice experience. In addition to your reflective writing it is useful to collect relevant policies, procedures and literature for your portfolio.

Case study: Adult

Pauline Scott is 56 years old and has had progressive multiple sclerosis for 30 years. She is unable to mobilize and is confined to a wheelchair for most of her day. She lives with her husband, John, who is a retired farmer and her main carer. They live in a rural area in an old farmhouse. The living area is comfortable and warm, but Pauline finds the bathroom and bedroom very cold in the winter and as a result is now washing and dressing in the kitchen, which she finds unsatisfactory.

- What factors would you need to consider when assessing Pauline's ability to maintain her body temperature?
- What advice would you give to Pauline and John about minimizing the risk of hypothermia?
- Find out what other agencies or members of the primary care team could help with this problem.

Case study: Learning disabilities

Malvika Singh is an 8-year-old girl with mild learning disability and profound physical disability. She attends a special needs school in a wheelchair which has been made to accommodate her needs. Malvika's posture is severely affected by scoliosis of her spine and her trunk deviates to the right; she is unable to sit upright. Over the last year she has had repeated chest infections, which have required antibiotic therapy.

- What are the factors that make Malvika at risk of recurrent chest infections?
- Decide on what observations you should take when Malvika has a chest infection and why.
- What could you do to minimize her risk of developing a chest infection?

Case study: Mental health

Paul Grey is a 47-year-old recently divorced man with three school-aged children who live with his wife. Paul has become increasingly anxious and unable to deal with his daily workload. The head of his department, who is aware of the stresses in Paul's personal life, has asked him to seek help through the occupational health unit. The occupational health nurse finds that Paul's blood pressure is elevated at 160/105 mmHg and he is 5 kg overweight. Paul and the nurse discuss his lifestyle and personal problems.

- Review the factors that might have led to the increase in Paul's blood pressure.
- Explore how lifestyle and life events can lead to hypertension (see also Ch. 9, 'Stress, relaxation and rest').
- Decide what ongoing monitoring and health promotion would be appropriate for Paul.

Case study: Child

Jade, a 9-month-old infant, has been admitted to the children's ward accompanied by her 18-year-old mother, Mandy, who lives at home with her mother and father. Jade looks flushed and has a pyrexia of 38°C; she has been crying and irritable and is not taking her feeds. Mandy is very tearful and worried about her baby.

- Decide on which 'vital signs' you need to assess and how often.
- What would you need to consider when assessing these 'vital signs' in Jade?
- Review possible nursing interventions that could be implemented to control Jade's temperature.

SUMMARY

This chapter has drawn together theoretical concepts relating to homeostasis and applied this knowledge in relation to the practice of caring for individuals. It has included:

1. The biological theoretical basis of thermoregulation, blood pressure maintenance, pulse and respiratory homeostasis, and the maintenance of feedback loops in maintaining homeostasis.
2. Behavioural, cultural and environmental influences that may affect an individual's ability to maintain homeostasis.
3. Consideration of factors influencing nurse decision making in monitoring and aiding maintenance of homeostasis for patients. These factors relate to the measurement, assessment and nursing management of body temperature, blood pressure and respiration.
4. Professional and ethical dimensions of patient consent, and nursing accountability in relation to the provision of nursing care.
5. Considerations relating to the use of medical technology in assessment.

Knowledge illuminated within this chapter has been combined with evidence from other referenced sources and applied within a range of situations. Suggestions have been made for portfolio development in relation to management of homeostasis. Further consideration of homeostasis can be found in Evolve 7.3.

7.3 – BIOLOGICAL ADAPTATION AND HOMEOSTASIS

- Revise general control mechanisms seen in living systems.
- Examine the role and function of the endocrine and nervous systems.
- Explore control of blood glucose levels as a further demonstration of a key homeostatic control mechanism.

ACKNOWLEDGEMENTS

The author would like to acknowledge the previous contributions of Helen Dobbins, Gary Adams and Diane Hewson to this chapter.

Annotated further reading and websites

Montague SE, Watson R, Herbert RA (eds) 2005 Physiology for nursing practice. Elsevier, Edinburgh

This excellent physiology textbook provides good back-up information in relation to the biological basis of the elements of homeostasis covered in this chapter.

Mallett J, Doughty L 2000 The Royal Marsden NHS Trust manual of clinical nursing procedures, 5th edn. Blackwell Science, Oxford

A good reference book about how to carry out the skills of measuring homeostasis. The rationale for each of the activities is provided.

Wong DL, Hockenberry MJ, Wilson D et al 2003 Whaley and Wong's Nursing care of infants and children, 7th edn. Mosby, St Louis

For students who wish to specialize in children's nursing, this book is a very comprehensive resource book for all aspects of infant, child and teenage care. See Chapter 1 on assessment of the child.

http://www.dh.gov.uk
From the Department of Health's web page you can access numerous useful web pages on public health policy and health education, National Service Frameworks and screening and environmental issues and health.

http://www.bhsoc.org/default.stm
Website of the British Hypertension Society. This is a good website with guidelines on measuring blood pressure.

References

Age Concern 2008 Older people in the United Kingdom: key facts and statistics 2007. Age Concern, London. Available online: http://www.ageconcern.org.uk/AgeConcern/Documents/Key_facts.pdf (accessed 17 August 2008)

Beevers G, Lip GH, O'Brien E 2001 ABC of hypertension, 4th edn. British Medical Journal, London

Bernard C, (ed) Dastre A 1878–9 Leçons sur les phénomènes de la vie communs aux animaux et aux végétaux. 2 vols. Baillière et fils, Paris

Carroll M 2000 An evaluation of temperature measurement. Nursing Standard 14(44):39–43

Cree L, Rischmiller 2001 Science in nursing, 4th edn. Harcourt, Sydney

Cutter J 1994 Recording patient temperature: are we getting it right? Professional Nurse 9(9):608–616

Department of Health 1997 The health of the nation, 2nd edn. HMSO, London

Department of Health 2001a Health effects of climate change. HMSO, London

Department of Health 2001b Good practice in consent: achieving the NHS plan commitment to patient-centred consent practice. HMSO, London

Durkin N 1979 An introduction to medical science: comprehensive guide to anatomy, biochemistry and physiology. MTP Press, Lancaster

Faulkner A 1985 Nursing: a creative approach. Baillière Tindall, London

Gift A 1990 Dyspnoea. Nursing Clinics of North America 25(4):955–965

Gilbert M, Barton A, Counsell C 2002 Comparison of oral and tympanic temperature in adult surgical patients. Applied Nursing Research 15(1):42–47

Goonasekera CDA, Dillon MJ 2000 Measurement and interpretation of blood pressure. Archives of Disease in Childhood 82:261–265

Health and Safety Commission 1988 The control of substances hazardous to health, regulations. HMSO, London

Helman CG 1994 Culture, health and illness, 3rd edn. Butterworth Heinemann, Oxford

Holtzclaw BJ 1993 Monitoring body temperature. Clinical Issues in Advanced Practice Acute and Clinical Care 4(1):44–55

Kleinman A 1980 Patients and healers in the context of culture. University of California Press, Berkeley

Lewis LW, Timby B 1993 Fundamental skills and concepts in patient care. Chapman & Hall, London

Marriner-Tomey A, Alligood M (eds) 1998 Nursing theorists and their work. Mosby, London

Martini F 2006 Fundamentals of anatomy and physiology. Pearson, San Francisco

Medicines and Healthcare products Regulatory Agency 2008 Mercury in medical devices. Available online: http://www.mhra.gov.uk/Safetyinformation/Generalsafetyinformationandadvice/Product-specificinformationandadvice/Mercuryinmedicaldevices/CON019599 (accessed 12 August 2008)

Mishler J 1981 Social contexts of health, illness and patient care. Cambridge University Press, Cambridge

Montague SE, Watson R, Herbert RA (eds) 2005 Physiology for nursing practice, 3rd edn. Elsevier, Edinburgh

Moran J, Peter J, Solomon P et al 2007 Tympanic temperature measurements: are they reliable in the critically ill? Critical Care Medicine 35(1):155–164

National Institute for Health and Clinical Excellence 2007 Feverish illness in children. NICE, London

Nursing and Midwifery Council 2008 The Code: standards of conduct, performance and ethics for nurses and midwives. Nursing and Midwifery Council, London

Oakey R, Slade V 2006 Physiological observation track and trigger system. Nursing Standard 20(27):48–54

O'Brien E, Waeber B, Parati G, Staessen J, Myers MG 2001 Blood pressure measuring devices: recommendations of the European Society of Hypertension. British Medical Journal 322:531–536

O'Brien ET, Petrie JC, Littler WA et al 1997 Blood pressure measurement: recommendations of the British Hypertension Society. British Medical Journal, London

Office of National Statistics 2006 Mortality in southern England during the 2003 heat wave by place of death. Office of National Statistics, London

Pickersgill J 2003 Temperature taking: children's preferences. Paediatric Nursing 15(2):21–25

Seeley RR, Stephens TD Tate P (eds) 2008 Anatomy and physiology. McGraw Hill, New York

Shmaefsky BR 2007 Applied anatomy and physiology: a case study approach. EMC/Paradigm Publishing, St Paul

Sorof JM, Portman RJ 2000 Ambulatory blood pressure monitoring in the pediatric patient. Journal of Pediatrics 136(5):578–586

Thomas C, Gebert G, Hambach V 1992 Textbook and colour atlas of the cardiovascular system. Chapman & Hall, London

Torrance C, Elley K 1997 Practical procedures for nurses. 3.1 Assessing pulse. Nursing Times 93(42, Suppl.): 1–2

Watson R 1996 Hypothermia. Elderly Care 8(6):25–28

Webster C 1995 Health and physical assessment. In: Heath H (ed) Foundations in nursing practice. Mosby, London, pp 71–102

Wong DL 1993 Whaley and Wong's Essentials of pediatric nursing, 4th edn. Mosby, St Louis

Woollons S 1996 Temperature measurement devices. Professional Nurse 11(8):541–547

Chapter 8

Nutrition

Lindsey Bellringer

KEY ISSUES

SUBJECT KNOWLEDGE

- Energy producing and non-energy producing food, what it is and why it is needed in the body
- The chemical structure of the different food groups
- Storage and use of food in the body
- How metabolism extracts energy from food
- Social and psychological influences on nutrition

CARE DELIVERY KNOWLEDGE

- Assessing nutritional status
- Calculation of body mass index and the healthy range
- Identification of different nutritional needs related to age
- Feeding patients
- Identification of appropriate alternative and supplementary methods of feeding when patients are unable to eat normally
- Alterations in nutritional status
- A review of common disorders of nutrition

PROFESSIONAL AND ETHICAL KNOWLEDGE

- Legal aspects of food safety
- Professional accountability
- Ethical dilemmas in feeding
- Patients' rights

PERSONAL AND REFLECTIVE KNOWLEDGE

- Explore your personal beliefs about nutrition
- Apply your knowledge to professional practice

INTRODUCTION

Food is essential for life; it provides the nutrients we need to maintain our bodies and is integral to our social and cultural life. In the UK there is a large range of affordable foods available so it should be possible to ensure the population as a whole does not suffer from diseases caused by lack of essential nutrients. Increasingly a healthy diet is implicated in the prevention of diseases such as coronary artery disease, bowel cancer and diabetes; there is no lack of information available about these facts. Why then are health professionals still dealing with impaired health and disease due to poor nutrition? Nurses should be able to explain the vast amount of occasionally conflicting information about diet to patients. They must give informed, up-to-date advice and ensure that patients are not left feeling guilty because they have not eaten all the right foods or that they have been unable to provide a healthy diet for their families.

The provision of nutritional care is a challenge to nurses in the institutional setting and also in the wider community. Despite the evidence that good nutrition is essential for individuals' health and recovery from illness, articles appear frequently in professional journals and newspapers highlighting deficiencies in the provision and delivery of food to patients in hospitals (Savage and Scott 2005, Holmes 2007).

There is no shortage of published material about nutritional assessment tools designed to identify patients at risk of malnutrition and provide recommendations for nutritional care planning (Green & Watson 2006, Johnstone et al 2006). The Department of Health produced the resource pack *Essence of Care* (Department of Health 2001) aimed at improving standards of care by using benchmarks of good practice. The food and nutrition benchmark requires that 'Patients/clients are enabled to consume food (orally) which meets their individual need'. Nurses are encouraged to compare practice in their clinical area to the benchmark of good practice and formulate action plans on how to improve the standard of care from initial assessment through to health promotion.

OVERVIEW

This chapter aims to provide you with core knowledge on good nutritional care, ways of providing food and the professional, ethical and legal responsibilities of the nurse in ensuring that patients are nourished.

Subject knowledge

This section deals with functions of food as a source of energy, growth and repair. It outlines the physiological processes of nutritional components and considers the physiological evidence against common contemporary dietary myths. Social and psychological factors and their influence on nutrition are discussed.

Care delivery knowledge

Assessment of the patient's nutritional status to include variation according to age, gender and lifestyle is included. Strategies for planning, implementing and evaluating nutritional care are discussed. Alternative methods of feeding when patients are unable to eat normally are explored.

Professional and ethical knowledge

Legislation, professional responsibility and ethical issues in the provision of food and drink are outlined.

Personal and reflective knowledge

This final part encourages you to reflect on what you have read, consider how you can put it to practice and produce evidence for your learning portfolio.

Four case studies are presented at the end of the chapter, each one relating to one of the nursing branch programmes.

SUBJECT KNOWLEDGE

BIOLOGICAL

ENERGY PRODUCING FOODS

All of the activities we undertake involve the expenditure of energy. Even at rest we require energy for physiological processes; this energy requirement is called basal metabolic rate (BMR) and it is variable between individuals. All of the energy for these processes is derived from food. The amount of food we need is controlled by our energy expenditure; this is called the energy balance.

Weight change = energy input less energy output

The amount of food we eat is determined to a large extent by appetite. The main control of appetite is physiological, involving two centres within the hypothalamus – the feeding (hunger) centre and the satiety (full) centre – which work in opposition to each other. The satiety centre is mainly controlled by the blood glucose concentration and functions to suppress the hunger centre. As the blood glucose level decreases the power of the satiety centre is lowered and the hunger centre becomes active giving rise to the feeling of hunger and the desire to eat. Other physiological influences on appetite are the body fat deposits and the distension of the gut. Psychosocial influences are also important as will be discussed later in this chapter. How the body uses energy producing foods, i.e. carbohydrate, proteins and fats, is discussed below.

Carbohydrates

Carbohydrates should account for more than half the energy intake in the diet. They have a general formula $(CH_2O)_n$ and are manufactured by plants from carbon dioxide, water and energy from sunlight through the process of photosynthesis. By this means the energy of the sun is trapped and made available to animals when they eat the plant.

The most simple carbohydrates, such as glucose, fructose and galactose, contain six carbon molecules and are called monosaccharides. These three monosaccharides all have the formula $C_6H_{12}O_6$ but the positions of the carbon atoms in relation to the oxygen atoms differ. These monosaccharides can combine to form pairs of molecules called disaccharides. This is achieved by the removal of a water molecule and is known as a condensation reaction. Depending on the combination of monosaccharides, different disaccharides are produced. For example:

- The disaccharide we are most familiar with is sucrose – table sugar – and this is simply one glucose molecule joined to one fructose molecule.
- Two molecules of glucose form maltose, which is a disaccharide.
- One molecule of glucose and one molecule of galactose form lactose.

Because of their relatively uncomplicated molecular structure, monosaccharides and disaccharides are quickly absorbed and utilized. They are also referred to as simple sugars. Many glucose molecules joined together form a polysaccharide called starch, which plants use as an energy store, for example the starch in potatoes and cereals. Foods containing these will therefore be high in complex carbohydrate.

Plants use another carbohydrate called cellulose to form their structure. Humans are unable to digest this structural carbohydrate, but ruminants such as cows or sheep are able to break it down and use it for energy.

Many people believe that some forms of simple carbohydrate are more natural and therefore healthier than others and these myths are exploited by the food industry who try to convince us that their products are more healthy than those of their competitors. It is worth remembering that from a nutritional viewpoint there is no difference between glucose, fructose and sucrose and certainly no advantage to cane sugar over beet sugar. Pure carbohydrate from whatever source releases 4.1 kcal/g when metabolized, although foods containing a higher proportion of water and cellulose will have a lower energy density.

Digestion, transport and storage of carbohydrates

All complex carbohydrates must be broken down by the digestive system into monosaccharides before they can be absorbed. The process begins with the action of salivary amylase, which converts starch into the disaccharide maltose. Other starches are split into disaccharides by the pancreatic amylase. The final step is for a series of enzymes in the small intestine to break down the disaccharides into monosaccharides. There is a specific enzyme for each disaccharide, but the names are easy to remember:

- maltose is split by maltase
- sucrose is split by sucrase
- lactose is split by lactase.

Splitting disaccharides also involves putting the water back, a process known as hydrolysis (from the Greek words 'hydro' meaning water, and 'lysis' meaning breaking down).

This is the opposite process to the condensation reaction, which removes water to join the two monosaccharide molecules. Once broken down to monosaccharides in the digestive system, carbohydrates are absorbed in the small intestine and transported via the portal vein to the liver. This raises the concentration of the plasma glucose and stimulates the secretion of insulin by the beta cells of the pancreas. This in turn increases the rate at which the large glucose molecules are able to pass through the cell walls into the cells where they will be broken down to provide energy.

Excessive plasma glucose can be converted into an insoluble carbohydrate, glycogen, which is similar to starch in plants, through the process of glycogenesis. Glycogen is stored mainly in the liver and the muscles and can be converted back to glucose (glycogenolysis) when the plasma glucose concentration falls. When glycogen stores are full any remaining glucose may be converted into fat and stored until it is needed. As the glucose in the blood is used up, insulin secretion decreases and glucagon secretion from the alpha cells of the pancreas increases. Glucagon converts glycogen back into glucose to restore the blood glucose concentration and mobilize the stored fat.

Decision-making exercise

The hormone glucagon is secreted by the alpha cells of the pancreas when the blood glucose concentration falls. This causes a reduction in glycogenesis and an increase in glycogenolysis, which leads to an increase in blood glucose concentration. Glucagon can also be manufactured synthetically and administered by injection.

- What are the indications for the use of synthetic glucagon?
- What is the usual dosage?
- What are the limitations of using synthetic glucagon?

Utilization of carbohydrate: respiration

Carbohydrates are made in the chloroplasts of plant cells through the action of photosynthesis as follows:

$$6H_2O + 6CO_2 + energy \rightarrow C_6H_{12}O_6 + 6O_2$$

When the equation is moving in this direction, energy from the sun is used to form carbohydrate. However, in the mitochondria of animal cells this action is reversed, in the process of respiration, as follows:

$$C_6H_{12}O_6 + 6O_2 \rightarrow 6H_2O + 6CO_2 + energy$$

The energy produced in respiration takes two forms, heat and chemical energy. The heat energy maintains the body temperature. This explains why we get hot when we exercise, as an increase in the metabolism of food in the muscles generates more heat. The chemical energy is used to join phosphate to another molecule to store energy for future use. The commonest example of this action is phosphate (P) joining adenosine diphosphate (ADP) to form adenosine triphosphate (ATP). When energy is required the phosphate bond is broken to revert back to ADP and P so releasing the stored energy.

The process of obtaining energy from glucose occurs in three stages:

1. The first stage, glycolysis, takes place in the cytoplasm of the cell. Here the six-carbon glucose molecule is split into two three-carbon pyruvate molecules. Glycolysis releases eight ATP molecules.
2. If there is no oxygen present (i.e. anaerobic conditions) pyruvate is converted to lactate, which will be reconverted to pyruvate when oxygen becomes available. This costs six ATP molecules. Therefore in the absence of adequate oxygen, the energy yield from glycolysis drops two molecules of ATP. In the presence of oxygen, however, the pyruvate is transported to the mitochondria where it is converted to carbon dioxide and acetyl coenzyme A (acetyl CoA). The acetyl CoA enters

the Krebs cycle where the hydrogen is removed and carbon dioxide is released (aerobic metabolism).

3. In the third stage of the process, called the electron transport chain, the energy is once more used to combine phosphate with ADP to produce ATP. The hydrogen is then combined with oxygen to form water.

The three stages of this glucose metabolism will release sufficient energy from one molecule of glucose to produce 38 molecules of ATP.

The more mitochondria there are in a cell the more reactions can take place and the greater the amount of energy available. The mitochondria increase in response to the energy demand made upon a cell. Consequently this increases the individual's basal metabolic rate. When there is less demand the number of mitochondria decrease. You may notice this effect if you decide to increase your fitness by regular exercise. You will notice that as you continue a programme of training the length of time you are able to engage in activity increases. You see yourself becoming fit. Cells are able to engage in more activity as the number of mitochondria increase in response to the demand made on them during training.

Fats

Fats are solid and oils are liquid, and they are referred to collectively as lipids. They are insoluble in water and have the general formula $CH_3(CH_2)_nCOOH$, which looks complicated but like carbohydrate they only contain carbon, hydrogen and oxygen. Most lipids in the diet are in the form of triglycerides. These are made up of three fatty acids, each attached to a glycerol molecule to form a structure like a letter E, with the glycerol being the vertical stroke. Fatty acids are a line of carbon atoms with hydrogen atoms attached. There are three different forms of fatty acids known as:

- Saturated fatty acids, which contain the maximum possible number of hydrogen atoms.
- Monounsaturated fatty acids, which have two hydrogen atoms missing from each molecule.
- Polyunsaturated fatty acids, which have more than two hydrogen atoms missing from each molecule.

Saturated fats are solid at room temperature whereas mono- and polyunsaturated fats are liquid oils. Generally animal fats are saturated and those from vegetables and fish are unsaturated (two exceptions to this rule are palm and coconut oil). Saturated fat in the diet tends to raise the concentration of the blood cholesterol level whereas monounsaturated fats such as olive oil tend to lower it. Because a high blood cholesterol concentration is linked to arterial disease, the current recommendation is to reduce the total amount of fat in the diet and to limit the

intake of saturated fat so that it constitutes not more than 10% of the energy intake (Food Standards Agency 2008a). Examples of fatty foods include butter, margarine, lard, cooking oil and the fat on meat.

Reflection and portfolio evidence

Read the Cochrane Review: Dietary advice for reducing cardiovascular risk (Brunner et al 2005)

- Reflect on your personal dietary habits and review whether there is a need for you to change your habits to maintain your health.
- Make notes on how you would advise a patient with a high risk of cardiac disease to achieve a healthy diet.
- Write a short information sheet explaining the differences between saturated fatty acids, monounsaturated fatty acids and polyunsaturated fatty acids.
- How would you explain the difference between high density and low density lipoprotein cholesterol?

Under supervision provide the above information to a patient/client at risk and complete for your portfolio of evidence.

Fats are often thought of as being bad but a certain amount is essential for our health and well-being. Fats are needed to make cell membranes, steroid hormones, prostaglandins and bile, and to store energy. However, because fats pack many calories into a small volume it is easy to take too many calories in a high fat diet.

Digestion, utilization, transport and storage of lipids

Lipids are insoluble and form large globules in water; therefore they need to be emulsified. This is achieved in the body by the action of bile (Fig. 8.1). Once emulsified the triglycerides are split by the enzyme lipase into fatty acids and monoglycerides. Short chain fatty acids are absorbed into the blood directly at this point. Most fatty acids are long chain (i.e. they have more than 12 carbon atoms) and these and the monoglycerides take a different pathway to the blood. By combining with bile salts, long chain fatty acids and the monoglycerides form micelles and in this form are then able to enter the epithelial cells of the villi. Once in the epithelial cells lipase acts on the monoglycerides to reduce them to glycerol and fatty acids. Here they are combined with cholesterol and phospholipids to form chylomicrons. These in turn are absorbed into the lacteals of the small intestine and transported through the lymphatic system to enter the blood at the subclavian vein.

As fats are insoluble, absorbed fats are either transported in the blood as chylomicrons or as free fatty acids attached to albumin. These transport molecules are also

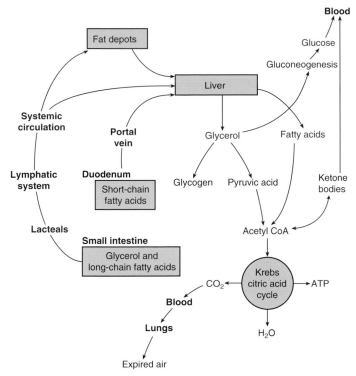

Figure 8.1 Diagram of fat metabolism (from Montague et al 2005, with kind permission of Elsevier)

known as lipoproteins. Because fat is lighter than water the higher the percentage of fat in a lipoprotein the lower the density. Low density lipoproteins (LDLs) carry a high percentage of cholesterol and are therefore associated with a risk to health. The high density lipoproteins (HDLs) on the other hand transport fat from the tissues to the liver to be excreted.

Lipids are either stored on adipose tissue as triglycerides or metabolized by the liver in a process called beta oxidation. The liver cells split pairs of carbon atoms from the fatty acids to form acetyl CoA, which can then enter the Krebs cycle. Excess acetyl CoA is converted into ketones and circulated to other tissues in the body where it is converted back to acetyl CoA and used for energy.

High cholesterol increases the risk of heart disease and strokes; for more information on diagnostic tests and treatment see Evolve 8.1.

8.1 – TESTING AND TREATMENT FOR HIGH CHOLESTEROL

- Define the constituents and functions of cholesterol.
- Differentiate between 'good' and 'bad' cholesterol.
- Outline conditions for accurate measurements.
- Describe how results are interpreted.
- Outline the use of statins.

Proteins

Chemical structure

Proteins share the same properties of fats and carbohydrates. They contain the same three chemicals – carbon, hydrogen and oxygen – but additionally all proteins contain nitrogen. Complex proteins are made up of amino acids linked together by a peptide bond. There is no general formula, but all amino acids have an amine group (NH_2) and an acidic carboxyl group (COOH) in common, with the remainder of the molecule varying depending on which amino acid it is. Although there are only 20 naturally occurring amino acids, the number of possible combinations to form proteins is almost infinite. One very important characteristic of proteins is that each one tends to fold itself into a particular shape which will determine its function. For example if the haemoglobin molecule does not assume its correct shape sickle cell anaemia results. The action of enzymes, which are proteins, also relies on their shape and if this is altered by heat or pH they will not function.

Sources

Many amino acids can be synthesized in the body; those that cannot are known as essential amino acids and must be taken in the diet. Many plants are deficient in one or more of the essential amino acids but a mixture of plant proteins is capable of supplying all the amino acids needed. Meat, fish, eggs and milk have high protein content. Plant sources rich in protein are seeds, with peas, beans and nuts particularly valuable. Cereals and potatoes have a comparatively low percentage of protein but because of the large amount in most diets they can make a significant contribution to total intake.

Decision-making exercise

A colleague has spent the weekend demonstrating against the export of live farm animals. She has decided to become a strict vegan. Of the 20 amino acids in the body it is only possible to synthesize 10 in adequate amounts and it is not possible to synthesize eight at all, nor is it possible to store protein in the body. Therefore if amino acids are to be synthesized it is only possible if combinations of foods containing the elements of amino acids are consumed together.

- What are the implications of protein synthesis for your colleague?
- Which foods contain essential amino acids?
- Which foods contain no essential amino acids?
- Using this knowledge, how would you help your colleague to devise a dietary plan to ensure she receives enough protein?

Utilization, transport and storage

Protein is unique in containing nitrogen so intake and the loss of protein from the body are termed nitrogen balance. Digestive enzymes split the proteins into individual amino acids which can then be absorbed. Once absorbed, the amino acids are used for repair and replacement of cells, and the manufacture of enzymes and hormones; any excess will be deaminated by the liver. This process involves splitting off the nitrogen and converting it into urea, which can then be excreted by the kidneys. The deaminated amino acid remnants can be used to form glucose (glucogenesis), stored as fats, or metabolized to provide energy.

NON ENERGY PRODUCING DIETARY COMPONENTS

The remaining components of the diet do not provide energy but are essential for health. These are water, vitamins, minerals and fibre.

Vitamins

Vitamins are a series of unrelated organic substances that are needed in very small amounts for normal body metabolism. They are divided into those that are fat soluble and those that are water soluble: see Tables 8.1 and 8.2.

Minerals

These inorganic salts are an essential part of the diet and are required for many processes. They include sodium, potassium, chlorine, iron, iodine, chloride, copper, cobalt, zinc, calcium and selenium. The most common minerals are shown in Table 8.3.

Fibre

Fibre is the indigestible part of the diet that comes from plants; it consists of bran, cellulose and other polysaccharides. Although fibre is not essential for life, deficiency is associated with a variety of diseases. Fibre passes unchanged into the colon adding bulk to the faeces, stimulating peristalsis which prevents constipation. Fibre may reduce the risk of bowel cancer by diluting any toxins and carcinogens in the faeces and reducing the length of time they are in contact with the colon.

PSYCHOSOCIAL

PSYCHOLOGICAL AND SOCIOCULTURAL ASPECTS OF NUTRITION

So far the physiology of nutrition has been considered. This assumes that people are rational dispassionate consumers who will choose to eat the quantity and type of foods

Table 8.1 Fat soluble vitamins

Vitamin and chemical name	Source	Functions	Recommended daily intake (adult)	Effects of deficiency
A *Retinol* (*provitamin carotene in plants*)	Milk, butter, cheese, egg yolk, fish liver, oils, yellow and green vegetables	Maintains healthy epithelial tissue, cornea and is required for the synthesis of visual purple	600–700 micrograms	Night blindness; atrophy and keratinization of the epithelium; increased infections of ear, sinuses, urinary and alimentary tracts; drying and ulceration of the cornea
D *Calciferol*	Can be synthesized by the action of ultraviolet light on 7-dehydrocholesterol in the skin; milk, butter, cheese, eggs, fish liver	Aids the absorption and utilization of calcium and phosphorus to promote healthy bones and teeth	10 micrograms	Rickets (in children), osteomalacia in adults
E *Tocopherol*	Egg yolk, nuts, seeds, olive and other vegetable oils, green vegetables	Prevents catabolism of polyunsaturated fats, needed for the structure of cell membranes	3–4 milligrams	Anaemia; ataxia; cystic fibrosis
K *Phylloquinone*	Dark green leafy vegetables, liver, fish	Needed for the formation of prothrombin and factors VII, IX and X	60–70 micrograms	Easy bruising and prolonged blood clotting time

Table 8.2 Water soluble vitamins

Vitamin and chemical name	Source	Functions	Recommended daily intake (adult)	Effects of deficiency
B₁ *Thiamine*	Yeast, liver, germ of cereals, nuts, pulses, egg yolk, legumes	Metabolism of carbohydrate and nutrition of nerve cells	0.8–1 milligram	Fatigue; neuropathy; loss of memory; beriberi
B₂ *Riboflavin*	Liver, yeast, milk, eggs, green vegetables, kidney and fish roe	Carbohydrate metabolism; maintains healthy skin and eyes	1–1.3 milligrams	Angular stomatitis; dermatitis; blurred vision
B₆ *Pyridoxine*	Meat, liver, fish, vegetables, bran of cereals	Protein metabolism; production of antibodies	1.2–1.4 milligrams	(Rare)
B₁₂ *Cyanocobalamin*	Liver, milk, poultry, fish; not found in plants	Maturation of the red blood cells, DNA synthesis	1.5 micrograms	Pernicious anaemia
B *Folic acid/folacin*	Synthesized in the colon; dark green vegetables, liver, kidney, eggs	Formation of red blood cells; DNA synthesis	200 micrograms	Anaemia; N.B. pregnant women need to take a supplement
B *Nicotinic acid/ niacin*	Synthesized in the body from tryptophan; yeast, offal, fish, pulses, wholemeal cereals, potatoes	Inhibits production of cholesterol; needed for cell respiration	12–17 milligrams	Prolonged deficiency causes pellagra
B *Pantothenic acid*	Meat, liver, yeast, fresh vegetables, egg yolk, grains	Amino acid metabolism	3–7 milligrams	Vague – loss of appetite, abdominal and limb pains; associated with alcoholic neuropathy
B *Biotin*	Yeasts, liver, kidney, pulses, nuts	Carbohydrate and fat metabolism (essential for Krebs cycle)	10–200 micrograms	Scaly skin; anorexia; elevated blood cholesterol levels
C *Ascorbic acid*	Citrus fruits, currants, berries, green vegetables, potatoes	Formation of collagen; absorption of iron from the gut; required to convert folic acid to its active form	40 milligrams	Slow wound healing; anaemia; scurvy

Table 8.3 Minerals

Mineral (chemical symbol)	Source	Importance in the body	Problems	
			Excess	Deficit
Sodium (Na)	Fish, table salt, cured meats, most other foods	The most common cation found in the extracellular fluid; principal electrolyte in maintaining osmotic pressure and water balance; essential for normal neuromuscular function	Implicated as a cause of hypertension	Nausea; abdominal and muscle cramps; convulsions
Potassium (K)	Most foods, especially fruit and vegetables	Helps maintain intracellular osmotic pressure; essential for normal nerve impulse conduction, muscle contraction, protein synthesis and glycogenesis	Cardiac arrhythmia; paraesthesia; muscular weakness	Cardiac arrhythmia; heart failure; muscular weakness; paralysis; nausea and vomiting
Calcium (Ca)	Milk, cheese, eggs, vegetables and shellfish	Required for the hardening of bones and teeth, blood clotting, transmission of nerve impulses and muscle contraction, normal heart rhythm	Impaired neural function; lethargy and confusion; muscle pain and weakness; calcium deposits in soft tissue; renal stones	Muscle tetany; osteoporosis; retarded growth and rickets in children

Continued

Table 8.3—cont'd

Mineral (chemical symbol)	Source	Importance in the body	Problems	
			Excess	Deficit
Chlorine (Cl)	Table salts	With sodium, helps maintain osmotic pressure and pH of extracellular fluid; required for the formation of hydrochloric acid in the stomach	Vomiting	Alkalosis; muscle cramps; apathy
Iron (Fe)	Red meat, liver, green vegetables, wholemeal bread, egg yolk	Essential for the formation of haemoglobin in the red blood cells and the oxidization of carbohydrate	Damage to heart, liver and pancreas	Iron deficiency anaemia; pallor, lethargy, anorexia
Iodine (I)	Salt water fish, cod liver oil, vegetables grown in iodine rich soil, iodized table salt	Required to form thyroid hormones T_3 and T_4 which help to regulate metabolic rate	Depressed synthesis of thyroid hormones	Myxoedema; impaired learning and motivation in children
Magnesium (Mg)	Nuts, fruit, leafy green vegetables, whole grains	Needed for normal neural function; lactation; oxidization of carbohydrates and protein hydrolysis	Appears to be linked to obsessive behaviour, hallucinations and violent behaviour	Not known
Zinc (Zn)	Seafood, meat, cereals, nuts, wheat germ, yeast	Required for normal growth, wound healing, taste, smell and sperm production	Ataxia, slurred speech, tremors	Loss of taste and smell; depressed immunity

best suited to maintaining their energy balance and supplying all the essential nutrients when they feel hungry. Nutritional value is only one of many things taken into account by the majority of people when faced with a choice of food. Sweet things may be associated with being given rewards or treats as a child and in buying them we may be rewarding ourselves for a job well done or comforting ourselves when feeling rejected.

Food plays a part in religion and culture, not only the type of food consumed but in the preparation and timing of meals. The taste and texture of food also influence the choice of foods. Fat, salt and sugar have a very widespread appeal as evidenced by the popularity of chips and crisps and chocolate.

Food advertising encourages us to eat the manufacturer's product whether we are hungry or not. This huge industry is very versatile and can respond to current fashion by targeting the consumer, for example with low fat, low calorie foods. Food cookery programmes appear on the television every day; few of these are aimed at low income groups though some demonstrate that interesting meals can be made quite cheaply. Much has changed in family life; often both parents are working and families may eat at different times of day with snacks in between. Ready meals that can be microwaved are often preferred to homemade meals, which take time and planning, despite being cheaper and usually tastier.

Current government guidelines recommend five portions of fruit and vegetables daily to help reduce the risk of death from chronic diseases such as heart disease, stroke and cancer (Food Standards Agency 2007a). However, achieving this can be difficult for those on a low income or for those working in areas that have restricted food available, for example out-of-town industrial estates (McKevith 2004). Schools throughout the country have been looking at ways of improving the diet of children supported by a variety of government initiatives (Department for Education and Skills 2003, 2004). Many innovative schemes and government initiatives are being tried: offering free fruit at infant schools; breakfast clubs; tokens issued for choosing healthy options to enable cheap access to sports centres; and inviting celebrity chefs to host cookery classes (Department of Health 2002, 2004). The Food in Schools website, a joint initiative of the DH/DfES which provides educational tools and guidance, has reports of pilots which can be accessed by teachers, parents and pupils (see Annotated Websites at end of chapter).

We live in a multicultural society and nurses need to have an awareness of dietary restrictions that may be part of a patient's culture or religion. For example the Islamic religion requires all healthy adults to fast (i.e. to take no food, drink or medication) from dawn to sunset during the month of Ramadan. People with diabetes would be able to refrain from fasting, as exceptions are made for those who are ill, but many people are reluctant to accept this concession (Khodabukus 2003). Nurses must be able to advise on how best to avoid or minimize the problems observing the fast might cause, while respecting the individual's right to observe his/her faith.

Institutions such as hospital and care homes must have a flexible menu available and be able to provide halal or kosher meals to clients that require them and facilitate any special requirements relating to the timing and way food is served. Many families wish to provide the food and will often wish to serve the client or help feed them.

CARE DELIVERY KNOWLEDGE

All the components of a healthy diet are required by everyone at all stages in the life cycle in both health and illness. However, nutritional needs change throughout the various stages of our lives. By carrying out a nutritional assessment on patients nurses can help individuals by educating them about diet and the part it plays in health and well-being. The following section gives a brief overview of special requirements at different stages in the life cycle.

NUTRITIONAL REQUIREMENTS THROUGH THE LIFE CYCLE

Pregnancy

Energy requirements increase during pregnancy to provide for the increase in tissue mass of the fetus and the mother. The energy requirement varies according to the trimester; extra food intake is only required in the latter stage of the pregnancy. The actual calorie requirement will vary in individuals but an increase of no more than 200 kcals is adequate for most well-nourished women (British Nutrition Foundation 2004a). A well-balanced diet provides most of the nutrients to maintain a healthy pregnancy, but evidence suggests that some supplements are advisable.

Lack of essential micronutrients (vitamins and minerals) is thought to be a cause of some birth defects and possible susceptibility to diseases later in life. Folic acid is particularly important as its deficiency is implicated in neural tube defects of the newborn. Most literature suggests that women should take a supplement of folic acid as it is difficult to achieve the recommended daily intake in pregnancy by diet alone. It is recommended that all women of child-bearing age who may become pregnant or who are planning a pregnancy should take a supplement that provides 400 micrograms of folic acid per day (Food Standards Agency 2008c). In May 2007 the Board of the Food Standards Agency (FSA 2007b) suggested that a form of mandatory fortification of food with folic acid be recommended to UK health ministers. It is suggested that adding folic acid to either flour or bread will not

only increase the folate intake of young women, reducing the number of pregnancies affected by neural tube defects, but will also improve the diets of 13 million people who currently do not eat enough folate.

Other supplements that may be required by some pregnant women include vitamin D and iron. Women of Asian origin or those that always cover up their skin when outside may be particularly short of vitamin D (Food Standards Agency 2007a, Scientific Advisory Committee on Nutrition 2007).

Pregnant women are also advised not to eat dishes containing raw or partially cooked eggs, soft or mould ripened cheeses, as these foods are possible sources of the bacteria *Salmonella* and *Listeria monocytogenes*. Current opinion is that liver and liver paté should be avoided during pregnancy as they contain high concentrations of vitamin A which may be teratogenic in high doses in early gestation (Goldberg 2003, Hale 2007).

Lactation

During lactation the extra energy required by a breastfeeding mother is approximately 450 kcal per day rising slightly as the baby gets older. To achieve these extra requirements only a small amount of extra food is needed as the mother can use energy from stores laid down during pregnancy.

Babies

In the first few months babies receive all their energy requirements of life from breast or formula milk. Breastfeeding is best for babies for the first 6 months of life but infant formulas are available for those who cannot or choose not to breastfeed. Cows' milk is not suitable for babies under a year old as it contains too much salt and protein. After about 6 months, milk no longer fulfils all the baby's nutritional needs and other foods should be introduced. It is currently recommended that this process, known as weaning, does not commence before the age of 6 months as the infant's gut is limited in the type of foods it can digest and absorb. The ideal time for weaning will vary as all babies have individual needs. Mothers should be advised that solid food should not be introduced until the baby is 17 weeks at the earliest and foods such as wheat, gluten, eggs, liver, citrus fruits and unpasteurised cheese should not be given (Department of Health 2005; Food Standards Agency 2008a). Infant diets need to be high in lipid for energy and for essential long chain fatty acids and fat soluble vitamins. Infants are also at risk of iron and zinc deficiency so it is important to ensure the diet has sufficient micronutrients. There is much evidence and continued research into the effects of a weaning diet on long-term health and health professionals need to be well informed about this aspect of child care.

Schoolchildren

A varied diet containing adequate energy and nutrients is essential for normal growth and development of children. They have a high energy requirement for their size so foods that are high in energy and also rich in nutrients should be eaten as part of small frequent meals. A good supply of protein, calcium, iron and vitamins A and D are also necessary as childhood is an important time for tooth and bone development (British Nutrition Foundation 2004b). Concern is growing over the increase in obesity among schoolchildren. The combined effect of an increased intake of high-fat snacks and sugary fizzy drinks with less physical activity has been cited in several papers (Haslam & James 2005, NICE 2006b). There is increasing evidence that overweight children and adolescents are being diagnosed with type 2 diabetes, a condition that is normally associated with adults over 40 (Pocock 2007).

Teenagers

Teenagers are particularly susceptible to media images which portray thinness as desirable. They are also at a stage where mood swings may be compensated for by comfort foods. As a result they can be prone to eating disorders which leave them short of nutrients and threaten their physical as well as mental health. Teenagers are the most common age group to suffer the disorders of anorexia nervosa and bulimia nervosa (Harris & Cumella 2006; see also later in this chapter).

Adults

Adults need to eat a well-balanced diet to maintain their optimum weight. A healthy diet contains a variety of types of food – fruit, vegetables, starchy foods, protein foods. A guide to the proportions of each type is shown below:

- Base your meals on starchy foods – bread, other cereals and potatoes 34%.
- Fruit and vegetables – five portions a day 33%.
- Milk and dairy foods 15%.
- Meat, fish and alternatives 12%.
- Cut down on saturated fats and sugary food 7%.
- Eat no more than 6 grams of salt a day.
- Drink 6–8 glasses of water a day (1.2 litres).

(Food Standards Agency 2007a, Truswell 2003)

Often activity decreases with age; if a middle aged person consumes the same amount of food as when an active teenager, weight gain will occur. The government's recommendation of eating five portions of fruit and vegetables daily and reducing intake of saturated fats has been linked with improved health benefits, especially in the prevention of heart disease and some cancers (British Nutrition Foundation 2004d).

Older people

Older people are particularly at risk of poor nutrition and its consequences. Between 30 and 50% of older people admitted to hospital are undernourished (Holmes 2006). There is a variety of causes including: loss of appetite due to decreased sense of taste and smell; poor dentition; lack of agility and mobility; social isolation and depression. Medical conditions or the side-effects of drugs can interfere with nutrient absorption and metabolism as well as suppressing appetite. Particularly at risk are patients with dementia as they often refuse food and exhibit choking behaviour when attempts to spoon-feed are made; this causes stress and poses ethical problems for the carers. Tube feeding may be used if tolerated but the risk of the procedure and issues surrounding informed consent need to thoroughly explored.

Whether in their own home, nursing or residential home or hospital, elderly people need to have a thorough nutritional assessment if presenting with an illness, as undernutrition has been demonstrated to increase morbidity and mortality, especially during the winter months.

When planning food intake for older people, the decline in basal metabolic rate (BMR) with age should be taken into account, as should the reduction of physical activity. Health professionals have the responsibility to ensure sufficient help and supervision are provided to enable meals to be eaten (NICE 2006a).

Evidence-based practice

Protein and energy supplementation in elderly people at risk from malnutrition: Cochrane Review (Milne et al 2003). The review of 31 trials (2464 participants) examines the evidence for improvement in nutritional status and clinical outcomes when protein and energy-rich sip feeds are provided. Supplementation appears to produce a small but consistent weight gain. There was a statistically significant beneficial effect on mortality and a shorter length of inpatient stay but more research is needed to provide conclusive evidence.

A more recent Cochrane Review (Baldwin et al 2007) concluded that dietary advice combined with oral nutritional supplements is more effective than dietary advice alone in improving weight and energy intake in people with illness-related malnutrition in the short term. There is not enough evidence to make conclusions about long-term and cost-effective benefits. It is recommended that a change in eating habits is more effective than relying on manufactured food supplements.

PATIENT/CLIENT ASSESSMENT

The extent of the nursing assessment will vary depending upon the client. The National Institute for Health and Clinical Excellence (NICE 2006a) issued guidance recommending that all hospital inpatients and all outpatients at their first clinic appointment should be nutritionally screened. It is essential that a validated tool is used for screening. The Malnutrition Universal Screening Tool (MUST) (MCae 2003) is recommended for use in practice by NICE (2006a).

The MUST tool is a five step screening tool to identify *adults* who are malnourished, at risk of malnutrition or obese. It also includes management guidelines which can be used to develop a care plan (Fig. 8.2).

Additional information required to complete a nutritional assessment may include:

- socioeconomic information
- cultural and religious beliefs.

Reflection and portfolio evidence

Conduct a literature search and identify four tools used for nutritional assessment. If your clinical area has an assessment tool in use include it. To help you choose criteria for reviewing tools see Malnutrition Advisory Group (2000)

- Critically review each tool using the same criteria.
- Identify one that you feel is most appropriate for your current clinical area.
- Does it fulfil the requirements of the NICE guidelines – *Nutrition Support in Adults* (2006a)?
- Record the results of your findings in your portfolio.

Calculating the body mass index (BMI)

Many clinical areas now have BMI charts in prominent positions to allow for a quick estimation of BMI. However, when dealing with patients in the community it is necessary to be able to calculate the BMI and to know the normal range and what risk deviations outside this range may have for the client.

To calculate the BMI you will need to measure the height of the patient/client in metres (m) and their weight in kilograms (kg).

The formula for calculating BMI is: weight in kilograms divided by height in metres squared.

For example, if a man weighs 70 kg and is 1.75 m tall the calculation is:

$$70/(1.75 \times 1.75) = 70/3.0625 = 22.8$$

Therefore this man's BMI is 22.8.

Is this man underweight, overweight or within the healthy weight range?

Table 8.4 gives the normal range for BMI and the meaning of BMI values outside the normal range. Figure 8.3 shows a ready reckoner for calculating BMI.

Assessment of physical conditions affecting the patient's ability to eat

Difficulties in eating may result from physical conditions such as arthritis, hemiplegia or dysphagia following a stroke, hand or arm injuries, and lack of motor skills in, for example, those with learning difficulties or very young children. Poor teeth, ill-fitting dentures or no dentures will all cause difficulty and may mean certain foods are avoided or need special preparation.

History

Taking a history from the client can reveal many conditions that affect their nutritional status.

- Medical conditions which may be related to diet.
- Medication that may affect nutritional status (e.g. thiazide and loop diuretics can cause potassium deficiency, corticosteroids can cause sodium and water retention and excessive vitamin and mineral intake can lead to toxicity).
- A history of constipation or self-medication with laxatives may indicate dietary fibre deficiency.
- A history of a high alcohol intake can cause vitamin deficiencies, particularly B_{12}, and lead to medical problems such as peripheral neuropathy.
- Unexplained weight loss in the recent past can indicate underlying disease.
- Cancer.

Socioeconomic information

It is important to take into account the client's living circumstances:

- Does the client live alone?
- Are they recently bereaved?
- Can they afford a balanced diet?
- Do they have adequate cooking facilities?
- Are there any agencies already involved in helping with shopping or delivering meals?

Cultural and religious beliefs about food and its preparation

Specific dietary requirements must be noted for each client. Food is an important part of religious observance and ritual for many different faiths including Christianity, Judaism, Islam, Hinduism and Buddhism. Individuals follow strict rules or interpret them according to their own beliefs and often concessions exist within religions to those that are ill or pregnant.

It is best to ask the client or relatives and not make assumptions; for instance, not all members of the Jewish faith follow the same strict dietary code (Collins 2002, Better Health Channel 2008).

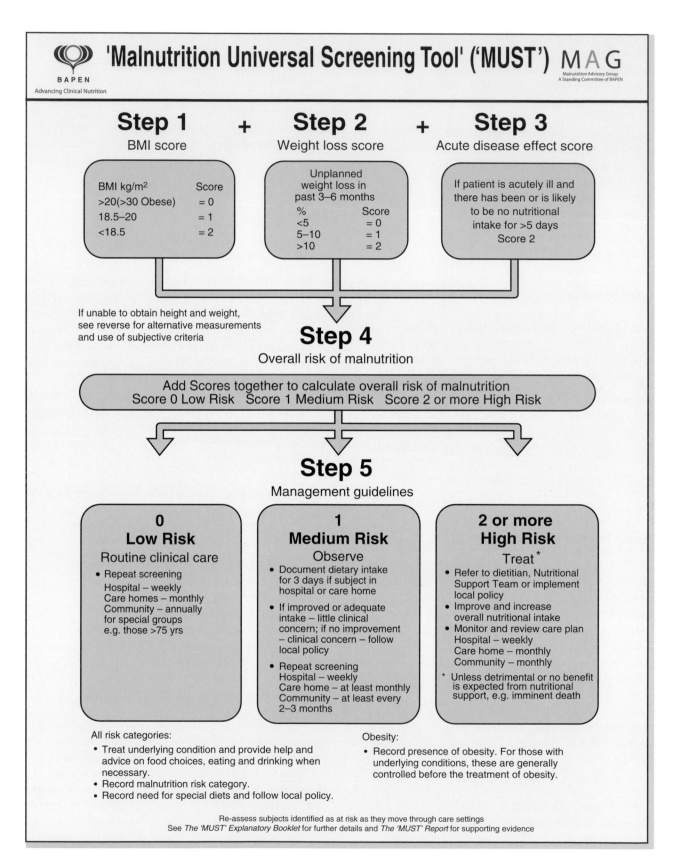

Figure 8.2 Malnutrition Universal Screening Tool (MUST) (reproduced by kind permission of BAPEN (British Association of Parenteral and Enteral Nutrition; www.bapen.org.uk)).

Table 8.4 Range of BMI

Less than 20	Underweight
20–24.9	Normal
25–29.9	Overweight
30 and over	Obese

PLANNING

The nursing assessment will indicate what particular dietary requirements and conditions the patient requires. In the institutional setting planning will ensure that the patient is provided with a diet that meets these requirements. In the community it may be necessary to plan information giving sessions to enable clients to select and prepare appropriate foods within their financial means and own preferences.

If clients wish to change their dietary patterns then a detailed planning procedure should be instituted. A useful strategy to promote is keeping a food diary for a week, making a note of what food is consumed and when. The health professional can then discuss this with the client and give advice on how to achieve a balanced diet, determine portion size, and tips on increasing physical activity (NICE 2006b). The client should aim to lose no more than 0.5–1 kg a week for sensible and sustainable weight loss. Clients with existing medical conditions such as diabetes should be monitored closely by healthcare professionals whether in the primary or secondary care setting.

INTERVENTION

In the institutional setting, nursing intervention may involve ensuring that patients are provided with food, and that they can reach it, cut it up and transfer it to their mouths, chew, swallow and digest it. The nurse must ensure that the food is accessible and patients are sitting up and able to feed themselves. Patients who have difficulty transferring the food to their mouths should be assessed by an occupational therapist who may be able to provide eating utensils that will make this easier.

The patient may be unable to eat orally due to a medical condition and this may necessitate feeding in a different way. Tube feeding, using the functioning gut, is known as enteral feeding. When the gut does not work, patients can be fed intravenously, i.e. directly into a large vein; this is known as parenteral feeding (see later in the chapter).

In the community setting, the client may need help with shopping or cooking and the nurse will liaise with social services in organizing the support services needed. Many large supermarkets now provide an ordering and delivery service using the Internet.

Mealtimes are a social event; in the institutional setting this is especially important as the day is usually structured around mealtimes. Mealtimes break the monotony, provide structure and are an opportunity to socialize. Food is often a common topic of conversation within hospital wards and in the busy setting it is easy to undervalue its social importance as well as its contribution to recovery and well-being. Ward staff should attempt to ensure that meal times are not interrupted by doctors' rounds, dressings or other routine tasks. Unpleasant sounds, sights and smells need to be minimized as they can destroy patients' appetite; ideally a separate dining area should be provided for those able to mobilize.

Reflection and portfolio evidence

Stress activates the sympathetic nervous system and releases epinephrine. This diverts blood from the digestive system and may cause anorexia and indigestion.

- What measures have you seen in your clinical areas to reduce stress and make mealtimes more relaxed and enjoyable?
- How do these compare to the standards on nutrition and the environment in the document *Essence of Care* (Department of Health 2001)?
- Can you think of any ways these measures could be improved?
- You may like to view the CD ROM Protected Mealtimes (NHS 2003).
- Record your findings in your portfolio.

FEEDING A CLIENT

Prior to feeding it should be noted whether the patient has any condition that may compromise swallowing. A full swallowing assessment by a speech therapist is needed for patients following a stroke or severe head injury. The care plan should include special instructions of how to position and feed the individual to ensure safety.

If patients require feeding they should be sat up in position where they can see the food and the method of feeding should be as normal as possible. The nurse should sit in a comfortable and relaxed manner to avoid any suggestion of hurry, and should be at the same eye level as the patient and in a position to make eye contact and observe the patient swallowing. Every effort should be made to maintain the dignity of the patient. Being unable to feed oneself is associated with early childhood and it is very easy to treat such patients as if they are children. The use of plastic bibs reinforces this image and they should be avoided; a

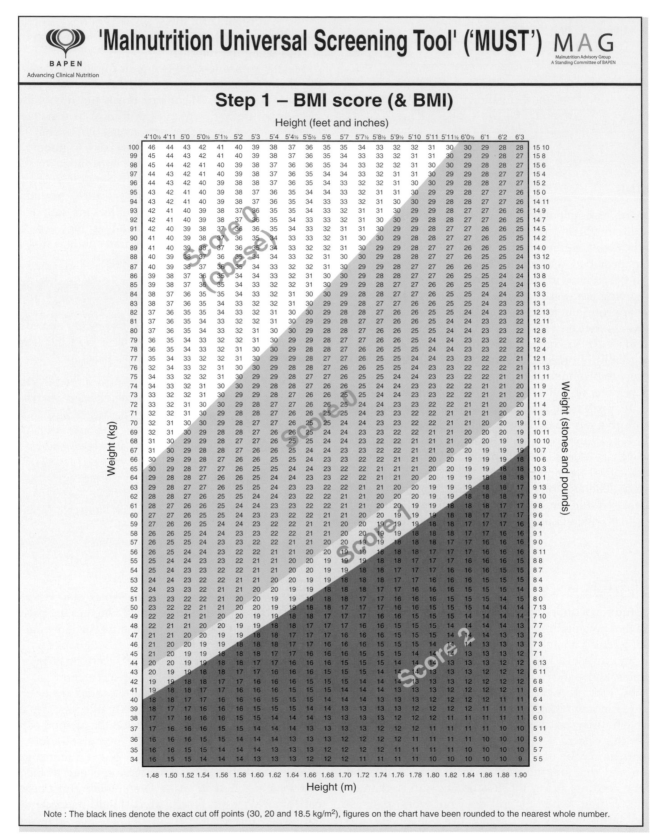

Figure 8.3 Ready reckoner for calculating BMI (reproduced by kind permission of BAPEN (British Association of Parenteral and Enteral Nutrition; www.bapen.org.uk)).

large napkin is preferable to protect the patient's clothing. Whenever possible the food should be cut up and given in the same way as the patients would eat it if they were able to feed themselves. The practice of cutting up all the food at once and then feeding the patient with a spoon should be avoided. Although feeding a patient is often left to the most junior staff it requires considerable skill and knowledge as well as sensitivity if it is to be done well.

> ### Decision-making exercise
>
> Children with learning difficulties often have muscle spasms that cause them to arch their back and scissor their legs and this can cause considerable problems when feeding them.
>
> - How would you position such a child when feeding him/ her from a spoon?
> - Check this with local protocols or guidelines.

Enteral feeding

Patients may not be able to take sufficient food orally to ensure adequate nourishment or they may be unable to swallow because of surgery, trauma or stroke. This may be a relatively short-term problem or it may be for life. As long as the digestive system is working normally, enteral feeding is a simple and, when managed correctly, safe method of providing nourishment.

Enteral feeding involves passing a feeding tube via the nose into the stomach or jejunum, or directly into the stomach or jejunum, by an X-ray guided or surgical procedure forming a gastrostomy or jejunostomy. Wide bore tubes used for aspirating stomach contents (e.g. a Ryles tube 10–12 Fr) are uncomfortable for patients and can cause complications such as rhinitis and they should not be used for feeding purposes (Best 2007). A fine-bore nasogastric tube size 6–8 should be used for enteral feeding as these are better tolerated by patients and less likely to cause damage to the nasal passages or oesophagus (Fig. 8.4). Fine-bore tubes do have some disadvantages: it is not as easy to check the correct position by testing gastric contents as aspiration of the tube can be difficult and an X-ray may be needed. The narrow lumen of the tube can block quite easily, especially if used for administering medication; however, when managed correctly they are used for long-term feeding in hospital and in the community.

A patient safety alert issued by the National Patient Safety Agency in 2005 stated that all NHS acute trusts and primary care organizations must provide staff and carers with information on the correct and incorrect methods of testing tube placement. The present recommendations (National Patient Safety Agency 2005) include:

- measuring the pH of aspirate by using pH indicator strips/paper
- radiography.

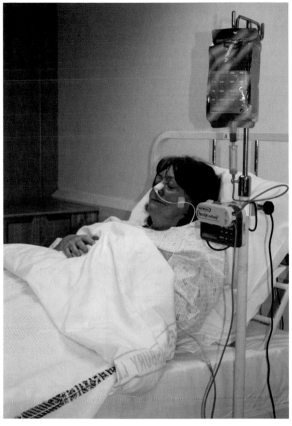

Figure 8.4 A 'patient' (the author) with fine-bore feeding tube and delivery pump (reproduced by kind permission of Salisbury Health Care NHS Trust).

Methods that should not be used include:

- auscultation of air insufflated through the feeding tube ('whoosh test')
- testing acid/alkalinity with blue litmus paper
- absence of respiratory distress
- monitoring bubbling at the end of the tube
- observing the appearance of aspirate.

Refer to Figure 8.5 and Evolve presentation 8.2 for further information.

8.2 – CONFIRMING THE POSITION OF NASOGASTRIC FEEDING TUBES

- List the times when position of an NG tube should be checked.
- List approved methods for testing position.
- Describe how to aspirate a NG feeding tube.
- Describe what to do if unable to obtain aspirate or if pH is 6.0.
- Outline developments for future safety testing of NG position.

Postoperative nutrition

Traditionally patients have been kept nil by mouth after surgery to reduce nausea and vomiting, to prevent paralytic ileus or to rest the bowel to allow an anastomosis to heal. There is no supportive evidence for these traditional approaches, whereas commencing early nutrition by resuming normal eating and drinking where possible or the use of sip feeds has been shown to have positive results on the recovery of patients (Scottish Intercollegiate Guidelines Network 2004, Gibney et al 2005).

Evidence-based practice

The role of early postoperative nutrition after gastrointestinal surgery is controversial. A review carried out by Anderson et al (2006) to evaluate whether early postoperative enteral nutrition (within 24 hours postoperatively) compared to traditional management is associated with fewer complications in patients undergoing gastrointestinal surgery. Thirteen randomized controlled trials with a total of 1173 patients were identified. The review examined whether there was a reduction in:

- wound infections, acute myocardial infarction, postoperative thrombosis or pneumonia
- anastamotic leakages
- lower mortality within 30 days postoperatively
- shorter length of hospital stay
- significant adverse side-effects.

The authors conclude that there is no obvious advantage in keeping patients nil by mouth post gastrointestinal surgery. However, they do acknowledge that the early nutrition is only part of the changes happening in surgery to improve patient outcomes.

DISORDERS OF NUTRITION

In everyday practice nurses, regardless of the specialist branch they undertake, are likely to be involved with children or adults with common dietary disorders. They are also likely to be exposed to malnutrition in the elderly both on admission to hospital or during their community placements and need to use their assessment skills and knowledge to promote an improved diet and outcome for these patients.

All nurses should have a working knowledge of the following conditions:

- obesity
- metabolic syndrome
- diabetes
- anorexia nervosa.

Obesity

Overweight (pre obese) is defined as a body mass index (BMI) of 25–29.9 and obesity as a body mass index of 30 or above. Being overweight is not considered to constitute a serious risk to health but may bring with it some restriction of mobility and social activities. However, being obese carries significant health risks such as heart disease, stroke, diabetes, high blood pressure, some cancers, osteoarthritis of weight bearing joints, gallstones, reproductive disorders and complications during and after pregnancy.

BMI does not distinguish between fat mass and muscle mass. It is now recommended that as well as calculating a client's BMI during nutritional assessment for adults, the waist circumference measurement should also be included (NICE 2006b). Obese patients can be described as apple or pear shaped. The apple shaped person has excess of visceral fat as demonstrated by the increased waist circumference. Current evidence suggests that individuals with increased visceral fat are most at risk of developing insulin resistance, type 2 diabetes, dyslipidaemia and coronary heart disease.

Waist circumference thresholds (general adult population UK; NICE 2006b).

Risk	Male	Female
Increased risk	94 cm (37 inches)	80 cm (31 inches)
Greatly increased risk	102 cm (40 inches)	88 cm (35 inches)

Waist circumference is not currently recommended as a means of diagnosing childhood obesity (National Heart Forum 2007).

Obesity predisposes people to a variety of health problems and an increased number of adults affected has significant cost implications for health service provision. The increase in obesity is not restricted to adults; children are also becoming obese and thus experiencing diseases that are normally associated with adults. Obesity among children aged 2–10 rose from 9.9% in 1995 to 16.7% in 2005 and among 11–15 year olds it rose from 14.4% in 1995 to 20.5 % in 2005 (NICE 2006b, National Heart Forum 2007).

It is unclear why obesity is increasing so rapidly, although a correlation with an increase in food consumed and a decrease in physical activity because of lifestyle changes in the developed countries of the world has been demonstrated (Department of Health et al 2007). In developed countries much of the energy expended by people at work and in the home has decreased. Many homes now have personal computers, and playing complicated and exciting games on the computer or getting information from the Internet uses much less energy than playing football or walking to a library.

Stigmas associated with being obese include laziness and gluttony which can significantly disadvantage individuals, who may then seek help. A walk round a bookshop reveals a plethora of self-help books aimed at helping people overcome obesity; some will be based on science and up-to-date nutritional principles, others claim novel and bizarre ways to lose weight. Most glossy magazines and many home web pages have celebrity diets, and supermarkets have low fat, low calorie, healthy-option foods intended to be used as part of a calorie controlled diet. Targeting the overweight and obese is big business and yet the incidence of obesity in the population continues to rise.

For every overweight kilogram, 7000 kcal of energy are stored and the only way to lose it, excluding surgery, is to metabolize it. This can only be achieved by decreasing energy intake and/or increasing energy output by the requisite amount. The amount of energy used during exercise is very little; for example using an exercise bicycle at a pedal load sustainable for any length of time by an unfit individual will use approximately 5 kcal/min. In other words it would take about 24 hours of cycling to lose 1 kg of weight. Exercise on its own is not an effective way of losing weight though it does have its own benefits, for example an individual who becomes fitter as a result of exercise is likely to be more active, benefiting heart, lungs, muscle and bones. To reduce weight effectively means cutting down on energy intake by altering the diet.

Fad diets, for instance a grapefruit or banana diet, will achieve weight loss but they are difficult to sustain and over time produce shortages in essential macro and micronutrients. Success depends on finding an acceptable diet that contains less energy than the individual is metabolizing. Slimming clubs help individuals to choose foods from a variety of categories to suit the individual's lifestyle and offer education and support. As a result the more reputable ones have notable successes; however, their services are not free and clubs do not appeal to everyone.

Many tools are available to help the nurse plan a weight loss programme with a client. One of the most comprehensive is the Care Pathway for the management of overweight and obesity designed to help health care professionals raise the issue of being overweight or obese with the client (Reddy 2006).

The general principles for successful weight loss are:

- Establish a realistic rate of weight loss – a target of 0.5–1 kg per week.
- Reduce overall calorie intake but base the diet on a healthy range of food (600 kcal/day deficit will achieve sustainable weight loss).
- Eat five or more portions of a range of fruit and vegetables daily.
- Base meals on starch foods such as pasta, rice, potatoes, whole meal bread.

- Reduce intake of foods high in fat and sugar.
- Grill or steam food – limit the addition of fat in cooking.
- Reduce alcohol intake.

In addition introduce lifestyle changes that reduce sedentary behaviour, for example use the stairs at work instead of lifts. Aim to achieve a minimum of 30 minutes of moderate activity, for example brisk walking on at least 5 days a week. Exercise will improve self-esteem and well-being and aids the loss of adipose tissue, not lean body mass.

In addition to dieting pharmacological treatment can be instigated for treating obesity in adults. Clients must be monitored closely and support from health professionals provided during treatment. Drug treatment is not recommended for children younger than 12 years of age unless there is life-threatening co-morbidity (e.g. raised intracranial pressure). Similar restrictions are in place for children over 12 years of age and all children should be treated in specialist paediatric settings. Currently, in the UK, the approved drugs for treating obesity are orlistat and sibutramine (NICE 2006b).

Decision-making exercise

Read NICE clinical guideline 43 – Obesity December 2006, available from www.nice.org.uk (NICE 2006b).

- Make notes on the rationale for prescribing orlistat or sibutramine for treating obese adults.
- Make short notes on each drug, how it acts and the side-effects.
- Are there any other anti-obesity drugs currently in use that you know of?
- What support should be available for individuals prescribed anti-obesity medication?

Bariatric surgery is recommended as a treatment option for people with obesity if they have a BMI of 40 kg/m^2 or more, or between 35 kg/m^2 and 40 kg/m^2 and with other significant disease. Surgery is also recommended as first line option for adults with a BMI of more than 50 kg/m^2 (NICE 2006b). However, bariatric surgery is not without risk and there are no long-term studies available as to its efficacy.

Metabolic syndrome

Although not a disease in itself, metabolic syndrome is described when an individual has three or more defining criteria:

- obesity with a waist measurement above 102 cm for men or 88 cm for women
- blood pressure of more than 130/85 mmHg
- fasting blood glucose of more than 6.1 and less than 7.0 mmol/L

- fasting plasma triglycerides of more than 1.7 mmol/L
- fasting plasma high density lipoprotein (HDL) less than 1.04 mmol/L men or less than 1.29 mmol/L women.

The importance of recognizing metabolic syndrome is that it predisposes the individual to serious disease, for example diabetes and cardiovascular. Restoring body weight to normal and increasing physical activity have been successful in reducing the progression to diabetes and cardiovascular disease (Marks 2003).

Diabetes mellitus

This common condition is characterized by an inability to control plasma glucose concentration. In type 1 diabetes mellitus no insulin is produced and glucose spills over into the urine (glycosuria) causing osmotic diuresis and dehydration. In addition the body metabolizes excessive amounts of fat, resulting in a rise in plasma ketone concentration which may be sufficient to cause acidosis and coma. Type 2 diabetes mellitus is when there is not enough insulin produced by the pancreas or when the insulin produced is ineffective; it usually results in hyperglycaemia, glycosuria and dehydration.

Both are serious medical conditions that require careful management to prevent long-term health problems. Diabetes mellitus of both types can be treated with medication but dietary management remains important. Patients will have an individual regime based on their basal metabolic requirements and level of physical activity. The principles of the diet are similar to those for any normal healthy diet but the amount, type and frequency of carbohydrate is controlled to allow a constant blood glucose concentration to be maintained (Pennock 2005).

The objectives of the diet are to:

- maintain or achieve desirable weight (BMI of 20–25)
- eat regular meals based on low glycaemic starchy foods such as pasta
- maintain a low fat intake of 30–35% of calories choosing monounsaturated fats, e.g. olive oil and rapeseed oil; use less butter, cheese and fatty meats; choose low fat dairy foods
- eat more fruit and vegetables – aim for five portions a day
- limit sugar and sugary foods; use sugar-free drinks and squashes
- drink alcohol in moderation only and never on a empty stomach
- reduce salt intake.

When planning the type of carbohydrate to include in the diet, the glycaemic index can be used. The index measures how blood glucose concentration is affected by eating a particular carbohydrate. Glucose itself has an index of 100 whereas the same amount of pasta will be absorbed more slowly, causing a smaller increase in the blood glucose concentration and consequently a lower score on the glycaemic scale. Combinations of high and low glycaemic index foods eaten together will cause a lower increase in blood glucose concentration than when a high index food is eaten alone.

One of the key factors in controlling diabetes mellitus is client education and the development of a partnership between the patients and those responsible for their care. Patients who do not understand their condition are less likely to comply with the diet and treatment thus risking the long-term complications of diabetes. Diabetic nurse specialists have made a valuable contribution to patient care by demonstrating that it is possible to tailor the diet and medication to suit the individual's lifestyle rather than the other way round. An approach to the management of type 1 diabetes is the Dose Adjustment For Normal Eating (DAFNE). This is an educational programme delivered by diabetes educators. The underlying principle is that insulin doses are adjusted to fit in with the food a person chooses to eat, at the time they choose to eat it. The aim is to improve glycaemic control and quality of life for those with type 1 diabetes (www.diabetes.org.uk).

Anorexia nervosa and bulimia nervosa

Eating disorders are common among adolescents and although more prevalent in females they can also affect males and all age groups (Harris & Cumella 2006).

Eating disorders are classified into three variants:

- anorexia nervosa – restricting and binge–purge anorexia
- bulimia nervosa – purging and non purging
- binge eating disorder

(Treasure and Murphy 2005).

Eating disorders are not always easy to diagnose: when would dieting become anorexia or obesity from over eating become binge eating disorder?

Anorexia

The generally accepted diagnostic criteria for anorexia are:

- Refusal to maintain body weight at or above a minimally normal weight for height and age (or failure to make expected weight gain during a period of growth).
- Intense fear of gaining weight or becoming fat, even when underweight.
- Disturbance in the way in which one's body weight or shape is experienced.
- Amenorrhea in females.

Patients with anorexia believe they are fat even when obviously emaciated. The desire to be thin is largely determined by culture. In affluent countries where food is easily available and affordable by the majority of society, being overweight becomes synonymous with sloth, self-indulgence and greed. Thinness conversely is associated with discipline and self-control; this tends to be reinforced by the media and advertising.

Many sufferers of eating disorders may have family problems, for instance being described as model children by parents may be associated with non-assertive behaviour and the eating disorder is a way of gaining control. This aspect of the disease can make it very difficult to treat as many patients see the disorder as part of their identity and may deny they have a problem or feign compliance.

Many patients with anorexia are treated as outpatients but admission to hospital will be necessary for the severely underweight who need intervention to ensure their survival. Treatment is aimed at correcting the physiological problems that are life threatening and feeding by enteral or parenteral routes may be necessary (NICE 2004). Once the patient is out of immediate physical danger, psychotherapy with or without drugs is commenced. Inpatient treatment is often based on behavioural interventions that use a combination of non-punitive reinforcement. The aim is to gain weight and restore normal eating patterns and body functions, aiming for a BMI of at least 18 in most individuals. Treatment is also aimed at teaching the client to understand and change dysfunctional behaviours and attitudes and to improve personal self-esteem; this may require family involvement and therapy but each plan of care will be unique to the individual. (See Evolve 8.4 for more detail.)

8.4 – EATING DISORDERS

- List key points about anorexia.
- Outline key features of bulimia nervosa.
- Describe binge eating disorder.
- Review the general guidelines as advocated by NICE (2004).

PROFESSIONAL AND ETHICAL KNOWLEDGE

FOOD SAFETY

The nurse should be aware of legislation regarding food, in particular the work of the Food Standards Agency, the Food Safety Act 1990 and the Food Standards Act 1999. The Food Safety Act is a wide ranging law that covers food safety and consumer protection throughout the UK. It affects everyone working in the production, processing, storage and distribution and sale of food. Hospitals are subject to the same rigorous rules as restaurants for storing, preparing and serving food. The Act also states that people handling food will need appropriate training in hygiene.

The Food Standards Act 1999 includes regulation on accurate labelling of foodstuffs. This is particularly important when buying processed food as many individuals are sensitive or allergic to certain food products. For example many products contain peanuts or peanut oil and can produce fatal anaphylaxis if ingested by individuals allergic to them.

Food poisoning may be defined as an illness caused by the ingestion of contaminated food. In the UK all clinicians have a statutory duty to notify the local authority of cases of food poisoning. The incidence of food poisoning is increasing at an alarming rate, although a true picture of the risk to health is difficult to obtain because many cases probably go unreported by individuals and clinicians. This increase could be due to changing behaviour, as more and more people in developed countries eat out, eat more convenience foods and buy food in bulk to store.

Decision-making exercise

Look at the evidence on one of the following topics: new variant Creutzfeldt–Jakob disease; *Campylobacter* contamination of food; genetically modified food.

- How is this reported in newspapers, in professional journals and in government reports?
- How easy was it to find the information?
- How accurate was the information from each source?
- How might a nurse working in a school use this information when advising an anxious mother on the safety of food?

A general outbreak of food poisoning is defined as one that affects members of more than one household or residents of an institution. Hospital catering departments have a duty to provide safe food for patients and their employees must adhere to strict codes of hygiene. When food arrives in ward areas it should be stored correctly and served at the correct temperature. Ward kitchens need to be inspected regularly and food kept in refrigerators should be dated and labelled. All members of staff, volunteers or relatives must wash their hands effectively before handling food for patients. Patients should be enabled to wash their hands prior to mealtimes. Nursing staff and housekeeping assistants should be trained in food hygiene and should be monitored by the clinical leader. Any outbreak of diarrhoea and vomiting within a hospital needs to be immediately managed by the infection control team. Isolating and barrier nursing the patients affected should be instigated immediately without waiting for confirmation from laboratory specimens. Any staff affected will need to stay off work and monitoring by the occupational health department may be necessary. (See Ch. 5, 'Infection prevention and control', and consult any documents in your practice learning placements for more detailed information.)

Institutions and businesses are controlled by strict laws relating to food production and consumption; however, many incidences of food poisoning are the result of poor personal and domestic hygiene. The principles of the advice given to the food industry are just as relevant to the domestic setting. Poor hygiene, the misuse of refrigerators, poor storage and inadequately heated food pose a risk to individuals in their own homes (see Evolve 8.5 for more detail).

8.5 – COMMON CAUSES OF FOOD POISONING

- Give a definition of food poisoning.
- List cause and symptoms of:
  - *Campylobacter*
  - *Salmonella*
  - *Clostridium perfringens*
  - *Listeria monocytogenes*
  - *E. coli*
  - Norovirus.
- Prevention and dealing with food poisoning.

PROFESSIONAL ACCOUNTABILITY

The Code: *Standards of Conduct, Performance and Ethics for Nurses and Midwives* (Nursing and Midwifery Council 2008) states that the people in your care must be able to trust you with their health and well-being. Consider how the standards in the code apply to the nutritional health and well-being of patients.

Involving the patients and their relatives in planning nutritional care will help to achieve compliance and co-operation that comes when individuals are consulted, informed and encouraged to address their own health needs. Communicating with all the agencies will ensure that your patients receive any help available to assist with the provision of nutritional needs, e.g. dietary information, Meals on Wheels, help with shopping. Maintaining good and collegiate relationships with dieticians, the catering department, ward housekeepers and kitchen porters benefits the patient by making the best use of all the team has to offer.

When caring for a patient with specific dietary needs (for example renal failure), if you have insufficient knowledge to give dietary advice to this patient or client you must consult or refer to a dietician or other suitably qualified practitioner.

To maintain your professional integrity when offering advice to patients care must be taken not to endorse particular products, for instance recommending a brand of slimming product or a particular slimming club or gym.

ETHICAL CONCERNS

Although nurses and all members of the multiprofessional team need to ensure that their patients' nutritional needs are met, there are ethical issues surrounding food and drink. Should nurses, as part of the multiprofessional team, be encouraging the use of invasive techniques like enteral feeding to ensure nutrition for the patients at all times? Consider the patient in a persistent vegetative state, a patient dying from incurable illness, or the patient with advanced dementia or anorexia.

Tony Bland was a victim of the 1989 Hillsborough Stadium disaster whose cerebral cortex was destroyed as a result of prolonged oxygen deprivation (Thompson et al 2000). In 1993 the Law Lords allowed the tube feeding of Tony Bland to be discontinued. Tube feeding is now regarded in law as a medical treatment. The judgment in the Tony Bland case was not that the tube should be withdrawn but that it was not in his best interest for it to be continued. The proposed action by the doctor to remove the tube was therefore ruled in a declaratory judgment not to be illegal, but it was still his decision whether or not to do so (*Airedale NHS Trust* v. *Bland* 1993).

Towards the end of life patients may refuse food and many of the ethical considerations in palliative care settings are concerned with feeding and providing adequate hydration to patients, elderly or otherwise, who have not long to live. These issues must be discussed with the multidisciplinary team, relatives and patients if they are able. The aim of palliative care is to provide comfort, support and relief of symptoms; persisting with diet and fluids or commencing a tube feed may not be appropriate. Local measures such as sips of fluid or ice to suck for comfort may be all the patient wants and enforcing fluids and nutrition is intrusive.

Patients with advanced dementia often refuse food and drink and exhibit dysphagia and choking symptoms; this makes it difficult and frightening for their carers when attempting to feed them. Patients with dementia should be encouraged to eat and drink for as long as possible with available specialist assessment and advice about swallowing and feeding (NICE 2006c). Tube feeding is not recommended in severe dementia if dysphagia or disinclination to eat is caused by the severity of the disease.

However tube feeding could be indicated and of benefit if the dysphagia is thought to be transient. Ethical and legal principles will have to be applied to discussion on withholding or withdrawing nutritional support and carers and patients should be involved in the decisions (NICE 2006c).

Decision-making exercise

Based on observations in practice and/or on debates with your peers, review how you would justify the decisions you might make in circumstances where there are obvious ethical dilemmas related to food and nutrition:

- In what circumstances should patients be able to refuse food?
- Does your decision alter according to the medical diagnosis?
- How does this integrate with the responsibilities of the nurse stated in the Code of Professional Conduct (Nursing and Midwifery Council 2008) and the Mental Capacity Act 2005?
- Should food ever be withheld from patients?

PERSONAL AND REFLECTIVE KNOWLEDGE

THE NURSE AS ROLE MODEL

In reflecting on your practice and in the knowledge gained from this chapter it is important that you manage your own personal nutritional needs, not only to maintain your health but also to provide a role model for your patients and clients. Meeting the nutritional needs of patients is a core function of nursing and there are many opportunities available to learn through your practice experience and the collection of evidence for your portfolio.

CASE STUDIES IN NUTRITION

To consolidate your learning from this chapter work through the following case studies.

Case study: Adult

Peter Dawson is a 58-year-old man who lives at home with his wife. He is very overweight, being 1.8m tall and weighing 100kg. He admits to drinking and smoking 'quite a bit' most evenings and says he has no time to exercise. He has recently been diagnosed as having non insulin dependent diabetes mellitus, for which he has been prescribed a hypoglycaemic drug and dietary advice.

- Calculate Peter's BMI. What grade of being overweight does this represent?
- What other measurement should be included in his nutritional assessment and why?
- Apart from reduced insulin sensitivity, why might his diabetes be made worse by his obesity, smoking and drinking of alcohol?
- What help and advice could Peter be given to improve his lifestyle?

Case study: Mental health

Sally, aged 17 years, lives at home with her mother, who is divorced. Sally start dieting 2 years ago, but continued to diet after reaching her target weight. She is now 20kg underweight but says she still feels fat. Sally's mother has always believed that her place was in the home looking after Sally and her younger brother, and is very worried because Sally looks so thin.

- Apart from lacking energy intake what other factors may be missing from Sally's diet?
- What sort of social pressures are there on young girls to account for the high incidence of eating disorders?
- Consider how Sally's school friends and her parents may have unwittingly contributed to her problems.

Case study: Child

- Marcus and Yvonne are strict vegans. Their son Jason has been breastfed for 5 months and they are seeking advice about weaning.
- What are the possible ramifications of Marcus' and Yvonne's dietary preferences on Jason's dietary needs?
- Plan a diet that is compatible with Marcus' and Yvonne's beliefs and Jason's nutritional needs.
- How could the nurse later assess that the diet is meeting all Jason's nutritional requirements?

Case study: Learning disabilities

Andrew is 38 years of age and suffers from a moderate learning disability. He attends a social centre on a daily basis but otherwise lives with his parents. Andrew is 1.76m tall and weighs 98kg. He enjoys his food and has a hearty appetite, eating a cooked breakfast every morning and a full dinner at night. This is supplemented by a cooked snack at the social centre every day and bars of chocolate. Andrew's parents feel that although he's a little over-weight he is otherwise happy. They have no time for special diets or 'rabbit food'.

- Calculate Andrew's BMI.

- What are the long-term physiological consequences for Andrew should this situation continue?
- How might the nurse help Andrew lose weight but continue to eat the food he and his family enjoy?

SUMMARY

This chapter has outlined knowledge needed for decision making in promoting health and providing good nutrition for patients/clients. It has included:

1. Information on the various components of a balanced diet, the common sources from which they may be obtained and the ways various foods are digested and used within the body.
2. An awareness of cultural differences and how food plays such an important part in psychological and social aspects of life.
3. A review of nutritional needs across the lifespan and knowledge of the key components of a nutritional assessment and the application of a variety of nutritional assessment tools.
4. The promotion of a healthy diet, ensuring that myths are dispelled and there is a balanced approach to media advertising.
5. A description of feeding techniques and methods that may be needed to support people with problems in meeting their own needs.
6. Acknowledgement that people with common nutritional problems are encountered in all branches of nursing practice, and provided information that is essential to give good quality advice and support.
7. Information on research to audit standards for evidence-based nutritional care for patients.
8. Legal aspects of food safety that need to be adhered to in order to prevent outbreaks of food poisoning at home or in healthcare institutions.
9. Ethical issues related to feeding which should be debated and decisions made based on patient, family and healthcare team participation.

ANNOTATED FURTHER READING AND WEBSITES

Gibney M, Elia M, Ljungqvist O and Dowsett J (eds) 2005 Clinical nutrition. Blackwell Science: Oxford

One of the Human Nutrition series, it complements the other texts by providing in-depth information on clinical nutrition; of particular interest are the illustrative cases which help the reader apply the knowledge in the chapters.

Eastwood M 2003 Principles of human nutrition, 2nd edn. Blackwell Science, Oxford

This comprehensive textbook examines human nutrition and encompasses traditional nutrition, evolving nutrition and complex concepts that will influence the future of nutrition. The chapter 'History of food around the world and the European diet' gives an insightful overview of how diets became so diverse and bound to culture. A chapter about nutrition in outer space provides facts for the nurse specialist who wants to plan an interesting career pathway!

Stockslager JL, Mayer BH, Munden J, Munson et al (eds) 2003 Nutrition made incredibly easy. Lippincott Williams and Wilkins, Philadelphia

This is a compact text on nutrition with a quiz to test your knowledge at the end of each chapter. Easy and enjoyable to read and broken down into manageable chunks. Well illustrated with extra memory joggers and helpful tips.

http://www.nutrition.org.uk
The British Nutrition Foundation (BNF) is an independent charity which provides reliable information on nutrition and related health matters to the public, press and health professionals. It produces leaflets and briefing papers and some books.

http://www.bapen.org.uk
The British Association for Parenteral and Enteral Nutrition is a registered charity whose aim is to improve the nutritional treatment of all sufferers from illness who have become or are likely to become malnourished. The association provides in depth reports and information for healthcare professionals and patients.

http://www.diabetes.org.uk
Diabetes UK runs this site which gives sensible and reliable information to diabetics, their carers and health professionals. It uses plain language in its advice sheets. Includes information on DAFNE and a link to the projects website.

http://www.food.gov.uk
The Food Standards Agency has been created to protect public health from risks that may arise in connection with the consumption of food. This is a useful site for information on food poisoning, genetically modified food, etc.

http://www.eatwell.gov.uk
This is a branch of the Food Standards Agency which deals with nutrition through life stages, food labelling and food hygiene. Well organized with links to other relevant websites and downloadable information sheets.

http://www.vegansociety.com/php
This website has food advice and recipes for vegans. It also lists events organized by the society and has comment on news items relating to food.

http://vegsoc.org/
This site caters for vegetarians with food advice.

www.endoflifecare.nhs.uk
This site covers a range of topics from care recommendations to ethical and legal decision making.

References

Airedale NHS Trust v. *Bland* 1993 Judgments of Family Division, Court of Appeal (Civil Division) and House of Lords. In: Fennel P, Harpwood V, Harpwood H et al (eds) Medico-legal reports: 12. Butterworth, London

Andersen HK, Lewis SJ, Thomas S 2006 Early enteral nutrition within 24 hours of colorectal surgery versus later commencement of feeding for post operative complications. Cochrane Database of Systematic Reviews Issue 4. ArtNo:CD004080.DOI:10.1002/14651858.CD004080.pub2

Baldwin C, ParsonsT, Logan S 2007 Dietary advice for illness related malnutrition in adults. Cochrane Database of Systematic Reviews Issue 1. Art.No:CD002008.DOI:10.10002/14651858.CD002008.pub2

Barndregt K, Soeters P 2005 In: Gibney MJ, Elia M, Ljungqvist O, Dowsett J (eds) 2005 Clinical nutrition. Blackwell Science, Oxford, ch 8, p 121

Best C. 2007 Nasogastric tube insertion in adults who require enteral feeding. Nursing Standard 21(40):39–43

Better Health Channel 2008 Food culture and religion. Available online: http://www.betterhealth.vic.gov.au/bhcv2/bhcarticles.nsf/pages/Food_culture_and_religion?OpenDocument (accessed 1 February 2008)

British Nutrition Foundation 2004a Maternal and infant nutrition. Available online: http://www.nutrition.org.uk/home.asp?siteId=43&sectionId=394&subSectionId=315 (accessed 7 February 2008)

British Nutrition Foundation 2004b Nutrition through life. School children. Available online: http://www.nutrition.org.uk/home.asp?siteId=43&sectionId=396&subSectionId=315 (accessed 7 February 2008)

British Nutrition Foundation 2004c Nutrition through life. Teenagers. Available online: http://www.nutrition.org.uk/home.asp?siteId=43&sectionId=397&subSectionId=315 (accessed 7 February 2008)

British Nutrition Foundation 2004d Heart disease and stroke. Available online: http://www.nutrition.org.uk/printArticle.asp?dataId=1374 (accessed 1 February 2008)

Brunner EJ, Thorogood M, Rees K, Hewitt G 2005 Dietary advice for reducing cardiovascular risk. Cochrane Database of Systematic Reviews. Issue 4. ArtNo:CD002128.DOI:10.1002/14651858.CD002128.pub2.

Collins A 2002 Nursing with dignity. Part 1: Judaism. Nursing Times 98(9):34–35

Davidson A 2005 Management and effects of parenteral nutrition. Nursing Times 101(42):28–31

Department for Education and Skills 2003 Food in schools. Stationery Office, London

Department for Education and Skills 2004 Every child matters: change for children. Stationery Office, London

Department of Health 2001 Essence of care: patient focused benchmarking for health practitioners. HMSO, London

Department of Health 2002 Healthy start: proposals for the reform of the welfare food scheme. HMSO, London

Department of Health 2004 Choosing a better diet: a food and health action plan. HMSO, London

Department of Health 2005 Weaning. Department of Health, London

Department of Health, MRD Human Nutrition Research, Jebb S, Steer T, Holmes C 2007 The healthy living social marketing initiative: a review of the evidence. Department of Health, London and MRD Human Nutrition Research, Cambridge

Food Safety Act 1990 HMSO, London

Food Standards Act 1999 HMSO, London

Food Standards Agency 2007a 8 tips for eating well. Available online: http://www.eatwell.gov.uk/healthydiet/eighttipssection/8tips (accessed 7 February 2008)

Food Standards Agency 2007b Board recommends mandatory fortification. Available online: http://www.food.gov.uk/news/newsarchive/2007/may/folatefort (accessed 7 February 2008)

Food Standards Agency 2008a Fats. Available online: http://www.eatwell.gov.uk/healthydiet/nutritionessentials/fatssugarssalt/fats/ (accessed 7 February 2008)

Food Standards Agency 2008b Eat well, be well. Weaning your baby. Available online: http://www.eatwell.gov.uk/agesandstages/baby/weaning/ (accessed 7 February 2008)

Food Standards Agency 2008c Folic acid fortification. Available online: http://www.eatwell.gov.uk/healthissues/factsbehindissues/folicacid/ (accessed 7 February 2008)

Gibney M, Elia M, Ljungqvist O, Dowsett J (eds) 2005 Clinical nutrition. Blackwell Science, Oxford, pp 319–321

Goldberg G 2003 Nutrition in pregnancy: the facts and the fallacies. Nursing Standard 17(19):39–42

Green S, Watson R 2006 Nutritional screening and assessment tools for older adults: literature review. Journal of Advanced Nursing 54(4):477–490

Hale R 2007 Maternal nutrition during pregnancy and folic acid. British Journal of Midwifery 15(3):167–170

Harris M, Cumella E 2006 Eating disorders across the lifespan. Journal of Psychosocial Nursing and Mental Health Services 44(4):21–26

Haslam D, James WPT 2005 Obesity. Lancet 366:1197–1209

Holmes S 2006 Barriers to effective nutritional care for older adults. Nursing Standard 21(3):50–54

Holmes S 2007 Eating for recovery. Nursing Standard 21(43):18–21

Johnstone C, Farley A, Hendry C 2006 Nurses' role in nutritional assessment and screening (part one). Nursing Times 102(49):28–29

Khodabukus R 2003 Advising patients with diabetes about fasting during Ramadhan. Nursing Times 99(28):26–27

MCae E 2003 The MUST report: nutritional screening of adults: a multidisciplinary responsibility. Development and use of the MUST Universal screening tool for adults. A report by the Malnutrition Advisory Group of the British Association of the Parenteral and Enteral Nutrition. BAPEN, Redditch

McKevith B 2004 The nation's diet: promoting healthy eating. Nursing Standard 18(48):45–52

Malnutrition Advisory Group 2000 Source of evidence and information for screening tool guidelines. In: Guidelines for the detection and management of malnutrition. British Association for Parenteral and Enteral Nutrition, Maidenhead, pp 19–27

Marks V 2003 The metabolic syndrome. Nursing Standard 17(49):37–44

Mental Capacity Act 2005 HMSO London

Microbiological Safety of Food 1990 Report of the Committee on the Microbiological Safety of Food: Part 1. HMSO, London

Milne AC, Potter J, Avenell A 2003 Protein and energy supplements in elderly people at risk from malnutrition. Cochrane Review. In: Cochrane Library, Issue 1, Update Software, Oxford

Montague SE, Watson R, Herbert RA (eds) 2005 Physiology for nursing practice, 3rd edn. Elsevier, Edinburgh

National Health Service 2003 Protected mealtimes: full instructional information for implementing 'Protected mealtimes on your ward'. National Health Service Estates, Leeds

National Heart Forum 2007 Lightening the load: tackling overweight and obesity. National Heart Forum, London

National Institute for Health and Clinical Excellence 2004 Clinical guideline 9. Eating disorders. Core interventions and management of anorexia nervosa, bulimia nervosa and related eating disorders. National Institute for Health and Clinical Excellence, London

National Institute for Health and Clinical Excellence 2006a Clinical guideline 32. Nutrition support in adults: oral nutrition support, enteral tube feeding and parenteral nutrition. National Institute for Health and Clinical Excellence, London

National Institute for Health and Clinical Excellence 2006b Clinical guideline 43. Obesity. Guidance on the prevention, identification, assessment and management of overweight and obesity in adults and children. National Institute for Health and Clinical Excellence, London

National Institute for Health and Clinical Excellence 2006c Clinical guideline 42. Dementia. National Institute for Health and Clinical Excellence, London

National Patient Safety Agency 2005 Patient safety alert: reducing the harm caused by misplaced nasogastric feeding tubes. National Patient Safety Agency, London

Nursing and Midwifery Council 2008 The Code: standards of conduct, performance and ethics for nurses and midwives. Nursing and Midwifery Council, London

Pennock T 2005 Diabetes and nutrition: the latest thinking on dietary management. Professional Nurse 20(8):27–30

Pocock N 2007 Rising incidence of type 2 diabetes in children in the UK. Diabetes Care 30:1097–1101

Reddy S 2006 Care pathway for the management of overweight and obesity. National Health Service, London

Royal College of Nursing 2005 Perioperative fasting in adults and children. Royal College of Nursing, London

Savage J, Scott C 2005 Patients' nutritional care in hospital: an ethnographic study of the nurse's role and patients' experience, final report. Royal College of Nursing, London

Scientific Advisory Committee on Nutrition 2007 Update on vitamin D. Stationery Office, London

Scottish Intercollegiate Guidelines Network 2004 77. Postoperative management in adults. Scottish Intercollegiate Guidelines Network, Edinburgh

Thompson I, Melia K, Boyd K 2000 Nursing ethics, 4th edn. Churchill Livingstone, Edinburgh

Treasure J, Murphy T 2005 Eating disorders. In: Gibney M, Elia M, Ljungqvist O, Dowsett J (eds) Clinical nutrition. Blackwell Science, Oxford, ch 6

Truswell AS 2003 ABC of nutrition, 4th edn. British Medical Journal, London, p 37

Chapter **9**

Stress, relaxation and rest

David Howard

INTRODUCTION

Although stress, relaxation and rest are separate concepts there is a high degree of interdependence. Fundamental to all, however, is the influence of psychological stress. Consequently, in this chapter emphasis has been placed on developing an awareness of recognizing and managing stress, as it is from this foundation that understanding of relaxation and rest can develop.

OVERVIEW

Subject knowledge

This section addresses the nature of stress, its effects on individuals and the role it plays in the lives of everyone, together with the physiological, psychological and social changes that occur in response. The consequences of exposure to very stressful events and prolonged exposure to stress are focused on when examining the conditions of burnout and post-traumatic stress disorder. Finally, the concepts of relaxation, rest and sleep are discussed and their relationship to stress is explored.

Care delivery knowledge

This section focuses on strategies that can be used in the assessment and management of both psychological stress and sleep. First stress in clients is addressed. The reasons why clients may suffer from stress help to identify what should be assessed and why, and these are examined in detail. Clients' carers are also likely to experience stress and common reasons why this is, and the signs that indicate this, are also explored.

The workplace is potentially a very stressful environment. This is probably first recognized by the effects on employees. Consequently, strategies for developing an awareness of your own level of stress, and also for identifying signs of stress in colleagues are discussed together with methods of management.

The final part of this section focuses on assessing sleep and examining ways that sleep can be promoted.

Professional and ethical knowledge

This section examines the context within which stress arises. As controlling stressors is a fundamental component of stress management, and with so many stressors outside individuals' control in health and social care, the ethical issues here examine the policy agenda and its implementation. This section begins by examining the relationship between policy, stress and employment in health and social care. Service users and carers have fewer rights and consequently less control over stressors than paid carers, however, so this section continues to examine the increasing number of demands, and their associated pressures, that are placed on service users and informal carers in contemporary society.

Personal and reflective knowledge

This chapter has been designed to enhance learning through developing self-awareness. The final part of this chapter looks at time management as a means of taking control of stressors and helps you to develop a stress management routine.

On pages 222–223 are four case studies, each relating to one of the branch programmes. You may find it helpful to read them before you start the chapter to use as a focus for your reflections.

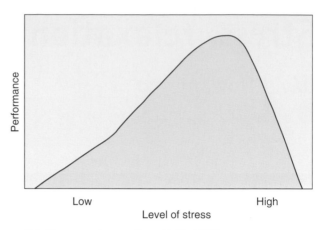

Figure 9.1 The arousal curve (from Hebb 1955).

SUBJECT KNOWLEDGE

Think about being stressed. Then think about being relaxed. Are they opposite ends of the same scale, or are they more difficult to define? Is stress always bad? Is being relaxed the same as resting? Can you relax and be active at the same time?

Answering these questions can be confusing as at face value the terms seem to be conflicting. So, to begin this chapter the concepts of stress, relaxation and rest will be examined in greater detail.

CONCEPTS OF STRESS

Most contemporary work into stress and stress management is influenced by the fundamental works of Seyle (1984) and Hebb (1955). It was Seyle's work that led medicine to become interested in stress (Pacak & Palkovits, 2001) and it is his definition of stress as 'the non-specific response of the body to any demand' (Seyle 1984: 74) that has become used widely in both research and practice.

In vernacular use the term stress is usually associated with negative feelings. This is not always correct though, as a certain amount of stress is a normal part of day-to-day life. Hebb (1955) originally demonstrated this in the arousal curve (Fig 9.1), where an individual's performance is seen to increase in proportion to the level of arousal. Once the individual's maximum capacity for arousal is exceeded

though, performance falls and adverse effects on an individual's health begin.

Although since surpassed by more complex models, what is important about Hebb's work is that it shows all individuals require a certain amount of stress to achieve optimal functioning. Once this point is exceeded though, an individual's ability to function deteriorates rapidly and this is also associated with negative effects in health. This explains why people in very demanding, high-pressure jobs are at risk of developing stress-related diseases.

Hebb's work explains the relationship between exposure to excessive stress, performance and illness; however, people who have jobs that offer little in the way of stimulation also develop stress-related diseases. This apparent contradiction to Hebb's arousal theory was proposed by Sutherland & Cooper (1990) and latterly by Zivnuska et al (2002). While they agreed with Hebb that over-stimulation caused excessive stress, they found that stress also could be caused by under-stimulation. This led to the evolution of Hebb's arousal curve into an inverted U which identified an optimal level of performance in the centre of excessive levels of stress characterized by under-stimulation and over-stimulation (Fig. 9.2) and shows that boredom is just as stressful as over-stimulation.

Seyle (1984) took a slightly different view on the nature of stress. He argued that stress could be positive or negative. Positive stress he named *eustress* (from the Greek word 'eu'; good) and it is associated with feelings of excitement or euphoria. Conversely, negative stress was named *distress* (from the Latin word 'dis'; bad). Although the body undergoes similar immediate physiological changes in both types of stress, it is the long-term effects of distress that are damaging. Seyle's definition integrates well with the inverted U hypothesis in that individuals require a certain amount of arousal to perform optimally (whether this occurs when working or when relaxing). This occurs in eustress stimulation. If the arousal becomes too great or too little, however, then eustress is replaced by distress.

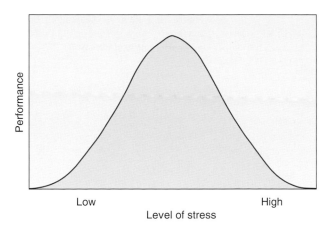

Figure 9.2 The inverted U curve (from Sutherland & Cooper 1990).

Often, whether stress is positive or negative is related to whether the individual has control of the stressor (the object triggering the stress). Stress that occurs where the individual retains control is positive and exhilarating. On the other hand, where the individual has little control of the threat then the experience is negative and damaging. This is referred to as the locus of control, a lack of which has been linked to poorer health outcomes (Schmitz et al 2000, Coyne 2006, Sjöström-Strand & Fridlund 2007). See Evolve 9.1 for more information and an exercise to develop your awareness of this.

9.1 – TAKING CONTROL

- Recognize the differences between eustress and distress.
- Be aware of the importance of control in stressful situations.

PHYSIOLOGICAL CHANGES IN STRESS

The General Adaptation Syndrome

Once a stressor is detected as a potential threat the hypothalamus is stimulated, which in turn invokes the General Adaptation Syndrome. This is a physiological response described by Seyle (1984), the framework of which continues to be accepted as valid. It occurs over three consecutive stages (Fig. 9.3).

1. Alarm reaction

This is a very rapid physiological response, activated by the sympathetic nervous system and adrenal medulla, which prepares the body for action. It causes an increase in the secretion of adrenaline (epinephrine) and noradrenaline (norepinephrine), invoking the fight or flight response causing the physiological changes summarized in Table 9.1, which prepare the body to either confront and fight, or to escape quickly from, the stressor.

2. Resistance reaction

The alarm reaction is followed by the resistance reaction. This is a long-term response brought about by a chain of hormones originating in the hypothalamus (see Fig. 9.3). It begins with the release of corticotrophin releasing hormone which stimulates the anterior pituitary gland to secrete adrenocorticotrophic hormone. In turn this stimulates the adrenal cortex to increase the secretion of cortisol. The action of cortisol increases glycogenesis and catabolism of body proteins leading to hyperglycaemia, which provides energy to sustain the response.

Cortisol also suppresses the inflammation response, enabling the body to continue this reaction if it becomes damaged. It also constricts the peripheral blood vessels and maintains blood pressure within the skeletal muscles and vital internal organs should blood loss occur though damage to the body surface.

Cortisol also suppresses reconstruction of connective tissue and the immune system though, which can have serious adverse consequences in the long term. In practice, this is likely to be of particular significance during recovery from illness or surgery.

3. Exhaustion

This is the final stage of the General Adaptation Syndrome. It occurs following prolonged exposure to stressors and, if continued, leads to illness and, eventually, death. Prolonged use of the General Adaptation Syndrome, as occurs in stressful environments where there is no escape, therefore has adverse consequences for the health of individuals.

THE STRESSFUL PERSONALITY

Some individuals consistently respond to stressors in similar ways. The most common classification is that of Friedman & Rosenman (1974) who identified two personality types: type A and type B (Fig. 9.4). The type A personality is characterized by extreme competitiveness and an inability to place stressors in perspective. They routinely work against the clock, find it difficult to say 'no' or to delegate, and consequently find themselves with multiple commitments. Consequently, they are unable to fit all their demands into the available time and they end up juggling tasks, switching from one to another, without completing any. This is

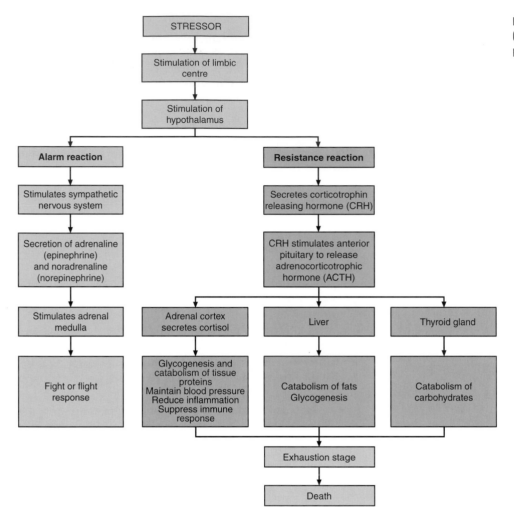

Figure 9.3 General Adaptation Syndrome (adapted from Seyle 1984 by kind permission of McGraw-Hill).

Table 9.1 Major physiological changes associated with the flight or fight response

System	Effect	Outcome
Circulatory system	Increased heart rate and force of contraction Peripheral vasoconstriction	Concentrates blood in the body core, increases blood pressure and increases the flow of blood to the large skeletal muscles that will be used either in fighting or running away
Respiratory system	Increase in respiration rate Dilation of bronchi	Increases oxygenation of the blood, providing the muscles with vast amounts of oxygen in anticipation of the increased aerobic respiration involved in major exertion
Eyes	Pupil dilation	Allows more light into the eyes, resulting in better vision
Skeletal muscles	Increased tension	Quicker response
Excretory system	Increased micturition	Removes excess fluid to reduce body weight and allow a quicker response
Digestive system	Diarrhoea Vomiting Dry mouth	Reduces weight Reduces weight Prevents eating and adding to weight
Skin	Sweat gland activation	Increases cooling in anticipation of muscle activity

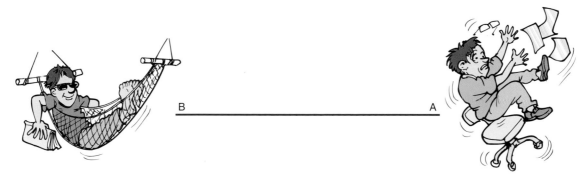

Figure 9.4 Type A and type B personalities.

worsened by a lack of direction. Rather than taking a systematic approach to problem solving, they attempt to solve problems without first identifying the goals. They are also fiercely competitive, leading them to appear aggressive, and they react to minor irritations in the form of temper tantrums. By way of contrast, the second personality type, type B, is the antithesis to type A. They are almost unconcerned when confronted by stressors.

Type A and type B are in reality two extreme points of a scale. Most people have traits of both personality types and fit on a point somewhere along it. Significantly though, Friedman & Rosenman, and latterly Myrtek (2001), found that people with more type B characteristics were less susceptible to coronary heart disease.

It is not just the circulatory system that is affected by continued exposure to stressful events though. Figure 9.3 shows that the action of cortisol suppresses the immune response. This was demonstrated by Brosschot et al (1998) and Segerstrom &Miller (2004), who found that when individuals were exposed to stressors they were unable to control, their immune systems became suppressed. Similarly, Pruessner et al (1999) reported that individuals who were in situations where they experienced high distress and low self-esteem had higher serum cortisol than would be expected, which in turn suppressed their immune systems. A suppressed immune system renders the individual less able to fight off disease. Often people find that when they are tired, such as when they have been working for a long time without a holiday break, they become more susceptible to minor infections such as colds, and that once they contract an infection it takes longer than usual to recover. Indeed, the incidence of sickness in the workplace is an indicator of employee stress.

The immune system also protects the body against more sinister diseases though. Following major life events an extreme stress response is invoked and it has been observed that for around a year afterwards people have an increased susceptibility to developing cancers (Lillberg et al 2003, Thaker et al 2007).

Evidence-based practice

Continued exposure to stressful events

One of the most obvious effects of continued exposure to stress occurs in the circulatory system. During the General Adaptation Syndrome, heart rate and blood pressure increase and after time this can damage the circulatory system as it tries to compensate. This was demonstrated in the fundamental research of Friedman & Rosenman (1974), although studies continue to report associations between high levels of psychological distress and coronary heart disease (Bosma et al 1997, Stansfeld et al 2002, Sjöström-Strand & Fridlund 2007).

Furthermore it has been identified that if type A behaviour is accompanied by hostile behaviour, then these individuals are the most likely develop coronary heart disease (Barefoot et al, 1995).

PSYCHO/SOCIAL RESPONSES TO STRESS

Psycho/social responses to stress vary according to the level of threat. A mild level of stimulation, where the individual remains in control (eustress), is accompanied by positive feelings. As the level of stress increases though, the pleasure changes to a feeling of being overwhelmed (distress). The ability to function effectively decreases and although individuals may be aware of what is happening, they find it difficult to engage in problem-solving thinking. Consequently, individuals find they have ever-increasing demands that they are unable to meet, which in turn perpetuates their distress.

Due to the fight or flight reaction that this invokes, individuals may become short tempered and aggressive, and often their social interactions will reflect this increased hostility where they may experience frequent arguments and become intolerant of others. In the long term, this causes their interpersonal relationships to deteriorate (Vernarec 2001), making things worse, and individuals can quickly find themselves locked into a stress cycle.

MENTAL DEFENCE MECHANISMS

Often, in response to stressors, individuals attempt to cope by using mental defence mechanisms (Table 9.2). These were originally identified by Freud (1934), who claimed

they provided a defence against conflict, and they have since been developed by many other psychologists. In the short term mental defence mechanisms are a healthy response and they buy time for the individual to adjust. As they do not alter the cause of the distress (they only alter an individual's interpretation of it) they involve a degree of self-deception and prevent the individual from addressing the problems. Consequently, prolonged use of mental defence mechanisms is unhealthy and potentially damaging.

Table 9.2 Mental defence mechanisms (Freud 1934)

Mechanism	Definition	Example
Denial	When reality is too unpleasant or painful to face then individuals may deny that it really exists. In some circumstances this is a healthy process as it allows the individual time to come to terms with the problem. Indeed it is the first stage of the grieving process (Kubler Ross 1975). In other situations denial may be more serious (see example)	A woman may deny that she could have a serious illness and may delay seeking medical help for a lump she has recently found in her breast
Displacement	When it is impossible to address the cause of stress then anger may be redirected on another, innocent but reachable object	You may have been given a hard time by your boss to whom you are unable to retaliate. When you return home you immediately have a blazing argument with your partner
Intellectualization	To use intellectual powers of thinking, analysis and reasoning to detach oneself from emotional issues	For people working in life or death situations, such as in high dependency units, this defence mechanism may be necessary for survival. If the emotional bluntness extends into other areas of the individuals' lives, however, then the mechanism becomes problematic
Projection	Blaming someone else for how you feel	The ward manager who is unable to manage the ward effectively may blame the situation on incompetent staff
Rationalization	To find an acceptable explanation for an act that you find unacceptable	'It's in the overall best interest' 'You have to be cruel to be kind' 'I don't really care that I lost the interview. I didn't really want the job anyway'
Reaction formation	To conceal what you really feel by thinking and acting in the opposite way	Some people who have an issue in their life about which they feel uncomfortable may campaign against the issue For example, individuals who have led promiscuous lives may campaign strongly for the sanctity of family values
Regression	Individuals engage in behaviours from an earlier, more secure, life stage	Losing your temper and engaging in tantrums when things go wrong Eating when feeling stressed
Repression	Painful thoughts are forced into the unconscious. Although they are out of the conscious they may resurface in dreams	An accident victim may utilize repression to have no recollection of the events surrounding the accident
Sublimation	To redirect the energy from unacceptable sexual or aggressive drives into another socially acceptable activity	Unacceptable aggressive energy focused into a sporting activity This may not always be a positive mechanism. For example, an ambitious manager may utilize sublimation to secure promotions at the expense of family and social commitments

POST-TRAUMATIC STRESS DISORDER

Post-traumatic stress disorder (PTSD) is a severe response to an extremely threatening or catastrophic event or situation (e.g. being a victim of a violent crime or witnessing a major disaster) that occurs within the 6 months of the triggering factor (World Health Organization 1992).

The main features of PTSD are:

- Flashbacks where individuals relive the experience during nightmares. Occasionally, when awake, they may also feel that the situation is about to recur.
- Emotional numbness and detachment from others.
- Hypervigilance and an enhanced startle reaction.
- Avoidance of anything resembling the triggering event.
- Confusion, anxiety and depression; there may be attempts to commit suicide.

Additionally, a number of other symptoms can occur including insomnia, headaches, ulcers and circulatory problems. Sometimes individuals blame themselves for the incident and suffer additional fear and guilt. Furthermore, to compensate individuals may abuse alcohol or other drugs, which may lead to dependence.

The most effective methods of treatment for PTSD are early supportive interventions that avoid focusing on the traumatic event. Following 1 month, however, all individuals involved in the event should be screened for PTSD. Those identified as suffering can then be offered targeted interventions, which should also include support for the sufferer's family (NICE 2005). Chapter 12, 'Aggression', contains further information on managing PTSD.

BURNOUT

When people are exposed to stressors for prolonged periods they can develop a condition called burnout. People suffering from burnout feel drained, emotionally blunt and cynical. As burnout is usually work-related; sufferers feel devalued by their employers and trivialize any achievements they make. Consequently their relationships within work deteriorate and the effects can also spill out of the workplace where they may struggle to maintain social contacts and partnerships (Leiter & Maslach, 2005).

Most employees in health and social care work with ill people for prolonged periods, often with inadequate resources or support. These are powerful sources of distress which predisposes to burnout (Schmitz et al 2000, Leiter & Maslach 2005).

Burnout is aggravated by the highly competitive, insecure workplaces that are common in contemporary society, where working long hours – frequently for low pay – are seen as normal (Leiter & Maslach, 2005). This leads individuals to feel that their feelings are as a result of weakness in their character, thus compounding their problem as they are reluctant to seek help (Payne 2001).

CAUSES OF STRESS

The causes of stress (stressors) are the result of an individual's interpretation of a phenomenon. Holmes & Rahe (1967) discovered that certain life events invoked differing amounts of stress and that their effects accumulated. Their classification of the significance of these stressors forms the Social Readjustment Rating Scale (SRRS) (Box 9.1), an instrument which is still commonly used. On this scale, according to the amount of stress invoked by a stressor, a greater weighting is ascribed to it.

To use the scale, each stressor that has occurred within the previous year is identified. By summating the rating ascribed to each it becomes possible to assess an individual's level of stress. For clinical work, Holmes & Rahe found that a score over 300 was associated with an increased risk of developing a stress-related disease.

Evidence-based practice

Following the loss of a partner, the surviving spouse often becomes ill and may die. Lichtenstein et al (1998) found people most at risk were those bereaved between 60 and 70 years. Similar findings were reported by Hart et al (2007) who found the mortality rate among surviving spouses of all ages to be raised significantly.

Within the context of stressful life events, surviving partners, particularly within the older age group, are likely to have: recently experienced retirement, a reduction in income, adjusted to their own ill health, supported the deceased partner and the demands of their illness, experienced the death of the partner, met the financial and family demands following the death and undergone their own grieving, from both the loss of their partner and, according to Narayanasamy (1996), from feeling abandoned by their spiritual beliefs.

Try using the SRRS to calculate the effect of the above stressors on an individual. You will find a web-based SRRS calculator in Evolve 9.2 on the Evolve website.

⊖volve learning system

9.2 – THE SOCIAL READJUSTMENT RATING SCALE

- Know the different stressful life events.
- Know how to estimate the level of stress in an individual's life.
- Know how to estimate the level of stress in your own life.

Even when experiencing similar stressors some individuals appear to be able to cope better than others. By using Hebb's model of arousal (Hebb 1955) in conjunction with the SRRS (Holmes & Rahe 1967), it is possible to see why one

Box 9.1 The Social Readjustment Rating Scale (from Holmes & Rahe 1967, by kind permission)

1. Death of spouse	100
2. Divorce	73
3. Marital separation	65
4. Jail term	65
5. Death of close family member	63
6. Personal injury or illness	53
7. Marriage	50
8. Loss of job	47
9. Marital reconciliation	45
10. Retirement	45
11. Change in health of family member	44
12. Pregnancy	40
13. Sex difficulties	39
14. Gain of new family member	39
15. Business readjustment	39
16. Change in financial state	38
17. Death of close friend	37
18. Change to different line of work	36
19. Change in number of arguments with spouse	35
20. Mortgage over $10 000	31
21. Foreclosure of mortgage or loan	30
22. Change in responsibilities at work	29
23. Son or daughter leaving home	29
24. Trouble with in-laws	29
25. Outstanding personal achievement	28
26. Wife begins or stops work	26
27. Begin or end school	26
28. Change in living conditions	25
29. Revision of personal habits	24
30. Trouble with boss	23
31. Change in work hours or conditions	20
32. Change in residence	20
33. Change in school	20
34. Change in recreation	19
35. Change in church activities	19
36. Change in social activities	18
37. Mortgage or loan of less than $10 000	17
38. Change in sleeping habits	16
39. Change in the number of family get-togethers	15
40. Change in eating habits	15
41. Holiday	13
42. Christmas	12
43. Minor violations of the law	11

A score over 300 is associated with an increased risk of developing a stress related disease (Holmes & Rahe 1967).

individual may be unaffected by an incident while to another individual the effect of the same incident may be catastrophic. By using the SRRS to review life events that occurred over the previous year, it could be found that one individual had an accumulation of many stressors while the other had comparatively few. Thus exposure to the same new stressor could push the first individual into overload whereas the other had sufficient coping reserve.

The SRRS was developed over 40 years ago and has been criticized for its inability to predict the specific type of illness and for relying on retrospective data. Despite this, it remains a reliable instrument and enjoys extensive contemporary use in practice and research (Scully at al 2000). There are two major limitations of the scale, however. First, it only addresses long-term stressors and fails to take into account short-term stressors such as being late for work or sitting in a traffic jam. Short-term stressors, or 'hassles', invoke a severe stress response but only for a short period (Lazarus et al 1985). Being out of the individual's control though, they invoke distress and have adverse effects on health.

The second shortcoming of the SRRS is forwarded by Le Fevre et al (2006), who argue that it is difficult to generalize individuals' esoteric experiences of stress. Holmes & Rahe (1967) assumed that a stressor causes the same amount of stress for everyone. This is the engineering model of stress and is demonstrated in Figure 9.5 where the spider is interpreted identically by subject A and subject B.

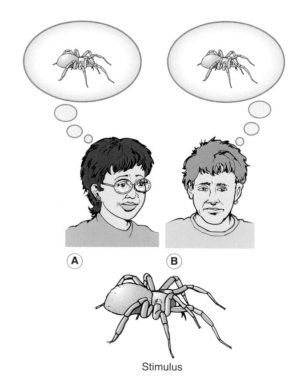

Figure 9.5 Interpreting the spider identically.

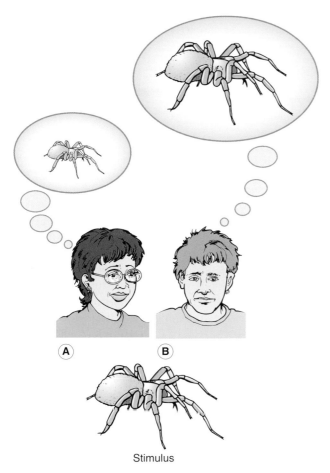

Figure 9.6 How each individual interprets the threat of the spider.

Le Fevre et al (2006) argue this model is too simplistic, and that to gain a true understanding of the nature of stress, the stressor must be appraised from the context of the perceived threat (or excitement) that it poses; i.e. the level of stress depends on the amount of threat the individual thinks it poses. This is represented in Figure 9.6 where subjects A and B are exposed to the same stressor as before but, because of the meaning subject B attaches to the spider in that particular context, the interpretation of threat is greater for subject B than subject A.

Therefore, to understand an individual's stress also requires measuring hassles and gaining an understanding of their interpretation of stressors (Lazarus et al 1985, Hahn & Smith 1999, Narayanasamy & Owens 2001, Le Fevre et al 2006). Applied to clinical practice, this suggests that the use of the SRRS to measure long-term stress is useful in so much as it identifies a baseline of background stressors. From this baseline, however, the effects of day-to-day stressors and the interpretation an individual attaches to the nature of stressful experiences must also be added.

RELAXATION AND REST

Relaxation and rest are linked strongly with stress. Sometimes relaxing is simply doing something different from work. Thus, relaxation can be active or recreational, for example walking or playing a sport (eustressful activities). At other times relaxing means reducing physical activity (such as sunbathing).

Relaxation is generally the precursor to rest. Rest is the period when the body does minimum activity; allowing restorative processes to happen and following which the individual feels refreshed or rested. Often this coincides with sleep.

Although there is a close relationship between stress and relaxation, they are not opposite ends of a scale. It depends on context and the amount of control the individual has over the situation. Sitting down and doing nothing in a quiet room at home may be relaxing; however, sitting and doing nothing in an airport because your flight has been delayed is far from restful! Similar to stress then, relaxation and rest need to be examined in context.

SLEEP

Sleep is associated with resting. It is a recurrent natural condition where consciousness is temporarily lost and bodily functions are partly suspended. It ends either by a natural return of consciousness or by external stimulation, for example by an alarm clock.

There are five stages in the sleep cycle (Box 9.2). Initially individuals move through stages 1 to 4. This is followed by a period of rapid eye movement (REM) sleep, a lighter level of sleep which is when dreaming occurs and is also when the individual will change position in bed. The sleep cycle then returns to stage 2 and repeats until the individual awakens. Each cycle lasts around 90 minutes in an adult, although the length of time spent at each stage alters throughout the night; during the early night the percentage spent in stages 3 and 4 is larger in comparison to REM sleep, while in the later hours of sleep the proportion of REM sleep increases.

Circadian rhythm

Why we feel tired at night and sleep when we do is largely controlled by the circadian rhythm. When deprived of light or other sources of time-keeping humans adopt a sleep–wake routine which cycles approximately every 25 hours. This is the circadian rhythm, although in real life it is modified in response to triggers called *zeitgebers* (time cues). These synchronize the circadian rhythm of an individual with the environment, and the most powerful of them are of an informative or social nature (Sharma & Chandrashekaran 2005). Examples are:

Box 9.2 The five stages of sleep (adapted from Horne 1988, by kind permission of Oxford University Press)

Stage 1	Falling asleep. The individual becomes drowsy and barely conscious, although any slight sound would arouse him or her. Electroencephalograph (EEG) recordings show alpha waves that are associated with being awake
Stage 2	The individual is now asleep. Skeletal muscles are relaxed and movements are still; however, the individual can be roused easily. The EEG shows the appearance of slow waves called K-complexes, as well as bursts of rapid waves known as sleep spindles (Borbely 1987). Stage 2 accounts for more than half the time spent asleep
Stage 3	The individual is completely relaxed and is difficult to arouse. Familiar noises, such as a child crying, can awaken the individual, however. EEG waves become slower and larger and are known as delta waves (Borbely 1987)
Stage 4	Deep sleep. The individual rarely moves and is difficult to awaken. An increase in the percentage of delta waves is noted on EEG recording
Stage 5	Rapid eye movement (REM) or paradoxical sleep. This is characterized by a period of light sleep during which dreaming is thought to mainly occur. For Freudian analysts, dreaming is a symbolic process where the unconscious conflicts are brought to the conscious for resolution

- the light/dark cycle
- knowledge of clock time
- the behaviour of others
- mealtimes.

Activity within circadian rhythm cycles also varies between two broad personality types:

- 'Larks' who awaken early and do their best work in the morning. However, they become tired by early evening and do not function as efficiently.
- 'Owls' who have difficulty rising in the morning, often have difficulty facing breakfast and do not really perform at their best until late afternoon and evening. Owls also tend to go to bed late.

Reflection and portfolio exercise

Are you a 'lark' or an 'owl'?

You can use this information when developing your time management programme, particularly when identifying the best time to study.

Patterns of sleep

Although sleeping once at night is normal in most North European countries, one type of sleep pattern is not relevant for all cultures. For example, in some Mediterranean cultures a siesta is taken in the hottest part of the day and in China workers are expected to have a sleep in the middle of the day as part of the lunchtime break. However, it is common in Western society for individuals to receive insufficient sleep. Taheri et al (2004) reported that this can lead to an endocrine imbalance resulting in an increased appetite and, in turn, weight gain; in nurses working rotational shifts, Muecke (2005) reported this resulted in a decrease in performance which in turn had ramifications on patients' safety.

The normal pattern of sleep also changes with age (Table 9.3). However, within these norms individuals' needs for sleep differ. It is therefore impossible to generalize exclusively from these data and it is the individual who best knows whether or not they are receiving enough sleep.

CARE DELIVERY KNOWLEDGE

Although individuals respond to stress in their own esoteric ways, some responses are universal. By measuring these it is possible to assess the degree of stress an individual is experiencing and to consider the ramifications on their ability to relax and rest. The first part of this section therefore begins by outlining tools to measure stress. This progresses to examine common causes of stress affecting clients, carers and care professionals and at the end of this section, strategies for managing stress are discussed.

The second part of Care Delivery Knowledge discusses how sleep may be assessed and outlines approaches to use to promote sleep.

METHODS OF ASSESSING STRESS

Physiological measures

Because of the relationship between psychological stress and physiological disturbance, demonstrated by the General Adaptation Syndrome (Seyle 1984), it is possible to

Table 9.3 Pattern of sleep according to age

Age	2 months	3 years	25 years	75 years
Amount of sleep	18 hours	13 hours	8 hours	5 hours in 24 hours
Pattern of sleep	Asleep between daytime feeds	Night sleep and day nap	Night sleep	Night sleep and day nap(s)

assess stress using physiological measures such as the electrical conductivity of the skin, heart rate and blood pressure. The disadvantage of physiological measures is that they do not *explain* why the individual feels stressed. Furthermore, the process of recording may be distressing for individuals and this may result in an inaccurate measurement (Gerin et al 2006). Therefore, although it is important to understand physiological indicators of stress, to understand the nature of the stress requires additional information.

Decision-making exercise

Immediately on admission most patients have their baseline observations recorded.

- Referring to the General Adaptation Syndrome, what are advantages and disadvantages of this?
- How might the disadvantages be addressed?
- Go to http://www.bpassoc.org.uk/BloodPressureandyou/Medicaltests/whitecoateffect and consider why nurses should take into account the 'white coat effect' when recording blood pressure.

The Social Readjustment Rating Scale

The SRRS (Holmes & Rahe 1967) was discussed in the Subject Knowledge section of this chapter. It is inappropriate to use only this instrument, as it may not record all the factors that are causing the current period of distress. Nor does it measure the amount of stress felt by the individual. However, this is an excellent instrument to gain insight into the background of an individual's situation, and to provide avenues for further exploration.

Stress scales and diaries

Because it is experienced by an individual, and not outwardly observable, stress is very difficult to measure. A very similar construct with equally difficult measurement is pain. Because of its subjective nature, the amount of pain patients experienced was frequently misjudged and in consequence they were given inadequate analgesia. This led to the development of pain scales where patients indicated the severity of pain they felt ranging from 'No pain' at one end to 'Unbearable pain' at the other. Although these are not decisive measures of pain, they indicate the effectiveness of pain management strategies, particularly if they include some form of scaling.

As stress is also a subjective phenomenon, to gain insight into stress from an individual's perspective, instruments should measure the nature, frequency and intensity of the experience. The combination of scales and diaries to indicate the time, nature and precipitating factors make these useful instruments to assess the nature of stress that clients experience.

Evidence-based practice

In research into the experiences of student nurses, a modification of pain scales proved a very effective measure. An instrument was designed around a 10-point scale. Prompts were included for guidance and ranged from 0, which indicated no stress at all, to 10 which indicated feeling totally overwhelmed, reflecting Seyle's (1984) model of stress with lower scores indicating eustress and higher scores distress. These were supplemented with brief diary notes and over a period of time stress profiles were generated for each student. Combining these data subsequently allowed identification of particularly stressful periods of the pre-registration nursing course which could be addressed in future course planning and provision of supportive services (Howard 2001).

IDENTIFYING COMMON SOURCES OF STRESS

For clarity, this section examines separately stress that occurs in clients, in their relatives and in the workplace.

Stress in clients

Stress that clients experience may be:

- a primary reason for referral
- a cause of, or a contributory factor to, an illness
- occurring as a consequence of an illness.

Stress as a primary reason for referral

Everybody's experience of stress is unique, depending on their interpretation of the stressors, the context of the stressors, and the number of stressors influencing the individual at any particular time. Similarly, individuals' responses to stress will vary. Although the fight or flight syndrome classifies specific stress response behaviours, some individuals present as very anxious and apprehensive, some become very dependent on others to the point of automatic compliance, whereas others react with anger. Consequently, to be able to assist individuals it is necessary to understand how they experience stress and why they react in that way. The purpose of assessment in this instance is to establish how the stress affects the individual's life and to identify recurrent patterns of events that act as triggers. From this baseline, interventions that are appropriate for that individual can be developed.

Stress as a cause of or a contributory factor to an illness

As was seen in subject knowledge on page 202, a high level of stress can adversely affect physical and mental health. Therefore, even though an illness may be physical, accompanying stress, if left unaddressed, may hinder recovery.

Individuals may also be referred for a condition that is exacerbated by stress – a stress related illness. The purpose of assessment in this instance is to identify what the precipitating stressor was (e.g. becoming unemployed), when it happened, the context in which it happened, what other issues occurred at the time, how quickly the illness developed, and to establish how the client feels able to cope with the issues arising.

Reflection and portfolio evidence

In your practice placements note:

- How often and for what conditions stress is referred to as a key factor in the development of the disease/illness.
- How knowledge of the part stress can play in the condition affects its management.
- What strategies are used to support the individual in managing stressors.

Record your findings in your portfolio of evidence.

Stress occurring as a consequence of illness

Clients may be concerned, for example, that they are going to die, that they are going to be in pain, that they may not wake up from an anaesthetic or that their prognosis is poor. To the nurse working on a busy ward these fears may appear unfounded. To the individual though, they are very real. It is very easy for nurses to become desensitized to clients' fears in a busy environment.

Waiting for results is a particularly stressful time. The insecurity inhibits positive thought processes, particularly if the tests are to confirm a life-threatening disease. Uncertainty therefore moves the stressor out of the individual's control and they become distressed which, due to the fight or flight response, may be shown as denial or an aggressive attitude. Although it is possible to plan how to cope with the consequences of the test, it is only when the results of tests are known that the stressor can be isolated and positive steps taken to secure control.

Clients going into hospital may also worry about their continuing responsibilities. They may have dependent relatives and be uncertain about how they will be cared for. They may have a pet that requires care. They may worry about loss of income. They may be concerned that they will be unable to work again. The nurse, on identifying these problems, must spend time with the client and explore the issues from the client's perspective. It may sound obvious, but it is only after problems have been identified that they can be addressed.

Clients may also experience spiritual distress, particularly when confronted with a poor prognosis. They may feel betrayed, asking 'Why me?', or may believe that they are being punished. Indeed, even in clients who do not have religious beliefs, often there is a need to make sense of their life and their situation, and it is this issue that provides a focus for nursing interventions (Lin & Bauer-Wu 2003).

Stress in clients' relatives

In a client's relatives, stress may result from concern about the client's illness, anger that the client is ill or guilt that they are unable to cope. Some carers demonstrate this by avoiding the client and rarely, if ever, visit. At face value this appears callous and uncaring. Within the context of individuals' reactions to stress though, this can result from the fight or *flight* reaction or the mental defence mechanism of denial.

Similarly, the *fight* or flight reaction explains why other relatives may react aggressively. Often their distress is projected on to the nurse and the relatives may be hostile and constantly find fault with care. In turn, the relative may be labelled 'troublesome', thus perpetuating the situation. Alternatively, relatives may feel excluded from caring for their sick relative. This compounds their guilt and may again increase hostility towards care staff. This emphasizes the importance of an understanding of the mechanisms of stress so as to recognize distress experienced by relatives and ameliorate their concerns. (For further information on managing hostility see Ch. 12, 'Aggression').

In the community, carers of clients may be distressed that they are unable to meet the client's needs, or that they experience too many demands on their time. According to the 2001 census (Office for National Statistics 2006) there are 5.1 million informal carers in the UK, and around half of these are in some form of employment in addition to their caring role. These demands generate considerable stress and this can eventually have considerable negative effects on their own health, particularly their mental health (Hirst 2004). Indeed, in some circumstances, when carers have insufficient support they have abused the person they are caring for. See Ch. 12, 'Aggression', for more information on the protection of vulnerable adults.

Stress in the workplace

Working in health and social care is a stressful occupation. Members of staff are expected to cope in traumatic situations. They work unsocial hours and are expected to do more with limited resources. Frequently their remuneration is minimal and many do not have the security of a permanent contract of employment. In addition to daytime shift work, many staff have to work periods of nights. Although research into circadian rhythms suggests that for short periods of time the body does not significantly alter its biological routines (Folkard 1991), it can lead to poor concentration and excessive tiredness (Muecke 2005); and it can be extremely disruptive to out-of-work commitments. In addition, care staff are exposed to physiological stressors such as chemicals, solvents, poor lighting, poor heating, inadequate ventilation and excessive noise.

Many inquiries into stress have focused on healthcare workers. Because of the wide range of staff working in health care, however, it is difficult to generalize findings obtained from one grade of staff to another. However, the core issues of mortality, workload and role conflict are consistently cited, and these are strongly associated with burnout (Quine 1998, Janssen et al 1999, Meadows et al 2000, Howard 2001, Payne 2001, Leiter & Maslach 2005).

Common indicators of excessive stress in the workplace are:

- bringing work home
- not being able to switch off from work
- feeling tense all of the time
- poor self-esteem
- difficulty in mixing with others
- deteriorating relationships
- an increase in arguments at work
- talking malevolently about colleagues
- feeling run down
- an increase in minor physical illnesses.

Individuals are often unaware of these signs, which can then develop into a more serious problem. However, using feedback from others, clinical supervision and developing greater self-awareness will help to identify these damaging events and plan actions to limit them.

STRESS MANAGEMENT STRATEGIES

Stress management strategies fall into proactive and reactive methods. Reactive methods are used following a stressful event to help to contain the problem. Consequently, they work on the assumption that there is stress to be managed in the first place. In contrast, proactive strategies are taken to prevent or to minimize the number of stressful events experienced. Most methods of stress management can be used either proactively or reactively; however, to manage stress effectively, the aim should be to use all strategies proactively.

Diet

Reactions to stress may lead to changes in eating habits such as under-eating or overeating. Commonly, when under prolonged stress (such as when completing assessments), individuals regress to a more secure developmental stage and engage in 'comfort eating' – consuming comfort foods which invariably contain high levels of sugar and fats. Additionally, many increase their consumption of alcohol. During the resistance stage of the General Adaptation Syndrome, the body also retains sodium by excreting high levels of potassium. Left unchecked this could lead to exhaustion and, eventually, death. Although this is an extreme example, because of the tendency to adopt unhealthy eating habits, a well-balanced diet is central to all stress management programmes.

> ### Reflection and portfolio evidence
>
> Keep a daily record of what you eat and drink, together with an indication of how stressed you feel. Use a scale of 0–10 where:
>
> - 0 = No stress
> - 1–4 = Positive stress
> - 5–7 = Becoming distressed
> - 8–9 = Very distressed
> - 10 = Totally overwhelmed
>
> You might also like to note what happened during the day to make you feel the way that you feel.

Continued

Reflection and portfolio evidence—cont'd

- Did your diet change as you became more stressed?
- How did it make you feel at the time?
- How does it make you feel now?
- How could you adopt a healthier pattern of eating when you feel stressed in the future?

Exercise

Exercise is often advocated as part of stress management and this commonly occurs in individual activities such as swimming, jogging, or gym work, or as sporting activity. Engaging in exercise means that attention is focused on the activity, thus diverting attention from the worrying recurrent thoughts that sustain the underlying stress. Exercise also provides a safe, socially acceptable outlet for the aggressive drives that manifest during the fight or flight syndrome.

When using exercise as part of stress management it needs to be remembered that the people who are most susceptible to the negative effects of stress are the highly competitive type A personality types (Friedman & Rosenman 1974). Consequently, in individual exercises, they are likely to set ever-increasing goals that they strive to achieve. Because of the underlying aggressiveness within their personality, when these individuals participate in sporting activities this effect is intensified if the end result involves defeating someone else. To counter this effect, some contemporary authors advocate engaging in non-competitive sports. As the nature of all sport is competition, however, the hollow 'politically correct' rhetoric of non-competitiveness is impossible to enact, and advocates of this strategy are understandably ridiculed. What is important is that individuals retain control of the competitive element of sport, playing for enjoyment as well as achievement, and enjoying the social benefits that accompany the activity.

Maintaining a realistic perspective on life

Time should be made for all aspects of life including work, leisure and personal relationships. When stress is excessive, individuals find that they have little time for anything other than meeting the demands of their stressors. This is a particular feature of work-related stress (Vernarec 2001, Leiter & Maslach 2005), and the difficulties are compounded should the individual work unsocial hours or shifts. In effective stress management, it is essential that individuals maintain their social contacts, for example friends and family, and take time to engage in leisure activities to retain an appropriate perspective on the impact of stressors within life. Indeed, many of the strategies that follow include helping the individual to maintain a normal perspective on their life and commitments.

Counselling

Earlier in this chapter it was seen that distress arises when individuals lose control of stressors. Counselling helps individuals to limit the amount of distress that stressors invoke by helping them to develop problem solving strategies for coping and gaining control (British Association of Counselling and Psychology 2007). At times, though, this appears unrealistic. For example, a man may be diagnosed with cancer. He is very likely to be extremely distressed regarding his condition and his prognosis and it is likely that this man would use mental defence mechanisms, particularly denial, at this time. Consequently, the initial focus of counselling would be to get him to accept the situation in which he finds himself. Once this is achieved a problem solving approach can be used to enable him to take control of events, as much as possible, which in turn will minimize his distress.

Cognitive behavioural therapy

The purpose of cognitive behavioural therapy (CBT) in stress management is to replace negative, destructive thoughts with those that are positive and constructive. CBT was developed as a treatment for negative thinking and low self-esteem in depression (Beck 1979). Similar to people with depression, however, individuals who feel overwhelmed through excessive stress also experience a low self-esteem, have negative thought processes and are often distracted by worrying thoughts. CBT can therefore be used successfully with these individuals and it forms part of many stress management programmes.

Rehearsal

A CBT technique that is often used in assertiveness training and is also very useful in the management of stress. It begins by defining the problem and considering the possible outcomes – desirable as well as undesirable. Individuals then consider strategies to achieve a desirable outcome from all alternatives. In this way, responses are practised, and confidence is developed, enabling the individual to take greater control of the situation when it happens in real life.

9.3 – REHEARSAL

- Know how to use the rehearsal technique to prepare for interviews.
- Know how to use rehearsal to help with difficult situations and relationships.

Group therapy

There are many variations of group therapy that can be used in stress management. Community mental health teams frequently run these and they commonly include the following:

Anxiety management groups

These utilize a combination of education, social skills and self-help techniques. Their aim is to provide individuals with an understanding of the nature of stress and anxiety, and to help them to develop more effective skills of coping.

Assertiveness groups

Low self-esteem is generally accompanied by poor assertiveness. Many individuals feel unable to refuse additional work, or fail to stand up for themselves, perpetuating their loss of control and leading to an increase in their level of stress. By developing skills of assertiveness individuals are prepared to take more control of their life. In turn this allows better management of commitments, and subsequently of their stress.

Assertiveness groups can also help people with type A personalities learn less aggressive and more assertive modes of interaction. Their presence in groups containing people with low self-esteem should be managed carefully, however, as type A individuals could become very dominant, and their actions become extremely destructive to other members of the group.

Social skills groups

Low self-esteem may contribute to individuals becoming socially isolated. Social skills groups are designed to help individuals to regain their skills of social interaction and frequently use rehearsal as a strategy. These groups are also useful for people with type A personality traits, who are often impatient and aggressive, to develop more appropriate skills of interaction.

Self-help groups

People with similar problems meet under the supervision of a trained facilitator. The intention of these groups is for members to support each other and to learn vicariously alternative ways of coping with their problems (Vernarec 2001).

Relaxation techniques

Relaxation techniques are used to control the symptoms of stress, predominantly increased muscle tension and recurrent worrying thoughts (Fisher & Durham 1999). Although this is a reactive measure, they are sometimes used to prevent a stressful period from developing into a crisis. They can also help to promote rest and prepare for sleep.

Meditation

The individual sits in a relaxed, balanced posture so that no muscular correction is needed to maintain position. Breathing is reduced to slow deep breaths, counteracting the increased shallow respirations that occur under stress. When the correct body posture is achieved, individuals try to empty their minds of all thoughts or they may focus on a single object, such as a lighted candle. In effect, this stops the recurrent worrying thoughts that occur when people feel distressed and which impair logical thought processes. Meditation enables a sense of calm, and it is from this state that individuals develop problem solving strategies to address their stressors.

Progressive muscle relaxation

In the fight or flight response, muscles contract in preparation for action. This leads to a feeling of tension which perpetuates the feeling of stress. The rationale underpinning progressive muscle relaxation is that stress and reduced muscle tone cannot coexist. Consequently this strategy focuses the individual's attention on relaxing groups of muscles. The individual is asked to contract a muscle group, and then to relax, and to compare the difference; remembering the feeling of relaxation. Each major muscle group is addressed in turn, leading to an overall reduction in muscle tone and, as relaxed muscles are incompatible with feelings of tension, the individual feels relaxed. Progressive muscle relaxation usually occurs when the individual is lying in a quiet room with relaxing background music. However, for individuals experiencing difficulty sleeping it may also be used when they retire to bed.

Relaxation in this way requires practice and clients are often given a tape to practise at home. It is usual for the initial sessions to be conducted by a trained therapist as some individuals may react against the feelings of relaxation with panic as they perceive it as a loss of control.

Massage

This is a method of muscle relaxation that is combined with touch. This is a form of non-verbal communication suggesting that the person performing the massage cares about the individual receiving the massage. Sometimes this is enhanced by the use of aromatic oils. Olfactory receptors are excited by these oils and in turn arouse the limbic centre (Cerrato 1998). In turn, the limbic centre stimulates the release of neurotransmitters, including endorphins, which produce a sense of well-being. The effect of massage often relaxes individuals sufficiently to enable them to discuss their main anxieties and from this foundation, problem solving strategies may be developed.

Biofeedback

This is a behavioural technique that uses operant conditioning to teach the individual how to manage the symptoms associated with stress. There are several variations to this method, all of which focus on the physiological symptoms of the fight or flight syndrome. At its simplest, patients are told to monitor their heart rate or to concentrate on their breathing. Utilizing techniques similar to those of meditation, individuals are asked to try to reduce their pulse or respiration rate. As these fall, so does the feeling of stress.

Acupuncture

In traditional Western medicine acupuncture is thought to work by the release of endorphins in a similar way to massage, and by suggestion. However, in traditional Chinese medicine acupuncture is an holistic treatment that is personalized for each individual. In traditional Chinese medicine, the body's energy (Qi) is comprised of two opposite forces (Yin and Yang). In times of illness Yin and Yang become imbalanced and the aim of acupuncture is to rebalance the flow of Qi. When used in stress management, this helps to resolve associated physical and mental problems. There are links to more information on acupuncture on Evolve 9.4 in the Evolve web resource.

evolve learning system

9.4 – ACUPUNCTURE WEBLINKS

- Access trusted web sources of information on the uses of acupuncture.
- Access trusted web sources of information on the value of acupuncture.
- Access trusted web sources of information on the regulation of acupuncture.

Drug therapies

Prescribed drugs

The routine use of drugs is not part of stress management. In severe instances where pathologies develop, however, the use of medication is helpful. Two categories of drugs are commonly prescribed: anxiolytics and antidepressants. Occasionally, medication may also be prescribed to aid sleep.

Anxiolytics

These include the drugs diazepam and lorazepam and provide immediate relief from the unpleasant feelings associated with stress. In a severe crisis they are prescribed for short periods to reduce the level of anxiety and facilitate the return of problem solving thinking. Should the underlying problems that caused the crisis not be addressed, however, the unpleasant feelings will return as the effects of the drugs wear off. The danger then is that the individual will continue to take the drug to relieve the symptoms, and this can lead rapidly to dependence.

Antidepressants

These drugs are prescribed when individuals experience prolonged periods of distress. Some types of antidepressants, such as amitriptyline, have sedative properties and can be used to reduce recurrent worrying thoughts or, if given as a single night-time dose, to aid sleep. When individuals experience prolonged periods of distress, however, they also experience low self-esteem and the main reason antidepressants are prescribed is to help to improve this, so enabling positive thinking to return and enable individuals to address their problems.

Non-prescribed drugs

Increasing use is being made of non-prescribed preparations, particularly herbal remedies. These are claimed to possess similar properties to traditionally prescribed medication but are available without prescription. Generally, herbal preparations have received little empirical research and their exact mode of action is unknown. Furthermore, the quality of herbal preparations is variable as the active ingredients are often mixed with other constituents, making it difficult to draw conclusions for the benefits or of side-effects (Wong 1998, Ernst 2002). In particular, the safety of these preparations in pregnancy and during lactation is unknown and it follows that women should not take them during these times. Despite these cautions, however, herbal remedies are popular and in the management of stress the two most common remedies are valerian and hypericum perforatum.

Valerian

Valerian is used as a sedative. However, it may also interact with other medication, particularly other sedatives, including alcohol. It is therefore, prudent to take similar precautions to other sedative medication (Wong 1998).

Hypericum perforatum (St John's wort)

Hypericum perforatum (St John's wort) has a long history of use as an antidepressant and is the most investigated herbal remedy (Wong 1998). It is thought to work in a similar way to selective serotonin reuptake inhibitor type antidepressants (SSRIs), and is often referred to as the 'herbal Prozac'. Indeed, it has been shown to be as effective as traditional antidepressants such as fluoxetene and amitriptyline in mild to moderate depression (Ernst 2002, Linde et al 2005). As part of a stress management system, the rationale for its use is similar to conventional antidepressants.

Other stress relieving substances

Many individuals use other substances to relieve stress. These include alcohol, nicotine and some street drugs. They are taken to provide immediate relief from the extreme unpleasant feelings associated with stress or to help induce sleep. This is a very short-term effect though and, as with all drugs, if the underlying problems that caused the distress are not addressed the unpleasant feelings will return as the effects of the drugs wear off. This may encourage the individual to take the drug again and a self-perpetuating cycle leading to dependence may quickly develop.

Decision-making exercise

Many people consume alcohol following stressful episodes. Meeting with friends over a drink is a socially useful outlet for discussion. What should be remembered, however, is that it is the discussion, not the alcohol, that is valuable. Furthermore, as more alcohol is consumed, conversations may turn to issues that have occurred at work.

- Do you ever meet up with friends from work for a drink?
- As conversations in pubs can be overheard by others, what steps do you take to maintain confidentiality?
- What would you do if a colleague began talking about a client in this situation?

SPIRITUAL DISTRESS

In providing spiritual care, Narayanasamy & Owens (2001) found that nurses adopted procedural and personal approaches. Procedural approaches ensured that clients' religious beliefs were recorded and involved arranging for the requirements of their faith to be observed. Personal approaches, where the nurse adopted a counselling type role, were the most valuable, however. Although the nurse could not provide solutions to clients' problems, by acting as a facilitator to help clients achieve realistic aims they could often realize an inner peace. Narayanasamy (1999) identified three skills for facilitating spiritual care:

- Communication – being non-judgemental and using active listening to encourage clients to unburden their thoughts.
- Trust building – promoting security by showing genuine concern and by keeping promises.
- Giving hope – supporting individuals struggling with questions of fear and faith by encouraging them to talk. Helping them to reflect on the memories of good things that had occurred in their lives, particularly when failure was defeated.

WORK-RELATED STRESS IN NURSING

Physical environmental stressors

These stressors should be addressed using the appropriate legislative framework such as the Health and Safety at Work Act 1974 and the Control of Substances Hazardous to Health Regulations. They are discussed more fully in Chapter 3.

Psycho-social stressors

Many issues that arise within professional practice can be managed with adequate peer support. This informal approach is excellent for most issues; however, it assumes that individuals have access to colleagues that they feel they can trust and that the incidents are addressed adequately by this method. This will not be the case all of the time and additional methods of support should be available for example; clinical supervision, line manager and counselling services.

Clinical supervision

Clinical supervision is a forum to discuss events that occur during clinical practice, to explore feelings towards them and to learn from the experience (Lindgren et al 2005). The supervisor is usually an experienced professional whose role is to facilitate reflection, consider alternative perspectives and help the supervisee to develop confidence and self-esteem. While this process helps to improve practice by maximizing control of stressors, it also assists in the management of stress (Meadows et al 2000). The emotional exhaustion that arises from continued exposure to stressful events is a major factor leading to the development of burnout (Leiter & Maslach 2005). Therefore, it follows that clinical supervision should be available to all practitioners and incorporated within working practice.

> ### Evidence-based practice
>
> Reporting on a major review on clinical supervision in the UK, Winstanley & White (2003) suggested that:
>
> - Longer sessions are better (60 minutes).
> - More frequent sessions are better (at least monthly).
> - Sessions should be away from the workplace.
> - Supervisor trust/rapport is higher if the supervisor is chosen by the supervisee.

Clinical supervision can be given in individual or group sessions. In individual supervision practitioner and supervisor meet at least monthly for around an hour to reflect on issues that have occurred since the last supervision and to plan a strategy for subsequent implementation. In group supervision an experienced supervisor will facilitate up to 10 professionals working in similar areas to reflect on their practice. The advantages of group supervision are that it is resource-efficient and that it makes it possible to draw from a broad range of expertise from practitioners who have similar experiences (Winstanley & White, 2003). These advantages are restricted, however, if a few powerful individuals monopolize the time. In addition, because of group dynamics and insecurities, individuals may not feel safe to disclose as much information in a group as they would during individual supervision. Ideally then, group supervision should be used to support rather than to replace individual supervision.

Evolve 9.5 contains an exercise that can be used to develop clinical supervision.

> ### 9.5 – CLINICAL SUPERVISION EXERCISE
>
> - Know the issues involved in clinical supervision.
> - Know how to use this in support of your own experience as supervisor or supervisee.

Time management

One of the problems that occur when individuals become overstressed is that organizational ability declines. Individuals attempt to accommodate an increasing workload; however, because there is a finite amount of time, they prioritize which tasks are to be given most energy and may end up leaving little time for family and social commitments. Life then loses structure and individuals become overwhelmed, a situation worsened by *procrastination* (Payne 2001).

Procrastination is avoidance. Engaging in the work means engaging in the additional stress required to complete it, so to avoid the additional stress, the individual avoids the task. For example a student may have an assignment to complete; however, when it is time to begin work on it other tasks such as housework, ironing, etc. suddenly take priority.

Procrastination worsens the situation as the task remains incomplete and has to be completed within an even more restricted time frame. It is addressed by an effective time management strategy that provides structure by setting goals, targets and dates. Time management is therefore a fundamental part of stress management. By allocating time for commitments, individuals gain control of stressors and prioritize what will (and will not) be achieved. An example of a time management strategy is given in the Personal and Reflective Knowledge section of this chapter.

ASSESSING SLEEP

An assessment of sleep should examine sleep habits and bedtime routines. It should include the individual's normal pattern of sleep, their current pattern of sleep and the activities usually undertaken prior to retiring to bed. Holcomb (2006) recommends the following as part of an assessment:

Bedtime:

- Time of retiring; whether it is dark.
- Bedroom environment (temperature, quietness).

- Pain.
- Partner snoring.
- Length of time from retiring to onset of sleep.

Sleep:

- Number of awakenings during the night.
- Why awakened.
- How long to get back to sleep.
- Waking too early.
- Nocturia.
- Pain, palpitations, difficulty in breathing, heartburn.
- Nightmares.
- Movement.
- Restless leg.
- Snoring.

Daytime functioning:

- Feel rested on arising.
- Driving ability.
- Attention/concentration.
- Daytime naps.
- Falling asleep when watching TV, when reading, or after a meal.

The onset of any changes in sleep (sudden or gradual) and possible triggering events such as illness, social changes (such as shift working) or anxiety should be identified. As assessments will be based on individuals' perceptions, they will be subjective. However, it is the clients who know whether they feel refreshed after sleep or not. On occasions, a sleep diary may be completed to establish an individual's pattern of sleep and the number of and reasons for awakenings.

An example of a sleep diary for use by children can be found at http://www.nhlbi.nih.gov/health/public/sleep/starslp/teachers/sleep_diary.htm.

AIDING SLEEP

Particularly on admission to hospital, clients can have great difficulty in sleeping. The following approaches are useful to consider when planning strategies to aid sleep:

- Darkness. In hospital it is difficult to provide darkness as dim light is needed at night to promote safety. Many people are used to sleeping in the dark though, and find that their pattern of sleep is disturbed by the light. In this situation, providing that safety is maintained and that the individual is able to tolerate them, blindfolds can be used to exclude unwanted light.
- Silence. Noise at night is a common problem which interrupts sleep. This can be addressed by turning down the volume of telephones and wearing quiet shoes. As a last resort, the use of earplugs may be helpful.

- Comfort. To be able to sleep, individuals need to be comfortable. Although most people can achieve this independently, for those who are partially or totally immobile assistance may need to be given. In addition, clients may be in pain. Analgesia should automatically be offered to such individuals rather than waiting for a request of pain relief after a period of distress (see Ch. 11, 'Pain').
- Not feeling tired. In illness, individuals who are used to being physically active may find that they are not tired and this can affect the time they take to settle to sleep. This may be compounded by anxiety, arising for example from their prognosis, or by separation from their loved ones.
- Food and drink. Many people settle to sleep following a light supper or snack, or are in the habit of taking a night-time drink. Provision of a suitable drink (including alcoholic if not contra-indicated) or a snack at an appropriate time can thus aid sleep.
- Temperature. People sleep less well if the ambient temperature is too warm or too cold. Although it is difficult to adjust the temperature, it can be compensated for by blankets and wearing appropriate nightclothes.
- Routines. The use of familiar bedtime routines can promote sleep. If a client is in hospital, retiring to bed at the usual time, having familiar objects from home (e.g. photographs or cuddly toys for children) and performing bedtime rituals may help to normalize the bedtime routine.
- Reading. Many people like to read before sleeping. While this may be unproblematic at home, in hospital this may be achieved by using bed lights that do not disturb others and ensuring the client has access to books and magazines.
- Pillows. Some individuals are used to sleeping with several pillows while others are not. Additionally, some people experience breathing difficulties if they have insufficient support. Consequently, the number of pillows needed should form part of the assessment and plan of care.
- Avoiding daytime naps. Often, if there is little stimulation during the day, it can be easy for clients to nap. In turn, though, this means that they will be less tired at bedtime and unable to sleep. This is particularly problematic for clients suffering from dementia who may reverse day and night time activities (see Ch. 17, 'Confusion').

Drugs to aid sleep

These fall into two main categories: hypnotics and anxiolytics. Hypnotics act on the central nervous system to induce sleep and include nitrazepam, temazepam and clomethiazole. Anxiolytics such as diazepam or lorazepam do not induce sleep but provide a sedative action from which sleep may develop. They are likely to be prescribed before major events such as surgery.

The sedative properties of some antidepressants, such as dosulepin or amitriptyline, can also be used to aid sleep. In this instance they will be prescribed as a single night-time dose.

PROFESSIONAL AND ETHICAL KNOWLEDGE

Health and social care policy within the UK has developed to use less institutional care and more care provided at home, placing a great reliance on informal (unpaid) carers and community support workers, resulting in a service based on contracting services from various providers. The effects of these policies have ramifications both for those working within health and social care and for those receiving care. Consequently, to place stress within health and social care into context, this section examines the socio-political context of caring within the UK.

THE TERMS AND CONDITIONS OF PAID CARERS

Health and social care services in the United Kingdom are based upon the principles of the marketplace. Services are commissioned by primary care trusts to meet local needs and performance targets, under the supervision of Strategic Health Authorities. These services are supplied by various health and social care providers, who may be NHS trusts or independent suppliers, and who in turn may subcontract services. Although contracts are set up for 3-year periods, local and national priorities can change rapidly and this results in a hurried change in focus by providers in order to retain business.

All purchasers and providers in health and social care have individual financial budgets which they must work within. As the cost of staff in health and social care is the largest expenditure, many employers have tried to obtain savings in this area. Frequently employers have failed to replace staff as they leave and according to Carvel (2007), in 2006/7 this strategy amounted to a loss of 22 300 posts. In addition, to further streamline costs some providers merged together resulting in a further reduction in posts; and Carvel noted that over the same period there were almost 1450 compulsory redundancies.

As an alternative cost-cutting strategy, when posts have become vacant employers have re-graded them to more junior positions which has allowed them to recruit less experienced staff or staff with fewer qualifications, with consequent lower salary costs. This strategy also justified a reduction of investment in post-qualification training and, as Carlisle (2007) reported, in 2006/7 this led to £117 million being diverted from NHS multiprofessional education and training (MPET) budgets to subsidize budgets in other areas.

Consequently, providers of contemporary health and social care services focus on meeting short-term, financial-led goals. While opportunities have been created for some staff, many others have been left with unclear career pathways, a requirement for 'flexible working' patterns and job insecurity. This deprives them of a significant amount of control over their lives at work and emphasizes the support that many will need to manage the additional stressors arising from the frequent changes in their workplaces.

EMPLOYMENT RELATED STRESS IN HEALTH AND SOCIAL CARE

It is easy for employers to claim that stress management is the responsibility of the individual. It must be remembered though that stress arises from the individual's reaction to the environment. Although the individual has some responsibility in managing their stress, managing stress also requires adaptation of the environment.

In addition to the adverse effects on front-line staff, the stressful workplace also affects the way in which line managers perform. Due to the competitive pressures within contemporary health and social care environments, managers may be hesitant to refuse extra work demands placed on already hard-pressed resources. In this situation staff subordinate to the manager are likely to find themselves pressurized and unable to control the situation. In the short term, productivity may appear to increase as staff draw on their reserve strengths to cope. Neglecting individual employees and promoting a stressful work environment leads to an increase in burnout, however (Payne 2001, Leiter & Maslach 2005), so in the long term this strategy becomes counterproductive as burned out staff result in decreased productivity.

In this type of environment it is easy for individual employees to become lost within the organization, feeling devalued and focusing on the negative aspects of work. This is compounded when managers concentrate on the underachievement of the organization rather than remembering to praise the good points (Meadows et al 2000, Leiter & Maslach 2005), a situation highlighted in *An Organisation with a Memory* (Department of Health 2000) where oppressive environments were shown to inhibit the reporting of, and learning from, adverse incidents.

One of the reasons that the stressful workplace has evolved, both in health and social care and in other areas of work, is that stress and stress induced diseases are not classified as industrial diseases. Although the Health and Safety Executive (2001) recommend that work related stress should be subject to risk assessment and managed like any other workplace hazard, because injuries are not usually measurable, or even directly attributable to the workplace, the ability for employees to seek redress from employers is limited.

Recently, the way stress induced diseases are viewed in law has altered. A number of claims against employers have been successful in securing compensation for stress induced diseases. Furthermore, since the implementation of the Employment Act 2002 it is possible for employees to write a letter of grievance to the employer setting out clearly instances of what had been going on in the workplace that resulted in them taking time off sick as a result of a stress related illness. If the employer does nothing to rectify the situation then this can be seen as a breach of the implied terms of mutual trust and confidence, and in turn forms grounds to resign and bring a claim for constructive unfair dismissal.

Workplace stress is estimated to cost £7 billion annually in lost working days and NHS costs (Cooper 2001). Indeed in 2005/6 workplace stress resulted in the loss of 10 537 000 working days in the UK (Health and Safety Executive 2006). Stressful workplaces also lead to a high attrition of staff and difficulty in recruiting replacements (Meadows et al 2000, Michie & Williams 2003). In turn, this exacerbates the situation for those who remain, who then become more likely to take time off with stress related illnesses, making it more difficult for employers to meet their targets. Ultimately, ignoring workplace stress has enormous potential costs for employers.

SERVICE USERS AND INFORMAL CARERS

Historically in the UK most health care, particularly for people with long-term conditions, was provided in NHS hospitals. Although community care was thought preferable, community services were seen as expensive luxuries that would divert funds from hospitals.

This view changed following the election of the Conservative administration in 1979 who saw community care as a cheaper option. Formal (state paid) care was replaced with informal (unpaid) care, and, following the recommendations of the Griffiths Report on Community Care (Department of Health and Social Security 1988) which were formalized within the National Health Service and Community Care Act 1990, the role of the health service changed to become a facilitator rather than a provider of care.

Since 1979 the number of hospital beds consequently fell from some 463 000 to 145 218 in 2004/5 (National Health Service Confederation 2006). Although some of these beds were absorbed by an increase in care home beds, they did not make up the shortfall and the remainder were placed into the community by using informal carers. Furthermore, since 1998 care home beds have also been falling by around 5% per annum (Netten et al 2005), the shortfall in care again being picked up by informal carers.

The contribution to care that informal carers make was first recognized by the New Labour government in 1997. They published *Caring About Carers: A National Strategy For Carers* (Department of Health 1999), in which they outlined specific measures to support unpaid carers. This was followed by further legislation:

- The Carers and Disabled Children Act 2000 gave carers the right to an assessment and introduced the direct payment scheme which enabled carers to purchase specific services.
- *Supporting People with Long Term Conditions: Liberating the Talents of Nurses who Care for People with Long Term Conditions* (Department of Health 2005) introduced case management to support people with chronic illnesses and their carers. Implemented by community matrons, it aimed to provide services to either prevent crises occurring, or if they did, to allow people to remain at home rather than be admitted to hospital.
- The Work and Families Act 2006 introduced the right to flexible working for carers. This allowed carers to alter their hours of work so that they could continue with their employment as well as provide care. However, if they were in receipt of the carers' allowance, and their earnings rose above £95.00 per week after deductions (in December 2007), they would no longer be able to claim the allowance.

What legislation has failed to address is whether informal carers actually want, or are able, to be carers. Unlike paid carers, informal carers provide care for 7 days a week and for 52 weeks a year. In *Caring About Carers: A National Strategy For Carers* (Department of Health 1999) it is stated that 855 000 carers provide care for more than 50 hours a week and in addition to the long hours spent caring, many carers also hold external employment (or in the case of young carers, attend school). Personal time for carers is therefore minimal and many become socially isolated.

Informal caring is potentially an extremely stressful experience which can have a detrimental effect on the carer's health (Hunt 2003). This may manifest in difficulties within family relationships, a deterioration of their own health, or neglect of, or occasionally abuse of, the person that they are caring for. Clearly, these have profound implications that must be assessed by professionals offering support within the community.

Reflection and portfolio evidence

How would you recognize if a client was suffering abuse? (Refer to POVA in Ch. 12, 'Aggression'.)

PERSONAL AND REFLECTIVE KNOWLEDGE

To consolidate the knowledge gained from this chapter you should become more aware of your own response to stress and develop your individual stress management programme, using the guidelines that follow, to include in your portfolio of learning. Becoming aware of your own stress and developing your own stress management programme will teach you many of the skills you need to help others during your professional practice. Finally, if you have not already done so, work through the reflective exercises.

TIME MANAGEMENT

Stress is intensified by losing control. In the Care Delivery Knowledge section it was shown how effective stress management programmes use problem solving approaches to enable individuals to take control of stressors. In personal stress management, this is underpinned by efficient time management. Essential equipment comprises:

- a diary
- a year planner
- a 'to do' list.

Make it a rule that you never make an appointment without your diary and when buying a diary it is important to choose one that will let you view at least one week at a time. Those that only allow you to see one or two days are of limited use in personal time management as you are unable to see new appointments within the context of existing commitments. Personal organizers are very useful in this respect as they often contain planners with monthly and yearly views affording comprehensive views of other commitments. Electronic organizers are also available and are included on many mobile telephones. Although these may seem an ideal solution, they should be synchronized with a PC frequently. Otherwise, should the organizer fail or get mislaid or stolen, all of your information will be lost.

The first items that should be entered into your diary and planner are holidays and time for yourself. These are the most important entries you will make and should not be altered – you will need to develop assertiveness skills here. All entries other than these will compete for the remaining space. Next enter dates and times that you know are committed into your diary; work days for example.

The second stage is to list all your objectives and construct a 'to do' list. It is also helpful to give each objective a priority rating. From this list identify end goals that will allow you to fulfil your objectives and the dates by which the goals must be achieved. Box 9.3 shows a completed list.

Take each goal statement and break it into smaller components. Set each component a target date for completion (Box 9.4).

Transfer these goals onto your planner. In your diary set aside time to achieve these goals. A completed diary page may then look like Box 9.5.

Things happen in life without warning and, due to its rigid structure, this approach to time management is sometimes criticized for being idealistic. Although this approach is highly structured, this is necessary as events can quickly get out of hand. However, once you are aware of what your commitments are, you are able to easily make adjustments to your schedule to accommodate alterations in demands on your time.

Box 9.3 Goal statements

Goal	To be completed by
Complete Physiology essay	10th October
Complete Sociology essay	21st October
Complete Psychology essay	7th November
Decorate kitchen	14th November
File holiday photos in album	20th November

Box 9.4 Target dates for smaller goal components

Physiology essay	To be completed by
Literature search	10th September
Write plan	15th September
First draft	25th September
Second draft	30th September
Read second draft	5th October
Final draft	10th October

Box 9.5 Completed diary page

September

Monday 11th
7.30–14.30 Early shift
19.30–21.00 Write plan for biology

Tuesday 12th
7.30–14.30 Early shift
19.30–21.00 Write plan for biology

Wednesday 13th
7.30–14.30 Early shift
19.30–21.00 Write plan for biology

September

Thursday 14th
Visit Mum and Dad for the day

Friday 15th
9.00–12.30 Finish plan for biology
Afternoon – gardening
21.00 Going out to pub

Saturday 16th
12.30–21.30 Late shift

Sunday 17th
7.30–14.30 Early shift

CASE STUDIES RELATED TO STRESS

Four case studies now follow. Use the knowledge you have gained from this chapter to answer the questions at the end of each.

Case study: Learning disability

Robin is 32 years of age and has a moderate learning disability which prevents him from managing daily activities of living independently. He lives with his elderly parents, attending a day centre twice a week and helping around the family home on other days. He is currently attending a well-man's clinic, run by the practice nurse who has been with the practice for over 20 years. The nurse notes that Robin has a BMI of 31 and a blood pressure of 142/90 mmHg. She curtly tells Robin that he is obese and that he should go on a diet and exercise more to lower his blood pressure.

Before the clinic, you happened to be talking to Robin's father. He had disclosed to you that both he and Robin's mother had been unwell and it had been arranged for Robin to go into respite care for a month. This will be the first time that Robin has been separated from his parents and he is not keen to go. You feel that the distress may be contributing to Robin's hypertension and mention this to the practice nurse. She replies, however, that she has no time for 'psychobabble'.

- What physiological processes would lead the current social circumstances to affect Robin's physical condition?
- How would you manage Robin's condition differently?
- Why do you think the practice nurse rejects the influence of psychosocial factors on Robin's condition?

Case study: Child

Jade is attending the health centre for examination of her baby, Britney, of 18 months. Jade's partner, Tyler, relies on casual work for the family income and this has led them to have severe financial problems. To worsen matters, Tyler has started to go out most evenings and drink heavily. In consequence they have got into debt and experienced several major arguments. Their relationship deteriorated to such an extent last week that Tyler walked out.

Jade complains to the nurse that Britney does not seem to feed properly and that she keeps waking up during the night. This means that Jade is not getting sufficient sleep and because of this she tends to become short tempered and ends up shouting at Britney. She feels unable to cope and finds looking after Britney, shopping, cooking and keeping the house tidy impossible to do on her own.

Weighing Britney at 12 months had shown that the target of treble birth weight had not been achieved. Regular weighing since then revealed a downward trend on the percentile scale. Britney is diagnosed as failing to thrive.

- Why do you think that Britney is failing to thrive?

- How would you assess Jade's level of stress?
- What strategies would you utilize to help Jade and Britney?

Case study: Adult

Following the advice from her occupational health nurse, Paula (aged 28) took up swimming once a week as a method of combating stress. She had always enjoyed swimming, and when she was younger had represented her school in swimming competitions.

Paula felt refreshed from swimming and found it a positive way of relieving her stress. One day she met an old school friend at the pool who suggested that she join her swimming club.

Paula joined the club and was soon persuaded to enter competitions where she was successful in winning trophies. Paula needed to train intensively to maintain her competitiveness, however, and soon found herself training for five evenings each week with competitions most weekends. In contrast to her initial intention to use swimming as a method of stress management, Paula now found that swimming was an additional stress in her life.

- At which stage was Paula experiencing eustress from her swimming activities?
- At which stage was Paula experiencing distress?
- What advice should the nurse give clients who decide to use sport as a stress relieving activity?

Case study: Mental health

Kathleen is 43 years of age and married with two daughters aged 16 and 14 years. Over the previous fortnight she has gradually become withdrawn and insular. She neglects her personal appearance and is sleeping for prolonged, irregular periods.

During the assessment the nurse used the Social Readjustment Rating Scale to explore what issues had occurred in Kathleen's life over the previous year. It emerged that Kathleen's husband, Wayne, who was employed as a fitter in the local garage, had been told that the garage was to close and that he would be made redundant. The time that the garage closure was announced coincided with the onset of Kathleen's latest relapse.

Stress is often seen to precipitate a relapse of depression (World Health Organization 1992). Wayne's redundancy was seen as a major life event resulting in stress (Holmes & Rahe 1967). This, in turn, contributed to the recurrence of Kathleen's illness.

Using the Social Readjustment Rating Scale the nurse was able to quickly focus on the Wayne's redundancy and, as she became able to engage in conversation, explore ways in which Kathleen and her family would cope.

- Is the stress of Wayne's redundancy eustress or distress?
- Think of other reasons that may be contributing to Kathleen's level of stress (which may or may not be listed on the scale).
- What are the disadvantages of the Social Readjustment Rating Scale?

SUMMARY

This chapter has examined the concepts of stress, relaxation and rest. It has included:

1. A demonstration that, although there is a relationship between them, they are independent concepts and in practice they need to be addressed as such.
2. Strategies for managing stress and promoting relaxation.
3. An exploration of the stressors encountered by professional and informal carers.
4. An examination of contemporary UK policy that provides the context for stress in health and social care.

Annotated further reading and websites

Back K, Back K 2005 Assertiveness at work: a practical guide to handling awkward situations, 3rd edn. McGraw Hill, New York

A self-training book that develops concepts of assertiveness and provides suggestions for nurturing assertiveness skills. Topics include negotiation skills, being able to say 'no', dealing with negative feelings, handling criticism and managing aggression from others. Although these skills are ideally developed in an assertiveness group (to which many universities and employers in health and social care offer access) this is an extremely useful book.

Bond M, Holland S 2005 Skills of clinical supervision for nurses. Open University Press, Milton Keynes

Meg Bond is a talented author who regularly manages to put complex issues into publications that are understood easily. This book, written jointly with Stevie Holland, begins by outlining the context of clinical supervision in nursing. However, it moves on quickly to discuss the skills and expectations of the supervisor and supervisee. This is an excellent book for nurses who want to set up and get the most out of their own clinical supervision system.

Martin P 2002 Counting sheep: the science and pleasures of sleep and dreams. Harper Collins, London

An examination of the processes of sleep and of the consequences of sleep deprivation. This is an easily read book that combines research with other literature to explore the nature of sleep and dreaming, and the possible consequences for an individual's health.

Espie CA 2006 Overcoming insomnia and sleep problems. Constable & Robinson, London

A book primarily written as a self-help text. This book uses a cognitive behavioural approach to learn healthy sleep hygiene and bedtime routines. There is also a section on learning to relax. This book is recommended by the Clinical Sleep Research Unit at Loughborough University.

Enter 'STRESS' or 'RELAXATION' into an internet search engine such as Google and you will receive pages and pages of links, many of which should be treated with extreme caution. Of those that are published by credible organizations, many are located in the USA. Although these contain interesting information, they tend to be USA specific and designed for access by US citizens. Consequently, should you want to obtain local services, you may need to restrict your search to sites within your own country.

9.6 – WEBLINKS FOR STRESS, RELAXATION AND SLEEP

- Know current web resources for information on managing stress and distress.
- Know current web resources for information on managing sleeplessness.

The following list is of established websites; however, these can go offline without notice. An up-to-date list can be found at Evolve 9.6 on the Evolve web resource.

http://www.lboro.ac.uk/departments/hu/groups/sleep/
The Loughborough Sleep Research Centre. Has information on sleep, and sleep research. Also links to other relevant websites.

http://www.mentalhealth.org.uk/
Home page of the Mental Health Foundation. This contains information and resources on a range of mental health issues and problems. It also has a good range of links.

http://www.samaritans.org
The website for Samaritans. It contains instructions for accessing services, resources and information. Samaritans is not a counselling service. What they do offer is to listen to people and hear their feelings in times of crisis, and they are available either on-line, by telephone 24 hours a day, or by a personal visit (within certain hours).

http://www.sleephomepages.org/
A comprehensive USA based site that has resources and links for sleep research and sleep disorders.

http://www.stress.org/
Home page of the American Institute of Stress. This organization was established in 1978 and contains a wealth of information on stress and stress-related diseases.

References

Barefoot JC, Larsen S, von der Lieth L, Schroll M 1995 Hostility, incidence of acute myocardial infarction, and mortality in a sample of older Danish men and women. American Journal of Epidemiology 142(5):477–484

Beck AT 1979 Cognitive theory of depression. Guilford Press, New York

Borbely A 1987 Secrets of sleep. Longman, Harlow

Bosma H, Marmor M, Hemingway H et al 1997 Low job control and the risk of coronary heart disease in Whitehall II (prospective cohort) study. British Medical Journal 314:558–565

British Association of Counselling and Psychology 2007 What is counselling? Available online. http://www.bacp.co.uk/education/ whatiscounselling.html (accessed 13 August 2008)

Brosschot JF, Godaert GLR, Benschop RJ et al 1998 Experimental stress and immunological reactivity: a closer look at perceived uncontrollability. Psychosomatic Medicine 60(3):359–361

Carlisle D 2007 Finance BMA and NHS employers hit out as strategic health authorities syphon off funds: SHA's £117m training raid attacked. Health Service Journal 31 May 2007, p 7

Carvel J 2007 NHS cutbacks leave £500m unspent. Available online: http://www.guardian.co.uk/society/2007/may/29/health.medicineandhealth1 (accessed 13 August 2008)

Cerrato P L 1998 Aromatherapy: is it for real? RN 61(6):51–52

Cooper C 2001 For pity's sake stop the work, I want to get off … Available online: http://www.jfo.org.uk/health/resources/cary1.htm (accessed 13 August 2008)

Coyne I 2006 Children's experiences of hospitalization. Journal of Child Health Care 10(4):326–336

Department of Health 1999 Caring about carers: a national strategy for carers. HMSO, London

Department of Health 2000 An organization with a memory: report of an expert group on learning from adverse events in the NHS. HMSO, London

Department of Health 2005 Supporting people with long term conditions: liberating the talents of nurses who care for people with long term conditions. HMSO, London

Department of Health and Social Security 1988 Community care: agenda for action (Griffiths Report). HMSO, London

Ernst E 2002 The risk–benefit profile of commonly used herbal therapies: ginko, St John's wort, ginseng, Echinacea, saw palmetto and kava. Annals of Internal Medicine 136:42–53

Fisher PL, Durham RC 1999 Recovery rates in generalized anxiety disorder following psychological therapy: an analysis of clinically significant change in the STAI-T across outcome studies since 1990. Psychological Medicine 29(6):1425–1434

Folkard S 1991 Circadian rhythms and hours of work. In: Warr P (ed) Psychology of work, 3rd edn. Penguin, Harmondsworth

Freud A 1934 The ego and the mechanisms of defence. Chatto & Windus, London

Friedman M, Rosenman RH 1974 Type A behaviour and your heart. Knopf, New York

Gerin W, Ogedegbe G, Schwartz JE et al 2006 Assessment of the white-coat effect. Journal of Hypertension 24(1):67–74

Hahn SE, Smith CS 1999 Daily hassles and chronic stressors conceptual and measurement issues. Stress Medicine 15(2):89–101

Hart CL, Hole DJ, Lawlor DA, Smith GD, Lever AF 2007 Effect of conjugal bereavement on mortality of the bereaved spouse in participants of the Renfrew/Paisley study. Journal of Epidemiology and Community Health 61(5):455–460

Health and Safety Executive 2001 Reducing risks, protecting people: HSE's decision-making process. HSE Books, Sudbury

Health and Safety Executive 2006 Health and safety statistics 2005/6. Sudbury National Statistics Office, Sudbury

Hebb DO 1955 Drives and the CNS (conceptual nervous system). Psychological Review 62(4):243–254

Hirst M 2004 Health inequalities and informal care. Social Policy Research Unit, University of York, York

Holcomb SS 2006 Recommendations for assessing insomnia. Nurse Practitioner 31(2):55–60

Holmes TH, Rahe RH 1967 The social readjustment rating scale. Journal of Psychosomatic Research 11:213–218

Horne JA 1988 Why we sleep: the functions of sleep in human and other mammals. Oxford University Press, Oxford

Howard D 2001 Changes in nursing students' out of college relationships arising from the Diploma of Higher Education in nursing. Active Learning in Higher Education 3(1):68–87

Hunt CK 2003 Concepts in caregiver research. Journal of Nursing Scholarship 35(1):27–32

Janssen PM, Schaufeli WB, Houkes I 1999 Work-related and individual determinants of the three burnout dimensions. Work and Stress 13(1):74–86

Kubler Ross E 1975 Death: the final stage of growth. Prentice Hall, London

Lazarus RS, Delongis A, Folkman S et al 1985 Stress and adaptational outcomes: the problem of confounded measures. American Psychologist 40:770–779

Le Fevre M, Gregory SK, Mathney J 2006, Eustress, distress and their interpretation in primary and secondary occupational stress management interventions: which way first? Journal of Managerial Psychology 21(6):547–565

Leiter MP, Maslach C 2005 How to avoid burnout: an action plan for career enhancement. Wiley, London

Lichtenstein P, Gatz M, Berg S 1998 A twin study of mortality after spousal bereavement. Psychological Medicine 28(3):635–643

Lillberg K, Verkasalo PK, Kaprio J, Teppo L, Helenius H, Koskenvuo M 2003 Stressful life events and risk of breast cancer in 10,808 women: a cohort study. American Journal of Epidemiology 157(5):415–423

Lin H-R, Bauer-Wu SM 2003 Psycho-spiritual well-being in patients with advanced cancer: an integrative review of the literature. Journal of Advanced Nursing 44(1):69–80

Linde K, Berner M, Egger M, Mulrow C 2005 St John's wort for depression: meta-analysis of randomised controlled trials. British Journal of Psychiatry 186:99–107

Lindgren B, Brulin C, Holmlund K, Athlin E 2005 Nursing students' perception of group supervision during clinical training. Journal of Clinical Nursing (14)7:822–829

Meadows S, Levenson R, Baeza J 2000 The last straw: explaining the NHS nurse shortage. King's Fund, London

Michie S, Williams S 2003 Reducing work related psychological ill health and sickness absence: a systematic literature review. Occupational and Environmental Medicine 60(1):3–9

Muecke S 2005 Effects of rotating night shifts: literature review. Journal of Advanced Nursing 50(4):433–439

Myrtek M 2001 Meta-analyses of prospective studies on coronary heart disease, type A personality, and hostility. International Journal of Cardiology 79:245–251

Narayanasamy A 1996 Spiritual care of chronically ill patients. British Journal of Nursing 5(7):411–416

Narayanasamy A 1999 ASSET: a model for actioning spirituality and spiritual care education and training in nursing. Nurse Education Today 19(4):274–285

Narayanasamy A, Owens J 2001 A critical incident study of nurses' responses to the spiritual needs of their patients. Journal of Advanced Nursing 33(4):446–455

National Health Service and Community Care Act 1990 HMSO, London

National Health Service Confederation 2006 Why we need fewer hospital beds. National Health Service Confederation, London

National Institute of Health and Clinical Excellence 2005 Post-traumatic stress disorder (PTSD) The management of PTSD in adults and children in primary and secondary care Clinical Guideline 26. National Institute for Health and Clinical Excellence, London

Netten A, Williams J, Darton R 2005 Care-home closures in England: causes and implications. Ageing and Society 25:319–338

Office for National Statistics 2006 Census 2001 Available online: http://www.statistics.gov.uk/CCI/nugget.asp?ID=925&Pos=&ColRank=1&Rank=374 (accessed 13 August 2008)

Pacák K, Palkovits M 2001 Stressor specificity of central neuroendocrine responses: implications for stress-related disorders. Endocrine Reviews 22(4):502–548

Payne N 2001 Occupational stressors and coping as determinants of burnout in female hospice nurses. Journal of Advanced Nursing 33(3):396–405

Pruessner JC, Hellhammer DH, Kirschbaum C 1999 Low self-esteem, induced failure and the adrenocortical stress response. Personality and Individual Differences 27(3):477–489

Quine L 1998 Effects of stress in an NHS trust: a study. Nursing Standard 13(3):36–41

Schmitz N, Neumann W, Oppermann R 2000 Stress, burnout and locus of control in German nurses. International Journal of Nursing Studies 37(2):95–99

Scully JA, Tosi H, Banning K 2000 Life event checklists: revisiting the social readjustment rating scale after 30 years. Educational and Psychological Measurement 60(6):864–876

Segerstrom SC, Miller GE 2004 Psychological stress and the human immune system: a meta-analytic study of 30 years of inquiry. Psychological Bulletin 130(4):601–630

Seyle H 1984 The stress of life. McGraw-Hill, New York

Sharma VK, Chandrashekaran MK 2005 Zeitgebers (time cues) for biological clocks. Current Science 89(7):1136–1146

Sjöström-Strand A, Fridlund B 2007 Stress in women's daily life before and after a myocardial infarction: a qualitative analysis. Scandinavian Journal of Caring Sciences 21(1):10–17

Stansfeld SA, Fuhrer R, Shipley MJ, Marmot MB 2002 Psychological distress as a risk factor for coronary heart disease in the Whitehall II study. International Journal of Epidemiology 31(1):248–255

Sutherland VJ, Cooper CL 1990 Understanding stress: a psychological perspective for health professionals. Chapman & Hall, London

Taheri S, Lin L, Austin D, Young T, Mignot E 2004 Short sleep duration is associated with reduced leptin, elevated ghrelin, and increased body mass index. Public Library of Science Medicine 1(3): Epub 2004 Dec 7. e62 doi:10.1371/journal.pmed.0010062

Thaker PH, Lutgendorf SK, Sood AK 2007 The neuroendocrine impact of chronic stress on cancer. Cell Cycle 6(4):430–433

Vernarec E 2001 How to cope with job stress. RN 64(3):44–46

Winstanley J, White E 2003 Clinical supervision: models, measures and best practice. Nurse Researcher 10(4)7–38

Wong AHC 1998 Herbal remedies in psychiatric practice. Archives of General Psychiatry 55(11):1033–1044

World Health Organization 1992 The ICD-10 classification of mental and behavioural disorder. World Health Organization, Geneva

Zivnuska S, Kiewitz C, Hochwater WA, Perrewe PL, Zellars KL 2002 What is too much or too little? The curvilinear effects of job tension on turnover intent, value attainment, and job satisfaction. Journal of Applied Social Psychology 32(7):1344–1360

Chapter 10

Medicines

Carol Hall

KEY ISSUES

SUBJECT KNOWLEDGE

- A nursing definition of 'medicine'
- The action of medicine upon the body
- Potential non-therapeutic action by medicines
- Calculation of medicine dosages
- Routes of medicine administration

CARE DELIVERY KNOWLEDGE

- Practice knowledge for safe medicines management using application of research evidence
- Assessing clients in relation to medicines management
- Planning to administer a medicine
- How medication administration can be evaluated

PROFESSIONAL AND ETHICAL KNOWLEDGE

- How medication errors can be effectively managed
- The legal acts governing the storage and administration of medicines in the UK
- Prescribing medicines
- Moral and ethical dilemmas that can arise within medicines management

PERSONAL AND REFLECTIVE KNOWLEDGE

- Application of principles of medicines administration across all branches of nursing
- Awareness of personal position in both the giving and the using of medicines

INTRODUCTION

In most healthcare settings, medicines need to be managed for some of the client group for whom there is responsibility. This chapter explores key information for nurse decision making about medicines management, including the practice of administering medicines. Associated elements related to licensing, prescribing and dispensing medicinal treatment will be explored and the related element of medicines dosage calculation will be addressed.

The broad concept of 'medicines management' is one which is multiprofessional. It is defined as: 'The clinical, cost effective and safe use of medicines to ensure patients get the maximum benefit from the medicines they need, while at the same time minimizing potential harm' (Medicines and Healthcare products Regulatory Agency 2004, cited by Nursing and Midwifery Council 2008b).

The safe management of medicines includes many component parts. Some examples are the purchase, supply and delivery, administration and evaluation across a range of situations, which have relevance for pharmacists and for medical and non-medical prescribers, including nurses. Without a wider consideration of care by others, such as pharmacists, the concerns of nurses in giving medicines safely and effectively would be impossible. However, this chapter intends to focus on nursing. The chapter will therefore address knowledge related to the preparation and follow-up required in giving a medicine within medicines management for nursing specifically, including knowledge for understanding the way medicines are able to enter the body and the effects that may occur both therapeutically and non-therapeutically as a result of treatment. Although it is not possible to offer comprehensive advice related to individual medications in this respect, some common groups of medicines will be considered. For more detail, annotated further reading is provided.

Effective management of medicines by nurses may involve educating other carers to give medicines or educating clients to self-administer medicines. There is also a role in health promotion with regard to the safe handling and storage of medicines in both hospital and community settings.

Finally, the nurse can facilitate understanding of the effects of the use of medicines socially, including public use of both 'over the counter' preparations and illegal substances. Legal and professional issues also need to be taken into consideration. The position of the nurse as both a professional and a member of the public is thus explored.

OVERVIEW

Subject knowledge

The physical aspects related to treatment with medicines are introduced, with a particular emphasis upon the mechanical and biological bases. Here, classification of medication by type is examined, followed by a consideration of the possible routes of administration, calculation of correct doses and examination of how the body deals with substances introduced to it. Further reading is offered and viewed as an essential development.

Wider psychosocial aspects of medicine use are included, with a consideration of the potential for abuse of medication and the societal impact of substance use today.

Care delivery knowledge

The role of the nurse in medicines management is explored. This discussion relates specifically to decision making in the assessment, planning, implementing and evaluation and recording of total care. It is intended that this section should lead to a deeper understanding of a nursing practice role.

Professional and ethical knowledge

This part addresses issues related to legality and accountability, as well as examining ethical issues in medicines management. Incidents such as errors in medication are explored and discussed in detail. Contemporary guidance relating to the eligibility of nurses to prescribe medicines is discussed, and resources are offered for further knowledge development in this area.

Personal and reflective knowledge

Throughout the chapter you are encouraged to think reflectively over issues related to the care that you give. It is anticipated that concepts raised throughout the chapter will be applied as a knowledge base for nursing practice. Throughout the chapter you will be invited to extend your thinking and knowledge further through consideration of evidence boxes, decision-making exercises and reflective points. 'Evolve' materials will be used to provide further information related to elements in the chapter.

On pages 246–247 there are four case studies with reflective questions, each relating to one of the branches of nursing. These can operate as a starting point for application of the principles identified within the chapter. You may find it helpful to read one of them before you start the chapter and use it as a focus for your reflections while reading. Of course, you should also explore examples from your own experience.

SUBJECT KNOWLEDGE

BIOLOGICAL

THE PHYSICAL BASIS OF MEDICINE ADMINISTRATION

Defining a medicine

When examining nursing issues related to the medicinal treatment of clients, there has been much debate about what constitutes a medicine, as well as what constitutes an appropriate role for nurses in treating their clients. Indeed, such has been the confusion over terminology and definition in this area of practice that both National and European regulatory bodies (Department of Health 1999; European Parliament and Council 2001, Article 1) have produced guidance to help facilitate a clear definition of what a medicine might be. The definition below is presented from the EC Directive above. It is useful to know about this definition because it is used by the Medications and Healthcare products Regulatory Agency (MHRA) in the UK when they consider whether a substance is to be classified as a medicine or not.

A medicine is:

(a) Any substance or combination of substances presented as having properties for treating or preventing disease in human beings;

or

(b) Any substance or combination of substances which may be used in or administered to human beings either with a view to restoring, correcting or modifying physiological functions by exerting a pharmacological, immunological or metabolic action, or to making a medical diagnosis.

(European Parliament and Council 2001/83/EC Article 1)

Marketing authorization

Medicinal products are currently regulated in the UK by the MHRA. They ensure that product licensing and monitoring concord with European Directives and UK law. Similar arrangements are in place elsewhere in Europe and the system is comparable with the rest of the world. Products are now issued with a marketing authorization which licenses them as safe for use. The marketing authorization includes a 'Summary of Product Characteristics' which stipulates safe routes of administration, dose strengths, constitution and the client group who can be considered (Medicines and Health Care Regulatory Agency 2008). Details of any summary of product characteristics can be found within the guidance details included in the medicine packaging, and these should be adhered to in order to ensure clients' safety. If a medicine is prescribed that has no national marketing authorization, or is exempted from this, then this is considered to be prescribed 'off licence'. If a medicine is prescribed 'outside of the summary of product characteristics' guidance included within the marketing authorization, then this is considered to be 'off label'. The use of off licence and off label medication is generally not advised and under current EU Directives will reduce significantly after a transitional period in place for some medicines until 2011. However, it is not illegal and is accepted by the medicine and pharmacy professions (Turner et al 2002) and the nursing regulatory body for nursing to be acceptable in some circumstances (Nursing and Midwifery Council 2008b). It is most likely to be found in the areas of neonatal nursing and paediatrics. There are implications in accepting this kind of prescribing, and these are addressed within professional issues later in this chapter.

In addition to the marketing authorization, all medications are issued with both a brand name and a British Approved Name or BAN. The brand name is the one by which the product is marketed, while the BAN is the generic name used in prescribing. Health carers should at all times use the BAN, while being mindful of different brands. Manufacturers must legally meet stringent requirements for labelling and provision of instructions relating to medicines. Though outside the scope of this chapter, this element is addressed thoroughly by Downie et al (2007) and their text is useful should you wish to extend your reading.

Classification of medicines

Medicines can be classified two ways. Firstly, there is the legal classification of medicines, which categorizes medicines according to requirements governing their supply to the general public. Contemporary legal classification continues to be derived from the Medicines Act 1968 and the Misuse of Drugs Act 1971, and will be addressed in more detail in the Professional Knowledge part of this chapter. Secondly, and less formally, medicines are classified into groups that indicate the effect on a body system, the symptoms relieved, or the desired effect of the medication (e.g. Waller et al 2005, Downie et al 2007). In fact it probably does not matter, and is as much personal preference as anything else.

A list of all medicines and their side-effects would be inappropriate in a chapter such as this so reference to formularies such as the British National Formulary (Joint Formulary Committee 2008) and the British National Formulary for Children (Paediatric Formularies Committee 2007) is recommended. However, it is acknowledged that a clear framework for categorizing drugs for further reference can be useful. The framework in Box 10.1 has been devised to assist nurses and students working and studying in practice. Although it must be emphasized that no nurse should give medications they are not familiar with, it is sometimes helpful to jot down notes about medications. By carrying this framework into the practice area, medicines may be noted down as you discover them in use, allowing access for revision and more in-depth study at a later date.

Box 10.1 A framework for classifying medicines

Type of treatment or area	Name of medicine and brief notes for future reference
Cardiovascular	
Respiratory	
Gastrointestinal tract	
Renal	
Central nervous system	
Analgesic	
Hypnotic	
Psychotropic	
Anaesthetic	
Blood	
Infection	
Antibiotic (or bactericidal/ bacteriostatic/antiseptic)	
Antifungal	
Antiviral	
Immunization	
Vitamin, fluid or electrolyte imbalance	
Hormone or endocrine imbalance	
Cytotoxic treatment	

Decision-making exercise

- In your practice identify one medicine used within each of the classifications in the framework in Box 10.1 and find out all you can about it using the references for further reading identified at the end of the chapter. If possible, reflect on the exercise with colleagues.
- Use your findings to discuss what factors may influence a nursing decision not to give an identified medicine to a client.

Although a useful way of identifying individual uses for medications, the above framework categories are not mutually exclusive. Looking at your list, can you identify any medication that may fit into more than one of the above categories? What does this tell you about using this drug therapeutically?

CALCULATING MEDICINE DOSES

Calculation of a therapeutic yet safe dose of any medication is achieved by weighing the client and determining a safe dose per kilogram or by calculating the client's body surface area. In critical care areas a nomogram (see example in Fig. 10.1) may be used to determine estimated surface area.

Medicines prescribed regularly in an adult setting may be appropriate for a wide range of clients and are often prescribed in a form that is held as stock by the pharmacist. For instance, an antibiotic such as ampicillin may be prescribed as a 250 milligram (mg) dose. The pharmacist sends capsules which have a strength of 250 mg per capsule so that the client requires one capsule. However, where children or the elderly are concerned, or where medication is particularly toxic, the dose can be calculated according to the weight of the client in milligrams per kilogram as recommended by the pharmaceutical company. This may not conveniently fall into a single unit dose such as one capsule. Once a dose has been ascertained, it is up to the nurse to decide that the prescription is correct and ensure that it is given. This means a further calculation may be necessary. A formula for calculating medicines is shown in Box 10.2.

Medicine doses are calculated using the Système International (SI) or metric system and are described in units of this system. When performing any calculation it is important that you ensure that the same SI unit is used for the stock and the prescribed dose. If the prescribed dose is in milligrams (mg) and the available medication is only available in grams (g), then one of these needs to be converted before a calculation can take place. It would be usual to convert grams to milligrams (see Annotated Further Reading for more information).

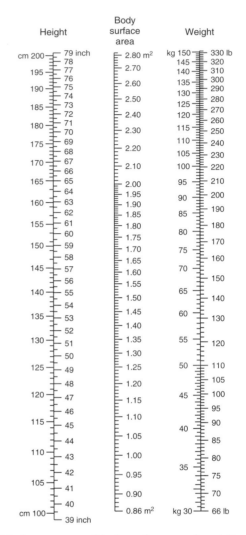

Figure 10.1 A nomogram of body surface area for adults. Directions: (1) find the patient's height; (2) find weight; (3) draw straight line connecting height and weight; (4) the point at which this line intersects the BSA column gives the patient's body surface area in square metres (reproduced with kind permission from Geigy Scientific Tables 1990, 8th edn, vol. 5, p. 105, © Novartis).

Box 10.2 Dose calculation formula

$$\frac{\text{What is required (prescribed dose)}}{\text{What is available (stock dose)}} \times \begin{array}{c} \text{Available dilution} \\ \text{(stock volume)} \end{array}$$

So if the dose prescribed is 500 mg of amoxicillin and the stock dose is 250 mg per one tablet (volume), the calculation is:

$$\frac{500}{250} \times 1 = 2, \text{ so two tablets are given}$$

In summary, it is essential to apply principles of numeracy in developing skills in administering medicines. Some elements that must be achieved effectively include:

- adding and subtracting
- multiplication and division
- conversion of SI units (e.g. converting from micrograms to milligrams)
- conversion of SI units to fractions
- estimation, proportion and rounding
- using formulae to calculate drug doses and milligrams of medication per kilogram body weight.

It is fair to say that many nurses find applied numeracy like this quite difficult, and it is critical that you ensure that you are competent in this area for your clients' safety. If you are a student nurse in the UK you will be expected to complete assessments relating to the use of numeracy in practice to help to demonstrate that you are a safe practitioner when you qualify. However, help is at hand. It is most important for a safe practitioner to be aware of their strengths and weaknesses and seek out help when necessary. Sources of help might include lecturers in university or mentors in placement, an online facility, such as that offered by learndirectuk or the Mathcentre (see section on websites at the end of the chapter) or one of the many text books written specifically for nurses (e.g. Lapham & Agar 2003, Gatford & Philips 2006, Chapelhow & Crouch 2007). Universities and colleges also have study support facilities that can be accessed by students.

Decision-making exercise

Mrs Johnson, an elderly lady, is found to be unwell while taking prescribed digoxin. The dose is reduced from 125 micrograms to 62.5 micrograms twice daily. The solution of digoxin provided for Mrs Johnson contains 50 micrograms per mL. Try to decide how much medicine Mrs Johnson should receive at one time.

10.1 – CALCULATING INTRAVENOUS INFUSION RATES

- Calculating flow rate.
- Calculating drops per minute (dpm).
- Practice examples to check your skills.

MEDICINES ADMINISTRATION

Routes of administration

Nurses have a useful contribution to make in their knowledge of what preparations of medication are available and appropriate for their clients, and due to their

Table 10.1 Routes for administration of medicine

Route	Notes
Oral	Including anything swallowed to the stomach or via nasogastric tubes
Sublingual/buccal	Allowed to dissolve under the tongue or in the cheek
Topical/local application	Including application into eyes, ears, or insertion into vagina, rectum
Transdermal	Through slow release patches adhered to the skin
Inhalation	Including via masks, nebulizers, breathing tubes
Intravenously/ intra-arterially	Administered into a vein or artery by a doctor or nurse with appropriate advanced qualifications
Subcutaneously/ subdermal	By injection under the cutaneous or dermal skin layers
Intramuscularly	By injection into muscle layers
Intrathecally	Administered by a doctor into the thecal cavity via a lumbar puncture procedure
Intraosseously	Administered by doctor into bone cavity (used for urgent access)
Other	It is possible for doctors to use other routes (e.g. into body cavities such as the pleural space or peritoneal cavity) in specific circumstances

assessment they are uniquely aware of their clients' needs. When selecting a route for administration nurses and doctors must work with the client to provide an optimum treatment programme that is safe and acceptable (Table 10.1).

Reflection and portfolio evidence

There are many different routes that can be selected for administration, as shown in Table 10.1. Think about a recent practice experience where a medication was given.

- What route was used?
- Was this the only possible way to give this medicine or could other routes have been selected?
- What are the issues if more than one route were possible?
- What did you learn from this exercise – record your findings in your portfolio.

Pharmacokinetics

The study of pharmacokinetics considers how a drug is processed as it passes through the body. The main phases of pharmacokinetic action are:

- absorption
- distribution
- metabolism
- excretion.

Absorption

Medication given is absorbed from the point of administration and into the cardiovascular system. Unless the medication is given by another route (thus bypassing this phase), nurses must be aware of the effects of the medicine in the effectiveness of absorption, and also the potential effect of the medicine at the site where it is being absorbed. With oral medication, consideration must include the effects of gastric secretion upon the efficacy of the drug and the potential effects of the medication upon the client's gastrointestinal tract.

With the administration of topical medications, there is usually an expectation that the desired effect will predominate at the local site. However, the potential for long-acting absorption of medication systemically is recognized in some situations. Transdermal patches are one example; these slowly release medications, for example progesterone and oestrogens for hormone replacement therapy, or nicotine to aid in the cessation of smoking. Nurses caring for patients using topically applied products must consider what effect (if any) the absorption of such medication may have upon a client's systemic well-being, especially if the intended action is purely a local one.

Distribution

Once in the cardiovascular circulation, the medication is carried to its site of action. Again, there are areas of nursing knowledge that are important for consideration. It is useful to understand how the treatment is carried in the blood, since many medicines are bound tightly to plasma proteins while others are not. If a medicine has a high affinity for plasma proteins it may be necessary to give a large dose of the medication to achieve a therapeutic effect since only the proportion of the medicine that is not bound to the plasma proteins can be used effectively. Commonly used medicines with a high affinity for plasma proteins (more than 80% bound) include the antidepressant amitriptyline, and the anxiolytic diazepam. Other medicines with a high affinity for plasma proteins are propanolol, warfarin, furosemide and the antibiotics erythromycin and rifampicin. A comprehensive review of protein bound medications is offered by Kee & Hayes (2005).

When planning to administer medicines, a factor that may affect the client's concentration of plasma proteins should be considered. This is because an individual with a reduced albumin concentration may be at risk of toxicity if a dose of medication with a high affinity for plasma protein is given. Other issues that should be considered in relation to the distribution of medication via the cardiovascular system include the rate and volume of perfusion to the desired area as any reduction in access to the required site may reduce the impact of the treatment offered. Additionally some areas of the body are protected from receiving many medications as a result of physiological barriers. The brain is one such area as the meninges around the central nervous system create a blood–brain barrier. Another area that selectively reduces the passage of substances is evident during pregnancy when the placenta offers a barrier between mother and baby. However, it should be noted that some substances may pass through these barriers. In nursing, the implications of the effectiveness of such barriers must be addressed when making informed decisions about nursing care. It is critical to assess the possibility of pregnancy in all premenopausal women who require medicinal treatment, with particular awareness of the potentially hazardous effects in causing fetal abnormalities of drugs such as phenytoin and tetracyclines, which can pass the placental barrier. Finally, the distribution of medication to infants via maternal breast milk must also be acknowledged. In some cases medication given to the mother may be safe for her, but can have toxic effects on the baby. For more information about the effects of specific medications in breastfeeding please refer to the Annotated Further Reading at the end of the chapter.

Decision-making exercise

Mr Jack Harvey, aged 85 years, is in hospital following a recent diagnosis of congestive cardiac failure. He has been prescribed propanolol, but after a few days his heart rate drops to less than 60 beats/min (compared to a more usual 80 beats/min) and he complains of feeling unwell.

- What could be wrong with Mr Harvey?
- Within coronary care, there is a variety of medicines that act upon the heart in different ways. Propanolol is a beta blocker. Find out how beta blockers work and compare their action with that of the digitalis group of medicines.
- What special considerations might you need to remember when administering medicines to clients who are elderly?

Metabolism

Metabolism (or breakdown) of any medication usually occurs in the liver (hepatic system). This may be therapeutic, in aiding the removal of active medication from the body by rendering it to inactive waste metabolites, or may hinder the effects of treatment, depending upon when such metabolism takes place. This issue is particularly pertinent when considering medicines that are administered orally, since much absorption via the gastrointestinal tract results in direct passage to the liver through the hepatic portal vein. In this situation the liver metabolizes a proportion of the medication (which varies between medications) before the medication reaches the cardiovascular circulation and is transported to the site of therapeutic benefit. This is known as 'first pass' metabolism, and although sometimes such a metabolism may be beneficial, as the metabolites themselves may have a therapeutic function, often it reduces the available therapeutic dose of medication by inactivating it. First pass metabolism is reduced in individuals with impaired hepatic function, and this is vital knowledge for nursing consideration in order to maintain the safety and well-being of the patient.

Finally, it is important to understand that it is possible to overload the liver with toxins resulting from the breakdown of medication as well as other substances such as alcohol, and this leads initially to an inability of the liver to cope effectively. If the liver continues to be overloaded with toxins over a prolonged period or is subjected to recurrent episodes of overload, damage may occur. This can create a permanently reduced hepatic function.

When considering administration to infants and young children, it is essential to recognize that in the young the ability to detoxify medicines is not mature, and therefore extreme caution should be taken when checking for an appropriate dose.

Excretion

After a variable period of time in the body the medication given to the client will be excreted. This is mostly via the kidneys, although other routes of excretion include the lungs, via bile into faeces, and in lactating mothers, breast milk. There may also be some excretion through sweat glands onto the skin surface (Downie et al 2007). Perhaps the most important factor in medicine excretion, however, is the speed at which it is lost from the body. The balance between absorption and excretion determines the half-life of a medicine. This is the time it takes for the concentration of the medicine in the plasma to fall by 50% (Downie et al 2007). Clearly, a medicine with a long half-life can accumulate easily within the plasma. Those medicines that are particularly problematic are monitored carefully through checking blood plasma levels to ensure that plasma levels do not become dangerously high.

An important consideration for nurses, therefore, relates to factors about the client that may affect the response and half-life of a medicine. For example, clients who are at the extremes of the age continuum or have renal impairment require particular consideration. The infant does not develop full renal and urinary tract function until after the first year of life, while the renal function of the elderly (over 80 years of age) deteriorates to about half the capacity of a young adult. Renal impairment can affect the excretion of medicines from the body, resulting in a build-up of metabolites, or in some instances medicines, in the circulation. A knowledge of such possibilities may alert you to making a decision to include specific points for observation related to medication in the client's plan of care. A full introduction to factors that may affect the response of medication can be found in Kee & Hayes (2005) or Downie et al (2007: Ch. 6).

Decision-making exercise

Simon is severely learning disabled and has difficulty in maintaining urinary continence due to poor bladder tone causing retention of urine and dribbling incontinence. He is cared for by his mother who maintains that clean intermittent catheterization techniques aid Simon's urinary continence, but he occasionally develops urinary tract infections. Simon's mother, while managing his infection, comments to the practice nurse that Simon's urine smells of the current antibiotic treatment and wonders why.

- How could you reassure Simon's mother that all is well?
- Find out how antibiotics work and what broad classifications can be identified.
- In a society that does not tolerate ill health, people are inclined to ask for antibiotics for minor infections. Reflect for a few minutes about the impact this may have in the long term.

Pharmacodynamics

Once a medicine has reached the site of therapeutic benefit it is able to exert a physiological effect before being excreted by the body. This is identified as pharmacodynamic action, and examination of this action of medicines in the body is comprehensively addressed within specific pharmacology texts such as Kee & Hayes (2005). A more detailed consideration is presented by Waller et al (2005). It is important to realize, however, that even with today's rapidly advancing understanding of medical science, the frontiers of clinical pharmacology are still being extended.

POTENTIAL ADVERSE EFFECTS OF ADMINISTERING MEDICINES TO CLIENTS

Although the aim of using medicinal treatments for clients may be therapeutic, diagnostic or preventive, it is simplistic to believe that all medicines given are completely therapeutic in all cases. For nursing, the aim has always been recognized as 'To do the client no harm' (Nightingale 1859). This next section will explore potential threats to such ideals.

Gaining a therapeutic dose

In order for medicine to be effective, the dose for your client must be sufficient to be effective, but not too much, in which case the client may risk toxicity or poisoning. Factors in achieving a therapeutic dose are related to nursing and medical skill in prescribing and calculating the correct dose of medication and also the pharmacokinetic and pharmacodynamic capacity of the client. This may be related to their age, lifestyle or health condition, as highlighted above. However, even with a therapeutically assessed dose of medication, the response of individual clients can vary significantly, and thus a potentially useful medicine may be harmful. Nurse decision making contributes to risk reduction associated with the administration of medicines, and the identification of potential adverse effects is essential. Some potential adverse effects arising when giving a therapeutic medication are identified in Table 10.2.

Table 10.2 Potential adverse effects of medicines

Adverse effect/side effect	Nature of reaction
Idiosyncrasy	Often genetically determined
Hypersensitivity/ allergy	May be life-threatening (anaphylaxis)
Skin reactions	Pruritus (itching) Urticaria (nettle rash) Erythematous eruptions (flushing and skin rashes) Skin peeling Eczematous lesions
Blood dyscrasias	Aplastic anaemia (due to bone marrow suppression) Thrombocytopenia (loss of platelets) Agranulocytosis (loss of white blood cells)
Gastrointestinal upset	Diarrhoea Dyspepsia Ulceration Nausea Vomiting Sore or dry mouth Anal pruritus Flatulence Abdominal pain
Central nervous system upset	Drowsiness Headache Dizziness Nausea Vomiting Tinnitus
Photosensitivity	Acute ocular sensitivity to light
Tolerance	The client responds increasingly less effectively to a regular dose of medication
Dependence	The client may become addicted to the medication

As well as the adverse effects of giving any single medication to an individual, external influences may also cause damage. Clients may already be taking other medications that could interact with new treatment, causing adverse effects or altering the pharmacokinetic or pharmacodynamic action of either medication. A common outcome is a reduced or halted action (antagonism), which may be useful for use as an antidote, preventing the action of a medication once it has been given, or a potentiated action (synergism). Other reactions are also possible and for a comprehensive listing of currently known interactions see the *British National Formulary* (British Medical Association 2007).

Polypharmacy

An interaction between different drugs, as described above, may not be restricted to two substances, but may involve a multiplicity of medical treatments. This type of interaction is known as 'polypharmacy', and is documented as a problem in the international healthcare literature, across many populations including the elderly, those with mental health problems and children and adolescents.

The role of the pharmacist

The responsibility of the pharmacist both in hospital and in the community is to ensure that any medications dispensed can be taken safely by the individual for whom they are prescribed. Within the hospital setting the pharmacist checks the client's prescription and can observe any possible effects of combining prescribed medications inappropriately. However, this is much more difficult within the community setting. Indeed, such is the concern in the UK that in 2005, the Department of Health initiated pharmacy based 'medicines use review' service for patients with chronic illness or those taking more than one prescribed medicine. This service is free to clients and is provided by primary care trusts through contracts with participating community pharmacies under the NHS (Pharmaceutical Services) (Amendment No 2) Regulations 2005 (SI 1501), which came into force on 5 July 2005 (National Health Services 2005). From a nursing point of view, however, it is essential that careful assessment of clients' medication and treatment is noted upon any assessment made, with care taken to monitor situations where polypharmacy occurs. Unfortunately, however, this service is limited by the number of reviews that may be contracted annually because of cost. This means that not everyone who may require a review will necessarily receive the opportunity. The service has also not been in existence for long enough for evaluation of its effectiveness to take place. Current evidence would suggest that a greater intervention may be required in order to achieve success in reducing the effects of polypharmacy.

Evidence-based practice

Royal et al (2006) systematically reviewed 17 research studies reporting pharmacist-led interventions in the prevention of misuse or overuse of medicines by clients in the community. They found that there was relatively weak evidence to indicate that pharmacist-led medication reviews were effective in reducing hospital admissions and suggested that more randomized controlled trials of primary care based pharmacist-led interventions are needed to decide whether or not this intervention is effective in reducing hospital admissions.

Decision-making exercise

Mrs Johnson was found to be nutritionally anaemic although she had been taking iron preparations prescribed by her general practitioner for some months. When informed about her anaemia, Mrs Johnson was adamant that she took her iron supplements and seemed quite angry that they did not appear to work. She complained that they gave her terrible indigestion leading her to take yet more medicine, and she showed her nurse a bottle of magnesium trisilicate, which she 'borrowed' from her husband as it worked well for him. Since she had not thought it to be a 'proper' medicine she had not mentioned its use.

- Identify the significance of the relationship between the two medicines taken by Mrs Johnson.
- How could you use this information to offer health education to Mrs Johnson?
- Reflect over the times when you have taken prescribed medications: have you ever taken 'home' treatments at the same time? Did you inform your doctor about what you were taking? Did your doctor or the dispensing pharmacist ask you if you were taking any other medicines?

Teratogenesis and iatrogenesis

When considering the possible effects of medicines on the body, it is not just the interaction between the client and medicine or between two medicines that can cause problems. Additionally there may be occasions when other factors such as the current health state of the client or issues associated with lifestyle may engender hidden dangers when combined with an otherwise acceptable treatment. The outcome of such problems may be described in two ways. First there is teratogenesis, which occurs in the treatment of women during or before pregnancy. The teratogenic outcome would be malformation or death of the unborn child. Perhaps the best known example of this situation was the treatment of women with the anti-emetic thalidomide in the early 1960s for morning sickness. Although a highly effective anti-emetic, thalidomide was found to cause amelia (absence of limbs) during fetal development, leading to tragedy for many families whose children suffered as a result of this treatment.

A second problem is iatrogenesis, or the causing of sickness or injury as a result of treatment. Any side-effect may be considered for inclusion, although usually more serious effects that may cause a need for treatment are highlighted. This situation may seem inconceivable to the nursing student who is advised about the benefits of treatment and assured that they should above all do no harm. However, this is a simplistic view of a complex issue and a balance of benefits versus harm may be a more reasonable stance to take. To ensure optimum safety and well-being for clients, you have a duty to understand the possible implications of treatment and to advise your clients so that they can make informed choices about proposed interventions.

Although nurses generally involve themselves in the use of prescription medicines for therapeutic, diagnostic or preventive benefit, many other substances may be used by clients. In this section, the use of substances that may not be prescribed by a medical practitioner are briefly explored, both in relation to the health of the individual and in relation to you as a nurse and as a member of society.

Decision-making exercise

Ahmed, aged 6 years, was diagnosed as having leukaemia and his family wished him to receive current medicinal treatment as a potentially life-saving measure, although Ahmed said that he felt 'all right' before his treatment. After his treatment, however, Ahmed was sick and miserable, and his mouth became ulcerated and sore for a while. The doctors prescribed Ahmed further medicinal treatment to help alleviate his symptoms.

- Was it right to offer Ahmed and his family treatment that would make him ill?
- What are your personal beliefs about treatment for Ahmed?
- How could your own personal beliefs affect the support you give Ahmed and his family through this difficult time in his treatment?

PSYCHOSOCIAL

CLIENT USE OF NON-PRESCRIBED SUBSTANCES

While a medicine has been identified within this chapter as something that is for therapeutic, diagnostic or preventative purposes, there is an issue concerning who decides on such benefits. In hospital settings, medications are prescribed by nursing and medical staff whose qualifications permit them to make an informed decision and offer their clients appropriate advice about their treatment.

In modern society, however, many substances are used by the public. These may be used unwittingly as part of a social norm or for a perceived therapeutic effect. Substances such as tobacco, coffee and alcohol, as well as over the counter preparations such as analgesics, cold cures, antihistamines or vitamins to name but a few, are used commonly by the public. Alternative therapies may also be adopted. These substances may pose a risk to the health of particular individuals or may interact with prescribed medical treatments (Cnattingius et al 2000). For nurses, pharmacists and doctors alike there is a challenge in ensuring that all clients receive health education about the medicines they receive and about the effects of interaction with other substances.

Reflection and portfolio exercise

Think back over the past week. How many times have you had:

- an alcoholic drink
- a cup of coffee or tea
- a cigarette
- a throat sweet or cough or cold cure
- an aspirin or paracetamol tablet
- a vitamin or iron tablet
- an oral contraceptive pill
- any non-prescription treatments?

Look at the above list. Reflect over which (if any) items:

1. Would be unsafe if inadvertently ingested by a child?
2. May, if taken in sustained amounts on a regular basis, eventually lead to physical damage to organs in the body?
3. May, if taken in sustained amounts on a regular basis, lead to psychological dependence?

Use the formularies to find out whether you are right. Make a summary for your portfolio.

Poisoning

In nursing children, it is perhaps particularly important to be aware of the presence of medicinal substances in the home. There are also a myriad of other substances such as cleaning agents, especially those containing caustic soda (e.g. dishwasher powder), fertilizers and weedkillers (e.g. paraquat) which could be extremely dangerous to a child if accessed inappropriately. Many children are admitted to hospital every year following the inappropriate use of common substances leading to poisoning. Children's nurses and health visitors have a role in educating parents and families about safety in home storage of substances hazardous to health and may manage the care of children who have been poisoned.

Overdose

When considering the issue of overdose, it should be stressed that it may occur either intentionally or accidentally. Accidental overdose may result from the client misreading or misunderstanding the prescription label or failing to realize that more than one medication contains the same drug. Taking medicines containing the same drug concurrently would result in an overdose. This is perhaps most common with over the counter cold cures, many of which contain paracetamol. Accidental overdose may occur by proxy in the form of a medication error if a nurse fails to record that a medication has been given, thus allowing the dose to be unintentionally repeated.

Intentional overdose

An area common to all areas of nursing is the intentional abuse of medicines, whether prescribed or not, with intent to cause injury or death to oneself or another. Nurses in practice may find themselves working with victims of para-suicide or with relatives of those who have committed suicide through overdose. The physical nursing needs of para-suicide clients depend very much upon the type of medication taken and require multidisciplinary team working between the nurses, pharmacists and medical team involved in each individual's care. In most para-suicide cases there is an additional referral to a liaison psychiatrist for risk assessment and planning future management. It is likely that the nurse's role would involve monitoring and assessment of the client. A clear understanding of the substance taken and its likely effects of toxicity is essential. Those involved in such sad situations will require counselling and support. This is addressed further in Chapter 13, 'End of life care'.

Reflection and portfolio exercise

For nurses caring for those who have attempted to either seek help by taking an overdose or who have attempted to take their own lives, caring can be emotionally difficult. Consider how you might feel in this situation.

- Would you feel cross that the person is taking up a bed by making themselves ill?
- Would you feel confused or unable to understand?
- Would you simply feel sorry for the person?
- Could your feelings affect your care for that person?
- Think about your own experience of caring for patients. Write a short reflective summary for your portfolio.

Use of illegal substances

A definition of an illegal substance is one that is classified within the schedules outlined in the Misuse of Drugs Act 1971 and is being manufactured, supplied or possessed by anyone not legally authorized to do so. The use of illegal substances cannot be ignored as there are important medical and psychosocial considerations, such as the impact of polypharmacy, or withdrawal if the substance is removed while treatment takes place. For drug-using pregnant women there is a particular concern about the impact of the substance on the fetus and the effect of withdrawal once the baby is born.

Evidence-based practice

Illegal drugs are a national and international problem within society. Within the UK, contemporary evidence has identified the following:

- Drug use amongst adults aged 16–59 has been falling since 2004/5.
- Cannabis use has declined, but cocaine use has increased.
- Data for Scotland are for 2004 and show the same downward trend in drug use identified in England and Wales in 2004/5.
- Among schoolchildren in England drug use has remained level since 2001 with a suggestion of a recent dip.
- The price of heroin, ecstasy and cocaine has fallen since 2004, while the price of cannabis, crack cocaine and LSD has remained stable; the price of amphetamines increased by more than 10% in 2005, having fallen in recent years. Reitox (2006). United Kingdom drug situation: annual report to the European Monitoring Centre for Drugs and Drug Addiction (EMCDDA).

Although it is not suggested that the use of illicit drugs should be encouraged or condoned by nurses, it is important to be aware of the nature and use of such substances by all clients in your care. Use must be assessed as part of the individual's lifestyle so that any prescribed medication can be given to best effect, since it is possible for non-prescription substances to interact with prescribed medications with serious consequences.

Assessment may reveal areas where individuals need help with managing the consumption of addictive substances, and nurses may have a role in helping find appropriate support and advice. However, issues associated with maintaining confidentiality when a client is pursuing an illegal activity are complex and extend beyond the remit of this chapter. Dimond (2004) explores these issues in more depth in her text *Legal Aspects of Nursing.*

Alternative or complementary therapies

The use of complementary or alternative medicines is within the rights of any client. However, the nurse must be aware of what is being used and must also be aware of any possible interactions between this and any proposed orthodox treatment. Nurses are able to use complementary therapies provided that they have successfully undertaken training to do so, take full professional accountability for their actions, have the informed consent of the client who is to receive such treatment, and have considered the appropriateness of the therapy to both the condition of the client and any coexisting treatments (Dimond 2004, Nursing and Midwifery Council 2008b).

Health promotion

Nurses have an important position in society in their capacity to offer appropriate health education to a wide range of individuals and to their families. A practice nurse's knowledge about the effects of smoking on the health of unborn children may be an essential contribution in helping a pregnant woman reduce the number of cigarettes she smokes (or better still stop smoking altogether), while the combined skills and knowledge employed by mental health nurses in drug and alcohol dependency units may offer a healthier future for their clients. Many more examples could be cited in relation to all nursing specialities. In relation to medicines advice, nurses form part of an interdisciplinary service where the delivery of information may promote the appropriate, and optimum use of medicines. This is vital in relation to the management of client discharge and in relation to home care, where clients must be prepared to self-administer medicinal treatment.

Reflection and portfolio evidence

Reflect upon a recent day in practice.

- Can you identify any times when you or your mentor were involved in an activity associated with administering medicines but not actually giving a medicine to a client?
- What aspects included assessment and planning for giving medicines to clients?
- Record what you learned from these situations in your portfolio and discuss with your mentor.

Finally, there is the issue of the use of non-prescribed medicines by nurses themselves. After all, in spite of professional accountability, health carers are human and part of the wider society in which we all live. Social use of 'medicines' and difficulties surrounding abuse of substances are a very real issue, particularly in the stressful occupation of nursing. Recognition of personal problems are all important for nurses and their professional colleagues. Indeed, as stated in the Nursing and Midwifery Council's Code there is an obligation for any nurse 'To act without delay if you believe that you, a colleague or anyone else may be putting someone at risk' (Nursing and Midwifery Council 2008a: Manage Risk Section).

CARE DELIVERY KNOWLEDGE

Nurses are accountable for the safe administration of medicines in whatever setting they may be working. To do this effectively they must be able to apply the knowledge discussed above according to the client's individual needs. Nursing skills are required that relate to assessment, planning of proposed nursing intervention, and the implementation and evaluation of any therapy prescribed. Additionally, the role of the nurse extends more broadly in ensuring the safety and well-being of clients when considered in relation to the guidance advocated within the Standards for Medicines Management (Nursing and Midwifery Council 2008b). This document assumes a much wider role for the nurse both before and after a medicine is actually given. It is useful to explore the subject knowledge about medicines and administration above in relation to the organizational context and the intertwined roles of the nurse, multidisciplinary team and the clients themselves.

ORGANIZING ADMINISTRATION OF MEDICINES

The role of the nurse may vary practically according to the type of nursing situation. For instance, in areas with responsibility for groups of dependent clients, a different role in medicines administration will operate as compared to a situation where clients are independent and able to self-administer their treatment. Nurses may directly give prescribed medicines, or be involved with administration through education and supervision of the clients or their carers. In some settings the nurse's remit will extend to a role that will include the prescription of medicines from the *Nurse Prescriber's Formulary* or through a supplementary agreement or a client group direction. This type of involvement is discussed further within the professional and ethical section of this chapter.

THE ROLE OF THE NURSE IN THE ADMINISTRATION OF MEDICINES TO CLIENTS

In practice, nurses are accountable for any medication they administer, and to do this safely they must use knowledge gained through education and experience in a personalized way with each of their clients. It is helpful to consider the nursing role systematically. This includes assessing, planning, implementing and evaluating care. This can be applied in conjunction with a conceptual framework in accordance with an individual practitioner's philosophy of care. Areas that may be addressed before giving a medicine to a client are revealed by the questions below:

- What is the age of the client?
- What is the client's weight and baseline observations?
- What is the client's past medical history?
- What is the diagnosis of the client?
- Has the client consented to this treatment?
- Is the client currently taking any medications? If so, what are they?
- Has the client taken this medication before? If so, was it tolerated and was it effective?
- How does the client prefer to take medication (i.e. can they take tablets?)?
- What is the preferred route for the medication prescribed?
- Is the client allergic to any medication?
- Does the client (and if appropriate, carer) understand why the medicine has been prescribed?
- Does the client (and carer) know about potential side-effects that may occur?
- Who is going to administer the medicine? Do they know how to do this to gain optimum benefit?
- Is there any reason why the client should not receive the medicine prescribed?

All of these considerations need to be taken into account when reviewing prescriptions and medicine administration records. Indeed, the nurse must ensure that such records contain all information relevant to the administration of a medication to the client, and that information is clearly documented without illegibility or ambiguity. This is recognized within government recommendations relating to safety in medicine administration practice, as a priority in maintaining a safe system (Department of Health 2000). The nurse must also ensure that the medicine administration record card is checked thoroughly prior to the administration of a medicine in accordance with local policy. This can be complex, as abbreviations and Latin terminology are used by prescribers despite recommendations that this is not acceptable (British Medical Association and Royal Pharmaceutical Society of Great Britain 2008). While some texts offer a range of abbreviations, it is advised that any prescription containing information that is not fully understood by the nurse should not be acted upon until it has been rewritten or appropriately clarified to the satisfaction of all parties. Poorly written prescriptions contribute to medicine administration error, and nurses should not administer any medication about which they are not fully informed. After a medication is administered the event must be recorded according to local policy.

Planning nursing care

When planning care, all the information derived from the medicines assessment by the nurse and other members of the multidisciplinary team needs to be combined. This information must be used to identify common goals for the administration of the medicine prescribed and outline an individualized plan of care for the client. This can be followed by implementing care that can be evaluated regularly to determine the effect of the intervention, as illustrated by the following case:

While in hospital for treatment of congestive cardiac failure, Mrs Johnson's needs are individually assessed by her nurses and a specific plan is made to assess the effects of her treatment:
- *The problem: Mrs Johnson has congestive heart failure which requires treatment with digoxin 62.5 micrograms/day.*
- *The outcome: Mrs Johnson will gain a steady pulse rate of 80–120 beats/min and appear well.*
- *Nursing action: Observe Mrs Johnson for a lowered pulse rate of less than 60 beats/min, coupling of heart beats (felt at the wrist as double beats) or nausea and vomiting. In the event of any of these, contact the medical staff for advice.*

In relation to planning, there may be other issues taken into account that are related more to individual preferences; for instance, if a medicine needs to be taken with food, when is the usual mealtime for the client? Although in hospital meals may be delivered at set times, mealtimes can vary widely for individuals in their own homes; and for neonates who are fed on demand, it would be difficult to write up a medication to be taken with food at a set time! With planning and negotiation between the client, nurse and medical staff, a solution to such problems may be reached that meets the needs of all parties in providing optimum treatment.

Planning also needs to take place within the work organization, and this requires knowledge and skill on behalf of the nurse. If a medicine needs to be given at a specific time, the nurse needs to ensure that both the medicines and the client are available and prepared. The medication may require retrieving from a locked cupboard, reconstituting (if it is a dry powder to be made into solution) and offered in an acceptable way for the client, according to the route for which it is prescribed. Procedures need to be followed and the medicine must be given in accordance with the law, local policy and *The Code: Standards of Conduct, Performance and Ethics for Nurses and Midwives* (Nursing and Midwifery Council 2008a) (see the Professional Knowledge section of this chapter). In the case of the client, skin may have to be prepared for topical creams or it may simply be necessary to ensure that the client has a drink ready to swallow tablets.

Safety in medicine administration

It is also important for the practice of medicine administration to be safe for the administrator. Since all medication is given for the therapeutic or diagnostic effect it is going to have on the client, it is important to remember that carelessness or inappropriate handling of medicine can lead to the nurse and (possibly others) inadvertently receiving treatment. Illustrations of this include the administration of skin creams. If the nurse does not wear gloves to protect the skin, then the cream will be applied to her hand as well as the client. Where medicines are drawn up in a syringe by nurses before administration to a client, carelessness can lead to aerosol inhalation during this activity. Many cytotoxic medicines are reconstituted by the pharmacist in laminar air flow cubicles to draw any particles of the medication away.

Finally, in the case of liquids care should be taken to avoid splashing the medicine, which could be absorbed through the skin or inhaled.

With all medicine administration, careful handwashing before and after the procedure is essential in order to avoid cross-infection contamination from the nurse's hand to the client and potential ingestion of particles of medicine by the nurse. Where medications are particularly toxic the pharmacist may advise extra protective measures when handling, such as safety glasses or a protective gown, and these should be adhered to.

Within this text it is inappropriate to dwell upon the many specific practical skills and procedures required in administering medicines. However, there are texts with a skills development focus that do this well; a particular example includes Dougherty & Lister (2006).

All of the above considerations require planning on the part of the nurse as an outcome of an informed assessment of the situation.

Planning for client discharge

There is a considerable role for the nurse in planning a client's discharge from the care setting. There is a responsibility to ensure that prescribed medications to take home are available by liaising with the pharmacy department. Additionally the nurse must ensure that the client or carer will be able to manage the prescribed treatment effectively once they return home.

The nurse's role may simply involve advising a client about the frequency with which tablets should be taken or it could be more complex, involving education and assessment of the ability to perform a skill such as the instillation of eye drops. In either case, the nurse must

evaluate the ability of those continuing care and be certain that care will continue after discharge. If this cannot be achieved alternative support may need to be planned, for instance a hospital based nurse discharging a client to the community may need to plan for intervention by the community nursing staff.

> **Evidence-based practice**
>
> Latter et al (2000) identified that nurses did not always perform their role in patient education related to medicine well. Communication is clearly a fundamental part of medicine administration practice and it is vital that both nursing practice and its effectiveness in client care are regularly evaluated.

> **Evidence-based practice**
>
> Wright et al (2002) evaluated self-administration in two children's wards. The researchers found that this method was well received by children and their families as well as nursing staff who reported improvements in facilitating care and improving comfort and access to medication.

Implementing nursing care

In the act of giving a medicine all the assessment, planning and background knowledge comes together to permit safe and accountable action. Additionally, the nurse has to acknowledge and respect the rights of the client in receiving their medication (as discussed in the professional knowledge section of this chapter).

Although delivery systems in nursing may differ, the nurse's responsibility in administering medicines to clients is constant. One starting point is identified by Hall (2002) within 'eight rights' in drug administration (Box 10.3). The Nursing and Midwifery Council (2008b) offers further advice relating to the professional accountability of the nurse administering a medicine, and it is wise to refer to this guidance also.

Although these references offer a useful start, the nurse may need to be flexible about how such guidance is achieved. For instance, it cannot be assumed that the nurse will always give a client his or her medicine. Self-medication by clients is recognized as one way of empowering clients and improving safety (Audit Commission 2002) and is found to be popular with patients (Wright et al 2002). In children's nursing, nurses work in partnership with parents and the children, and in the community, nurses may be responsible for overseeing their clients who are self-administering medicines in their own homes.

Box 10.3 The eight 'rights' of medicines administration

The nurse must ensure that:

THE RIGHT MEDICATION
is given to
THE RIGHT CLIENT
at
THE RIGHT TIME
on
THE RIGHT DATE
in
THE RIGHT DOSE
via
THE RIGHT ROUTE
in
THE RIGHT PREPARATION
and
THE RIGHT DOCUMENTATION
is completed

- How did the administration of this medicine integrate with the total care of the client and with the nurse's total role?
- What knowledge did the nurse need to have to ensure that the medicine was received safely?
- What new knowledge did you gain from the situation? Record your learning in your portfolio.

Evidence-based practice

A study of children's nurses' roles on administering medicine found that nurses identified 201 activities that were considered to be part of a nurse's role ensuring a medicine was to be administered safely (Hall 2002). Key themes that emerged in relation to these roles included client and family education and information, management and knowledge acquisition, and admission and discharge planning as well as more commonly acknowledged skills and practices associated with the rights of administering.

Practical considerations in giving medicines

Additionally, some practical issues fall outside the above rights and professional guidance, and must be addressed when implementing the administration of a medicine. Failure to acknowledge these would not perhaps be considered as a medication error, but would make the difference between unacceptable and optimum practice. Such issues are considered elsewhere in this book, but may include for instance the management of infection control (see Ch. 5), an issue that is particularly pertinent in relation to the administration of intravenous medication. If a client becomes septicaemic due to contamination during the administration of a medication, their safety could be as much compromised as if they were given the wrong dose.

A final aspect to consider is the nurse's knowledge of resuscitation techniques and equipment in the event of an anaphylactic reaction to a medication (see Ch. 4). When any medicine is given, it is the responsibility of the nurse to know what possible side-effects may occur and to observe for these once the medication has been administered. This aspect will be addressed further in the next section, on evaluation of care.

Reflection and portfolio evidence

In your practice placement, try to observe one situation where a nurse ensures that a client receives their medicines. Note in detail what you see, including the nurse's actions and the client's actions.

Evaluation of nursing care in relation to medicines management

For all clients, treatment with medication requires evaluation regarding its effect (beneficial or otherwise). A fundamental part of the nurse's decision making role with regard to medicine administration is related to identifying whether a medication is effective or sufficient for the client's needs. The nurse must use both general and clinical skills of observation as well as communication skills; the therapeutic effects of any medication given must be reviewed and any untoward reactions that may have occurred as a result of treatment must be managed. The nurse must also be able to record and communicate findings to other members of the interprofessional team appropriately. Within this, a major aspect is the evaluation and assessment of pain control (see Ch. 11). Evaluation may also require the use of many clinical monitoring skills (e.g. temperature assessment, respiratory rate, patient's colour, mood and behaviour) in determining outcomes.

All registered nurses are duty bound to administer medicines for therapeutic, diagnostic or preventive benefit, but there are many ways in which clients' optimum health and safety can be compromised in spite of the intentions behind the planned treatment with medicines. The qualified nurse therefore plays an important part in promoting the health and safety of clients with regard to the evaluation of the administration of their treatment as well as in the more recognized areas of health and safety already outlined and included in Chapter 3.

PROFESSIONAL AND ETHICAL KNOWLEDGE

In this section the nurse's role in the prescribing and administering of medicine is considered in relation to British law currently governing practice, *The Code: Standards of Conduct, Performance and Ethics for Nurses and Midwives* (Nursing and Midwifery Council 2008a), and the impact of local policy. Clients' rights will be considered regarding their consent to treatment and the right to refuse medicinal treatment will be explored. Finally, the nurse's role in the management of medication error is addressed.

LEGAL CONSIDERATIONS IN PRESCRIBING AND ADMINISTERING MEDICINES

In Britain, the manufacture, prescription, safe handling, storage and custody of medicines remain primarily subject to legislative control arising from two main Acts of parliament and a set of guiding regulations, as follows:

- Medicines Act 1968
- Misuse of Drugs Act 1971
- Misuse of Drugs Regulations 1985.

Each of the Acts determines different legal controls which must be observed by the nurse in daily practice.

Legal classification of medicines

Under the Medicines Act 1968 drugs are classified into three main groups:

1. Pharmacy-only products: those only to be sold through a registered pharmacy under the supervision of a pharmacist.
2. General sales list: medicines that may be sold from a retail outlet without a pharmacist or registration as a pharmacy, provided certain conditions relating to the security of the premises are adhered to.
3. Prescription-only medicines: medicines that are only available on a practitioner's prescription. This group is divided to identify those drugs that are simply to be prescribed by a practitioner and those that are further governed by additional requirements under the Misuse of Drugs Act 1971.

A clear knowledge of the classification of medications is essential for the nurse who has responsibility for ensuring the safe and legal administration of medicines to clients. Within the Misuse of Drugs Act 1971 and the Misuse of Drugs Regulations 1985, controlled drugs are identified and categorized according to requirements governing their import, export, supply, possession, prescribing and record keeping (Dimond 2004). However, following the enquiry into general practitioner and convicted mass murderer Harold Shipman, regulations relating to management of controlled drugs changed. Shipman was able to abuse his access to controlled drugs and administer lethal doses of these to patients. The five Shipman enquiry reports highlight how this was possible and made many recommendations which have been enacted in law within the Health Act 2006 (Part 3, Chapter 1).

Key changes relate to the determination of responsibility by care providers such as trusts, who have to identify an accountable person whose responsibility it is to ensure strict regulation of the whole process of controlled drug management. For nurses, knowledge regarding these Acts is essential in understanding the way controlled drugs are stored and handled in the practice setting. Strict regulations govern where a controlled drug should be kept, how it may be planned and transported from a pharmacy and by whom, where it must be kept, who holds the keys to access controlled medicines, and how the prescription checking and use of such drugs must be documented. The *Nursing and Midwifery Standards for Medicines Management* (Nursing and Midwifery Council 2008b) addresses the issues for nurses in some detail.

Decision-making exercise

You are working as a nurse in charge at a respite home for clients with severe learning disability. One morning, Simon, a short-stay client in the home, develops signs and symptoms of a urinary tract infection. You call Simon's general practitioner, but he is unable to see him until the afternoon. You know that another client has been prescribed antibiotics for a similar diagnosis. A colleague suggests that if you borrowed some of this client's antibiotics for Simon then he could begin treatment right away.

- How should you react to this suggestion?
- What knowledge and legal rationale would influence your response?

Reflection and portfolio evidence

In your practice, find a controlled drug prescription. Try to identify the following:

- How does a controlled medicine prescription differ from prescriptions that are not for controlled medicines?
- What is special about the cupboard where controlled medicines are stored? Who has the keys?
- What governs the administration and storage of controlled medicines?
- What does the nurse need to know in order to give a controlled drug safely?

- What is included in the controlled record of administration?
- Record your findings in your portfolio.

10.3 - RECORDING AND MEDICINES

- Signing the medicines chart.
- Writing prescriptions.
- Recording and controlled medicines.

NURSE AND NON-MEDICAL PRESCRIBING

Nurses and many non-medical staff can prescribe medicines, in accordance with government legislation. There are two main types of prescribing: 'independent prescribing' which can be performed by nurses and pharmacists who have undertaken specific training programmes, and supplementary prescribing which can be performed by nurses and pharmacists, physiotherapists, chiropodists/podiatrists, radiographers and optometrists provided appropriate training has been undertaken. Patients can also be prescribed medicines to be given under Patient Group Directions or under Patient Specific Directions. The range and scope of this legislation for each of the different professions allied to medicine and to nurses, midwives and health visitors is clearly and concisely explained in the Department of Health document *Medicines Matters* (2006) which is available on the Department of Health website. This section will focus entirely on exploring the different nursing roles and the impact of prescribing by nurses and others on the roles and practice of the nurse.

Types of prescriber

Independent prescribers

> From 1 May 2006 Nurse Independent Prescribing (formerly Extended Formulary Nurse Prescribing) was expanded. This allows nurses to prescribe any licensed medicine for any medical condition that a nurse prescriber is competent to treat, including some Controlled Drugs. It allows virtually any licensed medicine in the British National Formulary (see part XVIIB(ii) of the Drug Tariff) to be prescribed.   (Department of Health 2006: 7)

This consideration is expanded in the consideration of appropriateness of independent prescribing, where it is identified that nurse independent prescribing is most appropriate where:

- The nurse is competent to assess, diagnose and make treatment decisions for the patient.
- The condition is such that the nurse independent prescriber is competent to treat independently.
- The nurse works remotely from a doctor, seeing patients independently.

Supplementary prescribers

This category of prescribing was introduced in 2003 for nurses working with patients who have more complex conditions, and then expanded to include other professionals in 2005. Supplementary prescribers once again must complete an accredited post-registration training course. They can prescribe for a client once the client has been assessed by a doctor and a treatment plan has been established. They can alter dosages, frequency, and active ingredients of medication within the limits of the agreed treatment or clinical management plan.

Patient Specific Directions

This type of prescribing refers to the traditional type of prescribing where an independent prescriber provides a prescription for one named individual. While the independent prescriber may now be a doctor or a nurse or pharmacist, there are many situations where patient specific prescribing is a requirement.

Patient Group Directions

These directions enable nurses to supply prescription only medicines to clients under generalized directions of a doctor. Examples may include provision of vaccines, or specific medicines out of hours. Patient Group Directions are also used in hospital. An example might be the supply of topical anaesthetic creams prior to theatre admission or blood sampling. For further information about nurse prescribing see the section on websites at the end of this chapter, but the implications of this change in practice are profound. In nursing, there may be a range of individuals able to prescribe medicines for patients in different settings and it is important to appreciate the context in which care is taking place. For student nurses time will need to be taken exploring the contextual situations in placement in order to appreciate who is prescribing for the patient, and what the nature of the prescription might be.

Medicine administration and *The Code: Standards of Conduct, Performance and Ethics for Nurses and Midwives* (Nursing and Midwifery Council 2008a)

As well as working within the law and within professional training, the nurse is also accountable to the Nursing and

Midwifery Council, which is the nurses' governing body for professional practice. *The Code: Standard of Conduct, Performance and Ethics for Nurses and Midwives* and its supplementary guidance paper *Standards for Medicines Management* (Nursing and Midwifery Council 2008a, 2008b) assist the nurse in fulfilling the expectations the Council has of them as a professional body. Although the law will instigate criminal proceedings in the event of a breach, the Council's guidance adheres to the general principles of law and to regulations regarding the management of drugs.

The Nursing and Midwifery Council has the power to remove practitioners who fail to meet professional standards or protect the public from the professional register, thus removing an individual's right to practise as a nurse in the UK. The Nursing and Midwifery Council's regulations are more comprehensive and detailed in relation to nursing clients than those required by law, but they also assist the nurse in interpreting the law.

Local policies for medicines storage and administration

Local policies are established within individual health trusts and care settings and set the expectations of the employer with respect to their employed practitioners. Nurses must be aware of the contents of their local policy, because it is unlikely that an individual nurse who becomes involved in any legal action with a client would receive support or insurance if the employer's policy had been contravened during the incident. This would be irrespective of whether the practice is acceptable to the Nursing and Midwifery Council or legal standards. This is particularly important in relation to the administration of medicines because there are variations between individual employers in what is deemed to be acceptable practice. This is particularly well illustrated in relation to the checking of medicines by individual practitioners. The law holds an individual accountable for medicine administered irrespective of qualification, but the Nursing and Midwifery Council states that only a qualified practitioner can give medicines, and advocates that:

> *in the majority of circumstances a first level registered nurse, a midwife or a second level nurse, each of whom has demonstrated the necessary knowledge and competence, should be able to administer medicines without involving a second person.*

Local policies, however, vary with regard to how many (one or two) nurses are required to check a medicine, and where a second checker is required, there is variation as to who that person is to be. For nurses who change employment or who participate in agency employment, an awareness of local variations in policy is essential.

Clients' rights

As with any form of treatment all clients have a right to be fully informed about the medicines they receive and most have a right to refuse treatment if it is against their wishes. There are, however, some exceptions to this rule, and for nursing this has moral and ethical implications, which require consideration.

Treatment of children

In the treatment of children, it is incumbent upon the nurse to ensure that the child client and their family receive information about their treatment that is appropriate to their understanding. If it is considered that the child client is old enough and mature enough to understand the implications of his or her treatment then his or her decision should be allowed by the health carer. This is supported in law within the Fraser guidance (previously known as the Gillick competence in which a general practitioner won his case to prescribe a child under the age of 16 years contraceptive medication without recourse to her parents for permission). For a child who is under 16 years of age, however, any decision for treatment is usually made with the joint consent of the parents. This is commonly incorporated into hospital policy as a guideline for health carers. The Children Act 1989 also influenced treatment for children in stating that any course of treatment must be in the best interests of the child concerned. In a few cases this may have implications if a parent refuses to consent to treatment for a child where the child is too young to consent for themselves, and where the treatment is unanimously considered by medical professionals to be in the best interests of the child. As a last resort, the child may be made a ward of court in order to allow treatment to be given without parental consent. Similar assessments must be made for those with learning disabilities. The administration of medicines for children and those with learning disabilities can cause ethical dilemmas in practice.

Decision-making exercise

Six-year-old Ahmed is undergoing treatment for leukaemia. While you are in practice he is to have oral medication, which he hates intensely. On this particular occasion he refuses to take his medicine, which is a vital part of his treatment.

- Does Ahmed have any right to refuse his treatment?
- Discuss this with your peers and record the responses you conclude.

A second major consideration in children's nursing relates to the high number of medicines that are administered either off label or off licence. There are obvious ethical dilemmas here because it is the licensing restriction that contributes to ensuring the research tested safety of the medicine. Since in the past, access for research with children has been complex, many medicine licences have only been requested for use with adult clients. Over time, these medicines have become used within child health, although no licence has been agreed. This is a position children's nurses must be aware of, indeed in the *National Service Framework for Children's Hospital Services* (Department of Health 2003), a section is devoted to this problem. In a professional role, health carers should not have to choose to give medicines where the effects of their use is unknown. However, children's nurses may have the dilemma of choosing whether to administer a prescription off licence or off label, or refusing a child a treatment that may be therapeutic. If guidance from the Nursing and Midwifery Council (2008b) is taken into account, then the consideration may be to act in the best interests of the child, and to be fully aware of the evidence that would support administration of such medication.

Treatment of the mentally ill

Most mentally ill clients do have a right to consent to or refuse treatment. In some situations, however, treatment is obliged by law and is involuntary. This is usually because the client's illness indicates a risk to themselves or to the community unless treatment is maintained. Again issues may be raised regarding the rights of the client and the role of the nurse in protecting such rights, especially if the treatment given benefits the community rather than the client himself, for instance the use of medication to subdue noisy or aggressive clients.

Other considerations related to the management of all clients, but especially pertinent to those taking medicines for chronic illness, include the validity of an initial consent if a client changes his or her mind or wishes to stop treatment. Issues that require consideration include what rights a dangerously aggressive client has to stop treatment if the medication is successful. Many medications that affect mood also have side-effects, which may be uncomfortable or inconvenient to the client, but if treatment is stopped, will their aggression make them a danger to society? Do such clients have a right to refuse?

While there is both legal and ethical controversy surrounding the individual's rights versus the rights of the community for safety, the Nursing and Midwifery Council (2006) does identify for nurses that giving medication to patients without their knowledge and consent may occasionally be necessary. The Council's position statement acknowledges that while disguising medicine in the absence of informed consent must always be regarded as deception, a clear distinction should always be made between those who have the capacity to refuse medication and those who lack such a capacity. Within this distinction, they further identify that there are those who have not got the capacity to know they are receiving medicinal treatment and those who would have if they were not being deceived by covert administration. They advise that in any situation the nurse will need to be sure that 'what they are doing is in the best interests of the client and be accountable for this decision' (NMC position statement on the covert administration of medicines, 2006, overview).

Additionally, the effect of stopping medicines without planning must be considered, and clients should be advised if considering refusal. Medicines such as fluphenazine decanoate (Modecate) have a long-acting effect, which cannot be reversed quickly. There are also implications for withdrawing treatment where a medicine creates a dependence because it is addictive or it reduces the body's ability to produce a similar substance naturally (e.g. glucocorticosteroids). Rapid withdrawal of such substances could be dangerous or cause discomfort.

The client's position

Finally, when caring for individuals requiring treatment with medications there is also the possibility that they may not wish to disclose their use of other medicines. This may occur in all branches of nursing and for many different reasons. In children's nursing for instance, a teenage girl may not wish her family to know that she is taking oral contraceptives, or another situation may arise if a client is using a substance considered to be illegal. Many issues arise from these scenarios which merit reflection and discussion.

MANAGEMENT OF MEDICATION ERRORS

Medication errors occur in the event of a client not receiving their medicine when they should do (error of omission) or receiving it when there is reason to withhold it, or in a manner that is not appropriate (error of commission). When errors do occur, they may have a devastating effect; at the least they demonstrate the fallibility of systems and individuals, and at worst they can cause discomfort, pain or be potentially fatal for the clients involved. Given the seriousness of such errors, it is perhaps surprising to learn how commonly they occur (Department of Health 2000).

In the event of an error occurring, the nurse concerned must ensure the safety of the client and staff. This would usually involve immediately contacting members of medical and pharmacy teams and explaining what has happened in the incident so that an appropriate course of action can be taken. After the practical management of any error, the nurse must complete documentation to record the incident. The nature of further action then depends upon the type of error made and on whether the error is in contravention of *The Code: Standards of Conduct, Performance and Ethics for Nurses and Midwives* (Nursing and Midwifery Council 2008a) or the law, or local policy.

10.4 – MEDICATION ERROR

- Types of error
- Factors influencing error
- Support after error

PERSONAL AND REFLECTIVE KNOWLEDGE

AWARENESS OF PERSONAL POSITION IN EVERY ASPECT OF MEDICINES

In conclusion, this chapter has introduced you to many facets of knowledge required to make effective nursing decisions when planning the storage of and administration of medicines to clients. The chapter demonstrates the need for a wide range of nursing skills, from understanding the complexities of medicines law and physiological action to the more practical elements such as perceptual and communication skills required when working with both clients and other members of the nursing and multidisciplinary team. The safe and effective administration of medicine requires nurses to be knowledgeable, and importantly, vigilant in their practice, and as with other areas of practice highlighted in this book, also requires you to be aware of the latest developments in research related to of all the areas addressed. This chapter has introduced research-based evidence in medicine administration supporting rationale for the care to be offered. It is not intended to be a complete record of all applicable research or necessarily the most up to date and relevant to your own specific practice area, but it serves as an illustration of the work that is available and can be used to enhance care in practice.

CASE STUDIES RELATING TO THE USE OF MEDICINES

In summary, case studies are provided to enable the application of concepts presented in this chapter. In each one, issues will be raised that are meaningful to that individual situation, but may also be transferable to other settings with different clients.

Case study: Adult

Julia Hargreaves is 26 years old and lives alone in a flat in the centre of a large city. She moved 5 years ago from her parents' house in the country to find work after graduating from university. Julia is admitted to hospital after a car knocks her off her bike as she is cycling home one evening. On admission Julia is adamant that she wishes to have no treatment with medicines as she is in early pregnancy and does not wish to hurt her baby. Julia is found to have a compound fracture of her left tibia and is in considerable pain. Without antibiotics she risks seriously complicating her injury by developing osteomyelitis.

- What factors would you need to take into account when planning care for Julia?
- Discuss what you consider the nurse's role might be in the above situation?
- If Julia persisted in her request for no medical treatment, what dilemmas may face carers who are looking after her and her unborn child?

Case study: Mental health

Mohammed Shah is 20 years old and newly diagnosed as having mental illness, which requires long-term treatment with antipsychotic drugs to prevent deluded, aggressive and occasionally violent behaviour. He has been treated now for 6 months and feels that he is cured and no longer requires his fortnightly injections. Although Mohammed continues to attend the clinic for these, he is becoming increasingly dissatisfied with the nurses, and is starting to suggest that he may not come any more.

- As the practice nurse, how might you respond to Mohammed?
- What would be the dilemmas to be solved in making your response?
- Mohammed was being treated with the antipsychotic fluphenazine decanoate (Modecate). What are the therapeutic benefits and side-effects of antipsychotic medications such as this?

Case study: Child

Chloe Jackson is 6 years old and lives at home with her mother and father and 2-year-old brother Caspar. She has had severe eczema since she was a baby and this frequently becomes inflamed with open lesions. At a visit to the surgery Mrs Jackson is advised by her general practitioner to accept a prescription for glucocorticosteroid treatment for Chloe. Mrs Jackson is very anxious about the prospect of this treatment since she has heard that glucocorticosteroids have bad side-effects.

- What information should be offered to Mrs Jackson about the benefits and effects of glucocorticosteroid treatment?

- What advice should be given if Chloe is to receive glucocorticosteroid treatment for her eczema?
- The glucocorticosteroid treatment is to be administered at home in the form of a topical cream. What education should be included regarding administration and storage?
- Mrs Jackson comments that she has heard that alternative medicine is an effective way of managing eczema. She asks the practice nurse for an opinion. What advice could the practice nurse offer?

Case study: Learning disabilities

Sam Doppler is a 30-year-old man with mild learning disability. He manages to live alone and works as a kitchen assistant in a small cafe. One day he cuts his hand on an unwashed knife at work. After a few days the cut becomes inflamed and sore and Sam is unable to use his hand and so he attends his general practitioner. Sam is prescribed a course of oral antibiotics and advised not to return to work until his hand has healed.

- What advice should Sam receive about taking his antibiotics?
- Given his learning disability, what strategies may be employed to ensure that Sam understands the prescription he is given?
- Sam asks the practice nurse to explain why the doctor has given him tablets when it is his hand that is sore. Discuss the pharmacokinetic action of oral antibiotic treatment from taking the medication to its therapeutic action at the required site.

SUMMARY

This chapter has drawn together theoretical concepts relating to the use of medicines. It has applied this knowledge in relation to the practice of caring for individuals. The chapter has included:

1. An outline of medicinal action on the body, and also consideration of non-therapeutic action by medicines.
2. Consideration relating to the administration of medicines including the calculation of medicine dosages, routes by which medicines may be administered and knowledge for storage and administration of medicines in safety using application of research evidence.
3. Nursing care of clients who require medicines, including the assessment of clients in relation to medicine administration, planning to administer a medicine and how medication administration can be evaluated.
4. Professional and ethical knowledge relating to the legal acts governing the storage and administration of medicines in the UK. Moral and ethical dilemmas that can arise within the practice of medicines prescribing and administration.
5. Effective management of errors in administration.

Knowledge illuminated within this chapter has been combined with evidence from other referenced sources and applied within a range of situations. Suggestions have been made for portfolio development in relation to medicines management.

Annotated further reading and websites

Dimond B 2004 Legal aspects of nursing. Prentice Hall, New York

In a specific chapter on law as it applies to medicine administration, the nurse's duty of care to the client is considered.

Downie G, Mackenzie J, Williams A in association with Hind C, 2007 Pharmacology and drug management for nurses, 4th edn. Churchill Livingstone, Edinburgh

This book offers a comprehensive explanation of current theories regarding pharmacodynamics in a complete chapter on this subject.

http://www.bnf.org.uk/
The website of the British National Formulary produced by the British Medical Association. The most up-to-date evidence relating to medicines licensed within the UK can be accessed here.

http://www.nmc-uk.org/
The website of the Nursing and Midwifery Council, this offers professional guidance to nurses on their role in administering medicines.

http://www.dh.gov.uk/
This is the Department of Health website. It holds a wealth of information, and reports on all aspects of health. It contains current plans for extending and developing nurse prescribing.

http://www.npc.co.uk/
The website of the National Prescribing Centre. Although designed for nurses who are prescribers, it holds useful information for all interested in prescribing and administering medicines.

http://www.mathcentre.ac.uk
http://www.learndirect.co.uk
These are the websites of national maths education initiatives. They hold useful resources for numeracy assessment and development for nurses as well as others.

References

Audit Commission 2002 Medicines management. HMSO, London

British Medical Association 2007 Nurse prescriber's formulary. British Medical Association, London

British Medical Association and the Royal Pharmaceutical Society of Great Britain 2008 British national formulary 55. British Medical Association, London. Available online: http://www.bnf.org.uk/ (accessed 14 August 2008)

Chapelhow C, Crouch P 2007 Nursing numeracy: a new approach. Nelson Thornes, Cheltenham

Children Act 1989 HMSO, London

Cnattingius S, Signorello LB, Anneren G et al 2000 Caffeine intake and the risk of first-trimester spontaneous abortion. New England Journal of Medicine 343(25):1839–1845

Department of Health 1999 Review of prescribing, supply and administration of medicines. HMSO, London

Department of Health 2000 An organization with a memory. HMSO, London. Available online: http://www.dh.gov.uk/en/Publicationsandstatistics/Publications/PublicationsPolicyAndGuidance/DH_4065083 (accessed 14 August 2008)

Department of Health 2003 The national service framework for children: acute and hospital services. HMSO, London. Available online: http://www.dh.gov.uk/en/Healthcare/NationalServiceFrameworks/Children/DH_4089111#_4 (accessed 15 August 2008)

Department of Health 2006 Medicines matters. Stationery Office, London

Dimond B 2004 Legal aspects of nursing, 4th edn. Prentice Hall, New York

Dougherty L, Lister S 2006 The Royal Marsden manual of clinical nursing procedures, pocket edn (Royal Marsden NHS Trust). Blackwell Publishing, Oxford

Downie G, MacKenzie J, Williams A, in association with Hind C 2007 Pharmacology and drug management for nurses, 4th edn. Churchill Livingstone, Edinburgh

European Parliament and Council 2001 Directive 2001/83/EC on the Community code relating to medicinal products for human use. 6 November 2001. EC, Brussels

Gatford J D, Philips N 2006 Nursing calculations, 7th edn. Churchill Livingstone, Edinburgh

Hall C 2002 An evaluation of nurse preparation and practice in administering medicine to children. Unpublished PhD dissertation, School of Education, University of Nottingham, Nottingham

Health Act 2006 Part 3 Drugs, medicines and pharmacies. Chapter 1: Supervision of management and use of controlled drugs. Stationery Office, London. Available online: http://www.opsi.gov.uk/ACTS/acts2006/ukpga_20060028_en_1 (accessed 15 August 2008)

Joint Formulary Committee 2008 British national formulary, 55th edn. British Medical Association, Royal Pharmaceutical Society of Great Britain, London

Kee JL, Hayes ER 2005 Pharmacology: a nursing process approach, 2nd edn. Saunders, Philadelphia

Lapham RW, Agar H 2003 Drug calculations for nurses. Oxford University Press, Oxford

Latter S, Rycroft-Malone J, Yerrell P et al 2000 Evaluating education preparation for a health education in practice: the case of medication education. Journal of Advanced Nursing 32(5):1282–1290

Medicinal Products: Prescriptions by Nurses etc. Act 1992 HMSO, London

Medicines Act 1968 HMSO, London

Medicines and Health Care Regulatory Agency 2004 Cited by Nursing and Midwifery Council 2008b Standards for medicines management. Nursing and Midwifery Council, London

Medicines and Health Care Regulatory Agency 2008 Marketing authorisation. http://www.mhra.gov.uk/home/groups/pl-a/documents/publication/con1004417.pdf (accessed 3 May 2008)

Misuse of Drugs Act 1971 HMSO, London

Misuse of Drugs Regulations 1985 SI 1985/2066 HMSO, London

National Health Services (2005) (Pharmaceutical Services) (Amendment No 2) Regulations 2005 (SI 1501) HMSO, London

Nightingale F 1859 Notes on nursing: what it is and what it is not. Reprinted 1980. Churchill Livingstone, Edinburgh

Nursing and Midwifery Council 2006 Position statement on the covert administration of medicines. Nursing and Midwifery Council, London

Nursing and Midwifery Council 2008a The Code: standards of conduct, performance and ethics for nurses and midwives. Nursing and Midwifery Council, London

Nursing and Midwifery Council 2008b Standards for medicines management. Nursing and Midwifery Council, London

Paediatric Formularies Committee 2007 BNF for children ('BNFC'). British Medical Association, Royal Pharmaceutical Society of Great Britain, Royal College of Paediatrics and Child Health, Neonatal and Paediatric Pharmacists Group, London

Reitox 2006 United Kingdom drug situation: annual report to the European Monitoring Centre for Drugs and Drug Addiction (EMCDDA). EMCDDA, Lisbon

Royal S, Smeaton L, Avery AJ, Hurwitz B, Sheikh A 2006 Interventions in primary care to reduce medication related adverse events and hospital admissions: systematic review and meta-analysis. Quality and Safety in Health Care 15:23–31

Turner S, Longworth A, Nunn AJ, Choonara I 2002 Unlicensed and off label drug use in paediatric wards: prospective study. British Medical Journal 316(7128):343–345

Waller DG, Renwick AG, Hillier K 2005 Medical pharmacology and therapeutics, 2nd edn. Elsevier Saunders, Edinburgh

Wright A, Falconer J, Newman C 2002 Self-administration and re-use of medicines. Paediatric Nursing 14(6):14–17

Chapter 11

Pain

Karen L. Jackson

INTRODUCTION

Treating pain is a basic humanitarian concern (Park et al 2000). The desire to have one's pain eased has a long tradition (Loeser 2005). Pain therefore must be a key responsibility for the nurse as a member of a multidisciplinary team and up-to-date knowledge of pain is essential throughout your nursing career. Pain is a problem in its own right, but may be associated with other areas of care. For example it has been suggested that between 30% and 70% of all surgical patients experience considerable postoperative pain and also that assessment of pain and pain relief is inadequately completed by both physicians and nurses (Klopfenstein et al 2000).

Pain is also a symptom common to many illnesses and therefore nursing knowledge in this field is vital. It has been found that nurses often lack knowledge and awareness of the resources available for the effective management of pain. Such nurses are therefore unable to perform their role effectively. Successful pain management can be difficult, requiring approaches that need multiprofessional teamwork. Pain can have harmful effects on many aspects of the body's normal functioning and repair processes (Munafò & Trim 2000). Chronic changes within the nervous system can result from failure to control acute pain effectively; this can lead to neuropathic and chronic pain states (Woolf & Slater 2000). Chronic pain has many serious adverse effects and has been linked with suppressing immune function (McCaffery & Pasero 1999). This chapter will explore how pain might be experienced. Although most people can readily identify with the concept of physical pain, other areas such as the emotional, mental and psychological elements of pain are often overlooked.

This chapter is designed to further your knowledge and to encourage you to continue to explore this subject. The activities incorporated here are intended to act as a starting point for your development. It will help you explore the issues involved in the pain experience from a broad perspective. The approaches will encourage you to use other resources, including your personal and practical experience in various settings, library resources and interactions with your peers.

OVERVIEW

This chapter is divided into four parts, each with a specific focus in relation to pain.

Subject knowledge

This section considers the physiology of pain, pain transmission, physiological signs of pain, theories of pain, and psychosocial elements of pain.

Care delivery knowledge

This section considers the assessment of pain. Related symptoms relevant to pain assessment, the use of pain assessment tools, and the use of carers to aid assessment are also considered. Effective pain management, pharmacological interventions and modes of delivery, and non-pharmacological interventions are explored.

Professional and ethical knowledge

This section explores the nurse's role in effective pain care in a plural society. The nurse's specialist role and multidisciplinary team role in pain management are also examined. Ethical considerations around the delivery and management of pain are reviewed in the light of documents such as the Human Rights Act 1998, 2000 and the Children Act 1989/2004.

Personal and reflective knowledge

In this section you will bring together the issues covered by the previous three sections as well as your existing knowledge and experiences to explore the care of four individuals related to the specialist branches of nursing. It is also relevant to consider your personal gain in relation to your knowledge base and evidence of learning.

On pages 265–267 there are four case studies, each one relating to one of the branches of nursing. You may find it helpful to read one of them before you start the chapter and use it as a focus for your reflections while reading.

SUBJECT KNOWLEDGE

BIOLOGICAL

This section explores the physiology of pain. Theories of pain transmission are discussed and you are encouraged to apply these to your own experiences.

THE PHYSIOLOGY OF PAIN

It is necessary to consider several factors in relation to how pain is evoked and perceived. The relationships between the major components need to be understood and recognized. 'Pain is a physiological and sensory process that is influenced by each person's unique experience, culture and response' (Cranford 2001: 288). In 1970, Merskey offered a definition of pain as 'an unpleasant experience which we primarily associate with tissue damage or describe in terms of such damage or both.' This definition allows for the concept of pain to be evoked even if there is no direct indication of tissue damage, and seems to agree with the everyday definition of pain. The exact mechanism for the transmission of pain is unknown, but several theories have been put forward. It is a recent phenomenon that there is acceptance that pain occurs on many levels and is specific to each person's experience including genetics, current fears, past experience and their expectations of treatment (Jones 2001). It is important that you remember these are not facts but theories – a way that individuals can explore a concept.

Several theories of pain have evolved and guide the conceptualization of pain (Table 11.1).

Table 11.1 The evolution and major contributions of pain theories (adapted from Stevens & Johnston 1993)

Theory	Theorist	Major contribution
Specificity	Descartes (1664/1972)	Pain is a distinct sensation mediated by nerves designed for nociceptive processing with physiological specialization
Intensity	Erasmus Darwin (1794)	Pain is the result of intense stimulation of nerve fibres in any sensory organ
Pattern theories		Several conceptualizations of pain stimulus intensity and central summation are key concepts
(a) Central	Livingstone (1943)	Central mechanisms for summating peripheral summation pain impulses and pathological stimulation of sensory nerves initiates activity in reverberating circuits between central and peripheral processes

Table 11.1—cont'd

Theory	Theorist	Major contribution
(b) Sensory	Bishop (1946, 1959) Nordenbos (1959)	Rapidly conducting fibre systems excite, and inhibit, synaptic transmission in the slowly conducting system for pain. From this evolved the theories of myelinated and unmyelinated fibre systems, functions of nerve fibres, and the multisynaptic afferent system
Affect	Marshall (1894) Melzack & Wall (1965, 1973, 1982, 1988)	Emotional quality of pain distorts all sensory events. Global theory accounting for the sensory, affective and cognitive dimensions of pain – pain processing not rigid, but flexible

THE EVOLUTION OF PAIN THEORIES

Although pain theories enable some understanding of pain, an examination of how pain messages may be transmitted is necessary to develop further conceptualization.

Pain transmission

Pain fibres or nociceptors (noxious sensation receptors) are specialized neurones located throughout the body, particularly in the skin (Fig. 11.1). These specialized nerve endings recognize tissue damage. Pain results when the impulses from these nerves reach consciousness. The nerve endings can be stimulated by chemical, mechanical or thermal inputs. When the peripheral nerve fibres carrying impulses generated by the painful stimuli enter the spinal cord, they enter the dorsal horn of the spinal grey matter, passing through the dorsal root of the spinal nerve. When a nerve fibre ends it is involved in a synapse where the nerve message is chemically transmitted to the next nerve cell and its fibre. Many different chemicals are involved in transmission at different synapses and no one transmitter substance is confined to a single functional system. The primary actions and functions of some of these neurotransmitters are listed in Table 11.2. A useful introduction to pain perception/transmission can be found in Wood (2002).

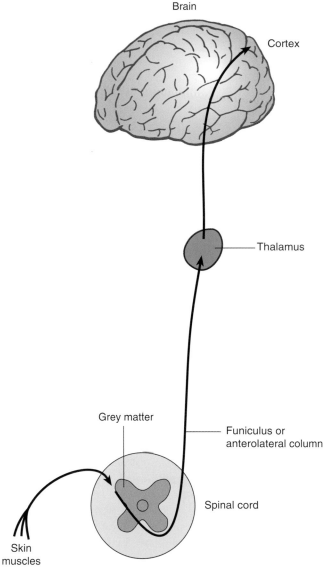

Figure 11.1 The central nervous system, structures and pathways.

Reflection and portfolio evidence

- Try to describe in your own words how you as an individual are able to perceive pain.
- Given this description, reflect upon factors that would affect your perception of pain. It may be helpful here to compare the differing perceptions of pain when 'banging your thumb' or having a headache or having a toothache.
- Use this exercise to write a short summary for your portfolio, demonstrating your understanding of your own pain experience.

Table 11.2 Functional relationships of neurotransmitters

Neurotransmitter	Action
Substance P	Is thought to be the neurotransmitter substance released that results in increasing pain perception
Enkephalins	Produce analgesia, euphoria and nausea
5-Hydroxytryptamine	Enhances pain transmission at local level, but inhibits pain when acting on central nervous system structures such as the dorsal horn
Beta endorphins	Probably responsible for dulling pain perception from injuries

Gate theory

One of the most widely accepted theories of pain, first suggested in 1965, is the gate theory, which proposed that pain is determined by interactions between three spinal cord systems (Melzack & Wall 1996). Simply it suggests that the 'transmission of pain from the periferal nerve through the spinal cord was subject to modulation by both intrinsic neurones and controls emanating from the brain' (Dickenson 2002: 755). It proposes that pain impulses arrive at a gate, thought to be the substantia gelatinosa (one of the most dense neuronal areas of the central nervous system). When open the impulses easily pass through; if partially open only some pain impulses can pass through; and if closed none can pass through. It further suggests that the gate position depends on the degree of small or large fibre firing. Accordingly, when large fibre firing predominates (non-noxious sensations), the gate closes, and when small fibre firing predominates (pain fibres) the pain message is transmitted (Fig. 11.2). For more detailed information see Wood (2002). It is now evident that the actuality is more complex than this explanation. Dubner in 1997 found that the nervous system has the ability to change its sensitivity following tissue

injury or nerve injury, termed plasticity. Gate theory also did not take into account the long-term changes that occur due to noxious stimuli or other external factors and also that there is not a single pain centre (Jones 2001).

Reflection and portfolio evidence

- Consider in everyday life an experience where it may be possible to close the gate on pain (e.g. what might be your immediate reaction on 'banging your thumb'?).
- Now consider where and when these mechanisms may be used in the practice of pain control in health care.
- Write a summary for inclusion in your portfolio.

PHYSIOLOGICAL SIGNS OF PAIN

In sudden acute pain certain physiological signs of pain may exist (Table 11.3); these are linked to the fight or flight mechanism of the adrenaline (epinephrine) and noradrenaline (norepinephrine) functions as an initial response to the experience of pain. However, over time the body seeks equilibrium physiologically as these responses cannot be maintained without causing physical harm. The major problem with physiological indicators of pain is that they may be due to other factors such as stress. Therefore although they may be indicators of acute and sudden pain, they are of little use as indicators of chronic pain. In chronic pain, lack of such signs may prompt the practitioner to inaccurately conclude that the patient does not look as if they are in pain (American Pain Society 1999) therefore they cannot be in pain.

Physiological manifestation of acute pain and adaptation

There are differences between acute and chronic pain and these impact upon the individual experiencing pain, since the physiological responses, psychological and social consequences differ. Acute pain is associated with a well-defined cause. There is an expectation that it is timebound and will disappear when healing has occurred. Chronic

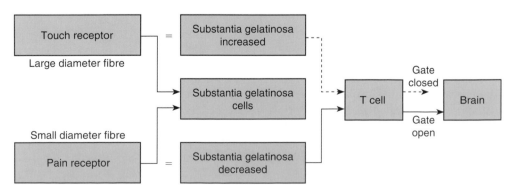

Figure 11.2 Gate theory of pain (adapted from Melzack & Wall 1965).

Table 11.3 Physiological manifestations of acute pain and adaptations

Physiological response to acute pain	Adaptation over time (chronic pain)
Increased blood pressure	Normal blood pressure
Increased pulse rate	Normal pulse rate
Increased respiration rate	Normal respiration rate
Dilated pupils	Normal pupil size
Perspiration	Dry skin

pain continues long after an injury has healed. It is a situation for the person experiencing it rather than an event (Munafò & Trim 2000).

Chronic pain can be further subdivided as either malignant or non-malignant. Chronic non-malignant pain is persistent and has no end point. It has far-reaching effects and may cause problems with partners, family, friends and employers. Loeser (2005) argued that chronic pain should be considered a disease in its own right. Treatment philosophies centre around helping patients to take responsibility for their pain and helping them to cope with it using a variety of strategies, such as in the care of a person with arthritis. Such strategies might include psychological interventions that focus on the behavioural, cognitive and emotional aspects of the illness, for example dealing with anxiety and depression, educating them about their condition and increasing the individual's control by teaching coping skills. In contrast, chronic malignant pain may have an end point; treatment approaches include sufficient analgesia to relieve pain and techniques such as relaxation. Such differences in definition reflect the multidimensional nature of the pain.

The International Association for the Study of Pain (IASP) has defined neuropathic pain as 'pain initiated or caused by a primary lesion or dysfunction of the nervous system' (Merskey & Bogduk 1994). However, this definition has more recently been criticized as being too vague. Because of the incidence of both malignant and non malignant diseases in an aging population and greater survival rates from cancer and its treatment, there is likely to be an increase in the occurrence of neuropathic pain (Dworkin 2002).

PSYCHOSOCIAL

PSYCHOSOCIAL ELEMENTS OF PAIN

In this section, definitions and ideologies are explored along with misconceptions of the experience of pain for the individual.

Pain is a difficult concept to understand. The assumption that there is a simple and direct relationship between a noxious stimulus and subsequent pain has been disputed by the realization that many environmental and internal factors modify pain perception (Main & Spanswick 2000). As has been previously stated, nociception is not pain until it is interpreted and perceived as pain. This pain perception is influenced by a range of factors. There are numerous causes of pain and these are not only physical. Also the terms 'pain threshold' and 'pain tolerance' (the greatest intensity of pain an individual can endure) are sometimes used synonymously. This leads to confusion since there are differences between them. There is also thought to be a link between a person's pain threshold and their risk of developing chronic pain and this may be because they have a mixture of genetic mutations that increase their sensitivity to pain (Couzin 2006).

This is further complicated by factors such as emotion, culture and previous experience, the end result being a unique experience for that individual. It is important then, that the nurse working with a person experiencing pain is able to accept that pain is both physical and psychological. Thus pain is both biologically and phenomenologically embodied. Moreover culture intercedes in the pain experience and therefore transcends the mind–body divide.

Some of the recognized behavioural responses to both acute and chronic pain are listed in Table 11.4. These may be used as cues by nurses in their quest to determine the pain experience of the patient.

Reflection and portfolio evidence

- In your own words try to define the term pain.
- Looking at this definition, explore how you view pain and from this try to consider on what your views are based. For example, you may have had a particularly painful experience that influences your views of pain or you may never have experienced pain.
- Consider whether these views affect your beliefs about other people in pain. If they do, in what way?
- Reflect on how your personal beliefs could affect your decision making when a patient or client requests pain relief.

BEHAVIOURAL RESPONSES TO ACUTE PAIN AND ADAPTATION

Pain has been defined as whatever the person experiencing it says it is, existing whenever the person says it does (McCaffery 1972). This definition allows for the complexity

Table 11.4 Behavioural responses to acute pain and adaptations

Behavioural response	Adaptation over time
Observable signs of discomfort	Decrease in observable signs, though pain intensity unchanged
Focuses on pain	Turns attention to things other than pain
Reports pain	No report of pain unless questioned
Cries and moans	Quiet; sleeps or rests
Rubs painful part	Physical inactivity or immobility
Frowns and grimaces	Blank or normal facial expression
Increased muscle tension	

Evidence-based practice

In 2004, Van Hulle Vincent & Denyes investigated nursing knowledge and attitudes relating to relieving children's pain. They found that the nurses in the study (n=67) had a moderately high ability to manage children's pain. The more experienced paediatric nurses reported greater capacity to overcome barriers to the best possible pain relief. There was a positive correlation between pain score and analgesic given which suggests that nurses respond differently to higher pain scores.

of pain, but in some ways limits its understanding. The literature indicates that the definition of pain depends upon the one person defining it. Wall's (1977) definition 'Pain is' allows freedom for the practitioner to consider the individual phenomenon but could also be considered problematic due to individual attitudes and beliefs about pain. Knowledge of individual behaviours and changes that occur with discomfort are useful in distinguishing pain from other causes (Herr et al 2006); carers therefore become valuable allies in discovering the usual behaviours of the individual.

Pain causes powerful emotions in its sufferers: fear, anxiety, anger and depression are frequently cited. These emotions have a great impact on the individual's understanding and control of the pain. Pain in any individual has to be judged by indirect evidence, and the appearance, non-verbal behaviour, physiological status and circumstance of the pain need to be interpreted (Fordham & Dunn 1994, Herr et al 2006). Many misconceptions can be problematic in the interpretation of pain. The amount of tissue damage is not an exact prediction of the intensity of pain. It is easy to suppose that individuals receiving the same surgery will experience the same pain. The evidence is that the pain experience is individual and varies from both person to person and situation to situation. An individual's reaction to pain is determined by past experiences, disposition, the cause of pain, their state of health and socialization, as well as factors such as the time of day and what else is going on around the person (Carr & Mann 2000).

In relation to behavioural responses to pain it is essential that vulnerable individuals, for whom behaviour may be a major characteristic, are considered. Vulnerable individuals would include young children and infants and people with impaired vocal or cognitive ability. A change in behaviour needs thorough evaluation of the likelihood of other sources of pain (Herr et al 2006).

Children may not have past experience of pain, but they learn quickly. Therefore an expression of distress in relation to tissue damage is of extreme importance to the infant's survival. Pain would logically become one of the first emotions to emerge. It has been found that tolerance to pain increases with age, so the child is more likely to have an intense pain experience. In relation to the neural system of infants, it is now believed that the process of myelination occurs before birth and by birth myelination of the sensory roots has begun. Therefore the ability to experience and perceive pain has been established.

Many factors influence the way pain is perceived by the individual. Past experience of pain, the personality of the individual experiencing the pain, anxiety related to the pain experience and cultural influences all affect the pain sensation. Often there are obstacles in pain assessment because of faulty perceptions that cause nurses to doubt others who indicate they have pain (Cranford 2001). We need to be aware of this and by this awareness prevent ourselves from acting on these misconceptions.

Any past experience of pain or pain relief can affect the intensity of the pain (Carr & Mann 2000, Main & Spanswick 2000). Pain can be influenced by the meaning it has to the individual. For example, the headache that you previously have dismissed as nothing may with a limited knowledge of medical theory be interpreted as being due to a brain tumour. This associated meaning will influence the way you perceive the pain. Anxiety, fear and depression can all increase pain sensation.

Evidence-based practice

Watt-Watson et al (2001) found in their study of 94 nurses that they had deficits in knowledge and misbeliefs about pain management; also that their knowledge scores were not significantly related to their patients' pain ratings. Patients reported moderate to severe pain but received only 47% of their prescribed analgesia.

PSYCHIATRIC/MENTAL PAIN

This complex issue has undergone considerable deliberation by many writers in recent years. The terms 'hysterical pain' and 'operant pain' have been used to describe the experience of patients who appear to be experiencing pain for psychological rather than physical reasons. It is important to consider that the patient's expression of pain is as real to them, as it is to those who have pain due to an accepted cause such as surgery or fractured bones. Wall & Melzack (1999) write that they 'have reservations of the use of this term in relation to its application to the theory of pain and psychological illness . . . Since those grouped under it include people whose pain is related to anxiety, depression and many psychiatric conditions' (Wall & Melzack 1999: 931). They further state that it is important to distinguish these phenomena in order to apply appropriate treatment, whether antidepressants, psychotherapy or rehabilitative measures.

CULTURAL AND SPIRITUAL INFLUENCES ON PAIN

The cultures within the profession of nursing or the institution of a hospital affect the way that pain is assessed, the way that decisions are made about the possible treatments, and the way that pain is managed.

Ethnicity in pain management is of particular significance in a multicultural country such as the UK. Each individual has intrinsic associations with culture: it socializes us to know what is expected of us and of others. Culture shapes beliefs and constrains behaviours. In such an environment the nurse must constantly be aware of professional issues in providing culturally appropriate care, and also of constraints on other practitioners due to their cultural beliefs and values. The process of the nurse–patient interaction occurs within the context of the demands and culture of the workplace (Walker et al 1995).

There are theological overtones in the pain experience as pain plays a central part in religious thought. The Christian concept is of pain as a paradox: Christ healed others in pain, but allowed himself to be crucified and endured agonizing pain. Pain is viewed as a challenge to be overcome. Buddha has been cited as a warrior, a saint and a victim. Examples of pain control can be found in many cultures, for example the Indian fakir who controls pain while lying on a bed of nails and the African tribes that practise lip or cheek piercing as ritualistic ceremonies do not appear to experience pain. Where stoicism is a cultural value, the behavioural expression of distress is generally less acceptable. Older people may view pain as a preliminary to death. Each culture has its own set of beliefs and attitudes with respect to the way people react to pain.

Care must be taken not to stereotype people, remembering that there is variability within cultures as well as between cultures. These misleading effects of cultural stereotypes, and the belief by nurses and doctors that they are the experts regarding the patient's pain, lead to problems in assessing the patient's pain. The under-treatment of pain, particularly among patients from racial and ethnic minorities, continues to be a problem in pain management (Green et al 2003, Burgess et al 2006). Also the ethnicity of both the individual in pain and those attempting to assess the pain clouds the perceptions of health professionals (Walker et al 1995, Burgess et al 2006). Professionals should consider the fact that the more difference there is between the patient and themselves the more difficult it is for them to assess and treat the patient.

Helman (2001) suggests that:

- Not all cultural or social groups respond to pain in the same way.
- Cultural background can influence how people perceive and respond to pain, both in themselves and others.
- Cultural factors can influence how and whether people reveal their pain to health professionals and others.

Gender is also an issue in the pain experience. Many of the debates around gender differences have focused on biological mechanisms, including genetic, hormonal and cardiovascular factors (Keogh & Herdenfeldt, 2002). Work by Kamp (2001) found that the men reported less severe pain than the women. Also that men's and women's pain experiences could relate to differences in their biology: the expectations and actions of healthcare professionals and society that treats the genders differently. Berkley (1998) found that females have lower thresholds of pain, greater abilities to discriminate pain, and higher pain ratings or less tolerance of noxious stimuli than males.

CARE DELIVERY KNOWLEDGE

In order to make the most of decision-making skills in practice, the nurse must access appropriate knowledge to support and rationalize these actions. This section applies knowledge about the areas of pain assessment and relief of pain to the practice of nursing. You are encouraged to examine and apply this knowledge to exercises that will help you develop decision-making skills.

Nurses are the gatekeepers of medication usage and as such have a responsibility to increase their knowledge in pharmacological as well as non-pharmacological techniques for pain management. Nurses can be instrumental in pain management in all settings. The prescribing of analgesia by physicians on an 'as required' basis leaves the responsibility for the decision to give analgesia firmly with the nurse (Carr & Mann 2000). The recent changes in prescribing practices that allow nurses with appropriate education and training to prescribe some medications for their patients as nurse independent prescribers (NIPs) should have made a difference to this element of pain care where nurses can respond more proactively to the needs of their patients. See Evolve 11.1 presentation of NIPs.

11.1 – NURSE INDEPENDENT PRESCRIBING IN PAIN MANAGEMENT

- Gain deeper appreciation of contemporary evidence surrounding pain assessment in children.
- Explore common misconceptions and beliefs around pain in children.
- Identify the role of parents and carers in assessing pain in children.

The routine and traditional practices of many care institutions can pose difficulties in the assessment of pain. The use of 'drug rounds' may cause patients to comply, accepting analgesia at this time and feeling unable to ask for it at a more appropriate time for them. Skilful assessment techniques will limit this problem, identifying both the individual nature of the pain and its recurrence at more frequent intervals than the 'drug round' timing. An awareness of pain should therefore be a routine matter in caring for patients. Because of its subjective nature, the individual in pain is the only one who can assess the pain accurately (Cranford 2001).

Reflection and portfolio evidence

Rituals in nursing practice can become entrenched, and in many healthcare institutions drugs are still administered via a 'drug round'.

- During your practice placements compare the experiences of patients on the unit or ward that links pain relief to drug rounds and those where self-administration of drugs is the norm.
- To what extent do drug round practices need to be modified to suit individual needs for pain relief?
- How might ritualistic practices affect your decision making in relation to pain management?

ASSESSMENT OF PAIN

Pain expression

Assessment is a process by which a conclusion is reached about the nature of a problem. Planning effective pain management is a crucial part of the nurse's role. In order to achieve this it is necessary to assess the level of the individual's discomfort in an attempt to identify a potential course of action. No single assessment strategy – e.g. interpretation of behaviours or estimates of pain by others – is sufficient by itself (Herr et al 2006). However, each element can be used in an endeavour to find a complete picture of the individual's pain experience. The nurse needs to be able to draw conclusions about the individual's pain to assess the level and intensity of the pain based on information from the patient. Once this has been achieved it is then possible to plan a course of action to alleviate the pain, implement this and evaluate the action. Although this is possible without the patient's cooperation, it is better to involve the individual in the assessment of their pain. Otherwise nurses are simply applying their own beliefs and values to the situation and making assumptions about patients' pain levels. Researchers suggest that the patient needs not only to be asked about their pain but also for their responses to be believed (Dahlman et al 1999). The nurse must be proactive and skilled in recognizing potentially painful situations, particularly in those instances where the patient may not be able to communicate verbally. To achieve this we need to ascertain whether pain assessment is an appropriate action, believe that the person has pain, and be committed to assessing the pain. This should lead to a clarification of the extent of pain and its treatment. In some circumstances this assessment will need to be not only accurate but also swift, for example when dealing with a patient suffering the pain of a myocardial infarction (heart attack), where the need for immediate and effective pain relief is a priority.

Although the nurse's role in this area is paramount, the only individual who is truly able to assess the pain is the person who is suffering it. The patient's spoken report of pain is the most reliable indication of pain (Cranford 2001). Wherever possible the patient should be assessing their pain rather than having it assessed by the nursing staff. In circumstances where the patient is unconscious, has a communication difficulty or is a baby, the nurse must make an informed decision based on the evidence presented by the patient, given that the family and other carers can be asked for further clarification.

Evidence-based practice

Kim et al (2005) found that when assessing postoperative pain the nurses in their study relied on criteria related to the patient's appearance and their past experience of the physical signs of pain rather than the report from the patient of their pain.

The accurate assessment of an individual's pain is an inherently difficult process. The nurse must be able to establish a trusting relationship with the patient and his or her family or carers. The nurse must also be aware of their own beliefs and prejudices about pain. Timing of pain

---

Box 11.1 Aspects of pain assessment

Pain	Nature, intensity and site
	Likely cause
	Precipitating factors and circumstances (e.g. time of day, movement, eating)
Examples of non-verbal pain behaviours	Facial expression
	Change in mood
	Crying, screaming, wailing, weeping
	Lack of appetite
	Nausea, vomiting
	Pale or flushed skin colour
	Reluctance to move
	Increased activity
	Unusual behaviour
	Unusual posture
	Holding, pressing on the part that hurts
Related symptoms	Nausea, anxiety, breathlessness
Resources	Patient's coping strategies
	Nursing knowledge and skills in using and teaching non-pharmacological methods of pain relief
	Medical and pharmacological knowledge and skills in both pharmacological and non-pharmacological methods of pain relief
	Availability of resources such as time, equipment, privacy and so on
Meaning and significance to patient	Purpose and consequences

assessment is very important and dependent upon many factors, not least of which is the desire of the patient to participate in the assessment, the severity of the pain and the potential pain treatment. Such assessment involves the skills of observation so that the non-verbal pain behaviours can be seen and recognized (Box 11.1). It must be remembered that these behaviours are influenced by the individual's social and cultural norms. Your interpretation will also be influenced by these factors. Therefore it is not possible to make assumptions based on the absence of a recognized non-verbal pain behaviour since each pain experience for the individual is unique.

The nurse may conclude that someone is in pain if they:

- state that this is the case
- demonstrate behaviour indicative of pain
- have undergone some experience that would be considered painful and they are unable to verbally report pain.

Decision-making exercise

Mrs Singh is an elderly widow living in a maisonette. Her family live close by and have regular contact with her. She is receiving treatment for glaucoma and the community nurse has been asked by her general practitioner to assess her needs as her family are unable to instil her eye drops at lunchtime. She speaks very little English and has limited mobility. When the nurse arrives Mrs Singh is accompanied by her niece who says she has just arrived and is worried about her aunt who does not appear to be herself today. On meeting Mrs Singh she is sitting hunched in a chair and is moaning and rocking back and forth slightly.

- Consider the appropriate nursing actions in this instance.
- Using the list of aspects related to pain assessment in Box 11.1, decide what factors you would take into account in Mrs Singh's case.
- Using a friend, role-playing Mrs Singh's niece, complete an assessment of her pain.
- What more do you need to know that might help you in effective decision making about Mrs Singh's care?

Related symptoms

An initial assessment should include some information about the history of the pain as follows:

1. Information about the initial onset of the pain. This includes a comparison of the medical history with the patient's own version and allows similarities and discrepancies to be addressed. This may be linked to surgery, illness, trauma or an unknown cause. The patient may believe that something totally unrelated to the identified clinical cause of the pain is responsible.
2. Position of the pain. A body outline may be used for this purpose and then used as a baseline to chart any improvement or deterioration in the pain.
3. A description of the pain. The patient should be encouraged to use his or her own words for this exercise. Children have a limited vocabulary and may well use words that an adult would not normally use, such as 'owie', 'squidgy' or a 'headache in my tummy'.
4. Elements affecting the pain. These can include position, eating, activity and time of day.
5. Previous treatment. The success or otherwise of past treatments helps the nurse plan effectively in this pain experience.
6. Any other medical history.

Psychological aspects

The possibility of stress, changes in lifestyle, depression or behavioural disorders in the individual and their relevance to the pain experience need to be considered, and specialist referral may be necessary (see also Ch. 9 covering stress and relaxation).

Social aspects

Information about the family, housing, employment and other interests are relevant in a pain assessment as often these positively or negatively influence a pain problem.

Observation

The most natural reactions are seen when observation is informal and carried out when the patient is unaware of being observed. Formal observation usually involves the use of some form of documentation or pain chart.

> **Decision-making exercise**
>
> Mrs Singh, whom you met in the earlier exercise, has now been assessed. There is nothing physically wrong with her. It transpires that she has received bad news from her family in India and a very dear nephew has been killed in a road traffic accident.
>
> - Reflect on whether this information would make a difference to your initial thoughts about your nursing actions.
> - Would the use of any of the pain assessment tools discussed below have been helpful in this case?
> - From information already covered in the section on Subject Knowledge, what might be the most important part of a pain management strategy for Mrs Singh?
> - How might you use this experience in caring for patients in practice?
> - Jot down your ideas for inclusion in your portfolio.

Use of pain assessment tools

There are many tools to aid in assessing the patient's pain, from simple to complex. For example the visual analogue scale asks the patient to rate the pain along a line between no pain and the worst pain imaginable (Fig. 11.3) giving an intensity rating. A verbal descriptor can also be used, in which case the patient picks the description that most closely relates to the pain they are experiencing (Fig. 11.4).

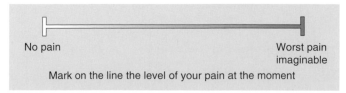

Figure 11.3 A visual analogue scale.

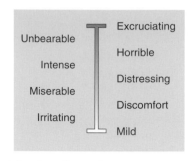

Figure 11.4 An intensity rating scale.

For clients in the community the use of a personal pain diary has been recommended. The patient records the pain, describes it and includes comments about how it has changed, if at all, how it affects their daily lifestyle and any effective pain relief. Writing down this information allows the opportunity to organize potential triggers and patterns of pain that emerge (Chaitow 2002). The patient needs to get into a routine of recording in this diary, since it is likely that more accurate information is achieved with the recent experience of pain. The patient therefore records the information as it occurs, if possible, within their normal lifestyle. Questions might include:

- Is the pain constant or intermittent?
- After what activities does it hurt?
- What sort of pain is it?
- Is there swelling, redness or heat in the area of pain?
- Is the pain affected by emotion?
- If you are female, is the pain made better or worse by aspects of your menstrual cycle?

The method of pain measurement should be bias-free and there must be a particular focus on practicality and versatility (Twycross et al 1998, Main & Spanswick 2000). However, although these are desirable aims they may be difficult to achieve. An array of pain assessment tools have been developed for adults, but most rely on communication and cognitive abilities not mastered by young children (Twycross et al 1998). Their use is also restricted for people with some learning disabilities or those who are unable to communicate verbally. These people continue to be especially vulnerable to poor pain management (Carter et al 2002). Herr et al (2006) have produced useful guidelines for clinical practice in assessing pain in the non verbal individual. Parents have been found to be the best proxy measure of pain assessment for children with cognitive impairment because of their in depth knowledge of the child's behaviours (Stallard et al 2002). Specific tools to assess the pain of young children and infants are available, e.g. the Liverpool infant distress score (LIDS) (Horgan et al 1996) and face, legs, activity, cry, consolability (FLACC) score (Merkel et al 1997). However nurses need to understand how such tools can be used.

11.2 – PAIN IN CHILDREN

- Gain deeper appreciation of contemporary evidence surrounding pain assessment in children.
- Explore common misconceptions and beliefs around pain in children.
- Identify the role of parents and carers in assessing pain in children.

Reflection and portfolio evidence

Pain assessment tools in the practice situation vary in use according to the client group and the evidence about their reliability and validity.

- Find out what pain assessment tools are available for use and review how they are used.
- Have any of these tools been tested as valid and reliable? You may have to look at the research literature to find this out.
- Using these practice experiences and the case studies at the end of this chapter decide which pain assessment tool is appropriate for each patient. Try to justify your choice.

PLANNING EFFECTIVE PAIN MANAGEMENT

Management of pain should be diverse enough to take account of the various dimensions of the pain experience; however, it has been found that nurses contribute to inadequate pain management (Richards & Hubbert 2007). Nurses are responsible for the administration of drugs to patients. They are also responsible for educating patients and their families or carers, as appropriate, in the management of their prescribed medications (see Ch. 10, 'Medicines'). A client–provider relationship that promotes open communication and is free of age related expectations is essential in meeting the complex issues of pain management (Davis et al 2002). The nurse can be instrumental in ensuring a more personalized approach to the individual's pain management, but to achieve this the nurse needs a sound knowledge of the various methods of managing pain.

Decision-making exercise

Mr Phil O'Reilly has been admitted suffering from chest pain. This is thought to be due to a severe angina attack. He is grey, sweating profusely and is complaining of chest and left arm pain. He is obviously frightened and has asked you to contact a priest as he is convinced that he is about to die. His partner has been contacted and is on the way to the hospital from work. Accurate and quick assessment is required in this case of acute pain.

- What areas of pain assessment would take priority in this case?
- Consider the additional information you would require from Mr O'Reilly's partner to enable you to liaise effectively between the patient and the doctor managing Mr O'Reilly's pain.
- Once adequate pain relief has been achieved what health promotion strategy would be necessary from the nurse to help Mr O'Reilly prevent or reduce the frequency of recurrence of the chest pain in the future?

Pharmacological interventions

The correct use of medication is essential for effective pain management, but has been shown to be an area where nurses often fail to excel. Most commonly problems occur due to inaccurate assessment of pain as the presenting problem and a lack of insight into which drugs to use in the treatment of different types of pain (Young et al 2006). Nurses who have successfully completed a nurse independent prescribing (NIP) course are able to prescribe any licensed medicine including some controlled drugs for any medical condition within their clinical competence.

Nurses need knowledge of the methods of administration of analgesia and how these drugs are applicable to the patient's pain experience. For example in relation to children, many report the pain of injections as the worst pain therefore the use of such routes should be minimized. Some medicines have been found to be more effective for certain types of pain. The nurse interacts with both the patient and the doctor and is therefore in an ideal position to influence appropriate prescribing. This will result in an individualized and consequently more effective regimen to aid the patient's pain management. A sound knowledge base and experience will enhance the recognition of the implications of the information yielded by the assessment (Duff et al 2001, Royal College of Nursing 2001, Twycross 2002, Dihle et al 2006). Also the patient should understand the medicines they are taking and the reasons they are taking them, particularly in cases of chronic pain management where the patient may have available to them a variety of analgesic agents.

Types of analgesia

There are three categories of analgesics: opioid drugs, non-opioid drugs and co-analgesic drugs, and their usage is generally based upon their method of action.

1. Opioid drugs (e.g. morphine, pethidine, codeine) mainly work in the brain and spinal cord to inhibit the transmission of pain. They are generally used to relieve severe pain and associated effects include a sense of well-being in the individual. They are therefore linked with a tendency to produce mental and physical dependence. They are subject to the Misuse of Drugs Act 1971.
2. Non-opioid drugs (e.g. aspirin, paracetamol, ibuprofen, indometacin) mainly work in the peripheral tissues by interfering with chemicals that stimulate pain endings. Useful in the relief of musculoskeletal pain and mild to moderate pain.
3. Co-analgesic drugs have a variety of actions, for example muscle relaxant or sedative (diazepam), antidepressant (amitriptyline), anticonvulsants (gabapentin), or suppressor of inflammatory reactions (corticosteroids).

A range of issues are relevant in considering appropriate analgesic therapy. While drugs can be used alone or in combination to produce pain relief, a multimodal approach is most effective as can be seen by the previous indicators. The intensity of pain should influence the type of analgesic prescribed. The effective dose varies for each individual and therefore the effect of the drug given should be carefully monitored. There is a ceiling with non-opioid drugs so that beyond a certain dose there will be no increased analgesic effect, but with opioid drugs the limitations of dosage appear to be the associated side-effects. Repeated administration of narcotic (opioid) drugs have been shown to cause tolerance and dependence. This is no deterrent, however, in the control of pain in terminal disease. Recommended practice is to adjust both the dose and the frequency of administration so that the patient never suffers pain.

Ideally, an optimum level of pain control is achieved by using analgesic agents. However, this may take time, and because of the uniqueness of the individual pain experience, pain relief should be constantly evaluated and updated. The duration of action of the analgesic is an important issue since the ideal is to maintain an acceptable level of pain relief for the patient. The nurse therefore needs an awareness of both the effectiveness of the drug and its duration. In this way the nurse will be able to limit the delay between the time when the patient needs pain relief and the time when the administered drug becomes effective. Analgesic ladders are frequently used in practice situations to achieve this aim (Fig. 11.5). Many nurses have been shown to have erroneous ideas that lead to obstacles in pain management; these include fear of opioid dependence, anxiety about tolerance to effects of these medications and concern about depression of respiratory effort (Cranford 2001).

Many routes are available for the administration of medicines (see also Ch. 10) and it is helpful to explore some of these routes in relation to the administration of analgesics. Opioid and non-opioid analgesics can be given by various routes.

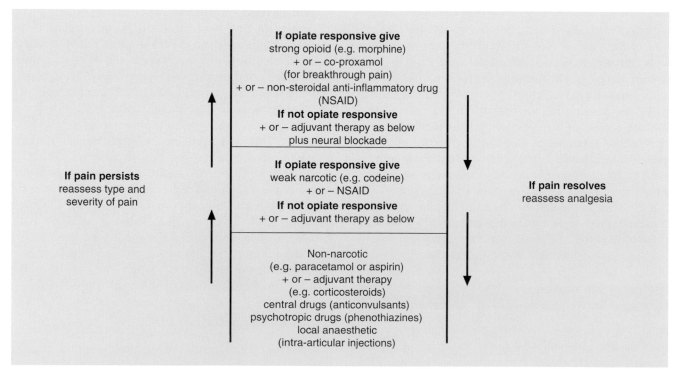

Figure 11.5 An analgesic ladder.

Infusion pumps are often used for the administration of analgesics and can be:

- intravenous (commonly used for acute postoperative pain)
- subcutaneous (commonly used for palliative care)
- epidural, that is, a nerve block (commonly used for labour pain).

Pumps can also be operated by the patient to provide patient controlled analgesia (PCA). The analgesic is prescribed as for the infusion pump and the nurse sets up the system as required. The patient is then able to take control of their pain in a positive way. There is usually a button control and when the patient depresses the button he or she receives a bolus dose of the analgesic to limit the pain. Each PCA pump has a 'lock out' time between doses so that the patient cannot overdose. There are also security features such as a key to lock the pump to limit the risk of interference once the prescribed rate has been set.

Whatever the mode of delivery a careful explanation is required for the patient and their family or carers as appropriate so that they can take an active part in the pain control.

Decision-making exercise

Using the example of Mr Phil O'Reilly from the earlier exercise, who was admitted with acute chest pain caused by angina:

- Explore the potential analgesia that may be used to help relieve his acute pain.
- Decide on an appropriate method of delivery for this choice and justify your decision.

Non-pharmacological interventions

There are many strategies that do not involve drugs that can be used to help relieve pain. Techniques that are commonly used include distraction, cutaneous stimulation, relaxation, deep breathing and meditation. Many people use such techniques informally, being told to take deep breaths when one is feeling nauseous for example. These non-pharmacological interventions can be used successfully with most client groups. For the infant, distraction can include holding and cuddling or using a dummy or comforter. Older children may be encouraged to count or talk about other more pleasant experiences to help distract them. Play therapy can also be useful in taking the child's mind away from the pain. Cutaneous stimulation includes gentle massage or rubbing of the skin, which may be used for all age groups. Relaxation techniques can be used effectively with older children who have the cognitive skills to understand instructions as well as with

adults and is a beneficial method in pain management (Main & Spanswick 2000). Deep breathing and counting can be used to take the focus off the pain and can result in a lessening of the pain experience. Meditation is one of the most effective means of counteracting the stress associated with pain and anxiety by producing a relaxation response (Chaitow 2002).

Visual stimuli have also been shown to be successful in increasing pain thresholds and pain tolerance. In 2002, Tse et al found that the use of visual stimuli could be a successful adjunct to pain relief. In their experiment they used a soundless video display of natural scenery, such as a mountainous area, river flow and a waterfall, which significantly increased both pain thresholds and pain tolerance in their subjects. In their conclusions they suggest that to help relieve anxiety and pain, the provision of windows with views for patients might be very useful within the hospital complex (Tse et al 2002).

Many forms of non pharmacological approaches are currently used as adjuncts in pain care management, some of which are explored here. However, as in the use of any therapy it is essential that the nurse remains cognizant of their professional role in practice and the boundaries within which they operate.

Complementary therapies

Complementary therapies are holistic natural therapies that may be used in conjunction with conventional medical or nursing treatments to enhance the physical and psychological well-being of the patient. The use of such therapy demands the practitioner to be autonomous in their practices. The practitioner in this instance need not necessarily be a nurse. The nurse in this situation will be answerable for the choices made in the treatment delivered and will be accountable under the Code of Professional Conduct (Nursing and Midwifery Council 2008a) for such actions. The therapies require a hands-on approach by the practitioner and the therapies need time as well as privacy in which the practitioner and patient can communicate. These approaches need careful handling, since some nurses may believe that they can learn all there is to learn about a complementary therapy in a half day's study. They may then go on to put the patient at risk because of a lack of competence.

11.3 – COMPLEMENTARY THERAPIES

- Gain an overview of types of therapy which may be used.
- Consider how therapies might be used.
- Identify some cautions in the use of these therapies.

Using the case study for Jordan Simpson, a 14-year-old boy admitted in acute pain due to a sickle cell crisis (see p. 266):

● Consider the non-pharmacological methods of pain relief that you might use to help Jordan deal with his pain.
● As Jordan's condition is long term, examine how these strategies can be developed to help him cope with future pain experiences.
● Explore how you would involve him in identifying the strategies that may help him cope with future pain experiences, and why certain non-pharmacological approaches may be more suitable for Jordan than others.

The Nursing and Midwifery Council's (2008b) advice about complementary and alternative therapies identifies that nurses must ensure that the introduction of these therapies is always in the best interests and safety of the patient. Further, they suggest a team approach where it should be part of professional teamwork to discuss the use of complementary therapies with medical and other members of the healthcare team. Furthermore, practitioners are reminded that we can be called to account for any activities carried out outside conventional practice.

These interventions can be grouped into categories (National Centre for Complementary and Alternative Medicine 2007).

● Alternative medical systems – such as homeopathic medicine.
● Mind–body interventions – such as cognitive behavioural therapy, relaxation or guided imagery.
● Biologically based therapies – substances found in nature such as herbs, or vitamins.
● Manipulative methods – such as chiropractic or massage therapies.
● Energy therapies – such as therapeutic touch or Reiki.

Evidence-based practice

Lin et al (2005) found that there is a high incidence of complementary and alternative medical therapies in paediatric pain management services in North America and advocated that further research into the safety and efficacy of such therapies is needed.

Wirth et al (2005) performed a literature search to investigate the efficacy of herbal treatments in pain care management. They found limited scientific evidence to support the use of herbal therapies to reduce pain. However the review also provides nurses with information to educate themselves about herbal therapies and so be more able to advise and treat patients who use herbal therapies.

Weidenhammer et al (2007) investigated the use of acupuncture for chronic low back pain in Germany. Their study involved 2564 patients and they concluded that acupuncture is associated with clinically relevant improvement.

Sharek et al (2006) found that comprehensive non-pharmacological postoperative pain management programmes in children receiving a liver transplant resulted in reduced pain scores, improved perception of pain by the parent, and an improved number of pain assessments in a 12 hour shift. There were also no increases in lengths of stay, time to extubation for the children, or total cost.

PROFESSIONAL AND ETHICAL KNOWLEDGE

This section explores the areas of decision making in relation to your future professional role in practice, specifically in relation to teamwork and the specialist role of the nurse. Legal and ethical areas are highlighted, but these are not exclusive and you should explore the multifaceted professional role further.

ROLE OF THE NURSE IN RELATION TO PAIN

The Nursing and Midwifery Council's (2008a) Code of Professional Conduct requires the nurse to 'protect and promote the health and well-being of those in your care' and also to 'have the knowledge and skills for safe and effective practice when working without direct supervision'. The nurse therefore has a responsibility to his or her patients and clients to increase their knowledge of pain and to use this knowledge in the implementation of pain care (Fig. 11.6). A conceptual framework is necessary if the complexity of pain is to be understood.

Pain is a complex phenomenon involving physical, psychological, emotional and spiritual components. It is therefore vital that the nurse views each individual's situation holistically. The nurse's sphere of responsibility may be within a hospital or other establishment or more widely in the community. The role includes teaching the patient, administering medications and using non-pharmacological pain relief methods (Nash et al 1999, Bucknall et al 2001, Watt-Watson et al 2001). Nurses should also take into account their own views about pain as these influence the way we interact with others. It is therefore necessary to attempt to have a positive attitude to the person in pain and to accept overall what he or she is able to tell you about their pain.

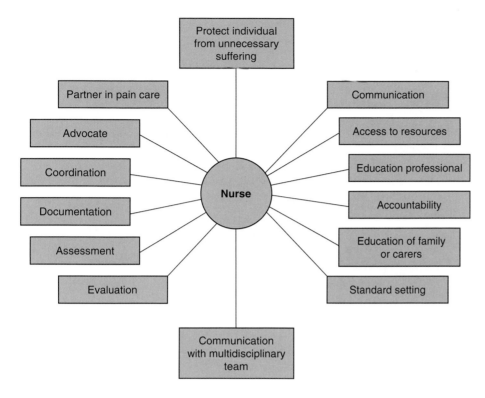

Figure 11.6 The role of the nurse in pain management.

Cranford (2001: 290) suggests six tips for nurses when managing patients in pain; these are:

- Always assess the level of pain.
- Base the amount of medication administered on individual patient needs.
- Stay flexible with the amount of medication administered.
- Assess and document the effects of medication.
- Maintain therapeutic blood levels of opioids.
- Remember that addiction is rare and therefore it should not be a major concern when caring for patients.

Evidence-based practice

Several studies (Bucknall et al 2001, Twycross 2002) have found that nurses give less priority to the relief of pain than other nursing duties; it is suggested that education would improve this situation. De Rond et al (2000) found that the implementation of a pain monitoring programme (PMP) consisting of two components – (1) education of nurses about pain, (2) assessment and management and implementing a daily pain assessment using a numerical scale – improved nurse assessment of patients' pain. It also improved the documentation of pain in the nursing records.

THE MULTIDISCIPLINARY TEAM IN PAIN MANAGEMENT

The nurse works as part of a team. Usually this team is working towards a common goal for the promotion of the ultimate good of the patient or client. In pain control many team members may be involved.

- the patient or client and their family, carers or significant others
- nurses – perhaps a specialist nurse with specific responsibility for pain management
- doctors – anaesthetists with their specialized skills in relation to local and regional block analgesia
- physiotherapists.

Frequently other individuals are involved in the pain care, particularly in cases of chronic or uncontrolled pain, for example:

- an occupational therapist
- a pharmacist
- a radiotherapist
- a complementary therapist
- a psychologist.

Since the environment of care is commonly a hospital or the patient's home, the nurse is in the ideal position to act as the coordinator of the team approach to pain control. Thus the importance of effective communication is further highlighted.

The patient and their family or carers have a greater responsibility and control of the pain plan when the patient is cared for in the community. The patient and their family or carers must therefore be adequately prepared to carry out this responsibility. While in hospital patients adopt a routine that is part of the hospital environment, but in their own home they need the support to facilitate their abilities to deal effectively with their pain. The teaching role of the nurse is a major factor in ensuring the patient is able to manage at home.

All nurses have a role in health promotion in relation to the use and abuse of analgesic drugs by the public. Mild analgesics can be obtained without a medical prescription and can be overused for minor ailments. Prolonged and continued use can be detrimental to the long-term health of the individual. The public are often not aware of the 'hidden drug' element when advertising promotes a product under a user friendly name such as 'Night Nurse'. The actual content of analgesia within the drug may not be noticed. People have inadvertently overdosed themselves because of this problem.

Easy to obtain analgesics were often those most readily at hand when someone wished to take an overdose, as in attempted suicide or deliberate self-harm (Davenport 1993, Carrigan 1994). The most dangerous drug in overdosage and also ironically one of the safest in its usual prescribed dose is paracetamol (Panadol). Because of its delayed effects on the liver a relatively small ingestion of this drug can have fatal consequences. However, since the introduction by the UK government in 1998 of legislation that limits the numbers of analgesics that can be bought over the counter there has been a reduction in deaths by suicide from paracetamol and salicylates (Hawton et al 2004).

THE ROLE OF THE SPECIALIST NURSE

The growth of the clinical nurse specialist role and specialist practitioners is a relatively recent phenomenon in the UK. The purpose is to promote autonomous practice sensitive to changing healthcare needs. Rouzan (2001) identified patient advocate as a vital and ethically important role for advanced practice nurses or specialist practitioners.

The pain specialist nursing role within a hospital or community unit has often been instigated within a multidisciplinary team. The pain specialist nurse gives advice to both healthcare professionals and the public on the effective management of pain. Thus health education and research are primary functions of such a team. The specialist nurse is a key member of the team and advises nurses, carers and the public, often through a system of links with individual representatives of a ward or unit or patient representative group. Through 'link nurse' schemes difficult individual cases can be referred directly to the specialist nurse for advice.

ETHICO–LEGAL ISSUES IN PAIN MANAGEMENT

'Ethically speaking, pain assessment and treatment is not an option but a necessity' (Rouzan 2001: 59). Moral thinking is primarily a matter of reflecting on past experiences and predicting future consequences (Kenworthy et al 2002). There are many moral dilemmas in pain management but currently there is much debate around the care of the dying and in the day-to-day decision making about adequate levels of analgesia.

Thompson et al (2000) suggest three models that the nurse may adopt in terms of professional role:

- Code based ethics – related to a code of conduct under which most nurses operate.
- Contractual ethics – usually apply where the patient or client approaches the carer before the start of treatment.
- Covenantal ethics – apply to long-term situations such as palliative care.

Providing prompt and adequate management of pain relief for adults is now a widely accepted philosophy, but there are still misconceptions in many care areas. Misconceptions about the effects of analgesia on children can seriously affect the care of children in pain. The nurse must have a clear understanding of the ways in which children and those with learning disabilities can experience and exhibit pain. Despite in some instances their limited ability to communicate we must recognize them as an authority about the nature and existence of their pain. A major role of the nurse must be to alleviate the individual's pain.

Problems also occur when there is confusion in understanding and acceptance of the patient's declaration of pain. Many researchers have found that nurses struggle to validate patient reports of pain and that nurses may not view pain as a problem requiring care (Cranford 2001, Dihle et al 2006, Stevenson et al 2006). It is recognized that pain may have an emotional or psychological origin, termed psychogenic pain, but many individuals caring for patients have difficulty with this distinction. This in turn can be a source of confusion and inappropriate care delivery when this pain 'in the mind' is considered made up or imaginary pain. Patients may be labelled as timewasters or attention seeking. Psychogenic pain may be defined as a localized sensation of pain caused solely by mental events, with no physical findings to initiate or sustain the pain (McCaffery & Beebe 1994, Sufka 2000). Conventional attitudes to pain make it difficult to believe that mental states can result in physically perceived symptoms and this in turn influences the care provided.

A further factor that influences nurses' medication practice is their ability to assess the level and intensity of pain and then to intervene to manage that pain. Ideally the individual should receive pain relief before they develop severe pain. The nurse has this responsibility in their professional role. With the arrival of quality mechanisms of clinical areas that provide charters to improve the wellbeing and increase the rights of individuals in hospital, freedom from pain should become a priority. Pain care should be a nursing priority for all client groups. But generally any vulnerable client, the person with learning disabilities, a mental health problem or a child, is at risk of poor pain care due to communication issues with healthcare professionals coordinating their pain care management

The rights of all patients, adult or child, are for high-quality care in all aspects of pain management. Nurses are accountable for their own individual level of knowledge, skills and attitudes. They will also, because of their position in the healthcare team, have a significant role in patient advocacy in relation to pain management (Mallik 1994, Royal College of Nursing 1995, Bucknall et al 2001, Rouzan 2001, Manias 2002, Herr et al 2006). In the broader professional arena the development of National Service Frameworks, Clinical Governance, standard setting and benchmarking are all moves toward equality in care provision and delivery.

Decision-making exercise

Charles is a 60-year-old retired miner who has been diagnosed with lung cancer and had surgery, but now has symptoms of spread of the cancer to the spine. He has been discharged home to the care of the primary healthcare team. The district nurse has noted that Charles's pain, despite regular doses of morphine, is not being controlled adequately. The general practitioner has been reluctant to increase the drug dosage any further and stated that he 'considered the dosage adequate for the stage of the disease'.

- Decide on how the district nurse should approach this situation if she is to remain accountable for providing Charles with adequate pain relief.
- Review the moral dilemma for the nurse if the general practitioner refuses to increase the dosage and review Charles's case in order to provide pain relief at this stage of his illness.

PERSONAL AND REFLECTIVE KNOWLEDGE

AWARENESS OF YOUR OWN BELIEFS AND VALUES ABOUT PAIN

To make effective decisions in relation to the patient in pain the nurse requires knowledge and skills in the area of pain management. An understanding of the theories of pain and pain transmission is necessary to help conceptualize the experience for the patient. Nurses have an important part to play in pain management by individualizing the assessment of pain and acting as advocates for their patients. They should be proactive and anticipatory in the care and assessment of their patients' pain. Involving the individual, if possible, and his or her family or carers in the assessment, management and evaluation of pain and using a partnership approach will provide holistic and theory based nursing care. To provide optimum care for your patient you must be aware of influences such as your own beliefs and values about pain, cultural norms, behaviours and stereotyping. This awareness should enable you to be less biased and lead to effective treatment of the patient's pain.

The experience you gain in practice is vitally important in your learning about pain management. Keeping a reflective diary will help you isolate those experiences that are relevant to the knowledge base provided by this chapter and the further reading necessary to solve specific problems you have encountered. Recording and analysing your experiences will also assist in developing your understanding and your portfolio development. The exercises throughout this chapter can prompt you to take a reflective and questioning approach to your practice experience.

CASE STUDIES IN PAIN MANAGEMENT

The following case studies will help you consolidate the knowledge gained from the chapter and further your reading and practice experience.

Case study: Adult

Miss Prudence Allison has been admitted for rehabilitative treatment after a fall at home. She has sustained a fractured right femur and a dislocation of her right shoulder. She has osteoporosis of the spine that has recently deteriorated. She has a great deal of pain and distress from this condition and she has frequently stated that she feels it's time her life came to an end. She has been prescribed analgesia of dihydrocodeine (DF118) on a *pro re nata* (PRN) basis. She has now been hospitalized for 4 weeks and has developed a chest infection.

The nurse is not in a position to address Miss Allison's request to end her life, but should seek to interpret the reason why this request may have been made. Miss Allison is in continual pain and lately her injuries and now her chest infection have combined to cause her added distress and discomfort.

Social, educational, racial, gender, religious and family circumstances can impact upon the behaviour and attitudes of the patient. The nurse should be aware of and able to judge the effect of these factors in assessing the patient and formulating the best approach to treatment.

- There are many areas within Miss Allison's care for an ethical debate. In the light of the information you have about Miss Allison, consider the request that she has made.
- What might be the reason for this request?
- How is your role as a nurse affected by the ethical and legal issues that surround this request?
- What might be considered the difference between effective pain relief for Miss Allison and her request to end her suffering?
- Miss Allison is suffering with her long-term condition. Consider the actions the nurse may be able to take to help Miss Allison cope more effectively with it.
- What advice and resources may be available to Miss Allison to limit her pain?

Case study: Mental health

Malique King is a 45-year-old man of no fixed address with an itinerant lifestyle. He suffers from schizophrenia and also has problems with alcohol. He has been brought into the accident and emergency department on several occasions in the last few weeks. He has usually been found collapsed in a drunken state in the street or park. Previously, despite attempts to refer Malique for appropriate mental health and medical consultation, he has disappeared from the department after a couple of hours. He has come into the department this evening of his own accord, smelling strongly of alcohol. He is dirty and unkempt and is complaining of 'bellyache'. His baseline observations of pulse and respiration are slightly elevated. The doctors have been informed, but they appear to believe that Malique is looking for a bed for the night. Malique has never complained of pain before when he has been brought into the department; in fact he has always appeared very unhappy at being in the department and has not been very communicative.

- Consider the reasons why the doctors may not believe Malique's complaints of pain.
- Consider the appropriate action that the nurse should take to assess Malique and to ensure his needs are met.
- What are the grounds for these actions?
- What are the responsibilities of the nurse?
- Write a short account of your actions in relation to the theory that supports the accountability role of the nurse in this

instance. This will help you to rationalize the decisions you have made in relation to Malique's needs.

Case study: Learning disabilities

Louise Freeman is 29 years old. She has cerebral palsy that arose as the result of trauma during her birth. She is quadriplegic with developmental delay and has very little communication, though is usually able to vocalize whether she is happy or sad. She has some difficulty swallowing and eating has always been difficult. She has been cared for at home by her elderly parents. Recently Louise has developed pressure sores on her buttocks and elbows and her parents are finding it increasingly difficult to maintain her normal eating pattern. She has been admitted to hospital to give some support to her parents and to assess the difficulty with feeding. She has recently lost weight and on admission she weighs 4 stone 10 lb (30 kg). Mrs Freeman tells you that she thinks Louise is not comfortable.

- You need to be able to assess the level of Louise's pain so that you can make decisions to carry out appropriate nursing care. Find out what tools are available to you and if they are suitable to assess Louise's pain.
- Consider the factors involved here so that the pain can be accurately assessed.
- What members of the multidisciplinary team may be involved in Louise's pain care and why would they be included?
- Louise is now able to return home. She has been prescribed pentazocine (Fortral) suppositories to help control her pain. Consider the information her parents will need about her analgesia to keep her pain under control.
- Louise's mother is reluctant to give her the analgesic as she does not want her to be sleepy in the daytime. How would you explain to her the way that the drug works and its effects?

Case study: Child

Jordan Simpson is 14 years old. He has sickle cell anaemia and has been admitted to the ward in crisis. Jordan is the eldest of three children and his mother, Joan, who is a single parent, relies on him to help with the care of his brother and sister. Joan works in a local public house and in the evenings Jordan babysits. Joan has had trouble paying the bills and Jordan has been very worried about this. It is felt that this stress has brought on the current crisis.

On admission Jordan is in severe pain. He is quiet and uncommunicative. His facial expression is a grimace. His mother has accompanied him, but she needs to return home very shortly to collect her other children from school. PCA has been commenced with a morphine infusion.

- Consider the care decisions that have to be made to achieve optimum pain relief for Jordan.

- Find out about sickle cell anaemia and the precipitating factors.
- Are there any special observations to be made when Jordan is receiving morphine?

- Make a decision about how you may be able to help Jordan and his family prevent further crises.
- Consider the various roles of the nurse here to provide Jordan with appropriate care and support.

SUMMARY

This chapter has drawn together theoretical concepts of pain and applied this knowledge in relation to the practice of caring for individuals. It has included:

1. Theories of pain and how pain is transmitted within the individual. Physiological and psychological signs and symptoms of the pain experience have also been examined.
2. Factors influencing decision making by nurses in relation to pain assessment and management have been considered.
3. The use of pain assessment tools in practice and different ways of reducing pain in an individual have been explored, including the use of pharmacological and non-pharmacological intervention and the inclusion of complementary therapies.
4. The professional role of the nurse in pain management has been discussed, both as an individual and as a member of a multidisciplinary team.
5. Knowledge illuminated within this chapter has been combined with evidence from other referenced sources and applied within a range of situations. Suggestions have been made for portfolio development in relation to pain management.

Annotated further reading and websites

Carter B (ed) 1998 Perspectives on pain: mapping the territory. Arnold, London

For an excellent account of the cultural aspects of pain, see the chapter 'Cultural dimensions of pain', by Bryn Davis.

Davis GC, Melinda LH, White TL 2002 Barriers to managing chronic pain in older adults with arthritis. Journal of Nursing Scholarship 34 (2):121–126

Explores the barriers to pain management experienced by older adults with arthritis. Nine themes were identified with a resulting model of personal decision making in pain management methods.

Dickenson AH 2002 [Editorial 1] Gate control theory of pain stands the test of time. British Journal of Anaesthesia 88(6):755–757

A useful article that helps to conceptualize the gate theory and developments since it was first put forward.

Jacob E, Miaskowski WC, Savedra M, Beyer JE, Treadwell JM, Styles L 2007 Quantification of analgesic use in children with sickle cell disease. Clinical Journal of Pain 23:8–14

This study aimed to 'quantify analgesic use in children with sickle cell disease who were hospitalized for a vaso-occlusive episode, using the Medication Quantification Scale (MQS) and to examine the relationships between pain intensity scores, number of painful areas marked on a body outline diagram, number of word descriptors of pain quality, and amount of analgesic medications administered.' The MQS was found to be a useful measure to quantify analgesic use.

Jones JB 2001 Pathophysiology of acute pain: implications for clinical management. Emergency Medicine 13:288–292

A useful article that considers the pathophysiology of pain and the various types of pain receptors, pathways and transmitters.

Lewandowski W, Good M, Draucker CB 2005 Changes in the meaning of pain with the use of guided imagery. Pain Management Nursing 6 (2):58–67

This study explores the efficacy of guided imagery with people experiencing chronic pain.

Sharek PJ, Wayman K, Lin E et al 2006 Improved pain management in pediatric postoperative liver transplant patients using parental education and non pharmacologic interventions. Pediatric Transplantation 10:172–177

An interesting article that explores the use of a patient specific pain plan of non pharmacologic interventions including hypnosis, positioning, swaddling, acupuncture and guided imagery for children who have undergone liver transplants. The authors conclude that such techniques have a positive effect on the children's pain experience.

Vadalouca A, Siafaka I, Argyra E, Vrachnou E, Moka E 2006 Therapeutic management of chronic neuropathic pain: an examination of pharmacologic treatment. Annals of the New York Academy of Sciences 1088:164–186

An exploration of the various pharmacological treatments of neuropathic pain with a consideration of the antecedents of these treatments and the current evidence for their use.

Wall PD, Melzack R 1999 Textbook of pain, 4th edn. Churchill Livingstone, Edinburgh

An excellent general textbook. See particularly the discussion on psychiatric/mental pain, pp 931–949.

Wang H-L, Keck JF 2004 Foot and hand massage as an intervention for postoperative pain. Pain Management Nursing 5(2):59–65

Explores the use of foot and hand massage as an adjunct to medication for postoperative pain; it was found to be beneficial to the patients.

Wirth JH, Hudgins JC, Paice JA 2005 Use of herbal therapies to relieve pain: a review of efficacy and adverse effects. Pain Management Nursing 6(4):145–167

This article summarizes the existing studies investigating the efficacy of herbal therapies as a treatment for pain. Possible side-effects, potential drug–herb interactions and information about common herbal therapies are also summarized. Uses, dosages, routes of administration and side-effects are summarized.

http://www.britishpainsociety.org/
This is the site of the British Chapter of the International Association for the Study of Pain. It includes recommendations of the society for nursing practice in pain management.

http://nmap.ac.uk/
This website contains resources related to many aspects of pain including management and assessment, but also relating to current evidence for practice in this area.

http://nccam.nih.gov/
This American website is the home of the National Centre for Complementary and Alternative Medicine and provides useful information of these strategies.

http://www.gosh.nhs.uk/factsheets/families/F050225/index.html
This website includes other useful children related fact sheets. This area looks at musculoskeletal chronic pain, and the mutidisciplinary team and practices in pain assessment in these children.

Science 13 July 2001:Vol. 293. no. 5528, pp. 311–315 DOI: 10.1126/science.1060952

http://www.sciencemag.org.ezproxy-m.lib.deakin.edu.au/cgi/content/short/293/5528/311 (accessed 12 April 2007)

References

American Pain Society 1999 Principles of analgesic use in the treatment of acute pain and cancer pain, 4th edn. American Medical Association, Glenview

Berkley KJ 1998 Sexual difference and pain: a constructive issue for the millennium. Available online: http://painconsortium.nih.gov/genderandpain/abstracts/KBerkley.htm (accessed May 2006)

Bishop G 1946 Neural mechanisms of cutaneous sense. Physiology Review 26:77–102

Bishop G 1959 The relationship between nerve fibre size and sensory modality: phylogenetic implications of the afferent innervation of the cortex. Journal of Nervous and Mental Disorders 128:89–114

Bucknall T, Manias E, Botti M 2001 Acute pain management: implications of scientific evidence for nursing practice in the postoperative context. International Journal of Nursing Practice 7:266–273

Burgess DJ, Van Ryn M, Crowley-Matoka M, Malat J 2006 Understanding the provider contribution to race/ethnicity disparities in pain treatment: insights from dual process models of stereotyping. Pain Medicine 7(2):119–134

Carr ECJ, Mann EM 2000 Pain: creative approaches to effective management. Macmillan, Basingstoke

Carrigan JT 1994 The psychosocial needs of patients who have attempted suicide by overdose. Journal of Advanced Nursing 20(4):635–642

Carter B (ed) 1998 Perspectives on pain: mapping the territory. Arnold, London

Carter B, McArthur E, Cunliffe M 2002 Dealing with uncertainty: parental assessment of pain in their children with profound special needs. Journal of Advanced Nursing 38(5):449–457

Chaitow L 2002 Conquer pain: the natural way. Duncan Baird, London

Children Act 1989/2004 HMSO, London

Couzin J 2006 Unraveling pain's DNA. Science 314:585–586. DOI: 10.1126/science.314.5799.585. Available online: www.sciencemag.org (accessed 12 April 2007)

Cranford JS 2001 Stay tuned for the next episode of pain. International Journal of Nursing Practice 7:288–291

Dahlman GB, Dykes AK, Elander G 1999 Patients' evaluation of pain and nurses' management of analgesics after surgery: the effect of a study day on the subject of pain for nurses working at the thorax surgery department. Journal of Advanced Nursing 30:866–874

Darwin E 1794 Cited in: Dallenbach K 1939 Pain: history and present status. Journal of Psychiatry 52:331–347

Davenport D 1993 Structured support at a time of crisis: treatment of paracetamol overdose. Professional Nurse 8(9):558–562

Davis GC, Hiemenz ML, White TL 2002 Barriers to managing chronic pain of older adults with arthritis. Journal of Nursing Scholarship 34(2):121–126

De Rond MEJ, De Wit R, Van Dam FSAM et al 2000 A pain monitoring programme for nurses: effects on communication, assessment and documentation of patients' pain. Journal of Pain and Symptom Management 20(6):424–439

Descartes R (1664/1972) Treatise on man (translated by M Foster). Harvard University Press, Cambridge

Dickenson AH 2002 Gate control theory of pain stands the test of time. British Journal of Anaesthesia 88(6):755–757

Dihle A, Bjølseth G, Helseth S 2006 The gap between saying and doing in postoperative pain management. Journal of Clinical Nursing 15:469–479

Dubner R 1997 Neural basis of persistent pain: sensory specialization, sensory modulation, and neuronal plasticity. In: Jensen TS, Turner JA, Wiesenfeld-Hallin Z (eds) Proceedings of the 8th world congress on pain. Progress in Pain Research and Management, vol. 8. IASP Press, Seattle, pp 243–257

Duff L, Louw G, Loftus-Hills A, Morrell C 2001 Clinical practice guidelines: the recognition and assessment of acute pain in children. Implementation guide. Royal College of Nursing, London

Dworkin RH 2002 An overview of neuropathic pain: syndromes, symptoms, signs, and several mechanisms. Clinical Journal of Pain 18:343–349

Fordham M, Dunn V 1994 Alongside the person in pain: holistic care and nursing practice. Baillière Tindall, London

Green CR, Anderson KO, Baker TA et al 2003 The unequal burden of pain: confronting racial and ethnic disparities in pain. Pain Medicine 4(3):277–294

Hawton K, Simkin S, Deeks J et al 2004 UK legislation on analgesic packs: before and after study of long term effect on poisonings. British Medical Journal 329:1076–1076

Helman C 2001 Culture, health and illness, 4th edn. Arnold, London

Herr K, Coyne PJ, Key T et al 2006 Pain assessment in the nonverbal patient: position statement with clinical practice recommendations. Pain Management Nursing 7(2):44–52

Horgan M, Choonara I, Al-Waidh Sambrookes J et al 1996 Measuring pain in neonates: an objective score. Paediatric Nursing 8(10):24–27

Human Rights Act 1998/2000 HMSO, London

Jones JB 2001 Pathophysiology of acute pain: implications for clinical management. Emergency Medicine 13:288–292

Kamp TE 2001 Survey reveals impact of pain may differ by gender. Pain and Central Nervous System Week 22(2):16–17

Kenworthy N, Snowley G, Gilling C (eds) 2002 Common foundation studies in nursing, 3rd edn. Churchill Livingstone, Edinburgh

Keogh E, Herdenfeldt M 2002 Gender, coping and the perception of pain. Pain 97(3):195–201

Kim HS, Schwartz-Barcott D, Tracy SM, Fortin JD, Sjöström B 2005 Strategies of pain assessment used by nurses on surgical units. Pain Management Nursing 6(1):3–9

Klopfenstein CE, Hermann FR, Mamie C, Van Gessel E, Forster A 2000 Pain intensity and pain relief after surgery: a comparison between patients' reported assessments and nurses' and physicians' observations. Acta Anaesthesiologica Scandinavica 44:58–62

Lin Y-C, Lee ACC, Kemper KJ, Berde CB 2005, Use of complementary and alternative medicine in pediatric pain management service: a survey. Pain Medicine 6(6):452–458

Livingstone W 1943 The mechanism of pain. Macmillan, New York

Loeser JD 2005 Pain: disease or dis-ease? The John Bonica lecture: presented at the third world congress of World Institute of Pain, Barcelona, 2004. Pain Practice 5(2):77–84

McCaffery M 1972 Nursing management of the patient in pain. Lippincott, Philadelphia

McCaffery M, Beebe A 1994 Pain: clinical manual for nursing practice, UK edn. Mosby, London

McCaffery M, Pasero C 1999 Pain: clinical manual, 2nd edn. Mosby, St Louis

Main CJ, Spanswick CC 2000 Pain management: an interdisciplinary approach. Churchill Livingstone, Edinburgh

Mallik M 1994 An impossible ideal? The role of the child advocate. Child Health 2(3):105–109

Manias E, Botti M, Bucknell T 2002 Observation of pain assessment and management – the complexities of clinical practice. Journal of Clinical Nursing 11:724–733

Mann E, Carr E 2006 Pain management. Blackwell Publishing, Oxford

Marshall H 1894 Pain, pleasure and aesthetics. Macmillan, London

Melzack R, Wall P 1965 Pain mechanisms: a new theory. Science 150:971–979

Melzack R, Wall P 1973 Psychophysiology of pain. International Anaesthesiology Clinics 8:3–34

Melzack R, Wall P 1982 The challenge of pain, vol. 1. Penguin, Harmondsworth

Melzack R, Wall P 1988 The challenge of pain, vol. 2. Penguin, Harmondsworth

Melzack R, Wall P 1996 The challenge of pain. Penguin, Harmondsworth

Merkel S, Voepel-Lewis T, Shayevitz J R et al 1997 The FLACC: a behavioural scale for scoring postoperative pain in young children. Pediatric Nursing 23(3):293–297

Merskey H 1970 On the development of pain. Headache 10:116–123

Merskey H, Bogduk N (eds) 1994 Classification of chronic pain, 2nd edn. IASP Press, Seattle

Misuse of Drugs Act 1971 HMSO, London

Munafò M, Trim J 2000 Chronic pain: a handbook for nurses. Butterworth-Heinemann, Oxford

Nash R, Yates P, Edwards H et al 1999 Pain and the administration of analgesia: what nurses say. Journal of Clinical Nursing 8:180–189

National Centre for Complementary and Alternative Medicine 2007 CAM basics. What is CAM? Available online: http://nccam.nih.gov/health/whatiscam/ (accessed 21 December 2007)

Nordenbos W 1959 Pain. Elsevier, Amsterdam

Nursing and Midwifery Council 2008a The Code: standards of conduct, performance and ethics for nurses and midwives. Nursing and Midwifery Council, London

Nursing and Midwifery Council 2008b Complementary alternative therapies and homeopathy. Nursing and Midwifery Council, London

Park G, Fulton B, Senthuran S 2000 The management of acute pain, 2nd edn. Oxford University Press, Oxford

Richards J, Hubbert AO 2007 Experiences of expert nurses in caring for patients with postoperative pain. Pain Management Nursing 8(1):17–24

Rouzan IA 2001 An analysis of research and clinical practice in neonatal pain management. Journal of the American Academy of Nurse Practitioners 13(2):57–60

Royal College of Nursing 1995 Advocacy and the nurse. Paper 22 – Issues in nursing. Royal College of Nursing, London

Royal College of Nursing 2001 The recognition and assessment of acute pain in children. Technical report. Royal College of Nursing, London

Sharek PJ, Wayman K, Lin E et al 2006 Improved pain management in pediatric postoperative liver transplant patients using parental education and non-pharmacologic interventions. Pediatric Transplantation 10:172–177

Stallard P, Williams L, Velleman R, Lenton S, McGrath PJ, Taylor G 2002 The development and evaluation of the pain indicator for communicatively impaired children (PICIC). Pain 98(1–2):145–149

Stevens B, Johnston CC 1993 Pain in the infant: theoretical and conceptual issues. Maternal Child Nursing Journal 21(1):3–14

Stevenson KM, Dahl JL, Berry PH, Beck SL, Griffie J 2006 Institutionalizing effective pain management practices: practice change programs to improve the quality of pain management in small health care organizations. Journal of Pain and Symptom Management 31(3):248–261

Sufka KJ 2000 Chronic pain explained. Brain and Mind 1:155–179

Thompson IE, Melia KM, Boyd KM 2000 Nursing ethics, 4th edn. Churchill Livingstone, Edinburgh

Tse MMY, Jacobus KF, Chung JWY et al 2002 The effect of visual stimuli on pain threshold and tolerance. Journal of Clinical Nursing 11:462–469

Twycross A 2002 Educating nurses about pain management: the way forward. Journal of Clinical Nursing 11:705–714

Twycross A, Moriarty A, Betts T 1998 Pediatric pain management: a multidisciplinary approach. Radcliffe Medical Press, Oxford

Van Hulle Vincent C, Denyes MJ 2004 Relieving children's pain: nurses' abilities and analgesic administration practices. Journal of Pediatric Nursing 19(1):40–50

Walker AC, Tan L, George S 1995 Impact of culture on pain management: an Australian nursing perspective. Holistic Nurse Practitioner 9(2):48–57

Wall PD 1977 Why do we not understand pain? In: Duncan R, Weston-Smith M (eds) The encyclopaedia of ignorance. Pergamon Press, Oxford, pp 361–368

Wall PD, Melzack R 1999 Textbook of pain, 4th edn. Churchill Livingstone, Edinburgh

Watt-Watson J, Stevens B, Garfinkel P, Streiner D, Gallop R 2001 Relationship between nurses' pain knowledge and pain management outcomes for their postoperative cardiac patients. Journal of Advanced Nursing 36(4):535–545

Weidenhammer W, Linde K, Streng A, Hoppe A, Melchart D 2007 Acupuncture for chronic low back pain in routine care: a multi center observational study. Clinical Journal of Pain 23(2):128–135

Wirth JH, Hudgins JC, Paice JA 2005 Use of herbal therapies to relieve pain: a review of efficacy and adverse effects. Pain Management Nursing 6(4):145–167

Wood S 2002 Special focus: Pain, part 1. Nursing Times 98(38):41–45

Woolf CJ, Slater MW 2000 Neuronal plasticity: increasing the gain in pain. Science 288:1765–1769

Young JL, Horton FM, Davidhizar R 2006 Nursing attitudes and beliefs in pain assessment and management. Journal of Advanced Nursing 53(4):412–421

Chapter 12

Aggression

Paul Linsley

INTRODUCTION

This chapter addresses the topic of aggression and how nurses respond to this danger. It does this by explaining aggression from its theoretical and practical aspects. An important feature of this chapter is the application of the concepts that are discussed to nursing practice.

OVERVIEW

Subject knowledge

This part of the chapter examines the term aggression and the situations where it occurs. The main focus of this section is on biological and psychological explanations of aggression.

Care delivery knowledge

This section addresses how to manage aggression. Models of aggression management are discussed and applied to clinical practice. Aggression management and methods to reduce the aggressive actions are key elements of this section.

Professional and ethical knowledge

Here there is a discussion of the professional issues that stem from aggression. This includes those arising from the management of aggression as well as legal, preventive and safety concerns.

Personal and reflective knowledge

Within this section is an extended exercise for you to complete, to increase awareness of your own responses to aggression and to provide you with evidence for your learning portfolio. In addition, this section contains four case studies (pp. 288–289) that explore issues of aggression management in each of the four branches of nursing. You may find it helpful to read one of them before you start the chapter and use it as a focus for your reflections while reading.

SUBJECT KNOWLEDGE

AGGRESSION AND VIOLENCE IN HEALTHCARE

One of the difficulties in addressing violence and aggression is that they are not easy to define. This is because they mean different things to different people. Behaviour that one person might find acceptable another might take offence at. It is because of this that healthcare organizations and staff groups have defined violence and aggression in different ways for different purposes. However, in order to recognize, address and prevent violence and aggression, healthcare staff must have a clear understanding of what these terms mean. This requires a description that encompasses the different forms that violence and aggression can take, while allowing for personal interpretation and understanding.

Aggression is any form of behaviour used with the intention to harm or injure another person (Health Services Advisory Committee 1997). This includes acts carried out with the intent to cause physical harm, directed either outwardly towards others or inwardly at the individual (self-mutilation). They range from verbal or emotional acts to serious physical harm (Shepherd 1994). This includes antisocial behaviour, for example lack of respect towards others; physical or verbal aggression where the intent is to injure; and assault with the intent being to cause the other person harm.

Bibby (1995) defined health-related aggressive actions as those occurring when a health worker feels threatened or abused or is assaulted by a member of the public during the course of their duties. Similarly the Counter Fraud and Security Management Service, a special health authority within the NHS who have overall responsibility for the management of violence and aggression within the healthcare sector, define aggression as: 'the intentional application of force to the person, without lawful justification, resulting in physical injury or personal discomfort' (CFSMS 2006).

These definitions however, fail to take into account unintentional violence resulting from illness or injury, or where a patient's mental capacity is impaired. Whatever definition of aggression is used, it should have meaning for those involved, and show recognition of the problem encountered as part of their work. Promoting the issue of violence and aggression within the healthcare setting is as important as defining it, if not more so.

Nurses frequently deal with people who are in desperate need of attention and care, which they may, through ill-health, age or other circumstances, be unable to provide for themselves. They work with people across the whole of society, in circumstances that may be difficult and demanding, and often work long and unsociable hours. Patients may be anxious and worried about coming into hospital and what might happen to them. Some may be predisposed towards violence and aggression as a means of coping. Likewise, it may be that their relatives or friends express frustration or distress through aggression. While these factors do not excuse aggression, it is understandable why nurses and those that they care for occasionally come into conflict. It is important to recognize at this point that aggression is very rarely purposeless. People are aggressive either because they want something to happen or because they want something to stop happening. In clinical settings, aggression and violence may be used by patients as a way of getting what they want. Violent acts may be used to force change or to gain control. Rewards from violence include attention from staff and status and prestige among the patient group. For example, the patient who behaves violently is observed more frequently and has more opportunities to discuss concerns with their doctor and nursing staff. Despite this nurses are often expected to face their assailants and even to continue to provide and care for them following an attack. This situation is likely to test the nurse's ability to cope with the psychological consequences of threats and assaults even further, and the cycle can become self-perpetuating.

Aggressive actions can also originate from colleagues. Many tensions can occur within work teams and in healthy organizational cultures; those tensions can be a valuable force for initiating change. Psychological violence is often perpetrated through repeated behaviour, of a type which may alone be relatively minor but which cumulatively can become a very serious form of violence. Although a single incident can suffice, psychological violence often consists of repeated, unwelcome, unreciprocated and imposed actions, which may have a devastating effect on their target. This is typical in bullying and harassment. Bullying turns to harassment when it is targeted repeatedly toward the same person or staff group and the chosen target is to some extent defenceless in the face of the perpetrator.

Bullying is a real problem within the health service, causing many staff to take sickness absence or early retirement and to leave the service altogether. Most organizations now have polices and procedures for dealing with bullying and harassment that outline what is and what is not acceptable behaviour. Penalties for transgression can result in dismissal. However, proving someone has been a bully is difficult, particularly if it has been done in a covert way.

The Evolve 12.1 resource provides further information on bullying in the workplace.

	12.1 – BULLYING AND HARASSMENT

- Understand what is meant by the terms.
- Know the forms they may take.
- Know when to seek help and support.

It would be wrong to rely solely on policies and procedures to protect the individual from aggression. One possible way of combating aggression such as bullying is to develop skills of assertiveness (RCN 2005). It is suggested that those people who are singled out for bullying and harassment are those that lack the ability to stand up for themselves and their rights. Linsley (2006) suggests that assertiveness is about the individual standing up for their rights in such a way as not to violate the rights of others. Being assertive can help the individual to develop a belief and confidence in herself or himself. The more that individuals stand up for their rights and act in a manner that is respectful of themselves and others, the higher their self-esteem. Assertiveness consequently can help a person to develop their self-confidence so that they can address threatening situations effectively.

THE VULNERABLE ADULT

A vulnerable adult is someone who, because of mental or other disability, age or illness, relies on the help and services of others in order to meet their needs. At times this can bring them into conflict with those that care for them, and in some cases this leads to conflict, exploitation and abuse. This is a growing area of concern and one that warrants the attention that it is only now getting.

Vulnerable adults may be abused by a wide range of people including relatives and family members, professional staff, paid care workers, volunteers, other service users, neighbours and friends. Abuse may be physical or psychological. It may simply be neglect or it may occur if the vulnerable person is forced to enter into an exploitative financial or sexual transaction to which he/she has not consented or cannot consent (Department of Health 2000).

When considering *physical abuse* it is important to consider the nature of the injury and whether this is in keeping with the history given. This should be balanced against what you know and observe of the patient; as in so many cases of abuse, the first real indicator is a change in the behaviour of the person.

Indicators of *sexual abuse* may include, along with changes in behaviour, bruising and bleeding around the sexual organs, and changes in personal hygiene, such as, wetting, soiling and a reluctance to undress.

Emotional abuse might result in the person becoming withdrawn; this can include physical changes such as weight loss and lack of sleep. The person might become watchful of others and their demeanour may change when a certain person is present. The abused may become withdrawn and lose interest in themselves and their surroundings.

Discriminatory abuse is perhaps one of the hardest forms of abuse to accept as it is perpetrated, sometimes through ignorance, by the very people who are meant to care. A lack of respect and a substandard level of service can be as emotionally and psychologically damaging as physical abuse. Denying a person the right to be involved in their own care; excluding them from opportunities such as health, education, employment and housing; explaining behaviour and medical symptoms solely in terms of the person's disability; viewing people on the grounds of race, culture, age and gender are further examples of this type of abuse.

The protection of adults raises a variety of complex issues; however, staff have a duty to report suspicions or disclosures made about any abuse. It is important to record events at the time they happened, with clarity and dispassion, separating fact from opinion. Other information should include: where and when the incident took place; if there were any witnesses; what was said and observed; what action was taken, if any. It is important that the member of staff report any concerns they have immediately to prevent further abuse occurring. The Safeguarding Vulnerable Groups Act 2000 introduces a new vetting and barring scheme for those who work with children and vulnerable adults (Department of Health 2006). At the heart of the scheme is the provision of a register that lists those that have been banned from working with vulnerable groups having neglected or otherwise harmed individuals in their care.

All trusts and voluntary agencies have policies on reporting abuse which should be in accordance with good practice and standards. Unfortunately though, many incidents and near misses go unreported (Ferns & Chojnacha 2005).

For further information see Evolve 12.2.

⊖volve *learning system* | **12.2 – THE VULNERABLE ADULT**

- Know what a 'vulnerable adult' is.
- Know forms of abuse.
- Recognize signs of abuse.

ABUSE OF CHILDREN

As with adult abuse, child abuse may consist of a single act or repeated acts. The abuse can be physical, sexual, emotional and/or psychological. If a child confides that they may have been abused, the following is advised (HM Government 2006):

- Remain calm, approachable and receptive.
- Listen carefully without interrupting.
- Make it clear that you are taking him/her seriously.
- Acknowledge how difficult this may be.

- Reassure him/her that he/she has done the right thing in telling.
- Let him/her know you will do everything you can to help him/her.
- Report on as per local policy.

What to avoid:

- Do not let any shock or distaste show.
- Do not probe (it is not your job to investigate but report).
- Do not suggest in any way to the child what may have happened. On occasions this may be done inadvertently by asking a leading question.
- Do not speculate or make assumptions.
- Do not make any negative comments about the alleged abuser.
- Do not make any promises you cannot keep.
- Do not promise to keep the information secret.

It is the responsibility of all staff to safeguard the welfare and well-being of those they look after and work with by protecting them from physical, emotional and sexual abuse, harm or neglect and supporting them if this occurs.

WHY AGGRESSION HAPPENS

Many theories of aggression have been developed, which suggests that there are many different causes of aggression. Each has its support and its criticism but although there is no unanimously accepted explanation, each theory helps to develop insight into the build up and display of aggression.

BIOLOGICAL THEORIES OF AGGRESSION

Biological theories focus upon somatic phenomena underpinning aggression. Three major theories are examined in this section: the role of neurotransmitters, the endocrine system and genetic influences.

Neurotransmitters

Two neurotransmitters, noradrenaline (norepinephrine) and serotonin, have been the prime focus of studies into aggression. Low serum concentrations of serotonin and high serum noradrenaline concentrations have been found in aggressive individuals (Hollin 1992). Unfortunately, though, a simple cause and effect relationship between these neurotransmitters and aggression has not in fact been found. So, while they do not cause aggression on their own, they may contribute to the severity of the aggressive episode (McElliskem 2004) (Fig. 12.1).

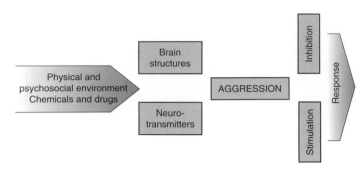

Figure 12.1 Neurological structure and function and the occurrence of aggression. This shows how environmental factors provide input to the brain structures and how the neurotransmitter state of the individual can give rise to aggression or inhibition of aggression.

The endocrine system

Most research into hormones and the aggressive response has concerned the sex hormones. These are thought to act at two levels:

- First, by predisposing the individual to become biologically developed in terms of muscular and other body systems to enable aggression to be used in the pursuit of sexual or other drives.
- Second, by the direct incitement to act aggressively under the influence of sexual hormones.

Owens & Ashcroft (1985) were among the first to note how the male sex hormone, androgen, influenced aggressive responses. They discussed how castrated rats became less aggressive – probably due to their removed androgen supply – and how monkeys with high serum androgen concentrations were associated with higher levels of aggressive responses. The problem is that it is difficult to replicate these findings in human subjects. Although it can be shown that males are more involved in violent and sexual crimes and that male delinquency is associated with the onset of puberty (Beresford et al 2006), attributing such behaviour to high androgen levels has not been proven in human subjects.

One other area of hormonal influence on aggressive behaviour is the role of hormones in the menstrual cycle (Hines & Kimberly 2003). This was promoted by women attributing violent or aggressive actions to the premenstrual stage of their menstrual cycle. Again problems establishing a definite causal linkage is the major issue and as yet this has not been established.

Genetic factors

Whilst the exact amount of influence that genetics have on aggressive behaviour is still questioned, studies on animals have shown that a tendency towards aggression is at least partly inherited. The main problem with biological research into aggressive behaviour is that it is difficult to separate factors like genetic make-up from the complex variables that make up human individuals.

Consequently, while biological theories throw an interesting light on the nature and severity of aggression, to adhere strictly to a biological causation of aggression is unsafe. Aggressive behaviour always occurs within a social context and it is this factor that must also be examined.

PSYCHOSOCIAL THEORIES OF AGGRESSION

The psychoanalytic theory

Freud's model of the person comprised a bipolar model (Frankl 1990):

- At one pole is an Eros drive – the instinct for life.
- At the other pole is a Thanatos drive – the death or destructive instinct.

The assumption behind this theory is that two primitive forces, the life and death instincts, oppose each other in our subconscious, and this incongruence is the origin of aggression. Freud asserted that this is a process void of thought patterns and is driven entirely by our instincts. This model would seem to have a crucial flaw, however; having defined the general aims of the life and death instincts, Freud failed to determine their source.

Frustration–aggression hypothesis

The frustration–aggression hypothesis was first set out in the 1930s by Dollard et al (1939). It proposes that aggression, rather than occurring spontaneously, is a response to the frustration of some goal-directed behaviour by an outside source. Goals may include such basic needs as food, water, sleep, sex, love and recognition. Contributions to frustration–aggression research further established that an environmental stimulus must produce not just frustration but anger in order for aggression to follow (e.g. Berkowitz 1990, Geen 2001), and that the anger can be the result of stimuli other than frustrating situations, such as verbal abuse (Cohen et al 1998). Anger will always lead to aggression, however, as anger can be displayed in a number of ways and conversely act as a motivator and medium for positive change (Berkowitz 2001).

Social learning theory

Social learning theory focuses on aggression as a learned behaviour. It analyses the roles of models (a behaviour displayed by another) in the acquisition of aggressive behaviour (e.g. Anderson & Dill 2000, Freedman 2002, Akert et al 2005).

Social learning has three principal components:

1. Behaviour: an observer sees a model perform a particular behaviour.
2. Learning or acquisition phase: the observer attends to important features of the behaviour, remembering what was seen and done.
3. Performance: imitates the behaviour at a later time.

Children learn many social skills through this process. It involves being attentive to the following: remembering, imitating and being rewarded by people, television, books and magazines (Bushman 1998). Reducing restraints on aggressive behaviour through modelling thus can in turn reduce the inhibitions against behaving aggressively by leading a person to believe that this is a typical or permissible way of solving problems or attaining goals, and in turn, distort their views about conflict resolution (Bushman 1995, 1998; Geen 2001).

The role of anger

While anger frequently precedes violent behaviour, it is important to recognize that anger does not always lead to violence. Anger is a negative emotion that arises when there is a threat or delay in achieving a goal, or a conflict between goals. It signals that something is wrong in oneself, in others, or in one's relationship(s) with others and the three possible targets of a person's anger are others, impersonal objects/life conditions, or oneself.

Sometimes it may be therapeutic to legitimize anger, perhaps if the standard of healthcare falls below what the individual expects. In fact, many people believe that anger is healthy and necessary. Hollinworth et al (2005) suggest that it is a common experience to become angry, and that expressing anger is a normal process. It is not the anger that is legitimate and right, but the stress that underlies the anger. Expressing anger is also a mechanism for enhancing self-respect, and a constructive action that can lead to correcting a perceived wrong.

CARE DELIVERY KNOWLEDGE

THE NATURE OF AGGRESSION

Aggression takes many different forms. Physical aggression inflicts harm through deed or act, whereas verbal aggression creates harm through words. Aggression can also be expressed directly or indirectly (Kaukiainen et al 2001). Direct means of aggression take place in face-to-face situations, whereas indirect aggression is delivered via the negative reactions of others (Buss 1995). Often, indirect aggression is a kind of social manipulation, like spreading malicious rumours about the target person or trying to persuade others not to associate with him or her. Bullying and harassment are two types of aggression commonly found in the workplace (Royal College of Nursing 2001) which encompass this type of behaviour. Not only are such behaviours upsetting for those directly involved, but also for those who witness and have to deal with it.

Reflection and portfolio exercise

As we have seen, aggression means different things to different people. Make a list of behaviours that *you* associate with aggression using the following headings:

Words and phrases
Behaviour
Moods and emotions
Body language.
- Which of these behaviours do you attribute to yourself?
- Which of these behaviours do you attribute to others?
- Are there similarities between the two lists?

MINIMIZING THE RISK OF AGGRESSION

Perhaps the biggest cause of aggression is interpersonal provocation (Berkowitz 1993, Geen 2001). Provocations include insults, slights, other forms of verbal aggression, physical aggression and interference with an individual's attempts to attain an important goal.

In some cases, the nature of a person's job might include multiple risk factors. Social workers provide an example of an occupation in which organizational, social and political factors can be found, including (Health and Safety Executive 2004):

- Allocation of scarce resources.
- Compulsory admission of some mentally ill and mentally impaired people to hospital.
- Removal of children from some homes against the wishes of the parents.
- Investigation of cases of non-accidental injury to children.
- Compulsory removal of some elderly people from home to hospital.
- Supervision in the community of men and women with a history of potential or actual violence, some with an associated mental disorder.

Violence and aggression then result as much from the characteristics of the healthcare worker and the organization in which they work as from the characteristics of the individual.

See also Tables 12.1 and 12.2.

Table 12.1 Prediction of aggression: the individual (adapted from Linsley 2006, Hinde 1993, Pollock et al 1989)

Prediction category	Examples
Personality factors	Low threshold of frustration or impulsivity Increased liability to become aroused An antisocial personality such as someone who is habitually aggressive or undercontrolled Substance abusers
Previous history of aggression or violence	An institutional record where violence has been a factor may mean an increased risk of violence A genetic constitution that tends towards a lack of control
Biological factors	Disinhibitory factors such as caused by brain damage, and some organic mental illnesses
Mental disorder	Psychotic individuals who experience a build-up of tension before a violent outburst Some depressed individuals may attempt to kill others for altruistic reasons, to relieve their supposed suffering Frustration, fear or pain may lead to aggressive responses

IDENTIFYING CUES THAT WARN OF IMMINENT AGGRESSION

At times, for whatever reason, interventions between service users and care staff go wrong. When this occurs, there are three possible types of outcome. The conflict may be resolved peacefully and may even result in positive learning and action; the conflict may be left unresolved and perhaps cause greater trouble at a later stage; or the conflict may escalate and result in some form of aggressive behaviour. Aggression places both clients and staff at risk, so it is essential that interventions are made before this occurs (DiMartino et al 2003).

Behaviour is the first warning of impending aggression in others. Box 12.1 lists a series of behaviours that are associated with aggression.

Staff may ignore such signals owing to a lack of confidence in their own skills to deal with the situation and fear that they could make matters worse rather than better. Unfortunately, avoidance of potential aggression is likely to increase the danger. Consequently, an awareness of the escalation of aggression is essential. Once the danger signals are recognized, limiting action can be taken, and there is consequently a greater probability of a satisfactory outcome.

Table 12.2 Prediction of aggression: the social environment (adapted from Pollock et al 1989, Hinde 1993 and Farrington 1994)

Prediction category	Examples
Peer influences and group pressures	Peer and group pressures to act aggressively may be exerted on individuals Certain geographical areas may process more aggressive cues than others School influences can occur with some schools processing relatively more offenders in their pupils compared with other schools Generally, the cultures that individuals may have been exposed to that do not denigrate aggression may predispose certain individuals to an aggressive response pattern
Economic, social and environmental influences	Economic and social deprivation tend to be associated with offending and sometimes aggressive responses There may be an association between situational influences and aggressive behaviour, such as the availability of weapons Additional social factors include extrafamilial roles, peer group and media influences Uncomfortable or stressful social or physical conditions can predispose to aggression
The presence of a victim	As a subject upon whom aggression is expressed is necessary, so victims are essential in the expression of aggression; the assertion is made here that aggression is not likely to occur without the presence of someone on whom to carry out the aggressive act

Decision-making exercise

Describe factors in each of the following that may contribute to the potential for violence and aggression in a care setting and identify how each might be addressed in your area of work:

- A client or their relatives/friends.
- A member of staff.
- The work environment.
- Event(s), e.g. keeping a client waiting too long.

Box 12.1 Behaviours associated with aggression (from Morrison 1992)

Motor agitation
Increased restlessness and an inability to sit still and concentrate
Rapid movement and change of position
Appearing tense
Foot tapping
Leg swinging
Departure from usual or previous posture
Increased respirations
Grinding of jaw
Sudden loss of colour
Closing hand to make a fist
Thumping fist or slapping hand on another object
Picking up objects
Pacing

Verbalizations
Verbal threats
Intrusive demands for attention
Pitch and volume changes
Shouting or muttering
Significant changes in the pace of speech delivery
Abrupt replies especially if accompanied by gesticulations
Speech directed in 'general' and not at individual
Evidence of delusional or paranoid thought content
Name calling, swearing or being deliberately provocative

Affect
Anger
Hostility
Noisiness increases generally
Sudden or unnatural quiet
Feeling of heightened tension

Level of consciousness
Confusion
Sudden change in mental health status
Disorientation
Memory impairment
Inability to be redirected

You might want to refer to Evolve 12.3 on risk assessment at this point.

12.3 – RISK ASSESSMENT AND RISK MANAGEMENT

- Develop an understanding of risk management within the clinical context

WAYS TO MANAGE AN AGGRESSIVE INCIDENT

What follows here is intended as a general guide. Specific interventions and procedures will be provided by individual employers and these should be used for final guidance.

Responding to violence and aggression

One of the major challenges facing modern health services is responding to violence and aggression but unfortunately there is no simple answer to the problem. During the last 10–15 years there have been a variety of strategies and recommendations, both from government agencies and experts in the management of violence; these have had varying degrees of success. Empirical research into the effectiveness of such actions is lacking and consequently there is confusion as to what constitutes best practice. It is difficult to predict exactly how someone will respond when faced with the threat of violence and aggression. For many staff their choice of response could greatly determine the safety not just of themselves but of everyone involved, and profoundly affect their relationship with those that they care for.

The immediate response to an aggressive incident

Personal safety is priority. Professional codes of conduct do not require individuals to jeopardize their own safety; it is better to leave and find an alternative safer way of containing the situation. If there is no choice but to intervene, however, as would happen if you were unable to remove yourself and needed to defend yourself, colleagues should be alerted via a panic button, call system, emergency telephone or panic alarm. Similarly, bystanders should be asked to leave the area and move to a place of safety.

Containing an aggressive incident: the assault cycle

If the point has been reached where an aggressive act is imminent, then the assault cycle is entered (Fig. 12.2).

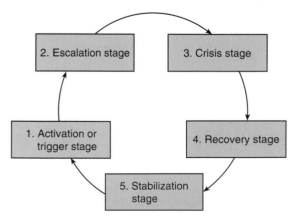

Figure 12.2 The assault cycle.

Using this model helps to identify how the aggression has occurred and the type of intervention that would be most appropriate.

Activation or trigger stage

In this stage some event or interpersonal situation arouses the person. It could be as the result of one thing or an accumulation of things.

> **Decision-making exercise**
>
> Judith woke up late for her morning shift. She went to the kitchen for coffee and breakfast and found that she had run out of milk. Hungry, she left the house, intending to buy a snack from the local shop, only to find when she arrived that she had forgotten her purse. As she could not do without her purse she had to return to her house to collect it. She was now very late and became entangled in morning traffic. Arriving late for work someone said the 'wrong thing' to her and she responded by 'biting their head off!'
>
> Referring to the fight or flight response and the effect of hassles (see Ch. 9, 'stress, relaxation and rest'), offer a possible explanation for Judith's reaction.

Escalation stage

Stress and frustration increase and calming interventions need to be used. Feelings, emotions, attitudes and posture all influence the way that people view and listen to each other. Explaining something to someone who is feeling upset, angry or indignant is difficult until the person's feelings have been relieved. Consequently, the person's feelings need to be recognized and acknowledged. A return to calm remains possible at this stage though and this should be the aim. However, in areas of low support, such as working in the community, the practitioner should aim to extract themselves from this situation and to return to base.

Crisis stage

Physical, emotional and psychological impulses are expressed. If escalation to the crisis stage occurs communication, although more difficult, is a priority intervention. If the situation continues to escalate, however, the personal safety of all is the prime concern and the area around the aggressive individual should be evacuated with help being sought from appropriately qualified staff in sufficient numbers to contain the situation.

Recovery stage

Agitation decreases, anxiety lessens, and communication becomes possible. At this stage the acute crisis has ended.

However, caution still needs to be maintained as the individual may feel upset at how they have been treated and can revert back to the crisis stage. Staff need to maintain control of the situation and contain the risk of further aggression. In some specialist areas, this may require the use of sedation or seclusion, in which case local policies for observation will need to be implemented. Other staff that were called to help may also need to maintain their presence. Alternatively, the individual may be detained by the police.

Stabilization

The client is able to regain control of outward behaviour. Often a post-crisis depression occurs and the individual becomes guarded and uncertain. At this stage he or she is most likely to be receptive to clinical interventions and may feel remorse, guilt or shame for their behaviour. It is important to maintain communication with the client and to find out why the crisis occurred. The client needs to know that he or she is still accepted and the focus should be on how aggression can be avoided in the future. The role of staff is not to judge or punish such clients, but to assist them to live more effective and less problematic lives.

FOLLOWING AN AGGRESSIVE INCIDENT

The nursing management following an aggressive incident falls into two areas: management immediately following the incident and post incident debriefing.

Management immediately following the incident

During this time it is important that things are allowed to return to normal. If appropriate, assistance should be given to get the victim home or to hospital, alerting significant others, retrieving possessions and the like. The immediate concerns of staff should be addressed as far as is possible, even if the incident seems to have been minor. Persistent low-level violence can produce psychological effects as damaging as more serious individual incidents. Likewise staff should be encouraged to fill out formal report forms, including those incidents that appear minor, as 'near misses' can be the precursors to more serious incidents.

Burton (1998) states that prompt and accurate recording of an aggressive incident is essential and should include every relevant detail, even from before the incident occurred. He provides a set of questions that are useful when writing up a report on an aggressive incident (Box 12.2).

While it is important to record an aggressive incident near the time it happened for purposes of accuracy, more important is the support of those involved in the incident itself. No member of staff should be should be left to go home alone as though nothing had happened. Violence

---

Box 12.2 Useful questions for writing a report (from Burton 1998)

- Who was involved?
- Where did it take place?
- What was/were the trigger factor(s)?
- What was the context?
- What was said, and by whom?
- What behaviours were displayed?
- What was the response of those intervening?
- How was the situation handled?
- What were the outcomes?
- What means finally ended the situation?
- What took place following the incident?
- What steps should be taken to prevent such an incident occurring again?

---

should not be seen as 'part of the job'; it cannot always be prevented or avoided, but it can be handled properly, with due regard for the safety and well-being of clients and staff alike. A violent confrontation or attack is an extremely upsetting experience, as well as being very frightening. It is only right that a great deal of thought goes into supporting people who have been subject of an aggressive incident.

Post incident debriefing

Healthcare staff who have encountered an aggressive incident can experience various feelings. Usually, there is a psychological numbing immediately following an attack in which the person begins to try and make sense of what they have just been through. This is followed by feelings of exhaustion, tension, anger and frustration which, over time, may develop into feelings of guilt about the incident. Often people ask 'Could I have done things differently?' or 'Was I to blame for the incident?' There may be a loss of confidence associated with feelings of fear, wariness and apprehension and an overestimation of future violence. In the long term the individual might experience flashbacks and intrusive memories of the event and may reach a state of burnout. There might be a loss of vocation and the person may go off sick or leave the profession altogether.

These feelings and thoughts are normal responses to abnormal circumstances and are generally short-lived. However, there is always the possibility that such feelings and thoughts could develop into something more disabling as in post-traumatic stress disorder. The disorder consists of three main types of symptoms, high arousal (e.g. irritability, startle response), avoidance (e.g. avoiding situations or people associated with an aggressive event) and re-experiencing (e.g.

upsetting and repeated thoughts of the event) (Wykes & Mezey 1994).

It is important that having been involved in a violent or aggressive incident, individuals are allowed to recover and receive practical help and support. Even after minor incidents, feelings may be difficult to control and may affect the ability to return to deal with further problems.

Reviewing the incident

While it is no longer recommended that individuals receive a full debriefing following an aggressive incident (National Institute for Health and Clinical Excellence 2005), it remains important to conduct a review of the situation. The purpose of a review is to take positive learning from the incident to reduce the likelihood of similar situations happening again and to see how such incidents could be managed more effectively, if at all. Littlechild (1996) suggests that strategies for managing aggression should exist at three levels: with practitioners, with managers and at an agency level. This structure should form the basis of a review:

1. At practitioner level opportunities are present for individuals to learn from their experience and they need to adopt different or modified personal strategies.
2. At manager level learning points can be identified and questions concerning issues such as the availability and skill of help provided and the speed of response should be asked.
3. At agency level issues of policy amendment or change may need to be addressed and the effectiveness and availability of post-incident support can be identified.

Decision-making exercise

Your colleague appears down during her clinical placement in the operating theatre. You ask what the problem is and she discloses that a particular consultant appears to be picking on her and ridiculing her for her inexperience at every opportunity. Recently he rapped her across the knuckles with a swab-holder because she held a retractor the wrong way during an operation. She has complained to the theatre manager but was told: 'He is like it with all new nurses until he gets to know them.'

- How does your trust/workplace/unit go about reporting incidences of violence and aggression?
- What constitutes an aggressive act on the part of a:
  – client?
  – relative?
  – member of staff?
- What would you advise your colleague to do next?

Evidence-based practice

In 2000 the Department of Health conducted a national survey into the reported incidences of violence and aggression in NHS trusts and authorities in England. A total number of 84 273 violent or abusive incidents were reported. This was an increase of some 24 000 over the previous year 1998/99 (the only other occasion on which this sort of information had been collected on a national basis).

The survey found that the number of violent incidents varied by trust type; for example, the average for mental health/learning disabilities trusts was two and a half times the average for all trusts. It found that there was a significant underreporting of violence directed at staff working in the NHS and that this was historical. The survey also found that there were differences in the way that data on violent incidents were collected. For example, the definition of a violent incident in one trust might include verbal abuse, and in another trust it might be excluded. Such information is vital if the true level of risk faced by NHS staff is to be identified.

SKILLS USED IN MANAGING AN AGGRESSIVE INCIDENT

So far the interventions have addressed dealing with an aggressor. The following section considers in greater depth the skills required of professionals managing aggression.

Communication skills

Reflection and portfolio exercise

The use of good communication skills when dealing with someone who is aggressive is highlighted throughout the chapter. Carry out a SWOT (strengths, weaknesses, opportunities, threats) analysis of your own communication skills to see where your strengths and weaknesses in communicating with clients lie, and identify the opportunities and threats which may aid or obstruct effective communication with an aggressive client. It is important that you are honest with yourself and again it might be interesting to ask a trusted colleague to complete a separate SWOT analysis of your communication skills, and to compare their perceptions with your own.

An aggressive person may be upset, frightened or confused. The immediate response to someone escalating towards violence is to communicate with them to try to restore calm and stabilize their emotional state.

Verbal communication

This is the initial step towards calming the individual's anger in an attempt to bring about a more rational discussion of the situation (Burton 1998, United Kingdom Central Council 2002). Several strategies can help here:

- Acknowledge the existence of the problem.
- Use active listening skills.
- Show genuine concern and understanding.
- Give reassurance and support as appropriate.

Supportiveness

Being supportive and avoiding defensiveness. Accept that the person is angry, and avoid retaliatory remarks. Ask questions that focus on the aggressor. For example: 'Tell me more about how you feel.' You must also be prepared to accept criticism, and you may even seek it by asking: 'What is it about my behaviour that is annoying you?' Allow the person time to express how they feel, and do not be in a hurry to resolve the encounter (Garnham 2001).

Certain phrases may be provocative and make an aggressive individual even angrier. Examples include: 'Now don't be silly', 'Pull yourself together', 'This is no way for an adult to behave', or even, 'You're not the only person with this problem!'. While the latter might seem an obvious thing not to do, it is surprising how many times the author has heard such phrases used in clinical practice, particularly when the member of staff has been under pressure or felt threatened.

Problem solving

When the situation is calmer, encourage the individual to identify and explain the nature of the problem, and to try and identify a solution. Do not agree or disagree and be careful not to get drawn into an argument, or to promise anything that cannot be delivered, as this could escalate the situation. This is a useful method of getting the person to take responsibility for their actions by promoting a sense of ownership and control over the situation, especially if you can get them to identify the best and most appropriate way forward.

Reflection and portfolio exercise

The meaning behind words is conveyed by the way in which they are spoken. We have a degree of control over what we say, but much less control over the way that we speak. If we are to appear calm in the face of an aggressor then we need to give some thought as to how we present

ourselves verbally to another. Consider the following non-verbal aspects of verbal communication:

- Clarity of speech – clear or indecipherable?
- Volume – too quiet or too loud?
- Tone – appropriate, soft, sarcastic?
- Modulation – adjustment of tone and pitch
- Stress – pressure and/or emphasis
- Silences – pauses and hesitations
- Respirations and sighing.

Information giving

This is a fundamental part of the role of all who work in health and social care, to the point that its importance is sometimes forgotten. Patients and their relatives can become agitated and threaten to harm staff when information is not forthcoming or is withheld. Confusion as to what is expected of the patient and not being involved in decisions relating to their care can provoke similar responses. The healthcare worker can determine what the patient's information needs are simply by asking.

When giving information, it is best to give important messages first in order that they are understood and retained. Repeating and stressing points is another strategy by which important information is emphasized. Also, try to be consistent in what you are saying and avoid confusing and conflicting messages. When giving information:

- Repeat and stress important points.
- Give important messages first.
- Try to be consistent, avoid confusing or conflicting messages.

Validation

Often, people who experience intense anger and rage feel isolated and may view themselves as alone in having these feelings. The healthcare worker can use past experience and knowledge to normalize the patient's reaction and validate the experience, and in turn bring control to the situation. For example, it may be appropriate to give the person 'permission' to use bad language as a means of expressing themselves, acknowledging that it is something you do when angry or frustrated.

Depersonalizing the situation

Depersonalize the issues in circumstances where you have no personal influence over decisions. Let the person know it is not your personal decision, but is due to the policy of the organization. Provide information about complaint procedures and alternative sources of help, if appropriate.

Personalizing the situation

This is the opposite of the above, where you take responsibility for your actions and decisions in an effort to promote dialogue and understanding of the matter. In doing so it allows the two of you to explore alternatives and engage on a much more personal level.

Exploring beliefs

It can be useful to explore the beliefs the patient has about the expression of anger. Discussion of beliefs that prevent the person from seeking alternative ways of handling the situation may help the patient to take charge of the situation. Interventions of this kind are designed to help the person in finding alternatives to the use of violence and aggression, and should be encouraged.

Listening to the patient's illness experience

Often patients and their family members are invited to provide details about past medical treatments, medication, hospitalizations and therapies. What is overlooked is the experience of the health problem or the experience of interactions with professionals. Inviting patients and their families to talk about their previous experiences with the healthcare system may highlight both their concerns and resources.

Non-verbal communication

Every time verbal communication takes place it is complemented with a complex repertoire of movements and gestures. Non-verbal communication helps to maintain the flow of communication and acts as a subtle indicator to show when a person has finished speaking. Appropriate use of non-verbal communication demonstrates interest and understanding of an individual's problems. Of particular use when working with aggressive individuals, correct interpretation of non-verbal communication provides considerable insight into the other person.

Not only is it important to be sensitive to the aggressor's non-verbal communication, but sensitivity to and awareness of our own body signals is also vital. Using body language appropriately in a helping relationship can help to facilitate an individual's trust and confidence. The use of tone of voice, eye contact, touch, facial expression and posture can convey the qualities of genuineness and warmth. Using non-verbal communication effectively can help the individual to relax and increase the likelihood of them

exploring their problems in a more constructive manner. The following section examines some of the common defusion strategies that can be employed using non-verbal communication when faced with an aggressor.

Mood matching

This is where the arousal level is matched between all people in the interaction. For example, in a conversation with someone who feels depressed, people attempt to be slightly 'downbeat'. Similarly, the mood is reasonably cheerful when talking to someone who is happy or excited about something.

In contrast, when talking to somebody who is agitated people attempt to be calm, so not to inflame the situation. The danger of this is that it can be misinterpreted as indifference. One option is to match the other person with a similar level of energy. However, in this instance, energy would not be a displayed as aggression. Rather it would be shown by concern, involvement and interest.

Mirroring

This is the physical equivalent of mood matching. Mirroring is exactly as it says: it is where one person physically reflects the way the other person is sitting or standing. Normally this occurs entirely spontaneously; if one person sits back then so does the other one, if one person comes forward then the other does likewise, and so forth. Observational research shows that people who are mirroring each other tend to get on better than those who do not ('getting on' being measured by the length of conversation they have) in spite of the fact that this is normally going on unconsciously. It is possible to utilize this phenomenon and use it to enhance the interactions with the aggressor. This needs to be done with some caution, however, as if exaggerated, it may be seen to be mimicking or mocking.

Eye contact

This is also an important and sometimes misunderstood area (Linsley 2006). In an escalating aggressive situation there are various types of exchange:

- Stage 1 is before any aggressive interaction has taken place and the eye contact is of an ordinary pattern.
- Stage 2 is where either or both parties sense that the conversation is gradually becoming more heated and one or both attempt to minimize eye contact.
- Stage 3 is where the situation is unambiguously aggressive and almost out of hand. This is where eye contact is of a long duration, high intensity, challenging and aversive.

The task therefore, is to try to maintain the pattern of ordinary eye contact, appropriate to stage 1, apparently not noticing any changes in eye contact demonstrated by the other person. If eye contact is too threatening, however, averting the gaze to the shoulders is effective as it signifies non-confrontational interest, but it also allows the aggressor to be kept in full view.

Touch

Touch in the common course of treatment can be a sign of positive communication; aggression is also primarily expressed through bodily contact and therefore it is recommended to avoid touching clients who are aroused or angry. Likewise, invading a person's personal space can be perceived as a threat. Encroachment of this by anyone who is uninvited creates feelings of uneasiness and crowding. This is important to remember when addressing an aggressive person as there is the danger of invading the aggressor's personal space and escalating the situation. Therefore a distance should be maintained between the nurse and the potential aggressor, mindful of the need to keep a safe means of exit.

Communicating assertively

Farrell & Gray (1992) made the observation that being assertive is an effective way of dealing with aggression. Assertive people are confident in and relaxed when dealing with others. They have a clear idea of their personal rights and do not allow others to infringe on them. They are able to say 'no' clearly and directly to other people, to ask for what they want, and to negotiate an equitable compromise in a difficult situation. They can respond to criticism realistically, accept complaints and handle put-downs.

The application of assertiveness in situations that threaten aggression assumes that people are attacked or victimized, or are in danger of becoming aggressive themselves, partly because they do not express their wishes or do so in a socially ineffective manner (McDonnell et al 1994). While assertiveness training may help people who are not confident to manage difficult situations more effectively, there are those that this approach does not suit and who are not comfortable with being assertive. Being assertive, like any other skill, needs to be practised and developed, and there is always the danger that if used inappropriately then it could exacerbate a situation rather than resolve it. A further drawback of this approach is that people may slip from being assertive to being aggressive (McDonnell et al 1994).

If nurses are to use assertiveness techniques then they need to be given proper training in their use. There are undoubtedly a number of benefits to be had from being assertive; however, in order to use such skills effectively, the nurse needs to appreciate and clearly understand the difference between being assertive and being aggressive.

> **Reflection and portfolio exercise**
>
> Experiment with assertive responses in situations that you find difficult. You could do this by the means of role play, enacting such situations with a colleague, trying out different responses and techniques. Likewise you could video the role play and make an analysis of your assertive skills with a view to bringing about change.

LIMITING THE NUMBER OF AGGRESSIVE INCIDENTS

Prevention

Prevention is always better than cure; however, it is impossible to eliminate incidents of aggression completely. Furthermore, it is impossible to generalize one approach to reduce aggression to all situations (Royal College of Nursing 1998). Prevention consequently uses all available information to minimize the risk of incidents occurring, including learning from the experiences of previous incidents. It is therefore essential that staff are encouraged to report identified risks to managers, as well as incidents that have occurred, so that learning can take place and appropriate action can be taken.

The physical environment has a significant effect on the likelihood of aggressive incidents occurring, and the ease with which people can respond to them. A poor environment suggests that neither patients nor staff are valued, which in turn can exacerbate frustration and aggression. Consequently, areas should be kept clean, hospitable, and above all welcoming, particularly reception and waiting rooms. All signs should be clear, simple and suitably visible, to direct people to the appropriate location, e.g. treatment rooms, toilets and other facilities.

Excessive time spent waiting to be seen can sometimes lead clients to become aggressive. The policy should therefore be to prevent waiting times as far as possible. Be honest about how long the person will have to wait. If you do not know how long it will be, then tell them so. Similarly, should additional delays suddenly occur, such as will happen in an emergency, explain the situation to those waiting and tell them how long a delay is expected. In many areas this is achieved by updating the expected waiting time for non-urgent cases on an electronic display system.

The design of facilities should also ensure uncrowded service conditions for staff. Rooms for interviewing clients should ensure privacy while avoiding isolation of the staff. In emergency departments, rooms are needed in which agitated patients or family may be separated safely to protect themselves, other clients and staff. A lack of space or a poor physical layout can create tensions between service users; this can lead to an increase in violence and aggression. Counselling or service rooms should be designed with two exits, if possible, and furniture should be arranged to prevent entrapment of staff. Doors should have unbreakable glass or plastic panels to enable colleagues to monitor the situation if there are concerns (such panels could be frosted to allow some degree of privacy). Consider the weight, size and construction of moveable objects within rooms. Access to staff counselling rooms, treatment rooms and other facility areas should be controlled. All doors from client waiting rooms should be locked from the inside, and outside doors locked from the outside (in accordance with fire codes) to prevent unauthorized entry. Lockable and secure bathrooms and other amenities should be provided for staff members, separate from client restrooms. All permanent and temporary employees who work in a secured area should be given keys to gain access or exit when on duty.

Access to buildings should be controlled and monitored and, where possible, they should have a single point of entry/exit. Patients and their relatives should not be left to wander aimlessly; a clear indication as to where they should proceed in order to seek help and assistance should be evident. Blind spots can make it difficult to observe patients and can lead to an increase in self-harming episodes. Therefore, the area should allow unimpeded sight lines with access points within sight of staff. To facilitate this, curved mirrors may be installed at hallway intersections or concealed areas.

Outside, bright and effective lighting systems should be installed. Parking for staff should be close to the building, lighted and free from heavy vegetation or anything that could conceal potential assailants. Where this is not possible, staff should make a point of not returning to their cars alone at the end of their shift, but to go with a colleague. Employers should also make provision for the safe escort of staff when required.

Reflection and portfolio exercise

Take a walk through the area which you are currently working.

- How safe is it?

RISK MANAGEMENT

Safe systems of work

The best approach to manage violence and aggression in the workplace is to minimize the opportunity of it occurring (risk prevention). However, if prevention is impossible, planning should focus on reducing the impact on the people, the workplace and the work processes (risk reduction and risk management). A safe system of work is a formal procedure, which results from a systematic examination of the task in order to identify all the hazards and assess the risks. It also identifies safe methods of work, to ensure that the hazards are eliminated or the remaining risks are minimized. While the student nurse may contribute in this process, it is for the more senior grades to ensure that such matters are instigated, put into action and their effectiveness monitored.

With the current focus on risk management there is an increased impetus for managers and clinicians to identify risk assessment practice and develop preventive strategies in the control and management of violence and aggression (Royal College of Psychiatrists 1999). Professional competence is demonstrated by making an assessment of risk factors and instigating appropriate interventions (Erskine 1991) utilizing a theory based framework (Allen 1997). Current trends indicate that a continuous risk management approach to aggression, to accommodate changes in risk, is likely to be the most effective (Paterson et al 1999).

Two important points must be borne in mind when designing a risk assessment. First, it should be integrated with other risk assessments within health and safety, and can generally draw on their logic and methods. Second, the risk assessment should be fit for the purpose for which it was designed. As yet there are no well worked out and validated systems of risk assessment for work-related violence that are easily available; however, risk from violence and aggression can be regarded as a function of four factors (Royal College of Nursing 1998):

- The frequency of potential conflict situations.
- The duration of the conflict situation.
- The likelihood of the individuals involved acting in a violent or aggressive manner.
- The magnitude of the harm caused.

One person alone cannot make an adequate risk assessment and information should be gathered from a number of sources. It should also be borne in mind that risk is dynamic and is largely dependent on circumstance, which can alter over a brief period of time. Because of this, risk assessment needs to be predominantly short term and subject to frequent review. Actions to reduce the identified risk can then be taken based on the findings of the risk assessment. These may include relatively small measures such as removing from a room ornaments that could be used as weapons to more major measures such as providing closed circuit television units (CCTV) and monitoring clinical areas.

The Royal College of Psychiatrists (1999) made a number of recommendations with reference to the structure and layout of rooms used to interview clients and their relatives. These are worth considering for all clinical areas and are as follows:

1. Healthcare workers should have safe working conditions and should not be expected to interview clients in isolated rooms. Interview rooms should be situated close to main staff areas.
2. All interview rooms should have a readily accessible panic button or an emergency call system, with policies for staff to respond rapidly to the alarm when it is activated.
3. The exit to all interview rooms should be unimpeded. Doors must not require a key to exit. Ideally doors should open outwards.
4. The furniture should be suitable and the room should be free from clutter.
5. It is advisable to have an internal inspection window, to permit viewing when the room is occupied.

Maintenance

General maintenance must be an integral part of any safety and security systems. Prompt repair and replacement of burned out lights, broken windows or locks, etc. is essential to maintain the system in safe operating condition. Delays in mending equipment, for instance broken televisions, can create tensions between patients that can lead to an increase in violence and aggression. An inability to ensure that clinical areas are maintained to an acceptable standard and that equipment is mended or replaced speedily can impact on the morale of staff and their ability to work effectively with patients (Linsley 2006). Any mechanical device utilized for security and safety should be routinely tested for effectiveness and maintained on a scheduled basis and in accord with manufacturers' recommendations. For example, to be effective, alarm systems, including personal alarm devices, must be tested and maintained according to manufacturer and facility policy. Batteries and operation of the alarm devices should be

checked by competent persons to ensure that the system functions properly.

PROFESSIONAL AND ETHICAL KNOWLEDGE

The management of violence and aggression makes explicit the need to have an understanding of legal principles and law. This helps staff to make decisions and leads to greater confidence when confronted with a challenging situation. Highlighted within the following section are areas of the law that require further consideration when dealing with violence and aggression within clinical practice.

Aggression is unacceptable and constitutes a fundamental violation of human and legal rights that can lead to criminal and civil law prosecution. Trusts, as employers, have duties, with respect to the management of work-related violent incidents, framed by both national and European health and safety legislation and in the UK by their common law duty of care (Royal College of Nursing 1998).

THE OBLIGATIONS OF EMPLOYERS

An employer must take reasonable care to protect employees from risk of foreseeable injury, disease or death at work. If an employer knows of a risk to the safety of their staff, and has failed to take reasonable steps to avoid or protect against the risk, he or she will be liable if a member of staff is injured or killed, or suffers illness as a result of the risk. The requirements on employers, under the health and safety legislation, have been summarized by the Health Services Advisory Committee (1997) and the Royal College of Nursing (1998) as follows:

The Health and Safety and Welfare at Work Act 1974

Employers must:

- protect the health and safety of their employees
- protect the health and safety of others who might be affected by the way they go about their work.

The Management of Health and Safety at Work Regulations 1999

Employers must:

- assess all risks to the health and safety of their employees
- identify the precautions needed
- make arrangements for the effective management of precautions

- appoint competent people to advise them on health and safety
- provide information and training to employees.

Regulation 13. Capabilities and Training

When allocating work to employees, employers should ensure that the demands of the job do not exceed the employees' abilities to carry out work without risk to themselves or others. This should take place during working hours and employees should not be required to pay for their own training.

Reporting of Injuries, Diseases and Dangerous Occurrences Regulations 1995 (RIDDOR 1995)

Employers must:

- report all cases in which employees have suffered death or major injury or have been off work for 3 days or more following an assault that has resulted in physical injury.

The Employment Rights Act 1996

Employees are also protected by the Employment Rights Act 1996, which says that they must not be disadvantaged or dismissed on particular health and safety grounds. These grounds include raising health and safety concerns with the employer and taking protective action such as leaving the workplace in the event of serious and imminent danger. For example, a community nurse is protected from any action by their employer if they leave a client's home because of abuse or violence from the client or a relative.

THE OBLIGATIONS OF EMPLOYEES

While it is the responsibility of the employing organization to provide safe systems of work, individuals also have a responsibility to follow safe working practices. In their everyday work, employees need to remain watchful for their own safety and that of their colleagues. However, the problem with the law is that it does not always explain how far staff may go in dealing with violent and aggressive acts. Any direct and intentional application of force to another person without lawful justification is battery, and in the healthcare setting this might include the use of restraint, sedation or forcibly searching a client.

As part of self-defence, any person can take reasonable steps to ensure that he or she does not come to any harm and that harm does not befall another; i.e. self-defence can be carried out on behalf of someone else. Self-defence can also be used to discourage or prevent unlawful force

and to avoid or escape from unlawful detention, although it is important to demonstrate to the aggressor that there is no desire to fight and a willingness to disengage.

The term 'reasonableness' in law means that the force used is actually necessary. Therefore, if a client could be dealt with by non-physical means, the use of physical restraint would constitute an assault. In addition, the force must be proportionate to the harm to be avoided and the degree and duration of force must be proportionate to the harm that is being avoided. This concept is complex, and it can only be determined in any particular instance in a court of law. However, it has been defined by Dimond (2005) as follows:

> the force used should be not more than was necessary to accomplish the object for which it is allowed (so retaliation, revenge and punishment are not permitted) and secondly, the reaction must be in proportion to the harm which is threatened in both degree and duration.

With the passing of the Crime and Disorder Act 1998, local authorities and police, in co-operation with other bodies such as NHS trusts and health authorities, are required to develop and implement crime and disorder strategies. Some trusts are actively involved with local crime prevention groups to share information, advice and intelligence on particular issues which might influence how best to manage difficult situations and we see evidence of this within the Zero Tolerance campaign highlighted below.

Zero Tolerance

In October 1999 the Department of Health launched the NHS Zero Tolerance campaign to inform the public that aggression, violence and threatening behaviour will not be tolerated by staff working in the health service. The guidance aims to balance staff protection with the duty to provide services, and states that care will be denied to those who abuse staff. However, the government also states that care is not to be denied to clients with severe mental health problems or other conditions that clinicians think leave the client incapable of taking responsibility for their actions.

The guidance is driven not just by health and safety requirements and the duty of care owed by employers but also by the Human Rights Act 1998 which seeks to protect the dignity and feelings of employees from 'inhuman' or 'degrading' treatment on the part of the employer (Article 3). In addition, the campaign has been backed by new prosecution procedures for both staff and service users resulting in closer working between NHS trusts and other local agencies such as the police and the Crown Prosecution Service, resulting in an increase of successful prosecutions against individuals for assaulting staff (Schwehr 2001).

Reporting incidents

Documentation of violent incidents in the workplace is part of preventive action. Collecting and analysing data (including near-misses) helps to establish whether there is a pattern of incidents, and to identify particular targets or practices at risk. Although reporting systems will be tailored to fit the organizational structure and the type of work undertaken, it is useful to record:

- the number of incidents
- when they occur
- the types of staff involved
- the categories of patients involved
- the environments or locations where incidents happen
- the level of injuries sustained
- the preventive measures recommended.

Burton (1998) stresses that prompt and accurate recording of an aggressive incident is essential and should include every relevant detail, including factors before the incident occurred. This allows investigation into the incident, and remedial action, to start quickly. Reporting incidents also helps to identify trends to assist in the process of review, and helps to inform risk assessments. The Reporting of Injuries, Diseases and Dangerous Occurrences Regulations 1995 (RIDDOR) require employers to notify their enforcing authority in the event of an accident at work to an employee. This includes any act of non-consensual physical violence done to a person at work. In addition to this, employers must also report cases in which employees have been off work for 3 working days or more following an assault that resulted in physical injury. Likewise, the Counter Fraud and Security Management Service (CFSMS) has also instigated a reporting system which managers are required to abide by in the event of a physical assault.

'Whistleblowing'

The Safety Representatives and Safety Committees Regulations 1997 and the Health and Safety (Consultation with Employees) Regulations (1996) state that employers must inform and consult with employees on matters relating to their health and safety (including possible violence and aggression), and that employee representatives may make representations to their employer on matters affecting their health and safety. However, some employers may choose to ignore employee concerns and this may lead employees to raise their concerns in a more public arena.

The Public Interest Disclosure Act 1998 protects whistleblowers from victimization and dismissal when they speak out, but their concerns must be genuine and must have been raised (unless there are very good reasons for not doing so) internally or with a specified person. It reflects public concern about the difficulties for workers to speak out when they believe something is seriously wrong in their workplace.

In order to be protected, the disclosure has to show one or more of the following has occurred:

- a criminal act
- a failure to comply with legal obligation (including negligence, breach of contract, including contract of employment, and breach of administrative law)
- a miscarriage of justice
- danger to health and safety
- damage to the environment
- an attempt to cover up any of these.

It is sufficient for the worker to have a reasonable belief that their information is correct; this means that the worker will not have to prove their disclosure is accurate, but they will need to demonstrate that they acted in good faith.

Special considerations: community care

Although the issues raised so far in the chapter also apply to community care, one important difference exists: that nurses working in the community often work on their own in clients' homes. To this end extra thought and consideration needs to be given to the issue of safety. To avoid being isolated in a client's home the community nurse should ensure that someone else within the team knows of their visit, both in terms of where they are going and when they should return. To this end it is also important to let colleagues know of any change in itinerary and what is expected of them in the event of the community nurse not returning at the designated time.

Where possible, the community nurse should arrange for contact with clients of particular concern to be made in a surgery or other health service premises where support staff will be available. Where a home visit cannot be avoided, however, the appointment should be scheduled for a time of day that affords extra security, such as the morning when parents are around taking their children to school and when drug activity and drunkenness should be at a minimum. If necessary, the community nurse should be prepared to take a colleague to accompany them and, if appropriate, ask the police for escort. In addition to this, the community nurse should be prepared to readdress the goals of their visit if the situation is not how they expected it to be and leave if they feel threatened or unsure. Consideration should be given over to the type of shoes and clothes that are worn by the community nurse. Shoes and clothes should not hinder movement or the nurse's ability to run.

While there has been an improvement to the network coverage enjoyed by mobile phone users within the British Isles, there are areas that receive a limited signal, particularly in buildings. It is important therefore that staff do not rely on mobile phones and ensure that other systems are in place to alert staff of possible difficulties. Likewise,

thought should be given to where the nurse has parked his or her car as it is likely that this will be the only means of escape if things go wrong. To this end the nurse should ensure that their vehicle has sufficient petrol, that it is well maintained, and that it is parked facing in the direction that will allow a rapid escape if required.

PERSONAL AND REFLECTIVE KNOWLEDGE

Reflection and portfolio evidence

Become aware of your own reactions to aggression

This exercise is intended to increase your analytical skills with regard to aggressive incidents. Using Johns' reflective model below, draw on your own experience or from peers or other professional nurses to look at an aggressive incident that took place in practice.

CHRISTOPHER JOHNS' MODEL FOR STRUCTURED REFLECTION

This model (Johns 1993) offers a series of questions for the nurse to help reflection on experience:

1. Can you describe your experience? What happened?
2. What caused the events to happen as they did?
3. What significant background factors were there? What was the context of the event?
4. Can you reflect on your experience? Try considering the following:
   (a) What were you trying to achieve?
   (b) Why did you intervene as you did?
   (c) What were the consequences for you, the client, relatives and colleagues?
   (d) How did you feel about the experience when it was happening?
   (e) How did the client feel about it and how do you know this?
   (f) What factors or knowledge influenced your decisions and actions?
5. Did you have any options and what would have been their consequences?
6. What have you learned from the experience? For example:
   (a) How do you feel about the experience *now*?
   (b) Could you have dealt better with the situation?
Once you have completed this exercise you can include it in your portfolio.

CASE STUDIES INVOLVING AGGRESSIVE BEHAVIOUR

There now follow four case studies, one from each branch of nursing. Using the evidence presented in this chapter, try to answer the questions at the end of each scenario.

Case study: Adult

Staff Nurse Clare Marsden works on a medical admission ward. Following the new admission of an elderly lady, the lady's husband requests to see Clare in private. The lady's husband explains that he has been looking after his wife since she had a stroke several months ago and that he had been 'forced into bringing her into hospital by their GP!' He becomes more and more angry as he relates to Clare his concerns for his wife's well-being. He is worried that his wife 'won't get the attention in hospital that she did at home', 'that she won't have company', 'that she'll be left to rot in bed', and that 'she would never get home again!' While expressing his concerns for his wife he invades Clare's personal space, making her feel ill at ease. He starts to raise his voice and becomes animated in both his speech and behaviour, punctuating his sentences with a pointing finger.

- What factors may underlie Mr Marsden's behaviour?
- What strategies could Clare possibly adopt to meet the situation?
- Should the incident be reported? If so, to whom and in what format?

Case study: Child

Max is aged 9 years. Following the recent death of his father in a car accident Max has become increasing hostile in his manner. He has physically fought with friends to the point that they will no longer play with him, and he now argues with his mother on a frequent basis.

On one occasion he spat at her and on another lashed out with his fists and feet. Max's mother confides in you during a visit to the Well Woman's clinic that she feels unable to control Max's behaviour and that he is 'escalating out of control!' She feels that 'she has not only lost her husband but her son as well'.

- How might Max's mother seek to address his anger and aggressive manner?
- What support could you offer Max's mother?
- What agencies within your local area could you refer Max and his mother to for more specialist help if needed?

Case study: Learning disabilities

Barbara is a woman in her early forties who had been resident in a long-stay hospital for people with learning disabilities. Although Barbara had a history of aggression, the incidences and severity of these outbursts were not as marked as they had been in the past. In fact everything seemed to be going well for Barbara until she was moved to a small community home run largely by mental health nurses following a merger of local healthcare services. Shortly after her transfer, Barbara's behaviour has deteriorated, resulting in her lashing out and striking a member of staff.

- With reference to knowledge gained in this chapter, offer possible explanations as to why Barbara's behaviour might have deteriorated.

- How could this situation have been better managed to prevent distress and aggression?
- What strategies might the staff of the new unit employ to bring the situation under control and address Barbara's needs?

Case study: Mental health

Mr Smith is a young man of 25 years. He has a medical diagnosis of paranoid personality disorder. He was 'persuaded' to come into hospital by the local community psychiatric nurse after he had voiced thoughts of harming his neighbours, who he believed to be 'out to get him'.

Following admission Mr Smith decides that he is not staying, as he now believes the nurses to be in league with his neighbours. On attempting to make his exit from the ward he threatens to 'punch the lights out' of a male staff nurse who tries to converse with him and encourage him to stay 'until he has seen the doctor'.

- What should the immediate actions of the staff nurse be?
- What factors should be taken into consideration when addressing Mr Smith's safety and well-being?
- What factors should be taken into consideration when addressing the needs of the other clients on the ward and staff members?

SUMMARY

This chapter has emphasized the need to be aware of potential outbursts of aggression in nursing practice. A wide range of issues relating to the management of aggression was explored, including:

1. Through various approaches, several challenging areas of nursing practice were highlighted in relation to the control and management of aggression, for example communication skills, assessment skills and practices, documentation requirements, policies and procedures and support available.
2. Key concepts include maintaining a therapeutic milieu, preventing escalation, identifying aggressive patterns of behaviour and using appropriate interventions.
3. Properly trained staff can improve the quality of life within the healthcare environment by decreasing frustration and fear for staff and clients alike.
4. Further recommendations include the need to adopt a risk management approach to working with potentially aggressive individuals, as well as the development of guidelines in aggressive management.
5. It is from this base that professional decision making can develop.

Annotated further reading and websites

Bibby P 1995 Personal safety for health care workers. Arena, Aldershot
The book on personal safety for healthcare workers by Pauline Bibby from the Suzy Lamplugh Trust offers a more personally orientated approach and gives advice for personal safety. Very useful chapters include assertiveness and practical steps to safety, as well as guidelines for travelling. This book also contains a chapter devoted to trainers in the management of violence.

Breakwell G 1995 General and specific clues and dangerousness checklist. In: Kidd B, Stark C (eds) Management of violence and aggression in health care. Gaskell, London
For a concise account of the current theories concerning aggression this chapter is an excellent resource of recent developments. The chapter also contains an account of the assault cycle.

Kidd B, Stark C 1995 Management of violence and aggression in health care. Gaskell, London
This book offers useful chapters on the practical management of aggression.

Royal College of Nursing 1998 Dealing with violence against nursing staff. Royal College of Nursing, London
This publication is concerned with the nature and management of violent incidents that NHS staff may encounter in the course of their work. Full of practical hints and advice.

Storr A 1992 Human aggression. Penguin, Harmondsworth
For a wider view of aggression in terms of social, individual and interpersonal factors, this book makes interesting and useful reading.

http://www.dh.gov.uk/en/Publicationsandstatistics/Publications/
PublicationsPolicyAndGuidance/DH_4007545

Department of Health 1999 NHS Zero Tolerance: we don't have to take this. HMSO, London

A useful resource that reminds the healthcare worker that they need not put up with violence and aggression in the workplace.

http://www.fnrh.freeserve.co.uk/index1.html
The Forensic Nursing Resource Homepage maintained by Phil Woods, Senior Lecturer in Forensic Mental Health Nursing, Florence Nightingale School of Nursing and Midwifery, King's College London. An excellent resource that includes research papers, articles, assessment tools and links to other relevant websites.

http://www.suzylamplugh.org/home/index.shtml
The Suzy Lamplugh Trust homepage. This contains links to resource packs, many of which need to be purchased. You can jump from this site to the trust's training department who can organize personal safety conferences. There is also a shop section selling personal safety equipment on-line.

**http://www.homeoffice.gov.uk/documents/keep-safe-booklet?
view=Binary**
Home Office guidance on personal safety. Advice for maintaining personal safety in a range of situations, and what to do if you have been attacked.

http://www.bullying.co.uk
A resource targeted at supporting those who suffer from workplace bullying. A useful resource; however, if you do feel that you are being bullied then your professional organization or union representative should be your first contact.

References

Akert MR, Aronson E, Wilson DT 2005 Social psychology, 5th edn. Pearson, Upper Saddle River

Allen J 1997 Assessing and managing risk and violence in the mentally disordered. Journal of Psychiatric and Mental Health Nursing 4:369–378

Anderson CA, Dill KE 2000 Video games and aggressive thoughts, feelings and behaviour in the laboratory and in life. Journal of Personality and Social Psychology 78:772–790

Beresford B, Coccaro EF, Minar P, Kaskow J, Geracioti T 2006 CSF testosterone: relationship to aggression, impulsivity and venturesomeness in adult males with personality disorder. Journal of Psychiatric Research 41(6):488–492

Berkowitz L 1990 On the formation and regulation of anger and aggression: a cognitive–neoassociationist analysis. American Psychologist 45:494–503

Berkowitz L 1993 Pain and aggression: some findings and implications. Psychological Bulletin 106:59–73

Berkowitz L 2001 Affect, aggression and antisocial behaviour. In: Davidson RJ, Scherer K, Goldsmith HH (eds) Handbook of affective sciences. Oxford University Press, Oxford

Bibby P 1995 Personal safety for health care workers. Arena, Aldershot

Burton R 1998 Violence and aggression in the workplace. Mental Health Care 2(3):105–108

Bushman BJ 1995 Moderating role of trait aggressiveness in the effects of violent media on aggression. Journal of Personal and Social Psychology 69:950–960

Bushman BJ 1998 Priming effects of violent media on the accessibility of aggressive constructs in the memory. Personality and Social Psychology Bulletin 24:537–545

Buss A 1995 Personality: temperament, social behaviour and the self. Allyn & Bacon, Boston

Cohen DJ, Eckhardt CI, Schagat KD 1998 Attention allocation and habituation to anger-related stimuli during a visual search task. Aggressive Behaviour 24:399–409

Counter Fraud and Security Management Services 2006 Tackling violence against staff. Counter Fraud Security Management Services, London

Department of Health 1999 We don't have to take this: NHS guidance on zero tolerance. Department of Health, London

Department of Health 2000 2000/2001 Survey of reported violent or abusive incidents, accidents involving staff and sickness absence in NHS authorities in England. Department of Health, London

Department of Health 2006 POVA guidance. Department of Health, London

DiMartino V, Hoel H, Cooper CL 2003 Preventing violence and harassment in the workplace. European Foundation for the Improvement of Living and Working Conditions, Dublin

Dimond B 2005 Legal aspects of nursing, 4th edn. Prentice Hall, London

Dollard J, Doob LW, Miller NE et al 1939 Frustration and aggression. Yale University Press, New Haven

Employment Rights Act 1996 HMSO, London

Erskine P 1991 Violence and mental illness. Heritage Publishing, Moruya, New South Wales

Farrell GA, Gray C 1992 Aggression: a nurse's guide to therapeutic management. Scutari Press, London

Farrington DP 1994 The causes and prevention of offending, with special reference to violence. In: Shepherd J (ed) Violence in health care: a practical guide to coping with violence and caring for victims. Oxford University Press, Oxford, pp 149–177

Ferns T, Chojnacha I 2005 Reporting incidents of violence and aggression towards NHS staff. Nursing Standard 19:51–60

Frankl G 1990 The unknown self. Open Gate Press, London

Freedman JL 2002 Media violence and its effect on aggression: assessing the scientific evidence. University of Toronto Press, Toronto

Garnham P 2001 Understanding and dealing with anger, aggression and violence. Nursing Standard 16(6):37–42

Geen RG 2001 Human aggression, 2nd edn. Taylor & Francis, London

Health and Safety and Welfare at Work Act 1974 HMSO, London

Health and Safety Executive 2004 Reducing risks – protecting people. HSE, London

Health Services Advisory Committee 1997 Violence and aggression to staff in health services: guidance on assessment and management. HSE Books, Sudbury

Hinde RA 1993 Aggression at different levels of social complexity. In: Taylor PJ (ed) Violence in society. Royal College of Physicians, London

Hines DA, Kimberly JS 2003 Gender differences in psychological, physical, and sexual aggression among college students using the revised conflict tactics scales. Violence and Victims 18(7):197–217

HM Government 2006 Working together to safeguard children: a guide to inter-agency working to safeguard and promote the welfare of children. HM Government, London

Hollin CR 1992 Criminal behaviour. Falmer Press, Brighton

Hollinworth H, Clark C, Harland R et al 2005 Understanding the arousal of anger: a patient centred approach. Nursing Standard 19:41–47

Human Rights Act 1998 HMSO, London

Johns C 1993 Professional supervision. Journal of Nursing Management 1(1):9–18

Kaukiainen A, Salmivalli C, Bjorkqvist K et al 2001 Overt and covert aggression in work settings in relation to the subjective well-being of employees. Aggressive Behaviour 27:360–371

Linsley P 2006 Violence and aggression in the workplace: a practical guide for all healthcare staff. Radcliffe Press, Oxford

Littlechild B 1996 The risk of violence and aggression to social work and social work staff. In: Kemshall H, Pritchard H (eds) Good practice in risk assessment and risk management. Jessica Kingsley, London

McDonnell A, McEvoy J, Dearden RL 1994 Coping with violent situations in the caring environment. In: Wykes T (ed) Violence and health care professionals. Chapman & Hall, London, pp 189–207

McElliskem JE 2004 Affective and predatory violence: a biomedical system of human aggression and violence. Aggression and Violent Behaviour 10:1–30

Management of Health and Safety at Work Regulations 1999 HMSO, London

Morrison E 1992 A hierarchy of aggressive and violent behaviours among psychiatric inpatients. Hospital and Community Psychiatry 43:505

National Institute for Health and Clinical Excellence 2005 Violence: the short term management of disturbed/violent behaviour in psychiatric in-patient and emergency departments – guidance. National Institute for Health and Clinical Excellence, London

Nursing and Midwifery Council 2008 The Code: standards of conduct, performance and ethics for nurses and midwives. Nursing and Midwifery Council, London

Owens RG, Ashcroft JB (eds) 1985 Violence: a guide for the caring professions. Croom Helm, London

Paterson BL, McCornish A, Bradley P 1999 Violence at work. Nursing Standard 13(21):43–46

Pollock N, McBain I, Webster CD 1989 Clinical decision making and the assessment of dangerousness. In: Howells K, Hollin CR (eds) Clinical approaches to violence. John Wiley, Chichester

Reporting of Injuries, Diseases and Dangerous Occurrences Regulations 1995 HMSO, London

Royal College of Nursing 1998 Safer working in the community: a guide for NHS managers and staff on reducing the risks of violence and aggression. Royal College of Nursing, London

Royal College of Nursing 2001 Challenging harassment and bullying: guidance for RCN representatives, stewards and officers. Royal College of Nursing, London

Royal College of Nursing 2005 Bullying and harassment at work: a good practice guide for RCN negotiators and health care managers. Royal College of Nursing, London

Royal College of Psychiatrists 1999 Safety for trainees in psychiatry. Council report CR78. Royal College of Psychiatrists, London

Schwehr B 2001 Zero tolerance: drawing the line in health and social care. Care and Health Guide, 9:25–26. Available online:http://www.CareandHealth.Com (accessed 24 June 2002)

Shepherd J (ed) 1994 Violence in health care: a practical guide to coping with violence and caring for victims. Oxford University Press, Oxford

United Kingdom Central Council for Nurses Midwives and Health Visitors 2002 The recognition, prevention and therapeutic management of violence in mental health care. United Kingdom Central Council, London

Wykes T, Mezey G 1994 Counselling for victims of violence. In: Wykes T (ed) 1994 Violence and healthcare professionals. Chapman & Hall, London, pp 207–225

Chapter 13

End of life care

Jane Seymour

INTRODUCTION

One of the only certainties in life is that we will all die, and the care and support of those reaching the end of their lives and of their companions is therefore a major public health challenge, especially in the light of the changing age structure of the countries in the developed world and the tragedies of the AIDS pandemic in the resource poor nations (Sepúlveda et al 2002). Since the Second World War, one particular philosophy of care at the end of life has gained international recognition: palliative and hospice care (Clark & Seymour 1999). There are many parallels between the emergence of nursing as a profession and the development of palliative and hospice care, with some arguing that the latter is a 'quintessential' example of the contribution that nurses can make to the relief of suffering (see for example Bradshaw 1996).

There are a number of challenges in providing good end of life care. At an individual level these include: identifying those patients who are in need of end of life care; assessing their needs and those of their companions and making plans to meet these; addressing frequently complex clinical, ethical and psychosocial problems; and accessing the health and social care services and informal support which make a difference to the quality of life for people approaching the end of life and their companions. At a societal level, governments and policy makers face huge challenges in making public health plans that can begin to address the scale of needs for end of life care. There are particularly acute challenges faced by policy makers in resource poor nations, where death is often precipitated by poverty, deprivation and lack of access to basic resources. The World Health Organization has promoted palliative care as one means of addressing these latter problems.

OVERVIEW

Subject knowledge

The aim of the first part of the chapter is to enable you to understand some of the historical roots of palliative and hospice care, and to reflect on the links between this model of care and the development of nursing. The chapter begins with an overview of the meanings of key terms related to end of life care and a sketch of key epidemiological trends which reveal the extent of need for end of life care worldwide. Dying and ageing are interlinked in the developed world, and this raises many challenges for individuals, society and nursing. To develop understanding of these issues you will be introduced to the concept of the 'dying trajectory' as a means of thinking about the heterogeneity of needs that people have as they approach the end of life, and have an opportunity to reflect on some differing definitions of death and the differences between bereavement, grief and mourning.

Care delivery knowledge

The second part of the chapter focuses on some common issues that you are likely to encounter in the care of patients who are approaching the end of life and their companions, and seeks to provide an overview of key concepts which comprise a framework to help you think about the vital contribution that your care makes to patients who are in need of end of life care and their companions. It also provides a brief guide to best practice in end of life care.

Professional and ethical knowledge

End of life care is associated increasingly with complex ethical issues, often associated with decision making, with the capacity of the person who is facing death, and polarized stances towards issues such as euthanasia and assisted dying. You will be introduced to some of these dilemmas and become aware of important trends in legislation and policy in the UK directed at addressing them.

Personal and reflective knowledge

Caring for those approaching the end of life can be emotionally demanding since it intersects with one's own worries and fears about illness, dying and death or personal experiences of bereavement. The final part of the chapter explores some of these issues, and presents some case studies to enable you to think about some of the challenges that you may face in end of life care across the four branches of nursing.

SUBJECT KNOWLEDGE

NURSING AND END OF LIFE CARE: A HISTORICAL OVERVIEW

Clark & Seymour (1999) have described how during the 19th century and in the context of: rising industrialization,

urbanization and the beginnings of a growth of hospital medicine directed at the curing and containing disease, there emerged a new social movement directed at the needs of the chronically sick, the aged, the dying and above all the poor. This group of people were somewhat neglected in the newly emergent voluntary hospitals and, as a consequence of the gradual disappearance of traditional models of community and family based care for the dying, found themselves in dire need of support. Homes for the dying, sometimes called 'hospices', began to be established during the 19th and early 20th centuries combining a focus on the care of the dying with attention to relieving poverty. Among the most famous is St Joseph's Hospice in London, which celebrated its centenary in 2005. In most cases, these institutions were founded by religious orders of women, such as the Sisters of Charity, who developed clinical practices in nursing which were to later have a major influence on the founder of the modern hospice movement, Cicely Saunders, and the related development of palliative care nursing. Saunders founded St Christopher's Hospice in Sydenham, London, in 1967. This was the first modern hospice in the world, which combined care with advanced clinical techniques to control complex symptoms. Saunders developed the notion of 'total pain' to capture an approach to care in which the focus is towards the person and their experience of illness: emotionally, spiritually, and socially, rather than just the body and its manifestations of disease (Clark 1999).

THE MEANING OF KEY TERMS

End of life care

'End of life care' is a broad term that encompasses more than the phase immediately before death. The term originates from North America, where it has been used particularly in the context of the care of older people and relates to an

> approach that treats, comforts and supports older individuals who are living with, or dying from, progressive or chronic life-threatening conditions. Such care is sensitive to personal, cultural and spiritual values, beliefs and practices and encompasses support for families and friends up to and including the period of bereavement.
> (Ross et al 2000: 9)

End of life care is an appropriate term to capture care given when a person is known to be in the last stages of their life but is not clearly 'dying'. In the UK, a document published by the NHS Confederation in 2005 gives the following analysis of the groups that will benefit from end of life care:

All patients with a chronic, progressive and generally fatal illness, or an advanced or irreversible disease, need high quality well organized end of life care. This group of patients includes patients with organ failure such as heart disease and chronic obstructive pulmonary disease, stroke, general frailty, dementia and other neurological conditions, as well as people with cancer.
(NHS Confederation, November 2005: 1)

In thinking about end of life care, certain associated terms have been used commonly in the UK policy and practice literature, sometimes rather loosely. Here a brief overview of the accepted meanings of some common terms is given.

Palliative care

The World Health Organization (2004) describes palliative care as an approach that improves the quality of life of individuals and their families facing the problems associated with life-threatening illness. This is enabled through the prevention and relief of suffering by means of early identification and impeccable assessment and treatment of pain and by addressing other associated physical, psychosocial and spiritual needs. Palliative care thus:

- Provides relief from pain and other distressing symptoms.
- Affirms life and regards dying as a normal process.
- Intends neither to hasten nor postpone death.
- Integrates the psychological and spiritual aspects of patient care.
- Offers a support system to help patients live as actively as possible until death.
- Offers a support system to help the family cope during the patient's illness and in their own bereavement.
- Uses a team approach to address the needs of patients and their families, including bereavement counselling, if indicated.
- Will enhance quality of life, and may also positively influence the course of illness.
- Is applicable early in the course of illness, in conjunction with other therapies that are intended to prolong life such as chemotherapy or radiation therapy, and includes those investigations needed to better understand and manage distressing clinical complications.

The World Health Organization adopted an explicitly public health orientation to the promotion of palliative care, and was concerned to distance this definition from the close association with cancer that had characterized earlier definitions. It thus promotes a broad vision of palliative care that is relevant to all with chronic illnesses, and their families, with the intention of informing policy decisions about minimum standards for comprehensive palliative care for all in need (Sepúlveda et al 2002).

General and specialist palliative care

Clearly, patients' families and other carers are often the most important source of day-to-day care for people with palliative care needs. The professionals involved in providing palliative care fall into two categories:

- Those providing general care to patients and their family carers, for example the GP or district nurse. General palliative care consists in a core set of knowledge and skills to be used by all health and social care staff involved in the care and support of those facing the end of life, and their companions.
- Those who specialize in palliative care (consultants in palliative medicine, or clinical nurse specialists in palliative care – some of these may be called Macmillan nurses). Specialist palliative care is necessary for people who have unresolved symptoms or complex psychosocial issues; complex end of life issues; or complex bereavement issues (NICE 2004). It can be delivered in hospices, hospitals, at home or in care homes, and is often provided as a consultancy or advice service.

Terminal care

Terminal care is part of palliative care, and usually refers to the management of patients' needs when it has become clear that they are in a progressive state of decline (National Council for Hospice and Specialist Palliative Care Services 1995). The term was used in the 1980s but has gone out of vogue with the trend towards viewing palliative care as a process and philosophy of care that is applicable from diagnosis until death and into bereavement. Although you may hear the term used by some professionals and the public, the guidance published during 2004 on improving supportive and palliative care for adults with cancer (NICE 2004) warns that the association of palliative care with dying that this term tends to encourage is one factor which has had negative implications for access and acceptability of palliative care services to those in need.

Supportive care

Supportive care is a term that has been introduced in the context of cancer care. It is an umbrella term for all services that can help people with cancer and their families to cope with cancer and its treatment – from pre-diagnosis, through the process of diagnosis and treatment, to cure, continuing illness or death and into bereavement. The key elements of supportive care have been derived from evidence about what people with cancer prioritize, namely: being treated with humanity, dignity and respect; good communication; clear information; symptom control; and psychological support (NICE 2004).

MORBIDITY AND MORTALITY: EPIDEMIOLOGICAL TRENDS

Worldwide, 56 million people die each year; with the majority of these deaths (some 40 million) occurring in resource-poor countries such as those in sub-Saharan Africa. It has been estimated that approximately 60% of those who die (i.e. 33 million people) could benefit from receiving some form of palliative care support as they approach the end of their lives. If we consider the companions or close family members of each of these 33 million people, this figure increases to 100 million people who might benefit from the provision of palliative care in its most basic form (Stjernswärd & Clark 2005: 1199).

Reflection and portfolio exercise

Think of a patient with whom you have had contact. Roughly estimate or guess how many people close to that person were affected by their illness and, if they have died, their death.

- Was it possible to assess the needs of these individuals and provide any sort of support to them?
- What sorts of services would need to be developed to do this well?

There are some major groups for whom support at the end of life is most necessary: this includes people affected by cancer, by AIDS related illnesses, and by long-term chronic or progressive terminal illness (Stjernswärd & Clark 2005: 1200). A report published by the Office of National Statistics in 2006 shows that in England and Wales during 2005, heart disease was the leading cause of death, followed by cerebrovascular disease and then cancer (all causes). Dementia is a rapidly increasing cause of death, but deaths from dementia are underrepresented in the statistics because of a tendency to record instead immediate causes of death, such as pneumonia, on death certificates.

One of the most common trajectories towards death in the developed world is associated with frailty and chronic illness among older people. The proportion of older people in the UK population is growing due to falling fertility rates, the post Second World War 'baby boom' and socio-economic, environmental and medical improvements that have resulted in the focus on death as an event at the end of a very long life. This has been a fundamental change from the situation common until the early 20th century when death commonly occurred in childhood or early adulthood and as a result of infectious disease.

Evidence-based practice

The Office of National Statistics provides a wealth of information about the population of England and Wales, including data on mortality trends over time. Their website notes that:

At the beginning of the 20th century over half of all deaths occurred under age 45. Infant mortality (at ages under one year) accounted for 25 per cent of deaths in 1901, but had fallen to 4 per cent of deaths by the middle of the century and is now less than 1 per cent. Childhood mortality has also declined, while decreases in the rates for young adults (15–44) were mainly seen in the first half of the century. In 2006, 4 per cent of deaths occurred at ages under 45. Deaths at age 75 and over comprised only 12 per cent of all deaths at the beginning of the last century. They rose to 39 per cent in 1951 and 66 per cent in 2006.

Source: Death registrations: Office for National Statistics. Available at: http://www.statistics.gov.uk/cci/nugget.asp?id=952 (accessed 15 October 2007).

In describing the essential elements of demographic change in the UK, the Royal Commission on Long Term Care (1999) and the Debate of the Age Study Group, established by Age Concern (1999) highlighted the following:

- 1 person in 6 in the UK is aged at least 65 and by 2031 this will be true of 1 in 4.
- Almost half of the older population is aged at least 75 and the most rapid increases are among the very oldest cohorts.
- Between 2001 and 2041 the number of people in the UK aged at least 85 is expected to double from 1.1 million to 2.3 million.

People in late old age are much more likely (in the current present cohort) than younger people to be disabled by physical or mental illness. This is due, in part, to the previous disadvantages in terms of life chances and environmental factors that they have faced.

Evidence-based practice

A report published in 2004 by the World Health Organization (Europe) about the palliative care needs of older people (Davies & Higginson 2004) draws attention to the following as being of particular importance:

- Many older people have multiple medical problems.

- The cumulative effects of these lead to greater impairment and needs for care than would be the case for any individual condition.
- Older people are at greater risk of complications from treatment, including adverse drug reactions.
- Older people who are ill are likely to have increased psychological distress.
- Older people may experience episodes of acute illness, against a backdrop of social isolation, physical or mental impairment, and economic hardship.

You can look at the report at: http://www.euro.who.int/document/E82933.pdf

DYING TRAJECTORIES

The notion of 'trajectories' of dying is useful to help us understand what might be the different experiences and needs of people as they approach death. They were first discussed by two sociologists working in the USA in the 1960s (Glaser & Strauss 1965). Depending on the cause of death and the type and availability of treatment, the trajectory of a dying process may be slow, sudden, or take the shape of a series of relapses and recoveries (Lynn & Adamson 2003). One conceptual model depicting different trajectories of dying has become popular over the last few years (Lynn & Adamson 2003): a hyperlink to this model is provided at the end of this chapter. This helps us to understand the similarities and differences among three groups of people who are likely to need palliative and end of life care: those who have a short period of decline before death, e.g. the typical case of a person dying from cancer; those who have long-term limitations with periods of relapse and remission before what is often a sudden death, for example as may be the case for people living with lung or heart disease; and 'prolonged dwindling' before death, as may be the case for older people living with extreme frailty or dementia.

DEATH AND ITS DEFINITIONS

While at first sight an obvious state, the definition of death has been subject to dispute and debate for thousands of years. There is no statutory definition of death in English law, and the diagnosis of death has to be determined by a medically qualified clinician on the basis of physical evidence, which in most cases will be complete cessation of respiration and heartbeat, together with fixed dilated pupils (De Cruz 2000). However, in some cases, patients who are at risk of dying or close to death will be artificially ventilated in intensive care units. The development of organ transplantation as technology has thrown up a need to define death differently in these circumstances and has resulted in the UK in a Department of Health code of practice which sets out criteria for brain stem death testing in adults and the clinical tests necessary for the diagnosis of brain stem death (Department of Health 1998). You can find a hyperlink which takes you to the code of practice at the end of this chapter and in the box below.

Evidence-based practice

The North Trent Critical Care Network provides the following useful information about brain stem death at their website http://www.ntccn.org.uk/Organ_Donation/o04brainstem-death.htm (accessed 16 October 2007).

- Brain stem death usually occurs secondary to severe head injury; intracranial bleed or other intracranial pathology leading to globally increased intracranial pressure (ICP) with subsequent infarction of the brain stem.
- Patients who become brain stem dead usually present deeply comatosed with or without respiratory effort. The initial management of these patients is no different to any other patient in that the objective of their treatment is to maintain life, determine the cause of a coma and to attempt to restore function.
- The concept of brain stem death may be difficult for relatives to understand. Indeed there is evidence that it is not always fully understood by healthcare professionals.
- Relatives need to understand that brain stem death is an irretrievable state, with somatic death an inevitable consequence, despite all available supportive measures. They also need to know that brainstem death is a legal definition of death in the UK.
- When this has been established the patient is dead, even though respiration and circulation can be maintained. The appropriate cause of action is then to withdraw artificial life support.
- If any of the dead patient's organs are still functioning it is appropriate to consider whether they can be made available for transplantation.
- The clinical diagnosis of brain stem death in the UK relies upon the lack of brain stem reflexes in a patient in apnoeic coma from a known, irreversible cause, with normal electrolytes, normothermia and in the absence of sedative drugs or muscle relaxants.

See also: Department of Health (1998) A code of practice for the diagnosis of brain stem death. Including guidelines for the identification and management of potential organ and

Continued

Apart from the special circumstances surrounding brain stem death, in everyday nursing practice it is probably more helpful to consider that death is a process rather than an event, in which the role of the nurse is to work with the multidisciplinary team to:

- Establish that the person is likely to be approaching the end of their life.
- Make any necessary decisions and plans that may be required to better manage the person's medical and nursing care in the promotion of their quality of life and comfort during the dying phase.
- Seek to provide the necessary support to the dying person's companions during the dying process and after the death.

We look in further detail at this later in this chapter.

GRIEF, BEREAVEMENT AND MOURNING

Bereavement is a virtually universal experience. Almost all of us will experience the loss through death of relatives, friends or colleagues. Each society marks the death of persons in a culturally determined manner through mourning ceremonies, which we often call 'funerals' (Clark & Seymour 1999). Mourning is thus a socially sanctioned behavioural response to bereavement but may not always reflect inner feelings.

Some bereavements may engender powerful feelings of grief and loss, in which those who were close to the dead person experience sadness and desolation. For some, grief is never fully eradicated and becomes a central part of everyday life. For others, grief is more transitory. Feelings of grief can also be associated with other types of loss, for example: retirement and the loss of meaningful employment; the loss of a family home; the diagnosis of a life limiting illness and consequent loss of plans and hopes for the future. The experience of bereavement will be influenced by a range of factors, including the nature of the bereaved individual's relationship with the dead person; the manner and timing of the death and whether the death was expected or unexpected. In affluent Western culture, the death of a child is one form of loss from which it may be particularly difficult to recover (Kohner & Henley 2001). In some circumstances, death may be associated with a sense of shame or stigma, which can make the expression of feelings of grief difficult and complicate bereavement. For example, death from suicide or as a result of the criminal activity of the deceased may engender confusing feelings that are difficult to resolve.

There is no right or wrong way to experience bereavement, although you may be aware of a number of stage models of grief – such as those put forward by Kubler Ross (1975) or Worden (1982) – that were popular during the 20th century. These tended to see the process of bereavement as a series of 'tasks' in which the person worked to 'detach' themselves from the dead person and to make a series of new attachments (for an overview, see Dickenson et al 2000). It has been suggested that such models represent the range of human experiences associated with bereavement poorly and have, in some cases, been applied uncritically in clinical practice with the result that bereaved people are sometimes expected to behave in certain 'typical' ways (Walter 1999).

CARE DELIVERY KNOWLEDGE

CONCEPTS OF SPECIAL RELEVANCE TO THE NURSING CARE OF THOSE APPROACHING THE END OF LIFE

Within the literature relevant to nursing care provision at the end of life it is possible to identify key elements. Among these are: teamwork; the relief of suffering; the promotion of quality of life and the promotion of dignity (Seymour 2004). Here, we explore these elements to enable you to think critically about the role of nursing and the contribution it can potentially make in end of life care.

Teamwork

In the NICE guidance for improving palliative and supportive care in adults with cancer (NICE 2004) the multidisciplinary team is defined as:

> A group of health and social care professionals from a range of disciplines who meet regularly to discuss and agree plans of treatment and care for people with a particular type of cancer or problem, or in a particular location. Includes primary care teams, site specific cancer teams and specialist palliative care teams.
>
> (NICE 2004: 200)

The guidance goes on to describe how the teams should seek to ensure effective interpersonal communication within the team and between them and other teams. One important aspect that contributes to the success of team working is that each member has respect and values the roles of other colleagues in the team; that leadership is not necessarily always ascribed to one particular professional group; and that decision making is openly shared, while each member accepts at the same time their professional accountability for the particular role they play within the team.

This is not always easy for nurses since, for historical reasons, many nurses can find it hard to make their voices heard during team working or may have a perspective on the needs of their patient that is not necessarily shared by others. Sometimes, stereotypes which we may all hold to a greater or lesser extent can get in the way of good team working. In the field of end of life care this has been a source of stress for nurses, which has been well described in the research literature (Vachon 2003). However, as Speck (2006) notes, 'in well functioning teams, protective attitudes to professional status and roles will not play a significant role' (p. 194). Moreover, in order to work within the framework of palliative care as defined by the WHO (Sepúlveda 2002), team working is imperative and is the only way to achieve 'early identification and impeccable assessment and treatment of pain and other problems, physical, psychosocial and spiritual' (Sepúlveda 2002). A commitment to team working is an important aspect of the professional duties of all of the clinical professions.

Reflection and portfolio exercise

Look at the Nursing and Midwifery Council's code of professional conduct for nurses (Nursing and Midwifery Council 2008) and find the paragraphs that refer to team working. In your experience, what helps team working to take place effectively during end of life care? What makes it difficult?

Suffering

In his study of suffering, the physician Eric Cassell argues that suffering is experienced when an impending destruction of the person is perceived and continues until the integrity of the person can be restored in some manner (Cassell 2004). Making sense of suffering and helping the person who is suffering involves understanding what may be a highly personal reaction to illness and distress. For some people, the experience of suffering is linked to a need to find meaning and to search for spiritual or religious explanations for questions that emerge from the experience of suffering: Why me? Why now? Why like this? However, we do not all seek to address such questions; nor is the role of the nurse always to provide a solution to suffering. Arguably, the nurse's role is to support the person until they reach a resolution in their own terms (Clark & Seymour 1999). Of course, the experience of suffering is not dependent upon or directly linked to the

severity of pain or the status of illness. Rather, it is dependent upon the meanings that illness and pain have for the person experiencing them. Kleinman (1988), in his seminal text *The Illness Narratives: Suffering, Healing and the Human Condition*, notes that: 'it is possible to talk to patients, even those who are most distressed, about the actual experience of illness, and that witnessing and helping to order that experience can be of therapeutic value' (Kleinman 1988: xii).

Sometimes it feels difficult to talk or to communicate with people who are suffering, particularly if you do not have years of experience or professional training behind you, but in these circumstances having the courage just to 'be with' the person can be experienced by them as deeply supportive.

Visit the first Evolve resource to learn more about the experiences of different people with serious and life limiting illnesses.

⊖volve   13.1 – INSIGHT INTO PALLIATIVE CARE ON THE WEB

- Access up-to-date resources on a variety of issues relevant to palliative care.
- Read personal accounts of living with dying and care.
- Think about the different ways suffering is experienced by individuals.

Quality of life

If you look back to the WHO definition of palliative care (Sepúlveda et al 2002) you will see that a key goal of palliative care is to enhance quality of life. In their detailed overview of the issues involved in evaluating quality of life, Kaasa & Loge (2004) noted that 'quality of life' was cited as one of the main goals of health care in Ancient Greece, which developed a system of health care and associated principles that now underpin the health care system in the modern West. Quality of life is essentially a subjectively defined phenomenon, which is difficult to assess or measure. In spite of this, there have been many attempts to operationalize and quantify 'quality of life' in palliative care research (Kaasa & Loge 2004).

Sometimes 'quality of life' has been related to the degree to which a person can live a 'normal' life or engage with the range of activities of daily living (Kaasa & Loge 2004), or meet the needs identified in Maslow's needs hierarchy – i.e. biological needs, needs for close relationships, needs for meaningful occupation and the need for change (Maslow 1970). However, these conceptualizations of quality of life do not fit well with the observation that many people living with quite severe illness, with its associated limitations and disabilities, may report a high quality of life. A more useful model is provided by the 'Gap' theory of Calman (1984) who argued that quality of life is related to the difference between an individual's expectations and their perception of any given situation. The wider the gap between expectation and perception, the less quality of life a person may have. It is important to remember that individual perceptions of what is a reasonable quality of life can change quite dramatically with changes in illness status: this is known as the 'response shift' phenomenon (Sprangers & Schwartz 1999). In end of life care practice, quality of life assessment is complex and encompasses all aspects of health and social care that people affected by life limiting illness require.

In the second evolve resource for this chapter is a reflective exercise to help you learn more about maximizing the quality of life in palliative and end of life care.

evolve

13.2 – MAXIMIZING QUALITY OF LIFE

- Be cognizant of the concept of quality of life in supportive and palliative care.
- Use this to review your own practice.

Dignity

Dignity relates to the respect of individuals and their bodies. Institutional structures and cultures are as critical to the preservation of dignity as individual nurse–patient relationships. De Raeve (1996: 71), suggests that we consider 'dignity' in terms of its contribution as a 'quality' or an aspect of nursing care given to people who are seriously ill or dying, and whose sense of innate dignity or personal, spiritual and physical integrity may be threatened. It is necessary therefore to consider what treating someone with dignity entails and what care practices maintain or compromise dignity.

In a study with patients and nurses in a hospital, Walsh & Kowanko (2002) show that nurses and patients agree on the key elements of dignity and the sorts of nursing care practices that support or detract from it (see Box 13.1).

Protection of dignity in the simple ways that Walsh & Kowanko (2002) describe is central to the palliative care approach (National Council for Hospice and Specialist Palliative Care Services 2001) and other studies confirm that the preservation of dignity is a prime issue for patients with palliative care needs and their carers (see for example Rogers et al 2000).

Communication issues in end of life care

Sheldon (2004) writes: 'Every moment that professionals spend with a person who is dying or their carers is spent

Box 13.1 Elements of 'dignity' identified by nurses and patients (adapted from Walsh & Kowanko 2002)

Nurses' descriptions of dignity	Patients' descriptions of dignity
Privacy of the body	Not being exposed
Private space	Being treated with discretion
Consideration of emotions	Consideration
Giving time	Having time/not being rushed
The patient as a person	Being seen as a person
The body as an object	The body as an object
Showing respect	Being acknowledged
Giving control	Having time to decide
Advocacy	

in communicating with them' (p. 9). She describes communication as a dialogue which is affected by a number of inter-relating factors:

- expectations
- family history and life experience
- beliefs
- meanings of illness.

By thinking about these factors it is possible to see how communication and its success or failure as an interaction can influence other key aspects of the experience of end of life care such as suffering, quality of life and making sense of one's situation. As well as skills of listening, of expressing genuine interest and concern and of empathy, nurses and other professionals responsible for communicating with patients and their companions need to nurture particular attitudes and values such as: being non judgemental; regarding patients as partners; and respecting the rights of patients to be self-determining according to their capacity to do so (Sheldon 2004: 15). This can take many years of experience but all are attributes that can be learned and honed through professional development. Some of them are related to the skills that a trained counsellor may provide but clearly it is neither necessary nor possible for all patients to see a counsellor; all professionals need to develop some basic counselling skills that they can draw upon in difficult communication situations. Of course, not all communication involves an interaction between patient and professional. Communication with multidisciplinary teams is also essential in delivering good end of life care.

Some situations require special skills and attention to the evidence surrounding the most appropriate way to handle them. The breaking of bad news (for example about the diagnosis of a serious illness or about death) is one example around which an extensive literature has developed in recognition of the need to do this gradually and to avoid traumatizing the patient and their family. Box 13.2 sets out the essential principles and steps involved.

Box 13.2 Breaking bad news

Preparation: find out from the patient as early as possible whether they are the sort of person who likes to know detailed information, and whether they would wish a family member to be with them when any information about their illness is given to them.

Get the environment right: finding a place where it is possible to sit in comfort and privacy is essential.

Giving a warning shot: rather than immediately launching into a detailed explanation, it is often better to warn the patient that you have some news that may not be good – 'we have your test results back and they are not as good as we had hoped'.

Find out how much the patient wishes to know and what they already understand about their illness.

Allow time for the patient to express their feelings.

Plan with the patient what will happen next and ensure that the person feels supported.

(Based on Buckman 1992, Sheldon, 2004)

The needs of the person approaching the end of their life and those of their companions

In the UK, guidance has been published by the National Institute for Health and Clinical Excellence on improving supportive and palliative care for adults with cancer. This is based on a review of the research evidence and provides a useful overview of the needs and concerns that patients with cancer and their close companions may have (NICE 2004). The National Council for Palliative Care (2006) provides a useful guide to palliative care principles based on research evidence (see Box 13.3).

Research examining the concerns and experiences of people with palliative care needs takes a variety of approaches.

Box 13.3 Principles of palliative care

1. Patient and family participation.
2. Collaborative multiprofessional approach by healthcare professionals.
3. Use of appropriate medications, tailored to each patient individually, given regularly to relieve and prevent symptoms.
4. Continued regular assessment and support, with emergency back-up available 24 hours per day.
5. Access and early referral to specialist palliative care services for patient and family support if needed.

From: National Council for Palliative Care 2006 Changing gear: guidelines for managing the last days of life in adults. National Council for Palliative Care, London.

One of the most common research techniques employed has been the surveying of the bereaved relatives of people who have died in order to ask them about the concerns and needs of the person close to them who has died.

Evidence-based practice

In the *Regional Study of the Care of the Dying*, Addington-Hall & McCarthy (1995) examined the prevalence of physical symptoms and pain among dying people and the type of services they received, publishing valuable information about the circumstances of people dying from cancer, heart disease, stroke and dementia. Although this study is now old, it was a model of conducting research into a difficult area and remains the largest body of evidence that we have about palliative and end of life care needs. Addington-Hall & McCarthy concluded one in six non-cancer patients experience symptoms such as pain and breathlessness which are similar to the most severely affected cancer patients.

One subset of the study involved data being gathered from the bereaved next of kin of 675 adults who had died of heart failure in 20 health districts (McCarthy et al 1996). Relatives were asked to report on the needs and symptoms of the person during their last year of life. Many patients were reported as having been unable to get adequate information about their condition, and of those who were thought to have known they were dying, 82% were reported to have worked this out for themselves. A wide range of symptoms were reported, including pain, breathlessness, low mood and anxiety. These were frequently distressing and lasted in many cases for longer than 6 months. For more than one quarter of patients, management in hospital brought no or little relief. At the time of death, 54% of patients died in hospital, 30% in their own home and 11% in a care home. More than one third of people died without their relative present.

Increasingly, this type of study is complemented by research which directly engages people with palliative care needs, usually by way of interviews. Work of this genre (for example Chapple et al 2004) has drawn attention to some key psychosocial aspects of the experience of becoming and being ill, which take us beyond assumptions that people who face loss through illness or death move through predictable 'stages'. These include:

- Serious or terminal illness as a crisis of identity.
- Experiences of loss of self or 'remaking' of self.
- Stigma and blame.
- Rejection of sick roles and search for 'normality'.
- The centrality of hope.
- The importance of 'difference' in terms of gender, culture, or ethnicity.

Evidence-based practice

In a study which involved in-depth interviews with people suffering from advanced lung cancer or heart failure, Murray et al (2002) revealed the similarities and differences between the two groups of patients. Those with cancer were able to make plans for the last stage of their lives: they knew that death was imminent and understood their diagnosis and prognosis. In contrast, the people with heart failure did not always see their disease as 'terminal', did not really understand what 'heart failure' was and had experienced gradual decline, punctuated by episodes of acute deterioration followed by partial improvement. This made planning and prediction difficult. People with heart failure often 'felt ill' but were told they 'looked well'. In contrast, people with lung cancer had initially 'felt well' but were told that they were 'seriously ill'. In terms of services, people with cancer found that they were able to access a range of specialist services, whereas people with heart failure found it difficult to find any specialist services to help them with their problems.

NURSING CARE AS DEATH APPROACHES

Signs that death is approaching

The National Council for Palliative Care (2006: 7) provides research-based guidance on the signs that may indicate that patients are in the last days of life. The guidance suggests that dying patients will manifest some or all of the following:

- Profound weakness:
  - usually bed bound
  - requiring assistance with all care.
- Gaunt physical appearance, particularly with cancer unless steroids have been taken (i.e. cushingoid appearance).
- Drowsiness or reduced cognition:
  - may be disoriented for time and place
  - extreme difficulty in concentrating
  - scarcely able to cooperate with carers.
- Diminished intake of food and fluids.
- Difficulty swallowing medications.

Usually, especially among patients with cancer, these signs appear gradually. A sudden and unexpected change must be investigated since it may indicate a reversible condition, such as an infection, rather than a being a sign of a person entering the terminal phase. In non cancer conditions entry into the terminal phase may be less clear and may mean that patients who are dying may receive interventionist medical treatment (such as cardiopulmonary resuscitation) which is inappropriate. There is increasing attention

being paid to the importance of ascertaining, before a loss of capacity, what people's wishes are with regard to end of life care treatment, through advance care planning (Henry & Seymour 2007). We look in more detail at this below.

Assessing and responding to needs

It can be very difficult to ask people who are near death what they are experiencing and which problems are the most distressing for them. They may have lost capacity, be confused or unable to communicate their needs. Family members and professional carers can often provide very useful information, but it is important to recognize that they may not see things in the same way that the patient might (National Council for Palliative Care 2006: 10). Therefore, very careful clinical assessment by the multidisciplinary team and good communication practices are essential to ensure that the needs of the person are anticipated, understood and well managed. Most of the time, management of the dying person's needs remains the responsibility of their core healthcare team. Sometimes it is necessary to refer to specialist palliative care services. This will always follow a careful assessment of the person's needs or the needs of their companions. Referral to specialist palliative care services may be indicated if:

- One or more distressing symptoms prove difficult to control.
- There is severe emotional distress associated with the patient's deterioration.
- Carers, particularly potentially vulnerable ones such as dependent children and/or elderly relatives, are experiencing severe distress.

(See National Council for Palliative Care 2006:10).

The most commonly reported symptoms in the terminal phase are:

- pain
- restlessness/agitation
- noisy breathing/respiratory tract secretions
- nausea/vomiting
- dyspnoea
- confusion
- urinary incontinence/retention
- dry/sore mouth
- extreme fatigue.

Other chapters in this book address these issues, but key principles are listed in Box 13.4.

The aim of all care and treatment at the end of life is to respond quickly and efficiently to the needs that patients and their companions may have, so that their comfort and quality of life is maximized as far as possible. Nursing care will include careful attention to skin integrity, mouth care and bladder and bowel care. It may be necessary for

---

Box 13.4 Key principles in the management of the terminal phase of illness

Current medications are assessed and non-essentials discontinued.

'As required' subcutaneous medication is prescribed according to an agreed protocol to manage pain, agitation, nausea and vomiting and respiratory tract secretions.

Decisions are taken to discontinue inappropriate interventions, including blood tests, intravenous fluids and observation of vital signs.

The ability of the patient, family and carers to communicate in their preferred language.

The insights of the patient, family and carers into the patient's condition are identified.

Religious and spiritual needs of the patient, family and carers are assessed.

Means of informing family and carers of the patient's impending death are identified.

The family and carers are given appropriate written information.

The GP practice is made aware of the patient's condition.

A plan of care is explained and discussed with the patient, family and carers.

Adapted from: National Institute for Health and Clinical Excellence 2004 Guidance on cancer services. improving supportive and palliative care for adults with cancer. NICE, London.

Box 13.5 Medications used in the last days of life

Analgesics – to relieve pain, e.g. morphine
Anxiolytics/sedatives – to relieve distress and breathlessness, e.g. midazolam
Anti-secretories – to relieve respiratory tract secretions, e.g. hyoscine hydrobromide
Anti-emetics – to relieve nausea and vomiting, e.g. cyclizine
For further details see: National Council for Palliative Care 2006: 12

---

well controlled (see for example Twycross & Wilcock 2002). Typical medications used at the end of life are summarized in Box 13.5.

As well as these common needs, some patients may have particular problems which require intervention either by their regular healthcare providers or by referral to specialists. Spiritual distress may be one example.

Caring for family and friends

One of the greatest concerns that a dying patient's companions may have is to know that he or she is being cared for as well as possible and is being kept as comfortable as possible (Kristjanson et al 2003). When care in the terminal phase of life is delivered well or badly, it can have a major impact on the way in which families and companions remember the death of a loved one, and major consequences therefore for the experience and outcomes of bereavement. (The third Evolve web resource contains a summary of the needs of family members at this time.) Sometimes family members will guess that a person is approaching death but do not know how to raise this suspicion with the healthcare team or with the person who is dying. They may be distressed if, in this situation, there is no integrated attempt to focus on the person's quality of life or on the immediate care arrangements needed to create the best possible experience of the death for the patient and their family but, rather, a persistence of a narrowly medically focused approach to care and treatment. One important role for the nurse is to act as an advocate for patients who may be dying and to facilitate communication between them and their family, and between the family and the wider clinical team about what plans need to be made to manage the last phase of a patient's life.

patients to be catheterized, but a decision about whether this is necessary will always be guided by what will most contribute to the person's comfort. It may not be in the person's best interests to give them artificial hydration and nutrition, but offers of sips of water or regular mouth care must be maintained.

Pharmacological treatment should be used to control troublesome symptoms such as pain or nausea, but unnecessary medications can be stopped by the responsible medical practitioner – following team discussion and consultation with the patient and their family where that is possible – if they are not contributing to the patient's comfort. One of the key principles of palliative care is particularly to attend to pain control, using the principles of the WHO three step ladder (WHO 1990) to systematically move from weak analgesics such as aspirin to strong opioids. The right dose and combination of analgesic therapy is that which relieves pain in the individual patient (see also Ch. 11, 'Pain').

It has been shown from more than 50 years of research that where opioids such as morphine are used according to standards of best practice and evidence, then they do not hasten death and can be used in increasing doses, along with appropriate adjuvant therapies, so that pain is

⊖volve

13.3 – THE NEEDS OF FAMILIES

- Know how the well-being of patients and their families is linked.
- Know the importance of nursing care to families of critically ill patients.

Providing bereavement support

Bereavement support has three major components, as outlined in the NICE guidelines on improving supportive and palliative care for adults with cancer (NICE 2004). These are:

- Grief is normal after bereavement but many bereaved people lack an understanding of grief and should therefore be offered information and how to access sources of support if needed.
- Some bereaved people may require a more formal opportunity to look at their experience. This need not involve professionals. Volunteer groups, self-help groups, faith groups and others can provide much support at this level.
- A minority of people may require specialist interventions and proper referral in these cases is essential.

The ways in which nurses and other health professionals interact with people who are bereaved, both before and in the immediate period after a death, can have long-term consequences on the experience of bereavement. It may influence the extent to which the bereaved person can adapt to their loss and thus their physical and mental well-being (Wiseman 1992). Providing sensitive support – which includes accurate and appropriately worded information about what will happen to the body of their dead relative, guidance about access to other services, as well as immediate compassionate help and comfort – to people who have been bereaved is thus a moral good, an issue of rights to correct information and a means of preventing morbidity associated with unresolved grief in the future (Department of Health 2005). In the UK, the importance of such support has been highlighted by events which occurred at the Bristol Royal Infirmary and Royal Liverpool Children's Hospital in relation to lack of informed consent about organ retention following post mortems. The inquiries of 2001 which investigated these issues resulted in a set of guidelines about supporting bereaved people that have wider applicability and which draw on evidence-based best practice (Department of Health 2005). The following key elements have been identified as good practice for health professionals who have to care for bereaved relatives of people who die in hospitals, although many of these are transferable to other care settings (Box 13.6).

In the days, weeks and months after a death, health professionals may have a role in assessing and providing appropriate support to those who have been bereaved. However, it should not be assumed that everyone will need intervention. Most people cope with bereavement through drawing on their own resources or with the help of their wider social or family networks. However, others may appreciate or need a level of support, which may range from a follow-up phone call to more intensive and specialist intervention. This may be because of social isolation or because of psychological morbidity due to some characteristic of the person who has been bereaved or the particular circumstances of the death. For example, the death of a child may be very traumatic. However, assumptions about what kinds of person or what kinds of death may lead to a need for intervention are not reliable.

Some of the approaches that might be employed by healthcare organizations that seek to provide support to the bereaved are as follows:

- Individual counselling and support.
- Group meetings for peer support: these may need to be organized according to age, gender or some special characteristic of the death (suicide or child death for example).
- Follow-up contact by way of a telephone call or card.
- Specific interventions for groups with special needs (people with learning disabilities, bereaved children, older people).
- Services of remembrance or other special events to mark loss associated with the institution.

Nurses are most commonly the professionals who are likely to come into contact with those who have been bereaved and have a key role in this important area of care, which should be planned, organized and critically reviewed with the same attention to detail as any other aspect of end of life care.

PROFESSIONAL AND ETHICAL KNOWLEDGE

THE UK POLICY CONTEXT

In the UK, policy and practice relating to end of life care reflects the socio-demographic changes described in the first part of this chapter, with attention increasingly focused on the challenges of supporting older people with chronic illnesses to live as well as possible as they approach the end of their lives. The NHS End of Life Care programme (EoLC), which was started in 2004, is one manifestation of this movement in policy. The key objective of the EoLC is to offer all adult patients nearing the end of life, regardless of their diagnosis, the choice and access to high quality end of life care in the place of care that they prefer (End of Life Care 2007). The programme draws upon a body of evidence which suggests that most people, when asked at any one time, will express a preference to be cared for and die at home during a final illness (Higginson 2003).

In enabling this objective, the programme encouraged the implementation of three 'end of life care tools' which were assessed by the National Institute for Health and Clinical Excellence (NICE 2004) as having the potential to

Box 13.6 Good practice in bereavement for hospital staff

When it is thought that a patient may die, the person or people closest to the patient should be kept informed and given the opportunity to be with their relative, child, partner or friend when he or she dies, if that is what they and the patient wish.

Provision of overnight accommodation could be considered where facilities allow.

When it is certain that a patient will die, issues may arise relating to the donation of organs or tissue for use in transplantation, therapy, education or research. Special training in communication skills will be necessary for staff to manage these situations. Formal, informed consent is needed for the donation of organs or tissue for further information, please see Department of Health 2005.

Staff should do all they can to maintain the dignity and privacy of the person who has died.

Ideally, people who are bereaved should be provided with a comfortable private room where, if they wish, they can spend time alone or with the body of the person who has died, immediately after the death. The specific needs of special groups such as children should be considered.

If the death is to be referred to the coroner it should be clear to all parties involved with the body what is to happen in respect of drips, tubes, lines or other equipment attached to the body.

In other cases and taking account of religious preferences, accommodating the wishes of the deceased's partner or family should be a priority, for example they may wish to clean the body of the person who has died, brush their hair or change their clothes.

Sources of support should be offered (for example, chaplaincy services) and it may be helpful to explain the kind of support that faith and other groups of people can offer.

Relevant professionals in the community (especially the GP) should be informed about the death as soon as possible.

Nothing should happen to or be done to the body of a person who has died without the knowledge of those closest to that person. Relatives and other close individuals may wish to be involved in laying out the body.

At an appropriate time after the death, the body should be moved to the hospital mortuary in a safe, respectful manner.

The possessions of the person who has died should be carefully sorted, cleaned and catalogued before being returned to their relatives.

The provision of written information (listing and describing sources of support, helplines and web-based information, for example) can help people who are bereaved manage the practical arrangements necessary after a death.

Written material should be sensitive to cultural values and religious beliefs and to the special needs of those who have lost a child or who have been bereaved through sudden or traumatic death.

Summarized from: Department of Health 2005 When a person dies. Advice on developing bereavement services in the NHS. London, HMSO.

aid coordination, communication and best practice in end of life care and to support care and death at home if this is what the patient and their family prefer. These are:

- The Gold Standards Framework.
- The Liverpool Care Pathway for the Care of the Dying.
- Preferred Priorities of Care (formerly Preferred Place of Care).

Reflection and portfolio exercise

Go to the NHS End of Life Care website at: http://www.endoflifecare.nhs.uk/eolc/ and follow the links to examine each of these tools. Compare and contrast the roles they may have in end of life care. Find out what the policy of your clinical area is with regard to implementation.

In 2007, the intention was announced in the UK to develop, for the first time, an 'End of Life Care Strategy' underpinned by a nationwide baseline review of services for people with end of life care needs to be undertaken by primary care trusts (Department of Health 2007a) and as part of a wider review of NHS services (Department of Health 2007b). This will involve assessing the population need for end of life care services, mapping current provision including its quality; comparing current provision with population need and identifying where service improvements are needed.

One key area where a great deal of development and policy focus is directed is at end of life care in care homes, where a number of well recognized problems exist and yet which are the place where more than 20% of people aged over the age of 65 die (Office of National Statistics 2000). Older people living in care homes will sometimes die having lived with multiple, often chronic conditions, often over a long period of time. There are also higher levels of mental confusion and impaired sight and hearing (National Council for Palliative Care 2004). Death in a care home therefore occurs typically after the person has had a gradual deterioration in their overall health over a long period which is punctuated by episodes of acute illness. Frequently, after death has occurred, it is possible to identify 'critical' events such as the onset of a chest infection or the reluctance of the person to drink and eat that pinpoint the beginning of a final stage. One of the major difficulties for residents' families, care home staff and visiting GPs in discussing and making appropriate care plans relates to anticipating the meaning and significance of such events as they occur. Highlighting this, one study of death and dying in care homes reports vividly how some extremely frail older people, who are fully expected to die, survive repeated episodes of acute illness and recover to live with a good quality of life for a number of weeks and months

(Froggatt 2001). End of life care planning is difficult in the context of such uncertainty and delivery of care to a high standard is frequently compromised by a lack of access in the home to adequate resources of knowledge, skills and outside support (National Council for Palliative Care 2004). There are a number of initiatives directed at finding ways to help residents, relatives and staff in care homes to work together with outside agencies to improve the quality of the environment of care homes as places within which to live and die. The *My Home Life* initiative is one example, which builds on a review of the evidence about promotion of quality of life in care homes (Help the Aged 2007).

ETHICAL ISSUES IN END OF LIFE CARE

As the means have become available to support life and to defer death for prolonged periods, so the moral and ethical complexities surrounding clinical practice at the end of life have multiplied. It is only possible to give a brief overview of some of these complex issues here. Some selected critical cases, which have either led to changes in the UK law or have led to widespread professional and public debate, are summarized in Box 13.7.

Killing or letting die?

As the medical technology exists increasingly not only to relieve the suffering associated with dying, but also to prolong life or to procure early death, the clarification of the distinction between 'killing' and 'letting die' is perhaps one of the most pressing concerns facing society today. In the UK, it is now recognized that where death is inevitable, then *life-prolonging* treatments such as resuscitation, artificial ventilation, dialysis, artificial nutrition and hydration can be withdrawn or withheld, and the goal of medicine redirected to the palliation of symptoms and the provision of '*basic care*' and comfort, which *must* be provided and can never be withheld (British Medical Association 2007). Basic care includes nursing care, pain relief and relief of other symptoms, the offer of oral nutrition and hydration. It is acknowledged that sometimes giving adequate symptom control or withholding or withdrawing life prolonging treatments may hasten a death that is already expected (British Medical Association 2007). It is important to note, however, that this is not euthanasia.

Euthanasia

There is a wide spectrum of views about euthanasia and there are many misunderstandings about it. A widely accepted (although subject to fierce debate) definition of euthanasia is the following: 'Euthanasia is killing on

Box 13.7 Critical cases

Anthony Bland*

'Since April 15, 1989, Anthony Bland has been in persistent vegetative state. He lies in Airedale General Hospital in Keighley, fed liquid food by a pump through a tube passing through his nose and down the back of his throat into the stomach. His bladder is emptied through a catheter inserted through his penis, which from time to time has caused infections requiring dressing and antibiotic treatment. His stiffened joints have caused his limbs to be rigidly contracted so that his arms are tightly flexed across his chest and his legs unnaturally contorted. Reflex movements in the throat cause him to vomit and dribble. Of all this, and the presence of members of his family who take turns to visit him, Anthony Bland has no consciousness at all. The parts of his brain which provided him with consciousness have turned to fluid. The darkness and oblivion which descended at Hillsborough will never depart. His body is alive, but he has no life in the sense that even the most pitifully handicapped but conscious human being has a life. But the advances of modern medicine permit him to be kept in this state for years, even perhaps for decades.'

(Extract from *Airedale NHS Trust* v. *Bland* (C.A.), 19 February 1993, 2 Weekly Law Reports, p. 350, of Hoffman's description of Bland. Cited in Singer 1994: 58.)

Diane Pretty

Diane Pretty was a woman of 43 who had late-stage motor neurone disease and applied during 2002 to the European Court of Human Rights to allow her husband to help her to commit assisted suicide. The application, which was rejected, was surrounded by publicity. Mrs Pretty eventually died in a hospice. It was widely reported that, in the days before her death, she had suffered the very symptoms she had feared, although these had eventually been well controlled. The case was supported by the Voluntary Euthanasia Society and the civil rights group 'Liberty'.

(BBC News, Monday, 13 May 2002: http://news.bbc.co.uk/1/hi/health/1983941.stm)

*Anthony Bland was fatally injured in the Hillsborough football stadium disaster of 1989 causing a persistent vegetative state. His feeding tube was withdrawn after a prolonged legal battle (Airedale Trust v. Bland [1993] 1 All ER 821 (HL)), and he died 10 days afterwards. Public concern about this case pushed forward the establishment of a House of Lords Select Committee on Medical Ethics, which reported in 1994. This committee ruled that Bland's death was a case of 'double-effect' in which death was an unintended, although not unforeseen, consequence of the removal of futile life-prolonging medical therapy (House of Lords 1993–94).

request and is defined as: a doctor intentionally killing a person by the administration of drugs at that person's voluntary and competent request' (Materstvedt et al. 2003: 98).

Euthanasia is illegal in the UK.

When considering euthanasia, we become aware of the conflicts that can exist between an individual's call to be released from suffering and society's efforts to protect and sustain life. Clinically, this tension becomes focused in the health professional's duty to provide beneficial care to those in need, to refrain from harming them, and to respect an individual's choices.

Periodically, there are attempts to change the law. In the UK during 2004–6, there were a number of attempts to change the law to permit assisted dying under consideration by parliament. In Belgium and the Netherlands, euthanasia at the voluntary request of a competent adult is legal under very tightly defined circumstances. The position taken by these countries is that under certain tightly defined conditions, ending the life of a terminally ill patient in extreme suffering is consistent with the ethic of beneficence in that it is a compassionate and merciful response that brings relief, and is also consistent with the ethic of autonomy, which allows people who competently request euthanasia to have their wish respected. In the UK, a beneficence approach has been dominant (Beauchamp & Childress 1994) in end of life care decision making, which emphasizes the need to act in the best interests of those who cannot speak for themselves (House of Lords 1993–94) and to protect vulnerable people from the potential for harm that legalizing euthanasia may bring.

Advance care planning

One of the key elements to support people at the end of their lives is to find out what their preferences and wishes are in relation to where they would like to be cared for and to help them to be involved, if they wish, in decisions about their care and treatment towards the end of life. Advance care planning (ACP), as highlighted in the NICE supportive and palliative care guidance for cancer patients (NICE 2004), is an important process in helping to ascertain this information (Box 13.8).

Do not attempt resuscitation orders (DNARs)

Nurses will often be involved in team discussions about cardiopulmonary resuscitation (CPR). One aspect of this may be an assessment of the risks and benefits of discussing this intervention with patients who have palliative care needs, in the light of evidence which shows that the survival rate after cardiorespiratory arrest and CPR is relatively low and carries a risk of adverse effects such as rib

---

Box 13.8 Advance care planning and associated terms

Advance care planning (ACP)

ACP is a process of discussion between an individual and their care providers irrespective of discipline. If the individual wishes, their family and friends may be included. With the individual's agreement, discussions should be:

- documented
- regularly reviewed
- communicated to key persons involved in their care.

Examples of what an ACP discussion might include are:

- the individual's concerns
- their important values or personal goals for care
- their understanding about their illness and prognosis, as well as particular preferences for types of care or treatment that may be beneficial in the future and the availability of these.

The difference between ACP and care planning more generally is that the process of ACP will usually take place in the context of an anticipated deterioration in the individual's condition in the future, with attendant loss of capacity to make decisions and/or ability to communicate wishes to others.

Statement of wishes and preferences

This is a summary term embracing a range of written and/or recorded oral expressions, by which people can, if they wish, write down or tell people about their wishes or preferences in relation to future treatment and care, or explain their feelings, beliefs and values that govern how they make decisions. They may cover medical and non-medical matters. They are not legally binding.

Advance decision

An advance decision must relate to a specific refusal of medical treatment and can specify circumstances. It will only come into effect when the individual has lost capacity to give or refuse consent. Careful assessment of the validity and applicability of an advance decision is essential before it is used in clinical practice. Valid advance decisions, which are refusals of treatment, are legally binding under the Mental Capacity Act 2005.

Lasting power of attorney

A lasting power of attorney (LPA) is a statutory form of power of attorney created by the Mental Capacity Act 2005. Anyone who has the capacity to do so may choose a person (an 'attorney') to take decisions on their behalf if they subsequently lose capacity.

Adapted from: Henry C, Seymour J 2007 Advance care planning: a guide for heath and social care professionals. NHS End of Life Care programme, Leicester. Available at:

http://www.endoflifecare.nhs.uk/eolc/acp/ (accessed 3 November 2007).

or sternal fractures, hepatic or splenic rupture, or potentially inappropriate life treatment in an intensive care unit (BMA, Resuscitation Council and RCN 2007).

Guidelines published in the UK in 2001 and revised during 2007 (BMA, Resuscitation Council and RCN 2007) suggest that where the outcome of resuscitation intervention is uncertain, anticipatory decisions should be sensitively explored with patients in question. Key points highlighted are the following:

- If there is a risk of cardiac or respiratory arrest it is desirable to make decisions about CPR in advance whenever possible.
- There should be a full clinical assessment of the chances of a successful outcome.
- Any CPR decision must be tailored to the individual circumstances of the patient.

- Decisions must not be made on the basis of assumptions based solely on factors such as the patient's age, disability, or on a professional's subjective view of a patient's quality of life.
- Advance care planning discussions must be led by someone with appropriate training and knowledge about the decision under examination.
- There will be some patients for whom attempting CPR is clearly inappropriate; for example a patient in the final stages of a terminal illness where death is imminent and unavoidable and CPR would not be successful, but for whom no formal DNAR decision has been made. In such circumstances, healthcare workers who make a considered decision not to commence CPR should be supported by their senior colleagues and employers.

PERSONAL AND REFLECTIVE KNOWLEDGE

Working with people who are approaching the end of life, or caring for the dying and the bereaved, raises significant personal questions about the meaning of life, and may at times raise fundamental anxieties about illness, dying and death. This is especially the case when something in one's personal life intersects with work life or when there are organizational problems which mean that you cannot provide the best care possible. Such work has long been known to induce considerable stress (Vachon 2003). Minimizing stress is crucial: to promote mental health and well-being, to prevent burnout and to ensure that one is in a position to support and help clients and colleagues appropriately and empathically. A key issue is how to contain powerful emotions while engaging in caring. 'Emotional labour' is a useful way of thinking about issues in achieving this balance (Seymour 2004). Similarly, Vachon (2003) draws attention to the importance of being aware of the idea of the 'wounded healer' (Nouwen 1972): a person who, possibly because of events experienced in their childhood or early adulthood, is drawn towards work which enables them to care for others in an unconscious attempt to heal themselves. Such people often have very high expectations of themselves in relation to helping others, but may not have insight into these, and may risk burnout or engage in patterns of behaviour at work or at home which ultimately stop them from being able to give the care that they wish. Of course, experiencing suffering oneself (which is a universal aspect of the human condition) means that one is perhaps better able to empathize with patients; however, it is necessary to 'tread lightly' between empathy and damaging over-identification if one is to survive long-term engagement in the field of end of life care. Looking after oneself is crucially important and will mean making sure that one gets enough rest, exercise and relaxation to maintain a good home–work life balance, as well as taking time to grieve losses that are experienced through work and finding time to discuss with others (either formally through clinical supervision or informally) events and issues which give rise to stress at work. The sections on clinical supervision and stress management in Chapter 9, 'Stress, relaxation and rest', are useful resources that can help here.

CASE STUDIES RELATED TO END OF LIFE CARE

The following fictional case studies are provided to help you reflect on issues involved providing care at the end of life.

Case study: adult

Mr Stewart is an ex shipyard worker aged 67 who has been investigated for the asbestos related disease mesothelioma. The investigations show that Mr Stewart does have mesothelioma, for which the prognosis is very poor.

- What should the healthcare team take into account as they prepare to disclose this news to Mr Stewart?
- What role will the nurse have who attends the meeting between Mr and Mrs Stewart and the consultant?
- What help can Mr Stewart and his family be provided with in the community?
- What issues may need to be taken into account in helping Mr Stewart engage with advance care planning?

Case study: Mental health

Mrs Adams is in her late 80s and has always had severe depression. She has recently also been diagnosed with vascular dementia, and tells the community psychiatric nurse who visits her that she wants to die. She asks the nurse to help her.

- What issues does the nurse need to consider to ensure Mrs Adam's safety?
- What help could the nurse call upon to ensure that Mrs Adam's receives the support she needs which may help her?

Case study: Learning disabilities

Tom is a 22-year-old man with severe learning disabilities and impaired communication abilities. He is dying of advanced cancer, and his parents tell you that they think he is in severe pain.

- How should you respond to the parents' concerns?

- What issues need to be thought about in assessing Tom's symptoms?
- Where can you go to get support to help assess whether Tom receiving the correct level of pain relief?

Case study: Child

Mary is 10 years old and has recently been bereaved of her mother following a long illness. Mary's father is concerned because Mary seems to want to try to forget about her mother and is always unwilling to talk about what has happened. However, Mary is having nightmares. Mary's school teacher is concerned because Mary has started to be disruptive in class, which is out of character. You are the school nurse.

- What issues do you need to consider in this situation?
- What sources of support are available to help Mary and her father cope with what has happened?

SUMMARY

This chapter has provided you with a wide-ranging overview of some key challenges in end of life care in the developed world:

1. The historical links between nursing and end of life care have been explored in the context of the rise of hospice and palliative care.
2. The consequences for end of life care of socio-demographic change have been reviewed, with particular emphasis on the tight links between ageing and the increase in long-term conditions.
3. The meanings of key terms and a concept analysis of key concepts have been provided.
4. Strategies and best practice in supporting people approaching the end of life and their companions have been reviewed.
5. Key aspects of UK policy developments have been described.
6. Ethical issues have been discussed, with special reference to advance care planning, decisions to withhold or withdraw treatment (including resuscitation) and euthanasia.

Annotated further reading and websites

British Medical Association 2007 Withholding and withdrawing life prolonging medical treatment: guidance for decision making, 3rd edn. BMA, London

This provides a summary of the current law regarding the withholding and withdrawal of life prolonging medical treatment, including information about the Mental Capacity Act 2005. Although it is a medically oriented publication, it is an excellent source of information for all health professionals.

British Medical Association, the Resuscitation Council (UK) and the Royal College of Nursing 2007 Decisions relating to cardiopulmonary resuscitation: a joint statement from the British Medical Association, the Resuscitation Council (UK) and the Royal College of Nursing. British Medical Association, London

This provides a comprehensive and detailed overview of all the issues that healthcare professionals should consider in relation to their practice with patients who may require cardiopulmonary resuscitation.

Davies E, Higginson I (eds) 2004 The solid facts: palliative care. World Health Organization Europe, Copenhagen

This is an excellent short evidence-based review of the key issues in palliative care.

http://www.endoflifecare.nhs.uk/eolc
The NHS End of Life Care programme website provides a useful overview of key issues in end of life care in England, and links to a wide range of other resources, including advance care planning, end of life care in care homes and innovations in practice.

http://www.ncpc.org.uk/
This website takes you to the National Council for Palliative Care, whose mission is to ensure that all those suffering from life-threatening conditions and who need palliative care receive it. The website has a useful list of publications on policy and practice, and a series of wide-ranging links to other organizations.

http://rand.org/pubs/white_papers/WP137/index2.html
This website allows you to read the report: Lynn J, Adamson DM 2003 Living well to the end of life: adapting health care to serious chronic illness in old age. Rand Health, Arlington VA. Lynn and Adamson put forward a model of 'trajectories' in end of life care which it is valuable to read.

http://www.dh.gov.uk/en/Publicationsandstatistics/Publications/PublicationsPolicyAndGuidance/DH_4009696
This website provides guidance on good practice relating to diagnosis of brain stem death and organ donation.

References

Addington-Hall JM, McCarthy M 1995 Regional study of care for the dying: methods and sample characteristics. Palliative Medicine 9:27–35

Age Concern, Debate of the Age Study Group 1999 The future of health and care of older people: the best is yet to come. The millennium papers. Age Concern, London

Beauchamp TL, Childress JF 1994 Principles of biomedical ethics. Oxford University Press, New York

Bradshaw A 1996 The spiritual dimension of hospice: the secularisation of an ideal. Social Science and Medicine 43(3):409–420

British Medical Association 2007 Withholding and withdrawing life prolonging medical treatment: guidance for decision making, 3rd edn. British Medical Association, London

British Medical Association, Resuscitation Council (UK), Royal College of Nursing 2007 Decisions relating to cardiopulmonary resuscitation: a joint statement from the British Medical Association, the Resuscitation Council (UK) and the Royal College of Nursing. British Medical Association, London

Buckman, R 1992 How to break bad news. Macmillan, London

Calman K 1984 Quality of life in cancer patients: an hypothesis. Journal of Medical Ethics 10(3):124–127

Cassell E 2004 The nature of suffering and the goals of medicine. Oxford University Press, Oxford

Chapple A, Ziebland S, McPherson A 2004 Stigma, shame and blame experienced by patients with lung cancer: qualitative study. British Medical Journal 328:1470

Clark D 1999 'Total pain,' disciplinary power and the body in the work of Cicely Saunders, 1958–1967. Social Science and Medicine 49:727–736

Clark D, Seymour J 1999 Reflections on palliative care. Open University Press, Buckingham

Davies E, Higginson I (eds) 2004 The solid facts: palliative care. World Health Organization Europe, Copenhagen

De Cruz P 2000 Comparative healthcare law. Routledge Cavendish, London

de Raeve L 1996 Dignity and integrity at the end of life. International Journal of Palliative Care Nursing 2(2):71–76

Department of Health 1998 A code of practice for the diagnosis of brain stem death: including guidelines for the identification and management of potential organ and tissue donors. Department of Health, London. Available online: **http://www.dh.gov.uk/en/ Publicationsandstatistics/Publications/PublicationsPolicyAnd Guidance/DH_4009696** (accessed 16 October, 2007)

Department of Health 2005 When a person dies: advice on developing bereavement services in the NHS. HMSO, London

Department of Health 2007a Operating framework 2007/08: PCT baseline review of services for end of life care. HMSO, London

Department of Health 2007b Our NHS, our future: NHS next stage review – interim report. HMSO, London

Dickenson D, Johnson M, Katz J 2000 Death, dying and bereavement, 2nd edn. Sage, London

End of Life Care 2007 Improving end of life care for adults. Available online: http://www.endoflifecare.nhs.uk/eolc/AboutUs/ (accessed 2 November 2007)

Froggatt K 2001 Palliative care and nursing homes: where next? Palliative Medicine 15:42–48

Glaser BG, Strauss AL 1965 Awareness of dying. Aldine, Chicago

Help the Aged 2007 My home life: quality of life in care homes. Help the Aged, London

Henry C, Seymour J 2007 Advance care planning: a guide for heath and social care professionals. NHS End of Life Care programme, Leicester. Available online: **http://www.endoflifecare.nhs.uk/eolc/acp/** (accessed 3 November 2007)

Higginson I 2003 Priorities and preferences for end of life care in England, Wales and Scotland. National Council for Hospice and Specialist Palliative Care Services, London

House of Lords 1993–94 Report of the Select Committee on Medical Ethics (HL Paper 21-I). HMSO, London

Kaasa S, Loge JH 2004 Quality of life in palliative care: principles and practice. In: Doyle D, Hanks G, Cherny N, Calman K (eds) Oxford textbook of palliative medicine, 3rd edn. Oxford University Press, Oxford, pp 196–210

Kleinman A 1988 The illness narratives: suffering, healing and the human condition. Basic Books, New York

Kohner N, Henley A 2001 When a baby dies: the experience of late miscarriage, stillbirth and neonatal death. Routledge, London

Kristjanson L, Hudson P, Oldham L 2003 Working with families. In: O'Connor M, Aranda S (eds) Palliative care nursing: a guide to practice. Radcliffe Medical Press, Abingdon

Kubler Ross E 1975 Death: the final stage of growth. Prentice Hall, Englewood Cliffs

Lynn J, Adamson DM 2003 Living well to the end of life: adapting health care to serious chronic illness in old age. Rand Health, Arlington

McCarthy M, Ley M, Addington-Hall J 1996 Dying from heart disease. Journal of Royal College of Physicians 30:325–328

Maslow A 1970 Motivation and personality. Harper, New York

Materstvedt LJ, Clark D, Ellershaw J et al 2003 Euthanasia and physician assisted suicide: a view from an EAPC ethics task force. Palliative Medicine 17(2):97–101

Murray SM, Boyd K, Kendall M et al 2002 Dying of lung cancer or cardiac failure: prospective qualitative interview study of patients and their carers in the community. British Medical Journal 325:929

National Council for Hospice and Specialist Palliative Care Services 1995 Specialist palliative care: a statement of definitions. National Council for Hospice and Specialist Palliative Care Services, London

National Council for Hospice and Specialist Palliative Care Services 2001 What do we mean by palliative care? A discussion paper. Briefing no. 9, May. National Council for Hospice and Specialist Palliative Care Services, London

National Council for Palliative Care 2004 Palliative care in care homes for older people. National Council for Palliative Care, London

National Council for Palliative Care 2006 Changing gear: guidelines for managing the last days of life in adults. National Council for Palliative Care, London

National Health Service Confederation 2005 Improving end of life care. Leading Edge 12(November):1–8

National Institute for Health and Clinical Excellence 2004 Guidance on cancer services: improving supportive and palliative care for adults with cancer. National Institute for Health and Clinical Excellence, London

Nouwen H 1972 The wounded healer. Doubleday, Garden City

Nursing and Midwifery Council 2008 The Code: standards of conduct, performance and ethics for nurses and midwives. Nursing and Midwifery Council, London

Office of National Statistics 2000 Mortality statistics general series. DH1 no. 33. Office of National Statistics, London

Office of National Statistics 2006 News release. Available online: http:// www.statistics.gov.uk/pdfdir/hsq0506.pdf (accessed 15 October 2007)

Office of National Statistics 2007 Death registrations in England and Wales in 2006. Available online: http://www.statistics.gov.uk/cci/ nugget.asp?id=952 (accessed 15 October 2007)

Rogers A, Karlsen S, Addington-Hall J 2000 'All the services were excellent. It is when the human element comes in that things go wrong': dissatisfaction with hospital care in the last year of life. Journal of Advanced Nursing 31(4):768–774

Ross MM, Fisher R, MacLean MJ 2000 A guide to end of life care for seniors. Health Canada, Ottawa

Royal Commission on Long-Term Care 1999 With respect to age: long-term care, rights and responsibilities. Stationery Office, London

Sepúlveda C, Marlin A, Yoshida T, Ullrich A 2002 Palliative care: the WHO global perspective. Journal of Pain and Symptom Management 24(2):91–96

Seymour JE 2004 What's in a name? A concept analysis of key terms in palliative care nursing. In: Payne S, Seymour JE, Ingleton C (eds) Palliative care nursing: principles and evidence for practice. Open University Press, Buckingham

Sheldon F 2004 Communication. In: Sykes N, Edmonds P, Wiles J (eds) Management of advanced disease, 4th edn. Arnold, London

Singer P 1994 Rethinking life and death: the collapse of our traditional ethics. Oxford University Press, Oxford

Speck P 2006 Teamwork in palliative care: fulfilling or frustrating? Oxford University Press, Oxford

Sprangers MA, Schwartz CE 1999 Integrating response shift into health-related quality of life research: a theoretical model. Social Science and Medicine 48:1507–1515

Stjernswärd J, Clark D 2005 Palliative medicine: a global perspective. In: Doyle D, Hanks G, Cherny N, Calman K (eds) Oxford textbook of palliative medicine, 3rd edn. Oxford University Press, Oxford, pp 1199–1224

Twycross R, Wilcock A 2002 Symptom management in advanced cancer, 3rd edn. Radcliffe Medical Press, Oxford

Vachon M 2003 Occupational stress in palliative care. In: O'Connor M, Aranda S (eds) Palliative nursing care: a guide to practice. Radcliffe Press, Abingdon

Walsh K, Kowanko I 2002 Nurses' and patients' perceptions of dignity. International Journal of Nursing Practice 8:143–151

Walter T 1999 On bereavement. Open University Press, Buckingham

Wiseman C 1992 Bereavement care in an acute ward. Nursing Times 88 (20):34–35

Worden W 1982 Grief counselling and grief therapy. Springer, New York

World Health Organization Expert Committee report 1990 Cancer pain relief and palliative care. Technical Report Series 804. World Health Organization, Geneva

World Health Organization 2004 WHO definition of palliative care. Available online: http://www.who.int/cancer/palliative/definition/en/ (accessed 6 May 2004)

Chapter 14

Hygiene

Maggie Mallik

KEY ISSUES

SUBJECT KNOWLEDGE
- Structure and functions of the skin, the mouth, the eyes, hair and nails as they relate to hygiene care
- History of hygiene care practices in society
- The impact of individual, cultural and spiritual beliefs on individual hygiene practices

CARE DELIVERY KNOWLEDGE
- Assessment of an individual's hygiene needs in relation to care of the body, mouth, hair and eyes
- Assessment tools and oral care
- Differing modes of delivery of hygiene care for all body parts

PROFESSIONAL AND ETHICAL KNOWLEDGE
- Ritualization of hygiene care
- Hygiene care and the image of the nurse
- Consent and privacy
- The politics of hygiene care

PERSONAL AND REFLECTIVE KNOWLEDGE
- Personal hygiene in the role of the nurse
- Reflection and experiential exercises
- Consolidation of learning through case studies

INTRODUCTION

Maintaining hygiene according to one's personal and cultural norms is a basic human need. Helping individuals maintain their own hygiene is recognized as a fundamental role for the nurse. In partnership with the client and/or carer, the nurse is the primary decision maker in this area of healthcare practice. Responsibility for promoting and maintaining excellence in the quality of hygiene care is a key function of nursing (Badham et al 2006). However, the role of the nurse in the actual delivery of care will alter depending upon the particular context in which hygiene care is provided and the specific needs of the individual. The term 'hygiene care', used throughout this chapter, is often employed interchangeably with the term 'personal care' or 'personal body care'.

Children and teenagers need varying levels of support and teaching to help them meet their hygiene needs. Health education for the child and the family is important in any context. Children and adults with deficits in learning ability need extra encouragement, time and teaching in order to meet their needs. For the person with a mental illness who has become demotivated about maintaining personal appearances and hygiene needs, the nurse needs to be highly sensitive to the client's personal wishes while still encouraging normal hygiene behaviour. Adults whose health status is compromised by acute or chronic illness need specific support within a continuum from total self-care to being totally dependent for hygiene care. The dignity and privacy of all clients, especially the elderly, needs to be facilitated and protected whatever the context of hygiene care delivery.

The content of this chapter outlines both the scientific and practice based knowledge needed to promote and deliver hygiene care.

OVERVIEW

Subject knowledge

Knowledge from the physical sciences is explored in relation to the skin, mouth, eyes, hair, nails and perineum. In each section the focus is on the applied knowledge needed to make decisions about hygiene care. The psychosocial knowledge base integrates these specific body parts in order to outline issues in hygiene care related to development and individuality. Historical and social dimensions of hygiene care and cultural and spiritual norms are explored.

Care delivery knowledge

This part follows a format similar to the Subject Knowledge section, but concentrates on the knowledge needed in the assessment and delivery of hygiene care to and with patients and clients.

Professional and ethical knowledge

The professional, ethical, political and social dimensions of hygiene care are addressed. Privacy and dignity issues are explored. Hygiene care as a ritual within nursing is discussed with a particular focus on the role of the nurse as the key decision maker in this area of healthcare practice.

Personal and reflective knowledge

There is a particular focus on the reflective experiences of students in the delivery of care that is intimate and private (Evolve 14.5). Case studies are used to help consolidate knowledge gained from practice and the chapter content.

On page 333 there are four case studies, each one relating to one of the branch programmes. You may find it helpful to read one of them before you start the chapter and use it as a focus for your reflections while reading.

SUBJECT KNOWLEDGE

BIOLOGICAL

STRUCTURE AND FUNCTION OF THE SKIN, HAIR, NAILS, PERINEUM, MOUTH AND EYES AS THEY RELATE TO HYGIENE CARE

The skin

The structure and functions of the skin are more fully outlined in Chapter 15, 'Skin integrity'. Reference will be made here to some of the specific structures that are pertinent to skin and body hygiene. A key function of the skin is protection. Its unique structures protect the body from:

- undue entry or loss of water
- pressure and friction
- microorganisms
- chemicals (weak acids and alkalis)
- most gases
- physical trauma (alpha rays, beta rays to a limited extent, and ultraviolet radiation) (Montague et al 2005).

The two layers of the skin (Fig. 14.1), the epidermis and dermis, function as a single layer. However, the outer layer, the epidermis, has five layers of cell types, each of which has its own unique function. The innermost cell layer of the epidermis (the stratum basale) is important in skin regeneration as the cells are constantly dividing and reproducing, the life cycle of skin cells being approximately 35 days (see Ch. 15). These new cells move through the epidermal layers to the surface of the skin. For the purposes of hygiene care, the stratum corneum, the outermost horny cell layer, is therefore of primary interest. The cells or squames of the stratum corneum are all dead and are constantly being shed from the surface of the body. According to Montague et al (2005), up to 1 million of these cells are shed every 40 minutes through the process of desquamation or exfoliation.

Keratin helps the epidermis form a tough protective barrier. The process of keratinization, which begins in the basal layer, means that the horny cells of the stratum corneum are filled with this protein. Keratin is most evident in areas of the skin exposed to stress, for example the palms of the hands and soles of the feet. Both psoriasis (a skin condition characterized by rapid and excessive production of keratin cells) and dandruff (hyperplasia of the scalp) result in the exfoliation of flakes of keratin (Montague et al 2005).

Certain bacteria are normally present on the skin's outer surface, for example *Staphylococcus epidermidis* and *Corynebacterium*. They are classified as normal flora (commensals) and are protective in function because they inhibit the multiplication of disease-causing organisms. These normal commensals, which inhabit the deeper layers of the stratum corneum, are not usually shed in exfoliation. Commensals use healthy skin scales as a source of food and also rely on the skin having a slightly acid pH in order to maintain their protective function in preventing disease (Montague et al 2005).

The dermis layer of the skin contains collagen and elastic fibres, nerve fibres, blood vessels, sweat glands, sebaceous glands and hair follicles. The last three are particularly significant in relation to hygiene care.

Decision-making exercise

Given that commensals are a normal feature of human skin investigate the following:

- What are the ingredients of soaps ?
- How might the use of soaps affect the skin and the activity of skin commensals?
- How will babies, born with no resident skin commensals, gain these normal commensals?
- What effect might alcoholic skin preparations extensively used in alcohol hand rubs and also in cosmetic skin cleansers have on the skin commensals?

(See Evolve 14.1.)

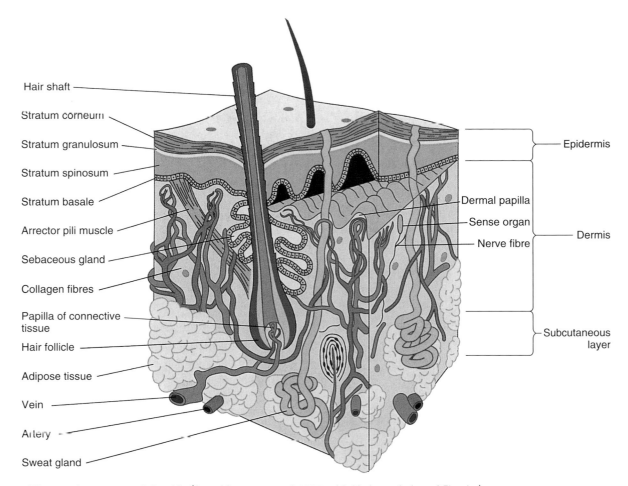

Figure 14.1 Microscopic structure of the skin (from Montague et al 2005, with kind permission of Elsevier).

14.1 – SOAP AND THE SKIN

- List the contents of different types of soaps.
- Describe the effects of soap on the skin.
- Explain the role of skin and its commensals as a protector against infection.
- Outline how hygiene care contributes to infection control.

Sweat glands

Eccrine (found throughout the body) and apocrine glands (responsible for odour and found at specific sites such as the pubis, genitalia, axillae) are two types of sweat (sudoriferous) glands; they are distributed throughout the skin and assist in temperature control. They produce sweat when the skin temperature rises above 35°C. Approximately 500 mL of sweat is produced each day in temperate climates. Secretion of sweat also occurs in response to stress and anxiety as well as to certain spicy foods. Both the production of sweat and its evaporation from the skin assist in heat loss from the body, and the rate of evaporation is particularly important in the patient with pyrexia (raised body temperature) (see Ch. 7, 'Homeostasis').

Sweat left on the skin, especially if from the apocrine glands of the axilla and genital areas, is responsible for body odour through the process of bacterial decomposition. The apocrine glands are dormant during childhood, but begin actively to secrete sweat during puberty and continue to do so throughout adult life. The widespread use of deodorants in developed countries is based on the principle that these solutions will kill the bacteria and mask any odour produced. Antiperspirant sprays block the openings of the ducts to the sweat glands with metal salts such as aluminium (Montague et al 2005).

Sebaceous glands

Sebaceous glands secrete sebum into the hair follicles. This sebum is an oily odourless fluid, containing cholesterol, triglycerides, waxes and paraffins, that lubricates the skin and keeps it supple and pliant. Sebum also has a role in waterproofing the skin and is inhibitory to many microorganisms. Sebaceous glands are found in highest numbers over the scalp and face, the middle of the back, the genitalia and in the auditory canal.

Babies and young children have relatively fewer and less active sebaceous glands and are therefore more prone to skin redness and excoriation in damp conditions, while the loss of sebaceous glands in old age also makes the skin of the elderly more vulnerable to damp conditions, redness and to breakdown. During the menarche (puberty in females), however, the secretion from sebaceous glands increases in response to an increase in adrenocortical hormones. The increasing output of sebum during the teenage years combined with hereditary factors can contribute to the development of acne vulgaris (common acne) (Hockenberry & Wilson 2007).

Hair

The hair follicle is situated in the dermis and is surrounded by its own nerve and blood supply. Sebaceous glands and sweat gland ducts open directly into the hair follicle causing the scalp to become moist and oily, particularly in a hot environment. The cycle of hair growth comprises a period of growth for up to 2 years followed by a rest period and then atrophy. About 70–100 scalp hairs are normally lost each day.

Certain factors affect the rate of normal hair growth and loss. These include:

- nutrition (hair loss in low calorie diets and starvation)
- hormones (puberty with increase in body hair)
- hereditary factors (baldness)
- age (decreased number of hairs with old age).

Most of the body is covered by hair, but it varies in type. Lanugo is the fine silky hair found on the fetus *in utero* and on premature babies, and which is lost from the body soon after birth. Vellus is colourless hair found on the female face. Terminal hair is found on the adult head and pubis and is the subject of hygiene care in relation to maintaining healthy hair covered later in this chapter.

Nails

Nails are keratinized plates resting on the highly vascular and sensitive nail bed. The external appearance of the nail bed is often used to indicate general health status as the shape, colour and condition of fingernails are easily observed. Toenails cause more problems for individuals than fingernails. Debilitated adults may have difficulties in maintaining adequate care and hygiene for their feet which will lead to their toenails becoming thick, brittle and prone to fungal infections. Children may have problems with ingrowing toenails because of difficulties in maintaining well-fitting shoes, especially in times of rapid growth such as during adolescence.

The perineum

The perineum is the area located between the thighs, extending from the anus (posterior) through to the top of the pubic bone (anterior). Anatomical structures in this area are concerned with the expression of sexuality, reproduction and elimination (see Ch. 16, 'Sexuality', and Ch. 18, 'Continence').

In the female, the external genitalia (vulva) consists of the mons pubis, clitoris, urethral and vaginal orifices, and the labia majora and minora. The normal moist environment around the vaginal orifice is maintained by secretions from Bartholin's glands, which are mucus-secreting glands in the lateral wall of the vagina. The slightly acid secretion varies in amount during the ovulation cycle, has a slight odour and helps to inhibit bacterial growth.

In the male, the perineal area includes the penis, the scrotum and the anus. The end of the penis (glans penis) through which the urethra opens in the centre is covered with a skin flap or foreskin in the uncircumcised male. Because the skin of both the penis and the scrotum is thin and hairless it is more easily irritated and injured than skin elsewhere.

The perineal areas of both men and women are prone to infections because they contain openings into the body and are also warm and moist environments. In both sexes, the urethral orifices lead to sterile bladders, but are in close proximity to the anus, which opens into the 'unclean' rectum. The main aim for hygiene care in this area is to prevent or eliminate infection. Prevention of odour is closely linked to the prevention of infection and is a cultural preoccupation in developed countries.

The mouth and teeth

The mouth has many physical and psychosocial functions that are important in supporting the health and well-being of an individual (Box 14.1). The mouth or oral cavity forms

---

Box 14.1 Functions of the mouth

- Ingestion and mastication of food
- Digestion of food
- Taste
- Formation of speech
- Social interaction – non-verbal expressions
- Psychosexual – expression of body image and intimacy

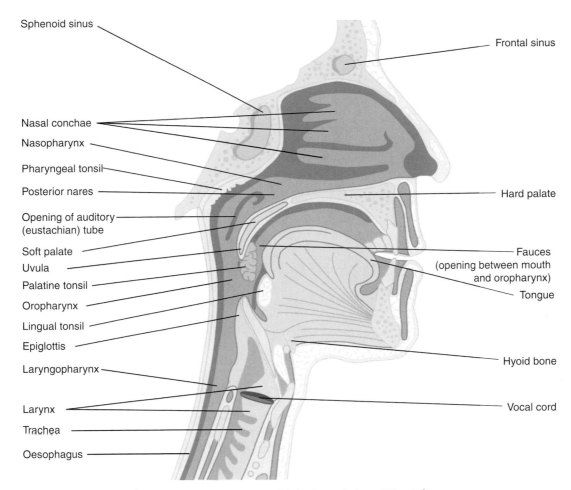

Sphenoid sinus

Frontal sinus

Nasal conchae

Nasopharynx

Pharyngeal tonsil

Posterior nares

Hard palate

Opening of auditory (eustachian) tube

Soft palate

Uvula

Palatine tonsil

Fauces (opening between mouth and oropharynx)

Tongue

Oropharynx

Lingual tonsil

Epiglottis

Hyoid bone

Laryngopharynx

Larynx

Vocal cord

Trachea

Oesophagus

Figure 14.2 Anatomy of the oral cavity (from Montague et al 2005, with kind permission of Elsevier).

the first part of the gastrointestinal tract (Fig. 14.2). It is lined by mucous membrane, which along with the three pairs of salivary glands – the parotid, sublingual and submandibular – secretes mucus and saliva to aid the mastication and digestion of food. The tongue is a large muscular organ involved in taste, speech and swallowing. There are numerous papillae and taste buds on the upper surface of the tongue. The teeth masticate food, help to shape the mouth and are involved in the formation of speech sounds. The deciduous teeth begin to erupt at between 5 and 8 months of age. In childhood there are normally 20 deciduous teeth. Gradual exfoliation of the deciduous teeth begins approximately from the age of 6. These teeth are replaced by 32 permanent teeth by the age of 18–25 years. A full complement of teeth has 16 in the lower and 16 in the upper jaw. Knowledge of the natural loss of teeth in childhood is important to the nurse caring for a child going for surgery under a general anaesthetic, as loose teeth may fall out and be inhaled during induction of anaesthesia.

The structure of the adult tooth contains three parts: the exposed section of the tooth is the crown (enamel), the root

(dentine) which is held in place in the jaw bone by cementum, and the pulp cavity, which contains the blood vessels and nerves (Fig. 14.3).

Dental hygiene

The two major types of oral problems in the normally healthy individual are periodontal disease and dental caries (cavities). Dental caries involve the calcified structures of the tooth. Bacterial enzymes combined with dental plaque produce organic acids, which decalcify both enamel and dentine. Cavities or caries begin to develop once the bacteria have access to the central matrix of the tooth.

Gingivitis is a reversible prevalent disease of the gingivae (gums) and in some cases can lead on to periodontal disease. Clinical features of gingivitis include red, swollen, bleeding gums. Periodontal disease is a chronic irreversible disease of the gingivae and supporting tissues of the tooth, i.e. the cementum, periodontal ligaments and underlying jawbone. Clinical features of periodontal disease (periodontitis) include chronic and/or acute gingivitis, gingival

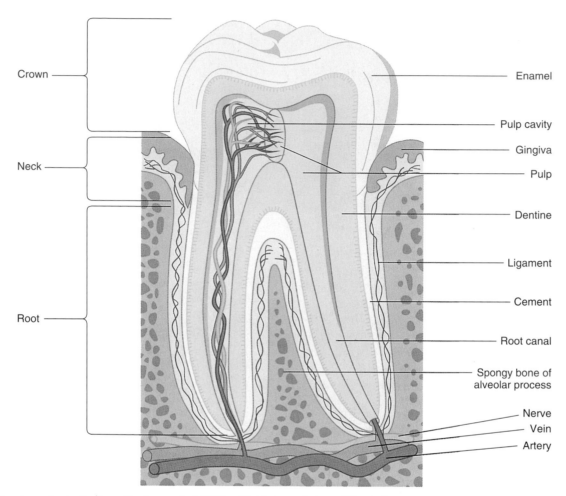

Figure 14.3 Structure of a tooth (from Montague et al 2005, with kind permission of Elsevier).

recession, leading to the root (dentine) becoming exposed in the oral cavity, severe bone loss, tooth mobility and ultimately premature tooth loss.

Saliva plays an essential role in maintaining a healthy mouth. Thin watery saliva flushes away some debris from around the gums and teeth and buffers any acids in the mouth. Thick sticky saliva will aid the formation of plaque and therefore increases the risk of periodontal disease and dental caries (Griffiths & Boyle 2005).

Halitosis ('bad breath'), also known as oral malodour or foetor oris, is a common complaint and has many causative factors which include strong spicy foods, coffee, smoking, alcohol, certain drugs and xerostomia (dry mouth). However, dental plaque is also a primary factor of halitosis due to its metabolic activity. Poor oral hygiene activity can lead to halitosis. People who stop cleaning their mouths will soon develop halitosis. Any form of oral sepsis such as gingivitis or periodontitis will produce a degree of halitosis. Rarer causes include diabetic ketoacidosis and severe renal or hepatic problems (Griffiths & Boyle 2005).

The prevention of peridontal disease and dental caries is necessary to control premature tooth loss throughout the lifespan. Particularly vulnerable times for tooth loss are during childhood and teenage years and the third age (over 50 years old). Pregnant women have a higher susceptibility to gum disease (pregnancy gingivitis) due to the increase of hormonal activity which exaggerates the way the gum tissues react to the bacteria in plaque. This results in an increased vulnerability to gum disease if there is not good control of plaque formation. It is important to note that it is the plaque and not the increased hormone levels that is the major cause of pregnancy gingivitis.

Health promotion strategies addressed to all ages must take into account the interaction between the oral environment of the individual and dental plaque. As soon as food and drink are ingested, the acidity in the mouth increases. The pH is lowered considerably by foods containing sugar and until the acidity is buffered by saliva there is a risk of demineralization of the teeth with subsequent decay. The mouth contains many varieties of bacteria, which do not cause problems if suspended in saliva. However, once these organisms attach themselves to the teeth, gums or tongue surfaces via a mucopolysaccharide glue they become insoluble in water and problems begin. The bacterial deposits cannot be rinsed away and dental plaque forms. Plaque takes 24 hours to develop. It causes periodontal disease and dental caries, which may eventually lead to systemic disease.

Reflection and portfolio evidence

You are undertaking a practice placement with the primary healthcare team and have had experiences working alongside the health visitor, the practice nurse and a school nurse. Reflect on the health promotion advice given by each of these three nurses in their particular roles and with their particular client groups.

- Note the questions asked by clients related to those areas that deal with all aspects of hygiene care to include skin care, oral and dental care and hair care.
- Note the specific advice given by these health professionals and how it relates to your current knowledge base.
- What health promotion strategies were being used to encourage compliance with advice given?
- Record your learning in your portfolio.

The eyes

The eye is a delicate organ with its own built-in mechanisms for protection and hygiene. The conjunctiva covers the exposed surface of the eye and the inner surface of the eyelids and helps to prevent drying of the eye. The eye produces tear fluid, which is washed across the eye by the regular blinking action of the eyelashes. Tear fluid contains salt, protein, oil from sebaceous glands and a bactericidal enzyme called lysozyme, which helps protect the eye against infection. Tears are produced by the lacrimal and accessory glands, which respond to reflexes and the autonomic nervous system. Tears need a drainage system if the eye is not to become 'watery' (epiphora). Drainage is normally via canaliculi at the inner end of the lid margin into the lacrimal sac and duct and finally into the nasal cavity. Any condition that interferes with these three protective mechanisms may cause problems:

- People who wear contact lenses, particularly in a dry centrally heated building for long periods, may be at risk of excessive drying of the cornea and subsequent inflammation (Montague et al 2005).

- The person who has had a stroke or is unconscious for any reason may be vulnerable to eye infections without adequate eye hygiene.
- Many elderly people suffer from 'watery eye' and may require surgery to prevent secondary infections (Montague et al 2005).
- Neonates and young children are prone to get what is known as 'sticky eyes', and the condition may be due to blockage or malformation of the lacrimal ducts and require surgery.
- *Chlamydia* infection passed from the mother to the baby during childbirth can cause serious eye infection in the neonate.
- Bacterial conjunctivitis can be a common problem in children's nurseries and schools, especially as children are prone to rub their eyes with dirty hands (Hockenberry & Wilson 2007).

PSYCHOSOCIAL

INDIVIDUAL ASPECTS OF HYGIENE CARE

Beliefs and attitudes to personal hygiene are developed during childhood and are strongly influenced by social and cultural norms. Nurses, aware of the scientific principles on which they base their beliefs about hygiene care, need to be sensitive to the family and cultural influences on their clients.

Historically, hygiene practices have been influenced by:

- social norms
- religious rituals
- the environment (accessibility of water for bathing)
- evolution of hygiene aids (e.g. showers, soaps, razors, electric toothbrushes, hair dryers).

Hygiene maintenance is a normal daily occupation and promotes a feeling of security and stability alongside well-being and self-esteem. An important stage in the development of independence in hygiene self-care in childhood occurs during the toddler and preschool phase (i.e. at 1–6 years of age). During this time children develop physically, learn to gain self-control and mastery over body functions, and become increasingly aware of their own dependence and independence (Hockenberry & Wilson 2007). The social and cultural beliefs of the family are of great importance in this preschool period in influencing attitudes and practices in hygiene care, and health promotion is usually directed through the parents/carers of the child. Peer influences become increasingly important through the school years and hygiene habits for both sexes may be influenced more by advertising, peer support and the wish to conform to group and sexual norms. Health promotion strategies by healthcare professionals during this phase of development need to consider these predominant social influences. During the late teenage years, values and attitudes become internalized and each individual justifies for themselves their choices in hygiene care. For adults, the influence of advertising which directs its message of responsibility to the family unit, particularly the mother, has an effect on patterns of hygiene practice in society (Aiello & Larson 2001). Anxiety in an individual can lead to an obsession with hygiene care expressed through frequent hand-washing and cleaning. Obsessive compulsive disorder (OCD) is relatively common within the general population and specialist help is needed to deal with the problem.

CULTURAL AND SPIRITUAL ASPECTS OF HYGIENE

Historically, bathing was an important social activity and public baths were a feature of ancient Greek, Egyptian and Roman society. The ancient Roman facilities included exercise rooms, hot, warm and cold baths, steam rooms and dressing rooms. These facilities are again very evident in Western societies with the growth in numbers of modern health and fitness centres which include saunas, steam rooms and jacuzzis. Sociologists have argued that this recent trend is linked with treating 'the body' as a consumer commodity that must be maintained and groomed to achieve maximum market value (Lupton 2003, Twigg 2006). Body maintenance in the interest of good health is linked with the desire to appear sexually attractive in both sexes, but more especially for women. However, cultural habits in hygiene care still demonstrate links with past beliefs, which are often expressed culturally (Helman 2007).

The early Christian church considered physical cleanliness as less important than spiritual purity and after the decline of moral standards in the Roman Empire discouraged public bathing. Bathing, even in private, came to be regarded as unhealthy and was considered an indulgence. In the Middle Ages, the use of water to clean the body was rare and the only areas that needed to be cleansed were those visible to others. Even then, the 'dry wash', which involved rubbing one's face and hands with a cloth, was considered healthy right up to the 17th century. The use of hot water was considered unhealthy as people believed that the pores of the skin would open and allow infection to penetrate the body, therefore being covered up meant that the body was protected from disease. Lay beliefs about how we become susceptible to colds can echo these earlier beliefs, e.g. 'allowing one's head to get wet', 'going outside after washing one's hair', 'getting one's feet wet', 'getting caught in the rain' (Helman 2007).

The relationship between bathing, body hygiene and becoming healthy changed with the Industrial Revolution when the body could then be compared with a machine; the use of cold water was seen as invigorating and helping to firm up the body and also became associated with moral austerity. With the scientific discovery of microbes, washing became important to rid the body of disease, touching of certain body parts considered 'dirty' became prohibited and more frequent washing was encouraged. At this time, buildings did not include bathing facilities and it was not until the level of dirt and disease increased after the Industrial Revolution that demand increased for good bathing facilities to reduce cross-infections such as cholera. By the late 19th century, private homes of the upper classes began to have separate rooms set aside for bathing, and municipal baths were built for the general public to use.

In developed countries today most private homes have their own bathroom facilities, which are often multiple as en suite bathrooms have become the norm in new housing at the end of the 20th century. There is now a more marked preoccupation with cleanliness and showers have become more commonplace, even in temperate climates.

Bathing has also been an integral part of the ritual cleansing of religious practices over many centuries. Baptism in Christianity and the mikvah in Orthodox Judaism are derived from bathing rituals, while bathing is an important part of Muslim and Hindu religious ceremonies. Muslims perform ablutions before prayer and are very particular that all bodily excretions are removed.

Culturally certain hygiene habits may appear distasteful and noisy to nurses in developed countries. Internal cleansing rituals such as sniffing water up into the nose and blowing it out into a basin may provoke disgust, but this can be a normal practice among Muslims and Hindus, while colonic irrigations are a method of internal cleansing of the gut among those who practise yoga.

The 'short back and sides' image of hair hygiene in developed countries is not relevant to a Sikh, to whom the hair (kes) is sacred and should not be cut, but should instead be kept covered by a turban. Rastafarians do not like to wash their long hair.

Items of clothing are also sacred in certain cultures and should not be removed during hygiene care. These can include neck threads (marriage thread for Hindu women), bangles and comb (kara and kasngha for Sikhs), nose jewels (wedding symbols for Bangladeshi women), and a stone or medallion around the neck (protection for Muslims). There are many other cultural and religious habits among different cultural and religious groups that have an important impact on the delivery of appropriate and sensitive hygiene care. It is important to be sensitive to any requests that may seem strange, but are in fact normal to the individual concerned (Hollins 2006). Knowledge and sensitivity to religious practices after death, when body care needs to be delivered according to certain rituals, is essential for the delivery of holistic care.

CARE DELIVERY KNOWLEDGE

Knowledge for the assessment of needs and implementation of care is the main focus for this section. Although in most instances hygiene care is delivered to meet the total needs of the patient, in order to incorporate the specific knowledge underpinning practice, the material in this section is presented under three headings as follows:

- body hygiene care, including reference to the perineal area, nails and eye care
- oral and dental hygiene
- hair care.

ASSESSMENT OF AN INDIVIDUAL'S HYGIENE NEEDS

Decision making around the delivery of hygiene care to a patient or client is dependent upon many factors, which include the patient's ability to self-care, the facilities available, including family members or informal carers, and the nurse's expertise and time. Accurate assessment of the individual patient's needs and level of participation should be encouraged wherever possible. Although there is still a need for the timing to be negotiated to fit organizational needs, the ritualization of bed bathing to the morning shift, whether in hospital, hostel or community, should be a thing of the past.

With children, infants and babies, bath times and routines in any healthcare facility should mimic as closely as possible the child's normal routine with the parents or significant carer being involved directly in providing care. Although the child may view hygiene rituals as unpleasant, they can be fun. There should be facilities both in time and the design of the environment that will maintain and encourage playtime for the infant and young child during the delivery of hygiene care. Children also need privacy, but there should be a balance between allowing them privacy and understanding how much help they require to be safe and to achieve the goals of good hygiene. A baby needs a warm environment and less exposure to prevent chilling. Teenagers will expect that facilities will allow them to maintain their privacy, while older adults may expect the nurse to respect their usual routines for bathing and not demand bathing as a daily ritual if their normal habit is to bath less frequently (Zeitz & McCutcheon 2005).

The ability to care for one's own hygiene needs is important to all individuals and is a prime motivating factor in focusing the nurse on teaching self-care to children or adults with intellectual disabilities. Goals set should be commensurate with the individual's intellectual ability and may need to be frequently revised in order to allow feelings of achievement if progress is slow. Being sensitive to the intimate nature of care and the need for personal control is important in facilitating privacy and dignity. Perceptions of lack of control can lead to the client being agitated and aggressive (Carnaby & Cambridge 2006).

The motivation to maintain personal hygiene as part of a personal self-image can be lost when a person is depressed or disturbed mentally. The nursing role is then focused on encouraging self-care through specific behaviour modification techniques or other counselling approaches that aim to improve the individual's feeling of self-esteem. Equally, the individual may be confused or have a loss of short-term memory and need constant direction in order to be encouraged to maintain his or her independence in hygiene care (Roe et al 2001).

ASSESSMENT FOR BODY HYGIENE CARE

If patients or clients need help from the nurse in meeting their hygiene needs, the following elements should be considered when making an assessment:

- Psychosocial needs: the need for privacy and dignity, personal habits and/or cultural background of the patient.
- Physical needs: level of dependence or independence, temporary or long-term dependence, therapeutic value of hygiene care.
- Facilities and time available: choice of method to deliver care, time of day (patient choice where possible), aids required and available.

The activity of washing removes sweat, sebum, dried skin scales, dust and microorganisms from the skin's surface. If not removed, microorganisms multiply and lead to body odour and infection. When people are ill, increased anxiety can lead to increased sweating and therefore the need to wash more frequently. In surgical patients, a preoperative shower or bath is essential; prevention of wound infection and cross-infection is a paramount consideration in decisions about how often and by what method to deliver hygiene care postoperatively. Patients who are incontinent will need more frequent and sensitive attention to their hygiene needs.

Aesthetically care should be given according to the norms of good taste and culturally specific values. The method selected should be effective in terms of the patient's and the nurse's time and energy. It should promote and maintain the patient's independence, enhance the nurse–patient relationship and provide an opportunity for two-way information processes such as health promotion activities. Body

hygiene care may also be therapeutic if part of a treatment regimen that includes the need for exercise of joints and muscle relaxation while the individual is submersed in warm water. Perineal hygiene care post childbirth also promotes wound healing in the mother who has perineal sutures (Spiby et al 2005).

Decision making around hygiene care is concerned with skilful adaptation of practice when the facilities within the context of care and the actual needs of the patient are incongruent.

Facilitating body hygiene care

There are many different ways of delivering body hygiene care (Box 14.2 and Evolve 14.2). Although nurses in multiple contexts use some or all of these methods on a daily basis, textbooks generally concentrate on the techniques of bed bathing the highly dependent patient (Nicol et al 2008). There has been a major shift in conventions around decision making in this area of total body hygiene as the emphasis is placed on patient independence in maintaining his or her own hygiene care.

Conventional methods of bed bathing are physically tiring for the patient and the nurse (Lomborg & Kirkevold 2005, Rader et al 2006). To overcome some of the disadvantages of bed bathing, towel bathing, disposable baths and Bag Bathing are now being used as an alternative way of delivering hygiene care (Hancock et al 2000, Collins & Hampton 2003, Larson et al 2004).

Bathing can also be used as therapy. Baths at skin temperature (37°C) are relaxing, those hotter or colder can be stimulating. Hot baths can help to relieve pain and discomfort and may control convulsions and induce sleep. Cold baths can be helpful in reducing fever and inflammation. All the body can be submerged or only a body part such as the feet in a foot bath or the perineum in a sitz bath. If any substance is added to the bath to have an effect on a disease, the bath can be termed as 'medicated', e.g. alkaline baths in the treatment of rheumatic conditions.

Box 14.2 Methods of delivery of body hygiene care

- Shower
- Bath
- Complete bed bath
- Towel bath
- Bag bath
- 'Top and tailing' in infants and small children
- Therapeutic bath

14.2 – METHODS FOR DELIVERING BODY HYGIENE CARE

- Describe resources to aid delivery of care to include specialist showers and baths.
- Outline differences between bed baths, towel baths and disposable (Bag Baths) baths.
- Give evidence base for use of disposable baths.
- Describe inflatable baths and basins.

Evidence-based practice

Hoeffer et al (2006) investigated whether certified nursing assistants (CNAs) who received training in a person-centred approach with showering and with the towel bath showed improved caregiving behaviours (gentleness and verbal support) and experienced greater preparedness (confidence and ease) and less distress (hassles) when assisting residents with bathing. The study conducted in the USA used a sample of 15 nursing homes, divided into three groups of five homes per group; two groups receiving training and the third acting as a control group. Observational and self report data were collected on five caregiving outcomes. Compared with the control group, treatment groups significantly improved in the use of gentleness and verbal support and in the perception of ease.

Special areas for care: the perineal area

Delivering care to the perineal area is often referred to as providing intimate care, needing extra sensitivity on the part of the nurse/carer. For babies and young children who are not yet toilet trained, this area needs extra hygiene care and the application of water repellent creams to prevent skin damage. Children should generally be encouraged to self-care, but in the older child there is a tendency to avoid cleaning this area (Hockenberry & Wilson 2007). For boys over 3 years of age who are not circumcised, the foreskin should be retracted and the exposed surface cleaned (except in circumstances where cultural beliefs will not allow this). However, care must be taken to retract the foreskin very gently as it may be tight (phimosis) and overstretching can create scarring, leading to sexual and micturition (passing urine) difficulties in the future.

In adults of both sexes who cannot maintain their own hygiene, extra sensitivity is needed in dealing with perineal care because of cultural and spiritual taboos in exposing this area of the body. Good quality perineal care in women following childbirth is essential, especially if there is a surgical wound in the area (Spiby et al 2005).

Special areas for care: nails

Most people can maintain hand nail hygiene according to their own particular standards and values. In children, hygiene care to keep hand nails clean is particularly important after outdoor play, toileting and before meals as the eggs from intestinal parasites or helminths (roundworms, hookworms, pinworms, threadworms or *Toxocara* from dogs or cats) can be ingested and the child then becomes infected (Hockenberry & Wilson 2007).

Foot nail care is also important in the elderly, and especially in any person who has diabetes mellitus as poor peripheral circulation makes this group of people vulnerable to skin breakdown with subsequent delayed healing. Specialist foot nail care is required through the expert skills of the chiropodist/podiatrist and the nurse's role is primarily in recognizing the need to refer clients and in providing preliminary care and advice.

Special areas for care: eyes

Eye hygiene is part of the process of maintaining personal hygiene and practices from washing the area around the eyes with a clean face flannel through to using commercial products for cleansing lids and lashes (e.g. Lid-Care by CIBA Vision) and the removal of eye cosmetics is a matter for individual choice. The normal defence mechanisms of blinking and washing tears over the eye are sufficient to maintain healthy eyes. However, in health care particular groups of people can be at risk and need special eye hygiene care. These include:

- the newborn
- the elderly who develop 'dry eye'
- the unconscious person
- people who have had an eye injury or surgery.

Although pupillary and corneal reflexes are present in the newborn infant, the tear glands do not begin to function properly until the infant is 2–4 weeks old. Particular risks for the newborn include ophthalmia neonatorum, an infectious conjunctivitis that needs specific treatment with antibiotic drops (guttae) or ointment (unguentum). The eyes are usually cleansed with sterile water before the insertion of drops or ointment. Conjunctivitis is common in infants and older children and the many different causes need specific treatments and eye hygiene measures (Hockenberry & Wilson 2007).

Dry eye in older people is a condition which has many causes and has varying degrees of severity. The complex tear film is made up of layers of oil, water and mucin, produced by the meibomian glands, main and accessory lacrimal glands, and by the goblet cells, respectively. Alteration in the normal function of any of these structures by disease, trauma or the environment can cause dysfunction of the tear film and result in the symptoms of dry eye. People will complain of varying degrees of a burning sensation, grittiness and blurred vision. Care is through good eyelid hygiene and providing the patient with artificial tears in the form of eye drops or eye ointment (Terry 2001).

In the unconscious person, the corneal reflex is lost and the eyes may tend to remain open and become dry. Drying of the eyes can lead to corneal abrasions and subsequent loss of sight. Regular cleaning of the lids and lashes, the installation of an eye lubricant, and keeping the eyes closed with a polyethylene film/cover are necessary to prevent damage to the eyes (Joyce 2002).

Following eye surgery or eye injury specific hygiene practices are usually instigated by the specialist ophthalmic nurse, but a key role is in health promotion in order to prepare the patient for continuing self-care following discharge. As the eye is such a sensitive organ, self-care is often difficult to achieve, especially by the elderly and those who have difficulty in remembering instructions or in manipulating the dropper or the ointment tube. It is important to know and practise the correct technique and be able to educate relatives and friends to deliver the care (see Nicol et al 2008 for details on eye care technique).

Principles of care

Whatever procedure is selected to deliver body hygiene, the principles of safety, prevention of cross-infection and promotion of privacy and dignity should be followed. Safety extends to promoting good back care and posture for the nurse or carer by encouraging the use of appropriate bathing aids (see Evolve 14.2). Children should never be left alone in the bath as there is always a danger of drowning regardless of the water level. People suffering from epilepsy or seizures (fits) of any kind need to keep bathroom doors unlocked to allow access.

The process of providing care should be methodical, logical and safe, taking into consideration the specific limits of the patient, whether temporary (for example post-surgery) or permanent (for example due to physical disability). Goals should be set for what the patient can realistically do without causing undue discomfort and exposure during the bathing process. Being sensitive and not taking over is important as most people are intrinsically motivated to participate in their own care and dislike any loss of dignity and freedom of action. Quality standards for the delivery of hygiene care can be audited or benchmarked using tools contained in the UK Department of Health document *Essence of Care* (Department of Health 2001a).

Giving hygiene care also allows the nurse to undertake other activities that are necessary for the overall decision making about care for the clients (Table 14.1). This particular aspect is often overlooked in skill mix debates when it is

Table 14.1 Nursing activities that can be incorporated into the delivery of hygiene care

Type of activity	Details
Observations	Observe for signs and symptoms of physical problems Note any non-verbal expressions of anxiety and fear
Interpersonal communication	Encourage disclosure by patient (intimate procedure) Time for mutual trust and building relationships Opportunity to offer empathy and support
Health promotion	Information giving about the immediate condition and its treatment Health promotion directly related to hygiene care practices Advice and support for self-care strategies on discharge or in the long term
Social interaction	Recognition of the influence of family, life and work on the patient Growth and development of the nurse as a person and a practitioner

argued that hygiene care does not need the skills of a registered nurse. The opportunity to make relevant observations, to initiate and sustain the nurse–patient relationship, to explore the patient's concerns and to promote a healthy lifestyle is a fundamental part of the delivery of body hygiene care.

ORAL HYGIENE

The focus in this section is on oral assessment and care primarily delivered in institutional health care settings.

Assessment

The nurse's role in the maintenance of oral and dental hygiene involves the use of general observation skills and specific assessment tools. Although it has been recognized that much of the responsibility for the delivery of oral care in an institutional setting has devolved to the junior or untrained nurse, the initial and ongoing assessment is the responsibility of the registered practitioner. Specific assessment tools should aid this process. However, to date, these tools are still not yet in common use and reliability is dependent upon the same nurse carrying out the assessment in order to reduce the subjective nature of the decision making about oral care.

It is important to encourage the use of an objective assessment tool that is valid, reliable and practical to use on a day-to-day basis. Many tools have been developed based on the reliable tool originally designed by Eilers et al (1988) for the prevention of oral mucositis (infection and ulceration of mucous tissue in the mouth most commonly caused by chemotherapy) in cancer patients (Eilers 2007). These tools have been revised and renamed to include such titles as: the OAG (oral assessment guide); OHAG (oral health assessment guide); THROAT(the holistic and reliable oral assessment tool); or JANET (joint assessment nursing education tool). Many of the tools have been designed for the assessment of particular client groups such as the older dependent adult, those in long care mental health settings, adults being nursed in critical care units, or patients undergoing cancer treatments such as chemotherapy and radiotherapy.

The content of the various oral assessment tools include:

- direct observation of areas of the oral cavity
- assessment of the functions of the mouth
- risk factors that have the potential to create oral problems.

The reliability of scoring systems that indicate the severity of the patient's oral condition have been questioned (Griffiths & Boyle 2005). Table 14.2 demonstrates the common features

Table 14.2 Common features of different oral assessment tools

Feature	Details
Observation of areas within mouth	Lips: colour, moisture, texture Tongue: colour, moisture, texture Gingiva: colour, moisture, haemorrhage, ulceration, oedema Teeth: shine, debris Palate: moisture, colour, ulceration
Functions within the mouth	Saliva: thin, watery, hypersalivation, scanty, absent, thick, ropy Voice: normal, deep, raspy, difficult or painful speech Swallow: normal, difficult, pain on swallowing fluids or solids, diminished or no gag reflex
Predisposing stressors	Mouth breathing Oxygen therapy Mechanical ventilation Restricted oral intake Chemotherapy or radiotherapy Drugs and concurrent diseases
Subjective data from patients	Taste changes Pain profile

of the various assessment tools presented in the literature. As it is important to use an objective measure, especially where care is being delegated to many (including junior) staff, the registered nurse should assess which of the tools, if used, will provide the most valid and reliable information for the particular client group.

A broader approach to oral assessment that includes the need to incorporate better interprofessional working with dentists, dental hygienists and clients themselves is advocated by Griffiths & Boyle (2005, Ch. 6). Tools should also include observation of the client's behaviour and involve clients themselves in expressing their own needs. Any tool used could be an adaptation of a number of approaches that will suit the particular client group and their health circumstances. There is also a need to ensure the use of these tools is consistent and regular audit of their implementation is essential to maintain quality of care.

Decision-making exercise

While on practice placement, observe the assessment and implementation of oral care. Remember that age groups, certain conditions and drug treatments can have an impact on oral health.

- Review the use/non use of an oral health assessment tool.
- Discuss the need for and/or selection of an oral assessment tool with your mentor.
- Debate whether this tool will cover all the needs of the patient/client group.
- Discuss your decision and how you could influence for change in current practice in order to improve the quality of care.

(Use the Department of Health (2001a) *Essence of Care: Patient-focused Benchmarking for Health Care Practitioners* and review the section on personal and oral hygiene to support your decisions.)

In the assessment of different client groups it is important to remember that specific predisposing factors may put them at considerable risk of developing oral problems. Children with Down's syndrome and other disabling conditions tend to have thick, ropy, sticky saliva that fails to 'wash' food debris away and adheres to the tooth surface. This process encourages the early formation of plaque (Griffiths & Boyle 2005, Ch. 10).

Teenagers wearing orthodontic appliances (braces) and those with an oral deformity such as a cleft lip or palate who have removable or fixed appliances will need special advice on how to maintain their oral hygiene, but may need encouragement from the nurse to sustain these practices (Griffiths & Boyle 2005).

For the older client, the ageing process leads to a decreased salivary flow. Although an increasing number of elderly people retain their own teeth, if the client is wearing dentures, these should be checked for fit to prevent trauma to the palate and gums. If the individual client has diminished neuromuscular control he or she may have difficulty in maintaining oral care through lack of hand to mouth coordination.

For the elderly mentally infirm, it may be the client's behaviour that needs to be targeted during rehabilitation so that the individual's coping strategies can be improved. This assessment will involve other members of the health-care team in order to measure the client's progress against preset short- and long-term goals. There are many risk factors to optimum oral health in the mentally ill. These arise from the condition itself or the drug treatment to control the symptoms of the illness (Chalmers & Pearson 2005) (Table 14.3).

Many other conditions, treatments and drugs can put the individual client at particular risk of developing oral problems. Some of these treatments are included in the risk assessment tools referred to earlier (see Table 14.2). Many drugs, regardless of their route of administration, have systemic effects on the body causing xerostomia (dry mouth) and damage to the normal defence and healing processes of the oral cavity and are detailed in Table 14.3.

Evidence-based practice

Talbot et al (2005), using a survey, investigated oral care provision in 71 stroke care settings in Scotland. 70 units responded with the following results; support from dental professionals was available to most units (64/70) on request; a third of units received oral care training in the previous year (23/70); use of oral care assessment tools and protocols was limited to 16/70 and 15/70 units respectively. Access to toothbrushes, toothpaste or chlorhexidine was not available to all units. For patients unable to perform oral care independently, senior nurses expected the patients' teeth or dentures to be cleaned at least twice a day in 59 of 70 and 49 of 70 units respectively. As with all survey results, what is reported by the respondents needs further validation in practice. However, the results provided baseline information to address improvement in services.

Facilitating oral care

In the delivery of oral care or health promotion to clients the nurse has many decisions to make concerning the most appropriate advice, tools and solutions to use. The single most effective method of promoting dental health is the daily removal of dental plaque. In addition the reduction of refined sugars in the diet is essential to maintain dental health; however, plaque is the primary cause of tooth and gum disease and not sugar.

The toothbrush is the most effective method for removing plaque. Ideally the design should include a small head with soft multitufted nylon bristles. Power brushes that are battery operated or rechargeable devices have an oscillating round brush head that is also efficient at removing plaque without causing damage to the gums (Heanue et al 2003). Manually, a good simple technique is to brush in small circles dividing the mouth up into sections and systematically brushing each section. Brushing gums is just as important as the area between the teeth and gums can trap plaque, which will lead to gingivitis. Single-tufted brushes with a pointed tip are useful for patients with trismus (limited mouth opening). The use of dental floss or tape is recommended to clean between the teeth. All the above tools are relatively easy to use when the client can understand how and can control their use. Problems arise when the client is dependent on the nurse for oral care.

Although toothbrushing is the method of choice, in the past, nurses have failed to use them with clients, particularly because they feared causing trauma and perceived them as unsuitable for an edentulous mouth. The choice of toothbrush and method for using it are of prime importance for different client groups.

Table 14.3 Drug groups that affect oral health (after Sreebny & Schwartz 1997)

Drug group	Mechanism of action
Antihistamines Antispasmodics Anticholinergics Antidepressants Antipsychotics Tranquillizers Anticonvulsants Narcotic analgesics	Reduce salivary production
Antibiotics	Alter the balance of commensal organisms so that candidal organisms can invade the mouth
Cytotoxics and chemotherapeutics	Reduce the autoimmune response and therefore allow easy growth of invading organisms
Corticosteroids	Reduce the healing properties of tissues
Diuretics	Potential dehydration resulting in a reduction in salivary flow

Young children need to have their teeth brushed for them; for the disabled child or adult, electric or specially adapted standard toothbrushes are necessary. As tooth brushing does not remove plaque from between the teeth, the use of dental floss or interdental brushes are now being recommended for regular use. Dental floss is available either waxed or unwaxed and is sometimes impregnated with fluoride. It does require skill to use dental floss in order to prevent damage to the gums and the teeth. It is recommended that children up to the age of 12 years approximately may not have the required level of dexterity to use dental floss safely and effectively (Griffiths & Boyle 2005, Ch. 3).

Toothpaste is the most common substance used to clean teeth and since the introduction of fluoride into toothpaste there has been a large reduction in dental decay, especially in children (Marinho et al 2003). The fluoridation of water has been widespread, although the ethical debates related to personal choice have prevented its implementation in some areas. Although special fluoride supplements (rinses, gels, tablets and drops) have been available for children, there is concern that with the increasing amounts of fluoride in toothpaste, there may be a danger of the child developing fluorosis (excessive fluoride can cause yellowing of teeth, white spots, and pitting or mottling of enamel). Ensuring that children do not swallow toothpaste and rinse their mouths carefully is important in order to prevent fluorosis. Fluoride supplements should only be used on the advice of a dentist.

Other solutions in common use are listed in Table 14.4. Overall chlorhexidine is the most effective anti-plaque agent (Imai 2006). There is a need to research more fully the effectiveness of some of the solutions that are still in common use in institutional healthcare settings. Commercially available solutions may contain alcohol, which has no benefit.

Other tools used for giving oral care to the dependent patient include foam sponges, swab on forceps and the swab on the finger technique. Foam sponges have the advantage of causing little oral trauma, but they are expensive and ineffective at removing debris from the surface or from between teeth (Griffiths & Boyle 2005). The swab on a forceps technique can be difficult to manipulate and may be more prone to causing trauma. The swab on the gloved finger, if used with a gentle sweeping action, can be effective in removing debris without causing undue trauma. However, in any dependent person with facial muscle weakness that affects the mouth (for example following a stroke), it is important that food and debris are not missed as the action of the swabbing may cause food to be compressed into one part of the mouth. Remember, the technique of the user is important in order to remove plaque regardless of tool used to deliver oral care.

Denture care

Dentures, both full and partial, are the most common oral appliance, especially among the elderly population, and need regular rinsing and cleaning, particularly after eating. Dentures should be removed at night and stored in plain water or a dental cleansing solution to prevent the development of oral candidiasis also called denture stomatitis (thrush). Plaque forming on dentures is not easily visible until eventually hard deposits of calculus (tartar) form in the plaque. The dentures develop rough surfaces that soon cause irritation and soft tissue damage.

As with teeth, the most effective method for removing plaque is through brushing and rinsing. Proprietary denture cleaners are available as solutions, brush-on cleaners or pastes, but all have some disadvantages such as staining, bleaching and corrosion of metal. Regular brushing with unperfumed household soap and water is considered one of the best methods of cleaning dentures (Griffiths & Boyle 2005).

A common problem may be loose-fitting dentures, especially if the wearer is ill and poor nutrition leads to physical deterioration. A temporary method to overcome this problem is to insert a soft lining until a new set of dentures can be made. A set of dentures should be checked and replaced

Table 14.4 Solutions in common use for oral hygiene: actions and limitations (after Griffiths & Boyle 2005)

Solution	Action	Limitations
Chlorhexidine gluconate (solution, gel, spray)	Effective antiplaque Well tolerated by most client groups	Reversible staining of teeth
Hexetidine and cetylpyridinium (mouthwash, gargle)	Antiplaque	Not as effective as chlorhexidine
Hydrogen peroxide and sodium perborate (diluted as mouthwash at 3%)	Mucosolvent that breaks down thick and viscous saliva	Unpleasant taste Short-term use only Incorrect dilution leads to chemical burns Risk of borate absorption
Sodium bicarbonate (powder diluted in water)	Mucosolvent Cleansing	Unpleasant taste Further research needed to ascertain how useful in practice
Thymol (mouthwash)	Antibacterial at high concentrations Refreshing taste	Little to no antibacterial action at low concentrations
Sodium chloride (mouthwash, gargle)	Effective cleansing agent Well tolerated	None indicated
Lemon and glycerine (impregnated swabs on a stick)	Lemon is a salivary stimulant Glycerine for lubrication	Overuse can lead to salivary gland exhaustion and increased xerostomia Low pH increases the risk of dental caries
Phenol (mouthwash, gargle, spray)	Cleansing	Epiglottic and laryngeal oedema Contraindicated in children Needs further research to test effects on plaque
Povidone–iodine 1% (mouthwash/gargle)	Cleansing	Mucosal irritation Hypersensitive reactions No antiplaque activity
Benzydamine hydrochloride (mouthwash, spray)	Relief of oral ulceration	Numbness or stinging

every 5 years and any soft linings used should be replaced every 2 years (Griffiths & Boyle 2005). In residential or nursing home care many of the elderly residents have dentures, but loss of dentures can now be prevented by labelling dentures when they are manufactured or using a commercially available naming kit (i.e. Indenture).

HAIR CARE

Hair styling and grooming feature very highly in maintaining physical and psychological health and a positive body image. Most people can and wish to maintain their own hair according to their own choice. In institutions where individuals are unable to care for themselves it is often therapeutic if a member of the family or a friend provides this aspect of hygiene care. Self-care is a significant goal to achieve for those with physical and mental disability.

Hair care among different ethnic groups can be part of deeply embedded beliefs that are cultural as well as religious, and these need to be respected. Hair care for black children or adults, if dependent, may need specific combs and techniques. Hair loss from the head, known as alopecia areata, can be a significant source of worry, especially if it occurs for no known cause in children and adolescents. Males and females are equally affected.

All of the above variations in hair care need to be taken into account in assessing and facilitating hygiene care. Resources, which include time, should be available to provide optimum hair care in any healthcare institution. Daily combing and brushing can usually be maintained through self-care, family support and nursing care. However, standards of care for shampooing can vary, and in the acute care setting may inevitably be given lower priority when resources are stretched. Many institutions for both acute and long-term care have back-up hairdressing services available, but often at a financial cost to clients.

Hair care also incorporates removing unwanted hair from the face in the male through regular shaving. For the dependent patient, nurses need to become skilled in using a razor and/or the use of an electric shaver (see Nicol et al 2008, Ch. 11). Shaving of hair from other parts of the body such as under the axilla is personal to the individual and their hygiene standards.

Hair infestation

Head lice are endemic worldwide and although they are not responsible for the spread of any disease, they are responsible for considerable social distress. They are cosmopolitan in that they can infest anybody and do not discriminate between class or cleanliness. Infestation with head lice can be quite debilitating if left untreated. However, this rarely happens today. The term 'feeling lousy' originates from feeling weak and 'nitwit' refers to poor performance at work due to untreated infestation.

School nurses, practice nurses and health visitors are key healthcare workers in dealing with head lice in children. Both education and public health acts make it mandatory for health professionals to monitor and diagnose the presence of head lice in schoolchildren, but it is then the responsibility of the parents to cleanse the head. Teachers often support parents through coordinated preventative activity during school time, to help reduce spread and the potential stigma of being an infested child. Free prescriptions for head lice preparations are available for children under 16 years of age and the UK Department of Health provides up-to date advice through their leaflets and website (Department of Health 2007). Most health districts now use a rotational policy for the main chemical treatments for head lice as there is evidence that resistance has developed (Hill 2006). All lotions used for treatments can cause undue irritation of the skin. Non-chemical approaches to the treatment of head lice, i.e. 'bug-busting', are becoming increasingly popular and are being more actively promoted.

As this area of health promotion and healthcare remains a problem for children and their parents world wide, you can access an exploration of the literature and the evidence on treatment choices via Evolve 14.3.

ⓔvolve | **14.3 – HAIR INFESTATION**
learning system

- List types of lice found on the body.
- Outline life cycle and methods of spread of head lice.
- List chemical treatments and their effect.
- Describe non-chemical treatments.
- List useful websites and references.

Decision-making exercise

On a recent placement the school nurse has asked you to help her with a health promotion session on the control of head lice that she is about to do for parents in a local primary school.

- Find out about the rotational system of treatment of head lice by chemical means in your area.
- Check the advice being given in your local area by the Health Education Authority/Department of Health about non-chemical treatments for head lice.
- Discuss the evidence for both types of treatment with your school nurse.
- Decide with the school nurse on the best approach to the proposed health promotion session.

PROFESSIONAL AND ETHICAL KNOWLEDGE

This section will explore the politics and imagery of hygiene care with a particular focus on the continuing role of nurses in decision making and controlling this area of their professional practice. Institutional care often removes choice and the patient's right to refuse care must be recognized despite creating ethical dilemmas in maintaining standards of care.

The words 'basic nursing care' have been adopted by nurses as synonymous with meeting the hygiene needs of patients. Dictionary meanings for the word 'basic' are given as 'forming the base or essence' or 'fundamental' (*Oxford English Dictionary* 1989). *The Essence of Care* is the title of the Department of Health's document outlining quality standards for care in core areas of nursing to include 'personal and oral hygiene' (Department of Health 2001a). The dictionary also acknowledges a meaning for 'basic' which implies having relatively little value. Professionalization of nursing seems to have permitted the word 'basic' to become synonymous with the notion of being 'simple' or 'easy', thus implying a hierarchy of skills with 'technical' nursing skills, where less body care is involved, having greater importance and status. Acceptance of the 'simple and easy' meaning allows this fundamental aspect of the professional nurse's role to be delegated to the most junior member of the nursing team or the unqualified nurse.

There is also a hierarchy in the organization of nursing work and its relationship to body care, with the lowest level of 'nursing' staff actually delivering hygiene care. Current preoccupations with cost-effectiveness in health care has put the division of labour into sharper focus with grading and skill mix reviews. This often means the allocation of technical and managerial work to the registered nurse with basic body care being assigned to semi-skilled care workers (Twigg 2006).

There is, however, a view that knowledge and control over these areas of body care are integral to a view of nursing as a distinct profession. The aim is to deliver quality holistic nursing care to help the individual patient live through their personal experience of pain and discomfort. Hygiene or body care is then fundamental as it offers the opportunity of closeness and the expression of care (Twigg 2006). By this argument, hygiene care remains an essential element and a core activity for the development of knowledge and decision making within the domain of nursing practice.

Reflection and portfolio evidence

There are debates in the professional and sociological literature around the role of the registered nurse in the delivery of hygiene care. Referring back to the content of this chapter and Chapter 1 and to your own personal experiences in practice

- Share with your fellow student nurses your experience in the assessment of need and the delivery of hygiene care to patient/client groups at home and/or in hospital.
- Debate how the care was organized, who was expected to deliver that care and how they/you have been educated and trained to deliver that care.
- Reflect and debate how or if you expect your role to change in relation to the delivery of hygiene/body care when you become a registered nurse.

HYGIENE CARE AND THE IMAGE OF THE NURSE

According to Foucault (1975), when an individual becomes ill and enters an institution for care the boundaries of what might be considered normal in society are breached. This contention has particular implications for the breaking of the rules of privacy associated with the delivery of hygiene care. The body of the individual becomes 'objectified' in a way that allows healthcare professionals to observe and treat the individual without seemingly having to consider the emotions that body exposure may arouse both in the patient and in the nurse (Lawler 1997, Wolf 1997).

Nursing is also considered as 'dirty work' because it deals with the 'body' and body products. It is viewed as acceptable that people of low status should do this work and it has been argued historically that women are best suited to this type of care giving. Paradoxically the women (nurses) who administered body care were expected to be both morally and physically pure (Wolf 1997). The notion that nurses should be female is an extension of their roles as wives and mothers and this gives permission for intimate care.

However, sexual stereotypes of female nurses are perpetuated by the media and by film and TV dramas. These stereotypes can be selected by male patients and instigated as part of the banter with female nurses, especially when having to subject themselves to the intimacy of hygiene care. Wearing a uniform may be important not just for cross-infection protection but also because it is symbolic in that it gives the nurse permission to administer intimate care (Seed 1995, Edwards 1998). In units where a uniform is not now worn, special garments such as plastic aprons may still be worn during the process of facilitating hygiene care.

There are equally powerful boundaries that the male nurse needs to cross in caring for female patients. The male nurse's role in giving hygiene care is more atypical of the accepted status quo in society in that nursing is seen in the context of 'motherhood', with a predominantly female profession giving intimate care. Therefore the need to seek permission may be more prominent when a male nurse seeks to give hygiene care to a female, especially if of a similar age. Seed (1995) found that male students were confronted with the feeling that they were doing something immoral in delivering intimate care to women.

According to Edwards (1998) age also has an impact, with the older person submitting to intimate care as they no longer regard themselves as a symbol of sexual taboo. Edwards (1998) also found that staff of both genders felt uneasy when giving intimate care to the opposite gender of a similar age. This was reported to be the case whether staff were aged 20 or 50.

Delivery of intimate and personal care to people with learning disabilities is a core part of daily care and has the potential to highlight the sexuality and sexual needs of the service users and also their carers. Adult protection and sexuality policies need to be clear about boundaries and approaches to care in order to protect both parties (Carnaby & Cambridge, 2006).

CONSENT AND PRIVACY

Respect for privacy, dignity and patient autonomy is central to giving good quality hygiene care. The processes for obtaining informed consent for treatment are well established in law and in health care. In accepting help with hygiene care, patients signify their implied consent through taking part in the process or submitting to the process. However, in the confused or intellectually impaired, nurses may make decisions for patients based on what they believe is in their best interest. Alternative approaches should be considered to ease the burden of discomfort and lack of control especially experienced by the confused elderly (Rader et al 2006).

Behavioural problems can occur when patients are frightened by the bathing process and feel out of control (Hoeffer et al 2006). The dying patient may wish to be left alone and not be subjected to the daily traditional bath. In some cases nurses, instead of being the patient's advocate, may deliver hygiene care despite lack of implied consent or even in the face of patient dissent in order to maintain the perceived professional standard of care (Lentz 2003).

Privacy and dignity are very important when giving intimate care especially with the sharing of facilities in an institution or even with interruptions of the process of giving hygiene care by other members of the multiprofessional team. Ensuring privacy is a key component in maintaining dignity. In a study on the meaning of dignity for patients and relatives, they indicated that being covered up and having the curtains drawn around during care activities is a very important example of ensuring individual respect and dignity (Gallagher & Seedhouse 2002).

For people with disabilities there is a policy focus on ensuring choice and person centred planning. Because of the widely differing needs of those with a learning and/or physical disability, there remain problems in the management of personal and intimate care that will allow adequate consent, privacy and autonomy for the individual concerned (Carnaby & Cambridge 2006).

Reflection and portfolio evidence

When in your practice placement in a healthcare institution, reflect on the approaches taken to meet patients'/clients' hygiene needs.

- Note whether all hygiene care is delivered at a set time during the patients' day.
- Observe how nursing staff deal with the patient who is reluctant or refuses hygiene care when offered.
- Monitor your own behaviour and communication skills when approaching patients to offer assistance with hygiene.
- Record any interruptions to the process of giving hygiene care and note how this is handled in relation to maintaining patient privacy and dignity.
- Record your reflections and debate the issues with your peer group.

THE POLITICS OF HYGIENE CARE

UK government health and social care policy focuses on the premise that where at all possible the disabled, those with long-term illnesses and the frail elderly should be cared for in their own homes (Department of Health 2001b, 2005).

Initial assessment of overall care needs was transferred to the social worker through the Community Care Act of 1990 and since 1996 (under the Community Care Direct Payments Act 1996) control of finances to purchase services has become more patient/client and/or carer centred. The aim of the 1996 Act was to promote independence through encouraging partnership processes in the allocation and spending of funding on care packages. Clients are empowered to make their own choices to meet their needs in innovative ways provided that these public funds are used effectively. Since 2005, there has been a major expansion of direct payments in the form of individual budgets for service users. This means that clients and/or their carers can select and pay directly for any services they need.

A large part of the overall workload of the professional nurse working in the community is the prioritization of patient needs often within a framework of diminishing resources. Generally, the actual delivery of hygiene care in the community, like institutions, is primarily undertaken by care assistants and is subject to strict budgetary limits. This often leaves the biggest burden of care with relatives and friends or informal carers; see Evolve 14.4 for more information.

⊖volve

14.4 – THE POLITICS OF PERSONAL (HYGIENE) CARE IN THE COMMUNITY

- Define community care.
- Debate the role of social services and health care services in providing personal care.
- Describe the impact of 'direct payments'.
- List the issues from the client perspective.

Attitudes to the importance of hygiene care are a factor in the allocation of resources. Assisted personal body care tends to be regarded as an unproblematic nursing activity with little professional challenge. In order to rationalize resources, care assistants (CA) have been widely employed in various settings to help improve efficiency and reduce healthcare costs. This reflects the view that personal care tasks, such as bathing, dressing, and bed making, can be allocated to care assistants, leaving the registered nurse

(RN) time to perform the more technical tasks such as assessment, drug administration and wound care. The nature of the RN role is all embracing and does not lend itself to being categorized into specific tasks (Perry et al 2003). However, in relation to the delivery of personal care, with current policy over costing in the UK there is a need to prioritize how RNs spend their time. The delegation of 'the task' of the delivery of hygiene care should not detract from the accountability of the RN for the overall assessment of need and the quality of care delivered to patients/clients. The level of training and support offered to CAs should also be commensurate with the complexity of situations they will need to deal with in the delivery of personal care (Carnaby & Cambridge 2006).

Decision-making exercise

When making decisions about the allocation of nursing support for hygiene care within a system where resources are limited what should be the priority for the care manager who has to make these decisions? Consider your answer by examining which of the following should take priority.

- Patient/client defined needs.
- The interprofessionals' perceptions of what the client needs.
- The resources available.
- Debate your findings and also the political role of the nurse in advocating for resources.

PERSONAL AND REFLECTIVE KNOWLEDGE

The delivery of high standards of hygiene care requires the nurse to have detailed knowledge and skills and to be able to take appropriate and sensitive decisions in facilitating hygiene care for each individual client. There is also a need to consider yourself in the role of a nurse as a role model for standards of hygiene, reflecting on your own personal standards in hygiene practices. Although a direct causal link between personal hygiene and infection cannot be made, maintaining a high standard of personal hygiene reduces the level of resident skin staphylococci. This reduction can be achieved by daily bathing, keeping nails short, tying the hair back and not wearing rings or other jewellery. These standards extend to ensuring that where a uniform is worn for the delivery of care, it is changed daily and adequately laundered (Wilson et al 2007 and cross reference with Ch. 5, 'Infection prevention and control').

It is important to reflect, integrate and consolidate the knowledge gained from this chapter with the knowledge gained from your practice experience. This can be achieved through reflection on your own personal experiences and those of your peer group of students and through the case study work, which you can complete on your own or which may form the basis for a group seminar.

Learning about all aspects of hygiene care for all client groups is a fundamental part of any nursing course. Much of your practice experience is gained directly with patients or clients in partnership with an assigned clinical supervisor or mentor. Expert nurses forget how embarrassed a student may feel when they first have to deliver

---

Reflection and portfolio evidence

Obtain and read a copy of O'Regan H, Tonks Fawcett J. 2006 Learning to nurse: reflections on bathing a patient. Nursing Standard 20(46):60–65.

- Reflect and compare the first author's experience of bathing a patient with your own experiences.
- Discuss the issues raised by her reflections on her learning with your fellow students.

---

intimate hygiene care to a client and take for granted their own knowledge and skills in the delivery of hygiene care. Reflective notes made in a personal learning diary will be useful so that you can discuss your feelings later if you wish. Problems faced by students in the delivery of hygiene care are often not discussed (Seed 1995, Wolf 1997). You may, however, get the opportunity to practise and reflect on your own personal feelings and reactions in the relatively safe environment of a 'practical room' or 'skills centre/laboratory'. Experiential exercises in assessing 'the normal' in your fellow students and in providing hygiene advice and care to your fellow students under different circumstances will help you gain confidence in your own ability before being exposed to patients and clients. Please see Evolve 14.5 for examples of these exercises.

14.5 – EXPERIENTIAL EXERCISES IN HYGIENE CARE

- Know and experience issues surrounding 'taken for granted' aspects of hygiene care delivery.
- Include your reflections in your journal or learning diary.

CASE STUDIES IN GIVING HYGIENE CARE

The following case studies will help you consolidate knowledge gained through studying this chapter.

Case study: Learning disabilities

David Hargreaves, aged 25 years, has recently been discharged from a long stay hospital to the care of his ageing parents. He has been in institutional care for most of his life because of a severe learning disability. He is also physically disabled and requires much support and encouragement in maintaining his own hygiene care. He can wash his face and clean his teeth regularly, but it needs two people to give him full body hygiene care. His parents will not be able to provide this care because of their age and lack of strength. Although they will have control over his care through being allocated a financial allowance, they had been waiting for a larger grant to make suitable alterations to their home that would allow them to have a purpose-designed shower unit built.

- Which members of the multidisciplinary team should be involved in providing support for David and his family?
- How should the team roles interact and collaborate to ensure a positive outcome for the family?
- Who do you think has the ultimate responsibility for decisions about resourcing the needs of this family?

Case study: Mental health (and child)

Li is a second generation member of a Vietnamese family who have settled in England. She has married a fellow Vietnamese and has recently given birth to her second child, a daughter. Her son is 2 years old. Li was depressed after the birth of her son and is beginning to show the same symptoms again. Her husband has become anxious as she is neglecting herself and the children. He has sought help from the health visitor (whom the family know) at the local health centre. Because her condition has deteriorated and it is difficult for her husband to cope with the newborn baby and his son, Li is admitted along with her two children to a special family unit that cares for women with postnatal depression.

- How might the needs of this family be assessed by the multidisciplinary team of the family unit?

- In relation to self-care, what strategies might be employed to encourage Li to care for her own hygiene needs initially?
- How much self-care might you expect Li's son to be able to perform for his stage of development?
- Are there any special cultural practices among Vietnamese people that the multidisciplinary team need to be sensitive to in relation to the hygiene practices of Li and her two children?
- On what basis might the multidisciplinary team make a decision that Li can return home with her two children?

Case study: Adult

John is a 75-year-old retired lecturer. He is married and has two sons who are also teachers. Three years ago he had a stroke, which has left him with weakness of the left arm and leg. He has been feeling weak and unwell for the past 3 months. He has lost his appetite and a considerable amount of weight. After a visit to his general practitioner he is admitted to an acute medical unit for investigation of his weight loss.

- What factors should be considered in assessing John's specific hygiene needs?
- When facilitating John's hygiene care, what other observations can be made by the nurse that will help with the overall assessment of John's problems?
- Because of weight loss, John's dentures are ill-fitting. Decide on the specific advice and care John may need in relation to his oral hygiene.

Case study: Child

Simon is 3 years old and has recently complained to his dad about pain on passing urine. He has not spoken at all about this to his mum and appeared acutely embarrassed when dad mentioned this problem. It is clear that Simon's mum will need to take him to see the family doctor since his dad will be unable to do this due to work commitments. Simon is diagnosed as having balinitis (infection under the foreskin). He is prescribed systemic antibiotics and his mother is advised to cleanse the area and apply an antiseptic cream. Simon is cared for by a childminder and his mum and dad.

- Initially what strategies could the mother be advised to use in order to introduce Simon to the idea of being seen and examined by the doctor? How would this advice relate to your role in dealing with children who need help with intimate hygiene care delivery in hospital?
- Consider the impact that this special hygiene care and treatment might have on Simon's privacy and dignity. How could he be helped to cope with the childminder administering this care?
- Simon becomes very interested in this 'new' aspect of hygiene and begins to retract his foreskin when using the toilet. How could his family manage this new habit?

SUMMARY

This chapter has sought to draw together the knowledge and practice underpinning the delivery of high quality hygiene care. It has included:

1. An overview of applied biology related to the skin, the mouth, eyes and hair.
2. Insight into individual, cultural and spiritual norms related to personal hygiene habits and care.
3. An outline of issues in the assessment of hygiene needs with particular reference to total body care, oral and dental hygiene, hair infestation, and eye care.
4. A review of current methods for the delivery of hygiene care with discussion on their evidence base.
5. A discussion of the professional, ethical and political issues surrounding patterns for the delivery of hygiene care in institutions and in the community.
6. Raising awareness of the personal feelings that may arise when undertaking the intimate work involved in providing hygiene care.

Annotated further reading and websites

Carnaby S, Cambridge P 2006 Intimate and personal care with people with learning disabilities. Jessica Kingsley, London

This focused book, which deals with intimate and personal care as it applies to a particular client group, provides sensitive and comprehensive information in this area of nursing care which is often neglected or given relatively little attention. The material presented is applicable across all vulnerable groups of people.

Griffiths J, Boyle S 2005 Holistic oral care – a guide for health professionals, 2nd edn. Stephen Hancocks, London

This is an excellent book for more in-depth information on all aspects of oral and dental hygiene. It is specifically written for all health professionals and includes much of the literature as it relates to nursing care. Chapters focus on different client groups and will be particularly useful when you move into your specialist branch of nursing.

Helman, C (2007) Culture, Health and Illness 5th revised edition, Hodder Arnold, London

The focus of the book is on explaining how different cultures view health and illness, the treatments they themselves believe in, and who they would seek help from when ill. It is an excellent background book for understanding individuals health believes and behavior.

Hollins S 2006 Religions, culture and healthcare – a practical guide for use in healthcare environments. Radcliffe Publishing, Oxford

A sensitive practical book providing more comprehensive information on the needs of people from differing religious groups which are applicable within healthcare settings.

http://www.dh.gov.uk/en/Publicationsandstatistics/Publications/
PublicationsPolicyAndGuidance/DH_4005475
The Department of Health site is useful as a key resource for all policy documents pertaining to health care in the UK. The *Essence of Care* document outlines the expected standards for quality practice. For this chapter refer to the two sections on personal and oral hygiene, and privacy and dignity.

http://www.patient.co.uk/showdoc/9/
From this site you can access many key sites, for example: the British Dental Association Fact Files; British Dental Health Association; British Fluoridation Society; British Society for Disability and Oral Health. All provide information to the public related to dental health care and policy in the UK.

http://www.podiatryonline.com
A very useful resource site for information on foot care and conditions. Check in particular 'Best practice' portal to obtain access to 'Free patient handouts'. All conditions are explained in the same format with diagrams and photographs to illustrate the text.

http://www.hairscientists.org/index.htm
Established by the Trichological Society in 1999, this site has a helpful menu that covers basic information on all conditions associated with hair health.

http://www.patient.co.uk/showdoc/26738784/#related_1
This site, managed by the Eyecare Trust, provides a portal of entry to many UK Eye Health websites. Each address is annotated with the type of material found in that particular site.

References

Aiello AE, Larson EL 2001 An analysis of 6 decades of hygiene-related advertising: 1940–2000. American Journal of Infection Control 29(6) (S1):383–388

Badham J, Wall D, Sinfield M, Lancaster J 2006 The essence of care in clinical governance. Clinical Governance: An International Journal 11 (1):22–29

Carnaby S, Cambridge P (eds) 2006 Intimate and personal care with people with learning disabilities. Jessica Kingsley, London

Chalmers J, Pearson A 2005 Oral hygiene care for residents with dementia: a literature review. Journal of Advanced Nursing 52(4): 410–419

Collins F, Hampton S 2003 The cost effective use of BagBath: a new concept in patient hygiene. British Journal of Nursing 12(16):984–990

Community Care Act 1990 HMSO, London

Community Care Direct Payments Act 1996 HMSO, London

Department of Health 2000 The NHS plan: a plan for investment, a plan for reform. Available online: http://www.dh.gov.uk/en/Publicationsandstatistics/Publications/PublicationsPolicyAndGuidance/DH_4002960 (accessed 19 August 2008)

Department of Health 2001a Essence of care: patient-focused benchmarking for health care practitioners. HMSO, London. Available online: http://www.dh.gov.uk/en/Publicationsandstatistics/Publications/PublicationsPolicyAndGuidance/DH_4005475 (accessed 19 August 2008)

Department of Health 2001b National service framework for older people. HMSO, London. Available online: http://www.dh.gov.uk/en/SocialCare/Deliveringadultsocialcare/Olderpeople/OlderpeoplesNSFstandards/index.htm (accessed 19 August 2008)

Department of Health 2005 The national service framework for long term conditions. Available online: http://www.dh.gov.uk/en/Publicationsandstatistics/Publications/PublicationsPolicyAndGuidance/DH_4105361 (accessed 28 August 2008)

Department of Health 2007 The prevention and treatment of head lice. Available online: http://www.dh.gov.uk/en/Publicationsandstatistics/Publications/PublicationsPolicyAndGuidance/DH_077269 (accessed 28 August 2008)

Edwards SC 1998 An anthropological interpretation of nurses' and patients' perceptions of the use of space and touch. Journal of Advanced Nursing 28(4):809–817

Eilers J 2007 Nursing interventions and supportive care for the prevention and treatment of oral mucositis associated with cancer treatment. Oncology Nursing Forum 31(Suppl. 4):13–23

Eilers J, Berger AM, Peterson MC 1988 Development, testing and application of the oral assessment guide. Oncology Nursing Forum 15(3):325–330

Foucault M 1975 The birth of the clinic: an archaeology of medical perception. Vintage, New York

Gallagher A, Seedhouse D 2002 Dignity in care: the views of patients and relatives. Nursing Times 98(43):38–40

Griffiths J, Boyle S 2005 Holistic oral care: a guide for health professionals. Stephan Hancocks, London

Hancock I, Bowman A, Prater D 2000 The day of the soft towel? Comparison of the current bed-bathing method with the soft towel bed-bathing method. International Journal of Nursing Practice 6(4):207–213

Helman C 2007 Culture, health and illness, 5th edn. Hodder Arnold, London

Hill N 2006 Control of head lice: past, present and future. Expert Review of Anti-Infective Therapy 4(5):887–894

Hockenberry MJ, Wilson D 2007 Wong's nursing care of infants and children, 8th edn. Mosby Elsevier, St Louis

Hoeffer B, Talerico KA, Rasin J et al 2006 Assisting cognitively impaired nursing home residents with bathing: effects of two bathing interventions on caregiving. Gerontologist 46(4):524–532

Hollins S 2006 Religions, culture and healthcare: a practical guide for use in healthcare environments. Radcliffe Publishing, Oxford

Imai P 2006 A review of the different methods of applying chlorhexidine in the oral cavity. Canadian Journal of Dental Hygiene 40(2):69–79

Joyce N 2002 Eye care for the intensive care patient: a systematic review. Review no. 21. Joanna Briggs Institute for Evidence Based Nursing and Midwifery, Royal Adelaide Hospital, Australia

Larson EL, Ciliberti T, Chantler C et al 2004 Comparison of traditional and disposable bed baths in critically ill patients. American Journal of Critical Care 13(3):235–241

Lawler J 1997 Knowing the body and embodiment: methodologies, discourses and nursing. In: Lawler J (ed) The body in nursing. Churchill Livingstone, Melbourne

Lentz J 2003 Daily baths: torment or comfort at end of life? Journal of Hospice and Palliative Nursing 5(1):34–39

Lomborg K, Kirkevold M 2005 Curtailing: handling the complexity of body care in people hospitalized with severe COPD. Scandinavian Journal of Caring Sciences 19(2):148–156

Lupton D 2003 Medicine as culture: illness, disease and the body in western societies, 2nd edn. Sage, London

Marinho VCC, Higgins JPT, Logan S, Sheiham A 2003 Fluoride toothpastes for preventing dental caries in children and adolescents. Cochrane Database of Systematic Reviews, Issue 1, art. no. CD002278. DOI: 10.1002/14651858.CD002278. Available online: http://www.cochrane.org/reviews/en/ab002278.html (accessed 28 August 2008)

Montague SE, Watson R, Herbert RA (eds) 2005 Physiology for nursing practice, 3rd edn. Elsevier, Edinburgh

Nicol M, Bavin C, Cronin P, Rawlings-Anderson K 2008 Essential nursing skills, 3rd edn. Elsevier, Edinburgh

O'Regan H, Tonks Fawcett J 2006 Learning to nurse: reflections on bathing a patient. Nursing Standard 20(46):60–65

Oxford English Dictionary 1989 2nd edn. Oxford University Press, Oxford. Available online: http://www.oed.com/

Perry M, Carpenter I, Challis D et al 2003 Understanding the roles of registered general nurses and care assistants in UK nursing homes. Journal of Advanced Nursing 42(5):497–505

Rader J, Barrick AL, Hoeffer B et al 2006 The bathing of older adults with dementia: easing the unnecessarily unpleasant aspects of assisted bathing. American Journal of Nursing 106(4):40–48

Robinson PG, Deacon SA, Deery C et al 2005 Manual versus powered toothbrushing for oral health. Cochrane Database of Systematic Reviews, Issue 1, art. no. CD002281. DOI: 10.1002/14651858. CD002281.pub2. Available online: http://www.cochrane.org/reviews/en/ab002281.html (accessed 28 August 2008)

Roe B, Whattam M, Young H et al 2001 Elders' perceptions of formal and informal care: aspects of getting and receiving help for their activities of daily living. Journal of Clinical Nursing 10(3):398–405

Seed A 1995 Crossing the boundaries: experiences of neophyte nurses. Journal of Advanced Nursing 21:1136–1143

Sheppard L 2006 Growing pains: a personal development program for students with intellectual and developmental disabilities in a specialist school. Journal of Intellectual Disabilities 10(2):121–142

Spiby H, Bratten C, Deane L, Wright G 2005 Incorporating evidence into practice to improve perineal care: a report to the Foundation of Nursing Studies. Foundation of Nursing Studies, Leeds Teaching Hospitals NHS Trust. Available online: http://www.fons.org/ahcp/completedprojects/pdfs/PerinealCareFinalReport.pdf (accessed 19 August 2008)

Talbot A, Brady M, Furlanetto D, Frenkel H, Williams BO 2005 Oral care and stroke units. Gerodontology 22(2):77–83

Terry M A 2001 Dry eye in the elderly: therapy in practice. Drugs and Aging 18(2):101–107

Twigg J 2006 The body in health and social care. Palgrave Macmillan, Basingstoke

Walters P, Campbell SL 2005 Five common misconceptions about power toothbrushes. RDH 25(10):82–84

Wilson JA, Loveday HP, Hoffman PN, Pratt RJ 2007 Uniform: an evidence review of the microbioligcal significance of uniforms and uniform policy in the prevention and control of healthcare-associated infections. Report to the Department of Health (England). Journal of Hospital Infection 66:301–307

Wolf ZR 1997 Nursing students' experience bathing patients for the first time. Nurse Educator 22(2):41–46

Zeitz K, McCutcheon H 2005 Tradition, rituals and standards, in a realm of evidence based nursing care. Contemporary Nurse 18(3):300–308

Chapter 15

Skin integrity

Kerry Lewis and Lorraine Roberts

INTRODUCTION

The skin or integument is a major organ of the body, providing a barrier between the internal and external environments. It is also an organ that is highly visible to others, and therefore any damage, alteration or deformity in its structure can cause not only physical but also psychological, social and environmental problems. Skin integrity is concerned with the maintenance of this barrier in its optimum condition.

The aim of this chapter is to provide the requisite knowledge and decision-making skills to enable nurses, within their role, to care for patients with skin problems, to reflect on current practice relating to skin care and encourage the maintenance of their own skin health.

OVERVIEW

Subject knowledge

The biological section covers basic anatomy and physiology of the skin. The process of skin healing is explored. The importance of appearance and its effect on self-image is highlighted in the psychosocial section. Cultural influences are included.

Care delivery knowledge

Assessment of the skin and knowledge, skills and understanding required to assess, plan, implement and evaluate the care of patients with wounds are addressed in broad terms. A more in-depth discussion of the management of three common types of wound is provided.

Professional and ethical knowledge

The contribution of nurses to the development of quality systems of care relating to skin integrity is explored. Opportunities available to nurses in the development of their knowledge and expertise in different aspects of skin care are examined. Clinical, educational, professional and ethical considerations for practice are highlighted.

Personal and reflective knowledge

On page 359 there are four case studies, each relating to one of the branch programmes. You may find it helpful to read one of them before you start the chapter, and use it as a focus for your reflections while reading.

SUBJECT KNOWLEDGE

BIOLOGICAL

STRUCTURE OF THE SKIN

The skin is one of the largest organs in the body. An adult's skin covers an area of about 2 m^2 and weighs approximately 4.5–5 kg. Every square centimetre of skin contains approximately 125 sweat glands, 25 sebaceous glands, 250 nerve endings, 50 sensors to pain, pressure, heat and cold, approximately 1 m blood vessels, and millions of cells. Skin is made up of three main structures (Fig. 15.1):

- the epidermis or outer layer
- the dermis or base layer
- the skin appendages such as hairs, nails and glands.

These structures are also termed the integumentary system.

Epidermis

The epidermis is the outer or cuticle layer of the skin, and consists of several layers of cells. It contains no blood vessels or nerve endings and its main function is to protect the underlying dermis. It has four or five different layers of cells depending on its location. From the deepest to the most superficial these are the:

- stratum basale (or germinating layer)
- stratum spinosum
- stratum granulosum
- stratum lucidum (not present on hairy skin)
- stratum corneum (or cornified layer).

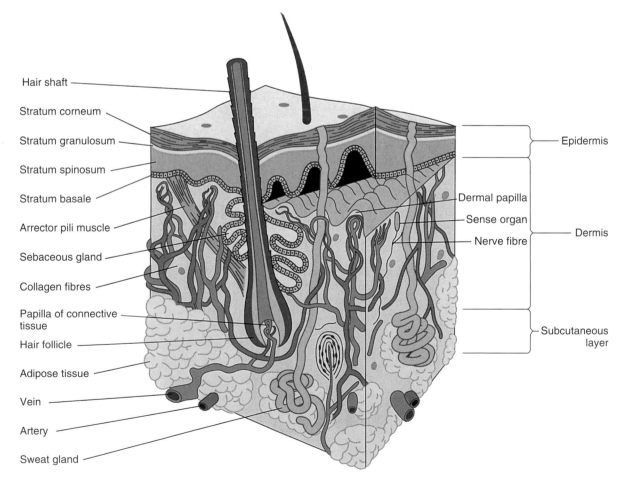

Figure 15.1 Microscopic structure of the skin. The epidermis is raised at one end to show the dermal papillae (from Montague et al 2005, with kind permission of Elsevier).

The cells in the stratum basale undergo mitosis and reproduce themselves. This enables the skin to repair itself when injured, and ensures an effective barrier against infection. As new cells are produced, they migrate to the surface of the skin. During this movement the cells' normal cytoplasm is replaced by keratin, a waterproof substance which gives the external layer of skin, the stratum corneum, its tough protective quality.

The greater part of the epidermis is made up of keratinocytes, the cells that produce the outer surface of the skin. Scattered among these cells are two other types of cells known as melanocytes and Langerhans cells.

Melanocytes are responsible for producing melanin, which produces the skin's pigmentation or colouring. White and black skinned people have the same number of melanocytes per unit of surface area, but in black skinned people the melanocytes are more active and produce pigment at a faster rate. Melanin protects other cells of the skin against the damaging effects of strong sunlight. Exposure of the skin to the sun stimulates the melanocytes to produce more melanin. This reaction causes the characteristic darkening of the skin (suntan). Black skinned people are therefore better protected against the sun's ultraviolet rays.

Overexposure to sunlight can cause sunburn and skin cancers such as malignant melanomas and non-melanotic skin cancers (NMSC), primarily basal cell and squamous cell cancers. The number of people developing skin cancers in England has been rising rapidly in recent years. Cancer Research UK (2005) state that malignant melanomas are diagnosed in approximately 8000 people each year in the UK and the incidence has quadrupled in British males between 1975 and 2001 and tripled in females. The increase in incidence is thought to be due to intermittent sun exposure of untanned skin during holidays and other outside activities. However, there is increasing concern and evidence regarding the use of sun beds and the development of malignant melanoma (Diffey 2007). A number of skin cancer and skin damage prevention campaigns and activities are important, including Sun Smart campaign (Cancer Research UK 2007). The National Institute of Health and Clinical Excellence (NICE 2006) guidelines provide advice on how healthcare services for individuals with skin tumours should be organized.

Evidence-based practice

Diffey (2002) questioned the belief that the daily use of sunscreens all year round reduces chronic skin changes associated with sun exposure in the UK. Findings of the study showed that the use of sun protection products during the summer months could reduce the lifetime (70 years) UV exposure of a person by an equivalent of almost 40 years' unprotected exposure, but there was almost no benefit from using the products between October and March in the UK.

Langerhans cells are thought to be important in the body's immune responses. They absorb small particles of foreign material such as nickel in jewellery and are responsible for setting up the allergic reaction common in contact allergic eczema (dermatitis). The resultant rash usually clears up within 1 week following removal of the irritant once it has been identified. Key to managing this condition, in the long term, lies in identifying and avoiding contact with the allergen.

Dermis

The dermis is the deepest layer of the skin. It is composed mainly of connective tissue and contains fewer cells than the epidermis, the main ones being fibroblasts, which produce collagen, a protein that attaches the skin layers to the rest of the body with tiny elastic fibres. These fibres give the skin its suppleness and ability to stretch. The upper part of the dermis contains rows of projections known as dermal papillae, which bind the two layers of skin together at the dermal–epidermal junction. The dermis contains a good blood supply and is responsible for nourishing and maintaining the epidermis, which does not have its own blood supply. The dermis also contains sensory receptors to heat, cold, touch and pain.

Glands

Three types of glands are present in the skin:

- Sebaceous or oil glands secrete an oily substance known as sebum, which lubricates and protects hair and skin.
- Sudoriferous or sweat glands assist in the regulation of body temperature through evaporation.
- Ceruminous glands produce cerumen or wax, which is found within the outer ear where it protects the ear by preventing the entry of foreign bodies.

Information on hair and nails can be found in Chapter 14, 'Hygiene'.

FUNCTIONS OF THE SKIN

The skin has five main functions.

Regulation of temperature

The production of sweat by the sudoriferous glands during hot weather helps reduce the body temperature through a process of evaporation. Changes in blood flow also occur. During hot weather peripheral blood vessels dilate, enabling heat loss by radiation. Conversely, in cold weather peripheral blood vessels constrict in order to maintain vital organs at an optimum temperature for functioning (see Ch. 7, 'Homeostasis').

Protection

The skin provides a physical barrier against harm, protecting the underlying tissues from abrasion and bacterial invasion. The melanin prevents damage from the sun's ultraviolet rays and the waterproof quality of the skin stops excessive loss of body fluid.

Excretion

Sweat contains water, salts, urea, ammonia and several other compounds. During sweating small amounts of these substances are excreted.

Stimuli reception

The skin contains many different types of receptors. The most common are receptors to temperature, pain and touch. These provide information about the external environment.

Synthesis of vitamin D

The skin aids in the synthesis of vitamin D. The precursor to vitamin D, 7-dehydrocholesterol, is present in the skin and is converted to cholecalciferol in the presence of ultraviolet light. After further conversion in the liver and then the kidneys, 1,25-dihydroxycalciferol is produced. This aids in the absorption of calcium from the dietary intake.

Tortora & Grabowski (2003) identify two further functions of the skin: immunity, due to the action of the Langerhans cells; and as a blood reservoir, due to the ability to divert blood to muscles during exercise through vasoconstriction.

AGEING AND THE SKIN

During an individual's lifespan, changes occur in the physical properties of the skin. In order to maintain healthy skin different requirements must be met at different stages of an individual's life. For instance, during infancy the skin is delicate and until the child is continent the skin requires protection from the damaging effects of urine and faeces. Similarly, during adolescence skin changes result in increased perspiration and oil production, sometimes leading to the development of acne.

During pregnancy there is an increase in activity of the sebaceous glands and melanocytes, resulting in increased oil production and patches of darker pigmentation on the skin – commonly the linea nigra, which is a pigmented line down the abdomen, and chloasma, which are darker areas on the face often referred to as the 'mask of pregnancy'. Although the skin has the ability to stretch, during pregnancy the increase in size of the abdomen can be so great that the collagen fibres rupture, leaving visible scars. These are known as striae gravidarum or 'stretch marks'.

In old age, the production of cells slows down and they become smaller and thinner. The collagen and elastic fibres lose their shape and elasticity, and the amount of fat stored in the subcutaneous tissues lessens, resulting in skin wrinkles. There is a decrease in the number and an increase in the size of active melanocytes, producing concentrated areas of pigment commonly known as liver spots. There is also a reduction in the amount of intracellular fluid resulting in dry skin, which can lead to itching or 'senile pruritus', and increased skin fragility. The use of moisturizers or emollients can help to prevent excessive flakiness of skin.

For many people the desire to preserve a youthful complexion brings with it the necessity of a continued battle against the ageing process. There are two distinct types of skin ageing. Chronological or intrinsic ageing is the normal ageing process that occurs over time in all organs of the body. Photoageing or extrinsic ageing is connected to environmental factors, mainly ultraviolet light induced (Ma et al 2001). Photoaged skin is characterized by 'wrinkling, sagging, mottled hyperpigmentation and yellowing' (Sator et al 2002: 292). Although creams and lotions may result in a superficial improvement in skin texture altered by normal ageing, cosmetic surgery is becoming more and more popular. Protection of the skin against sun damage from an early age is the only way to combat photoageing. Prevention is better than a cure.

Decision-making exercise

Liza Gordon is an 18-year-old student who enjoys holidays abroad with her friends. She also tops up her tan by using a sun bed regularly. She has been admitted to the day care ward for a biopsy of a 'suspicious' mole, which turned out to be benign. Liza is very concerned about her appearance and is anxious to protect her skin against sun damage and the long-term effects of ageing.

- What skin care advice would you give to Liza before discharge?
- Apart from advice to individuals, what other strategies are or could be put in place to reduce the effects of ultraviolet light/sun damage?
- Compare your answers with the Cancer Research UK (2007) Sun Smart campaign and the Sun Know How campaign developed by the Health Education Authority and the BBC (2000).

SKIN HEALING

Should the skin become cut or damaged, creating a wound, the process of healing has four distinct phases:

- coagulation
- inflammation

- regeneration
- maturation.

Skin heals by primary or secondary intention.

Primary intention

This type of healing occurs when the edges of the wound are opposed, as in a surgical incision. Healing tends to be rapid due to the close proximity of the wound edges (Fig. 15.2), and involves:

- Coagulation – within 8 hours following surgery the cut surfaces become inflamed, a blood clot fills the incision track, and phagocytes and fibroblasts migrate into the area.
- Inflammation – phagocytes begin to break down the clot, and cell debris and collagen fibres are produced by the fibroblasts and begin to bind the two surfaces together.
- Regeneration – after 3–4 days epithelial cells spread across the incision track, the section of clot above the new cells becomes a scab, the clot in the incision track is absorbed, and myofibroblasts draw the edges of the wound together by a process of contraction.
- Maturation – epithelial cells continue to be laid down until the full thickness of skin is restored.

Secondary intention

This type of healing occurs where there is a significant loss of tissue or where the skin edges are not opposed, as in an ulcer. Healing tends to be slower, but the exact time will depend on the extent of the damage (Fig. 15.3). It involves:

- Coagulation – the surface of the wound becomes acutely inflamed and phagocytes start to break down the necrotic tissue.
- Inflammation – granulation tissue develops at the base of the wound and starts to grow up towards the wound surface.

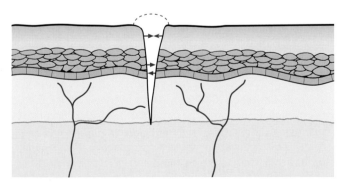

Figure 15.2 Wound healing by primary intention. The wound edges are in close proximity (often brought together by sutures). Healing occurs rapidly along the length of the wound.

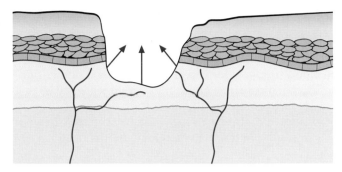

Figure 15.3 Wound healing by secondary intention. The wound edges are distanced due to crater formation. Healing is slower and begins at the bottom of the crater

- Regeneration – phagocytosis causes the necrotic tissue to separate, exposing a new layer of epidermal cells, and contraction occurs to reduce the size of the wound (as wound contraction is a normal process, it is important not to pack the wound with dressings unless specifically indicated, for example for a wound sinus, as it interferes with this process).
- Maturation – when granulation tissue fills the wound cavity and reaches the level of the dermis, epithelial cells migrate across the wound towards the centre, forming a single layer of cells. Epithelialization continues until full-thickness skin is restored.

Tissue viability experts are now using a slightly different definition of wound healing involving four major stages – inflammation, proliferation re-epithelialization and matrix formation/remodelling (Calvin 1998). These terms are not yet commonly used in physiology and tissue viability text but are terms to look for in the future.

Benbow (2005) uses the term 'tertiary healing' to describe a wound where there is a significant delay between injury and wound closure; for example, extensive tissue loss or dehiscence. Bale & Jones (2006) use a similar term, 'healing by third intention', to identify a wound containing a foreign body or infection that is left open until the problem has been resolved.

THE OPTIMUM ENVIRONMENT FOR WOUND HEALING

A variety of factors need to be present to create the optimum environment for wound healing to take place. These include:

- a good blood supply
- optimum temperature
- appropriate moisture
- oxygen
- freedom from contaminants and necrotic tissue
- freedom from infection.

Blood supply

Healing requires an integral blood supply to provide oxygen and nutrients to the developing cells. Reconstitution of the blood supply is termed angiogenesis and occurs during the regeneration phase of healing. Care must be taken not to disturb this process by the inappropriate use of dressings; for example dry dressings such as gauze can stick to wound beds, resulting in trauma when they are removed.

Evidence-based practice

Thomas (2003), reviewing the literature, indicates that pain and trauma relating to the removal of dressings is a major concern to patients and health care professionals. There is confusion between the terms 'adherent' and 'adhesive', which are often used interchangeably. 'Adherence' should describe the interaction between the dressing and wound and, 'adhesive' should describe the interaction between the dressing and intact peri-wound skin. Thomas advocates the use of a new term – 'atraumatic dressings' – to describe wound products that, on removal, do not cause trauma to the wound site or the peri-wound skin. Dressings coated with soft silicone could be described as 'atraumatic'.

Temperature

The optimum temperature for human cell growth is 37 °C. Wounds kept at a constant temperature of 37 °C will heal faster than those exposed to thermal shock (i.e. extreme changes in temperature). To keep wounds at a constant temperature, unnecessary wound cleansing and dressing changes should be avoided.

Moisture

The exudate produced by wounds, other than non-healing chronic wounds, contains nutrients, enzymes and growth factors that can aid the healing process. Lytic enzymes found in the exudate autolyse (break down) any necrotic tissue present, and growth factors increase the development rate of cells and result in less scarring. In such wounds, a moist wound environment facilitates wound healing, reduces the amount of tissue inflammation, produces less scarring and results in less pain for the patient. If the wound is allowed to dry out, a scab or eschar forms. This impedes cell migration and consequently slows down the healing process. Excessive exudate needs to be contained to prevent damage to the surrounding skin.

Exudate in non-healing chronic wounds is different in nature to that from acute wounds and has potentially harmful constituents which may inhibit wound healing (Vowden & Vowden 2003). Management of such exudate is part of an overall wound management approach to these chronic wounds, namely wound bed management (see Care Delivery Knowledge). An understanding of the role of exudate in the wound healing process is essential (see section on Annotated Further Reading: Vowden & Vowden 2003)

Oxygen

All cells require oxygen in order to develop and mature. An integral blood supply is therefore essential to ensure that cells receive an adequate oxygen supply in order to remain viable. The external administration of oxygen to the wound site, for example via an oxygen mask and tubing, will not benefit tissue perfusion, but will dry the wound site and delay wound healing.

Freedom from contaminants and necrotic tissue

The presence of foreign bodies and dead or devitalized tissue delays wound healing and provides a focus for infection, which will in turn also delay wound healing.

Freedom from infection

Wounds may be contaminated transiently or colonized by bacteria which do not affect wound healing adversely. Moore & Cowman (2007) suggest that whether or not an infection develops depends on the individual host's response to bacteria present and the virulence of the bacteria. If wounds become infected, the bacteria present in the wound cause host damage and delay healing (see section on Annotated Further Reading: Benbow 2005). However, there is a stage called critical colonization that precedes clinical infection, causing delayed healing and subtle signs of infection (Collier 2002). Early diagnosis and prompt treatment of critical colonization to prevent overt clinical infection presents a challenge to health care professionals.

Evidence-based practice

Moore & Cowman (2007) provide an overview of the European Management Association's (2005) position document *Identifying Criteria for Wound Infection* and discuss its relevance and application to clinical practice. While they acknowledge that assessing the presence of infection is not an easy task, they consider that early recognition of wound infections is essential in the development of effective treatment strategies.

PSYCHOSOCIAL

THE IMPORTANCE OF APPEARANCE

Physical appearance is important to most people. As the skin is visible to others, its condition often influences how an individual feels about him or herself. People who feel attractive often feel positive about themselves.

Images in the media of suntanned, high profile individuals such as fashion models may help to encourage the idea that a suntan is both healthy and desirable. Accordingly, suntanned skin can promote a sense of psychological well-being. As a consequence, despite current health education concerning the dangerous effects of ultraviolet light, sunbathing – in either natural or artificial sunlight – remains a popular pastime. Naidoo & Wills (2005) recognize the challenges for health promoters in that the message to reduce exposure to sunlight is at odds with lay beliefs that sunlight is beneficial. It is necessary to address the conflict between the improvement to psychological health and its detrimental effect on an individual's physical health. Gross (2005: 418) examines Festinger's theory of cognitive dissonance. Cognitive dissonance is a state of 'psychological discomfort and tension' caused by a person knowing that an action may cause harm, but at the same time participating in that action. Festinger's theory can be useful for choosing between two activities that are equally attractive. This involves highlighting the undesirable features of each activity in order to help with the decision making process. Although this may help in deciding whether or not to sunbathe, it must be acknowledged that an individual may still decide that the psychological benefits of sunbathing are more important and therefore continue the activity.

Reflection and portfolio evidence

You may wish to extend your personal reflection here into a debate with your fellow students on the choices to be made.

- Is an individual's psychological or physical health more important?
- If it is necessary to make one dimension of health a priority, which would take priority for you at a personal level? Justify your decision.
- In your practice placement review the above debate in relation to one patient or client.
- Record key points in your debate and your conclusions in your portfolio.

Just as a healthy skin can help to promote a positive self-image, a skin disorder can have a detrimental effect. For thousands of years skin disorders have been regarded as unclean: lepers, for instance, have often been treated as social outcasts. It may be argued that certain more common skin disorders continue to evoke a less than compassionate reaction nowadays, particularly those that are visible, such as eczema or psoriasis. The impact of a skin disorder on a person's self-image can depend very much on the individual's ability to cope. If the disorder affects the person's ability to carry out and meet their self-care needs, or if it causes stress to the individual or the family, it can seriously undermine their self-regard. The disorder can come to be viewed in a way that is out of all proportion to the problem itself and overshadow the individual's entire life.

Self-image

It is important to understand that the nurse's approach can have a significant effect on how the client responds to a skin disorder. Any signs of disgust, alarm or even fear may encourage the client to view their condition as offensive to others. Furthermore, the nurse needs to be aware of any signals that may be conveyed to the client. With thought, the nurse can project and encourage a more positive self-image. If the skin disorder is not infectious and does not require the use of gloves when handling, the client's self-image can be enhanced if the nurse touches the affected area with unprotected hands. In addition, the client will benefit from being able to discuss any feelings about the condition with both relatives and the nurse. Moreover, a simple explanation of the aetiology (cause), and prognosis (probable course) of the condition may help the client to accept it.

Some conditions of the skin, for example burns, ulceration and extensive surgery, can cause great distress to both the client and the nurse. In order to help the client accept the condition, the nurse will first need to come to terms with it him or herself. Nurses often do not feel they have the skills required to provide the level of psychological support that clients may require (Clarke & Cooper 2001). Although these skills can be provided by training, this is an area where lay-led or voluntary service may be useful. Changing Faces is a charity set up to support facially disfigured people and their families (www.changingfaces.org.uk). (See Ch. 19, 'Rehabilitation and recovery', for information on dealing with body image changes.)

Evidence-based practice

Rumsey et al (2004) surveyed 458 participants with visible disfigurements including burns, tattoos and skin conditions in order to establish their psychological needs. The results highlighted high levels of psychological distress when compared with normative values. 71% ($n=325$) expressed a moderate or strong desire for access to professionals with appropriate training to help them to deal with their appearance related concerns.

CULTURE AND APPEARANCE

Different cultures have very different approaches to and ideas about physical appearance. What is considered to be attractive in one culture may be regarded as physically unattractive in another. While a suntanned appearance may be desirable in Western culture, some eastern cultures, notably Japan, may favour an altogether paler complexion. The traditional 'geisha' look was originally achieved using face-whitening powder from dried nightingale droppings.

Some cultures use skin decoration to produce the opposite effect. The Tuareg paint their skin with turmeric to make themselves less desirable and therefore less vulnerable to evil spirits. In Ethiopia, the Surma women insert clay discs into their lower lip to cause it to protrude. It is thought that this was first done to make the women less desirable to slave traders.

Beauty is a matter of subjective judgement (i.e. 'beauty is in the eye of the beholder'). To some extent, the skin plays an important part in the perception of an individual's attractiveness, and for hundreds of years has been decorated in many ways to enhance or diminish its appeal (see Evolve 15.1).

15.1 – THE IMPORTANCE OF APPEARANCE

• Reflective exercises on impact of appearance.
• Evidence-based practice on impact of appearance on the care a patient receives.

Cosmetics

These are used to accentuate attractive facial features and disguise imperfections. Cosmetics can have religious or cultural significance; for example, the bindhi is traditionally a red or maroon dot worn on the forehead of Hindu women. It is customarily worn by married women to symbolize their marriage and myth is that it protects them from the 'bad eye' of people (Mehta Products 2007).

Tribal markings

These are a form of tattooing where patterns are cut directly into the skin. They often hold religious significance or show membership of a particular tribe or group. They are deemed to be an essential feature of some cultures and are considered attractive in both males and females.

Piercing

There has been a huge increase in the popularity of body piercing. Ears, nose, navel, eyebrows and nipples have all been subject to this trend and have become fashion statements, particularly among teenagers and young adults

Skin adornments, particularly tattoos and body piercing, have implications for healthcare workers (see Evolve 15.2).

15.2 – TATTOOS AND PIERCINGS: IMPLICATIONS FOR HEALTH CARE

• Stereotyping and impact on health care
• Case study and discussion on effects on disgnostic imaging (MRI scans)

CARE DELIVERY KNOWLEDGE

Problems affecting skin integrity are wide-ranging, varying from nappy rash to disfiguring wounds. The role of the nurse will differ according to the type and extent of the skin problem. For instance, when caring for an adult with a chronic skin condition such as atopic eczema, the focus of the nurse's role will primarily be that of a health promoter, empowering the individual to manage and live with his or her condition.

The wide range of conditions and possible therapeutic interventions prohibit detailed discussion of every example. Instead, the following discussion focuses on a general assessment of skin, and then on one of the common problems of skin integrity, namely wounds.

ASSESSMENT OF THE SKIN

Assessment of the skin not only gives an indication of the condition of the skin itself, but can also help in identifying the client's physical health, emotional state and lifestyle. Assessment requires close observation of the skin and includes visual inspection, palpation and noting skin odour. In addition, it is important to ask the client questions about his or her skin. Good illumination is necessary, and if there is any discharge from skin lesions, the nurse should wear disposable examination gloves. Above all, it is important that the nurse employs a sensitive approach and respects the dignity and privacy of the client. Holloway & Jones (2005) stress the need for a regular structured and systematic approach to skin assessments of clients.

Assessment of the skin should include observation of each of the following aspects of the skin:

• colour
• temperature
• moisture
• texture
• thickness
• turgor
• the presence of blemishes and lesions.

Colour and areas of discoloration

Skin colour varies between individuals, most obviously between people of different ethnic origins. There are several aspects of wound assessment and management that need to be addressed for patients with darkly pigmented skin (see Annotated Further Reading: Bethell 2005). There are also differences in skin colour in different parts of the body of each individual. Nipples and areolae of the breasts are darker than the rest of the skin, particularly in women during pregnancy. Similarly, areas that are exposed to sunlight, such as the face and arms, tend to be darker due to increased melanin concentration. These differences aside, and with the exception of older people in whom pigmentation can increase unevenly, skin colour is usually uniform.

An assessment of skin colour involves examining areas that are not generally exposed to sunlight, such as the palm of the hand. For the first few days of life the hands and feet of newborn babies are a bluish colour, termed acrocyanosis, due to inadequate peripheral vasculature. Assessment thereafter should involve looking for specific changes in skin colour, for instance:

- cyanosis (a bluish colour)
- pallor (a decrease of colour)
- jaundice (a yellow–orange colour)
- erythema (redness).

These changes in colour are most obvious in certain parts of the body. Cyanosis and pallor are particularly evident at the nail beds and buccal (mouth) mucosa. It is especially important to look at these areas in dark-skinned clients, as changes in general skin colour are less evident. Asian children may have Mongolian blue spots, which are very common and normal. The nurse should note any bruising. Although bruising can be normal, extensive or fingertip-type bruising can be a sign of abuse and should be investigated further, following agreed protocols.

Temperature

Feeling the client's skin with the back of your hand best assesses skin temperature. The temperature of the skin increases or decreases with an increase or decrease in the circulation of blood through the dermis. Hands and feet are normally colder than the rest of the body when exposed to a cold environment due to reduced peripheral blood flow. Localized areas of increased or decreased temperature may indicate a problem. Hot, inflamed, red and painful skin surrounding a wound indicates the presence of infection. Similarly, if an unexposed limb is cold and pale, there may be circulatory impairment. When clients have had vascular surgery or a plaster cast or bandages applied to a limb, it is important to assess for skin changes that indicate impaired blood flow.

Moisture

Moisture refers to the wetness and oiliness of skin. It is related to the level of hydration and general condition of the skin. Normally the skin is smooth and dry except in the folds of the skin where it is moist. An increase in skin temperature arising from a hot environment or exercise is accompanied by perspiration, and is a normal phenomenon. However, when a client has a fever resulting from, for example, an infection, the skin may initially feel dry and hot but become damp from perspiration as the fever breaks. In older people dry skin, which is often accompanied by itchiness, can be a problem.

Texture

Usually the skin is smooth, soft and flexible, although in older people it sometimes becomes wrinkled and leathery. Skin thickness varies in different parts of the body: for example, skin is thickest on the palms of the hands and soles of the feet. Assess skin texture by stroking and palpating the skin with the fingertips; the nurse can gauge smoothness, thickness, suppleness and softness. Localized areas of changes to skin texture may indicate previous trauma or lesions. Should such changes be apparent, the nurse should ask the client about them. Rough and dry skin can also be due to exposure to cold weather or overwashing.

Turgor

Turgor refers to the elasticity of the skin, which is normally elastic and taut. It can be assessed by gentle pinching, lifting and letting go of an area of skin, usually on the back of the hand. Normally, the skin should quickly return to its former position. If it does not, it indicates that the client is dehydrated. However, some loss of skin elasticity is normal in older individuals. Excessive accumulation of fluid in the tissue – termed oedema – gives the skin a taut shiny appearance. It results from either direct trauma to the skin or an underlying condition. The presence of oedema increases susceptibility to further skin damage and delays wound healing.

Blemishes and lesions

Many skin blemishes and lesions are normal, for instance birthmarks, moles and freckles, and minor cuts, abrasions and blisters. Equally, nappy rash and heat rash are common among babies and children and mild acne is not uncommon in adults. Other blemishes and lesions, however, require further investigation and it may be necessary to refer the client to a doctor. For example, changes in an existing mole may indicate the development of a malignant melanoma.

Rashes may be caused by infection, such as a postviral rash, chickenpox, meningitis and shingles, or an allergic response, for example to particular chemicals, food products or medication. Other lesions may arise from skin infestations such as scabies, as a result of accidental or intentional trauma to the skin, or as a result of skin disease such as psoriasis or eczema (see Evolve 15.3). When abnormal blemishes, including scars or lesions, are detected, their colour, size, location and specific characteristics and, where appropriate, distribution and grouping should be noted. Clients should be asked about such blemishes, in particular to determine their cause.

 15.3 – ATOPIC ECZEMA

- Possible causes of eczema.
- Effects of eczema on client and family.
- Treatment options available.
- Management – focusing on the nurse's role.

CLASSIFICATION OF WOUNDS

Wounds can be classified in a variety of different ways. They can be classified according to:

- cause (e.g. stab wound)
- status of skin integrity (e.g. open or closed wound)
- cleanliness of wound (e.g. presence or absence of infection or foreign bodies)
- the characteristics of the wound bed of open wounds
- extent of skin damage (e.g. full-thickness burn).

However, Westaby (1985) suggests that there are really only two types of wound:

- wounds characterized by skin loss
- wounds where there is no skin loss.

In practice, wound classification systems are often incomplete and overlap; for example, a surgically closed infected wound and an open, chronic, sloughy, bacterially contaminated wound. A simple wound classification system is given in Figure 15.4.

Acute wounds result from surgery or accidents. However, in some instances acute wounds progress to chronic wounds as a result of complications. Acute surgical wounds tend to be surgically closed and clean while accidental wounds may be either clean or infected and can also be open or closed. Chronic wounds usually result from underlying diseases and tend to be open, as in the case of pressure ulcers and leg ulcers. Chronic wounds are more likely to be colonized or infected.

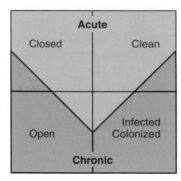

Figure 15.4 Wound classification diagram.

Open wounds can be further classified according to the observable characteristics of the wound bed:

- epithelializing (pink)
- granulating (red)
- infected (green)
- sloughy (yellow)
- necrotic (black).

Severity of skin damage

It is not always easy to determine the extent of skin damage: that is, whether there is superficial, partial or full-thickness damage. Burns and pressure ulcers are often graded and described in such terms. The European Pressure Ulcer Advisory Panel (2003) suggests grading damage by the amount of tissue involvement (Box 15.1).

Box 15.1 Classification of pressure ulcers (reproduced by kind permission of European Pressure Ulcer Advisory Panel 2003)

Grade one: Non-blanchable erythema of intact skin. Discoloration of the skin, warmth, oedema, induration or hardness may also be used as indicators, particularly on individuals with darker skin

Grade two: Partial thickness skin loss involving epidermis, dermis, or both. The ulcer is superficial and presents clinically as an abrasion or blister

Grade three: Full-thickness skin loss involving damage to or necrosis of subcutaneous tissue that may extend down to, but not through, underlying fascia

Grade four: Extensive destruction, tissue necrosis, or damage to muscle, bone, or supporting structures with or without full-thickness skin loss

(EPUAP 2003)

Despite the limitations of wound classification, it is nonetheless useful as it helps to identify both the potential complications of a given wound and the implications for wound care in each case, and this can guide decision making when planning wound care. Algorithms or flow charts based on the classification of wounds aid in identifying priorities in wound care, and have been devised to guide nursing decisions and actions in wound management.

Reflection and portfolio evidence

During your next practice placement select one patient who has been allocated to you who has sustained a wound of any type. Reflect on the need for a holistic assessment of the care needed for that person. Involve the patient as a partner in your assessment.

- Using Morison's (2004) model to facilitate the assessment and care planning for a patient with a wound, decide what aspects you would focus on during assessment to enable you to provide appropriate holistic care to meet that patient's immediate and long-term health needs.
- Record a summary of your experiences and a commentary on your learning in your portfolio.

WOUND MANAGEMENT

The management of wounds will be discussed in general terms, followed by a more in-depth discussion of three specific types of wounds, namely accidental wounds, closed surgical wounds and chronic wounds.

Assessment of a person with a wound

When undertaking an assessment of a person with a wound, it is necessary to consider the person as a whole and not just to focus attention on the wound itself. Morison (2004) (Fig. 15.5) has produced a model to facilitate the assessment and care planning of a patient with a wound. The model addresses the following aspects:

- Immediate cause of the wound.
- Any underlying pathophysiology.
- Other medical conditions that may impair wound healing.
- Local problems at the wound site.
- Risk of further tissue breakdown.
- Consequences for the patient's quality of life now – physical functioning, pain, social role/functions and emotional and spiritual well-being.
- Patient's social circumstances and optimum settings for care.
- Patient's needs for longer term rehabilitation.

Morison's (2004) approach allows the nurse to:

- Determine whether any health promotion activity is necessary to prevent a recurrence of the wound (e.g. advice on how to prevent sunburn).
- Consider any factors that may retard wound healing and take measures to overcome these (e.g. inadequate nutrition).
- Plan and provide holistic care that meets the needs of a person with a wound, both in the short term and longer term, rather than just treating a wound per se.

To meet the immediate and longer-term care of a patient with a wound an holistic assessment and understanding of the consequences of a wound for the patient is required. Other members of the multidisciplinary team will be involved in the care of a patient with a wound. Good communication between team members to facilitate the sharing of information is essential for achieving agreed goals.

Assessment of the wound site

When assessing the wound site, the following should be noted:

- the location of the wound
- the size and shape of the wound
- the characteristics of the wound bed (in open wounds), wound margin and any undermining or sinuses
- the quantity and quality of exudate
- the presence of infection (Box 15.2)
- odour from the wound
- pain
- the condition of the surrounding skin
- signs of other specific complications such as a haematoma
- where appropriate, the presence of foreign bodies, the type of skin closure and the presence of drains and details of drainage.

Open wounds can be traced on to plastic film to obtain a visual record of the wound size. These films can be annotated to show areas of the wound bed with different characteristics. Maximum wound dimensions can be taken from the tracing. Wound depth can be measured using sterile probes. Serial photographs can also be taken to show wound changes over time, which will give some indication of the effectiveness or otherwise of treatment regimens. The use of colour digital image processing is likely to become used more frequently for the assessment of wounds once these products become more refined.

If patients have existing wounds or have received wound care in the past, it is important during assessment to establish whether the patient has had any allergies to wound care products. Details of existing wound care should be recorded. Patch testing for allergies to any proposed wound

OPEN WOUND ASSESSMENT CHART

Type of wound (e.g. pressure sore, fungating carcinoma, etc.) ....

Location ....

How long has wound been open? ....

General patient factors which may delay healing (e.g. malnourished, diabetic, chronic infection) ....

Allergies to wound care products ....

Previous treatments tried (comment on success/problems) ....

Special aids in current use (e.g. pressure-relieving bed, cushion) ....

....

....

TRACE THE WOUND WEEKLY, ANNOTATING TRACING WITH NATURE OF WOUND BED, ORIENTATION OF WOUND, POSITION/EXTENT OF SINUSES, AND UNDERMINING OF SURROUNDING SKIN

All other parameters should be assessed at every dressing change.

Wound factors/Date								
1. **NATURE OF WOUND BED** a. healthy granulation b. epithelialization c. slough d. black/brown necrotic tissue e. other (specify)								
2. **EXUDATE** a. colour b. type c. approximate amount								
3. **ODOUR** Offensive/some/none								
4. **PAIN (SITE)** a. at wound site b. elsewhere (specify)								
5. **PAIN (FREQUENCY)** Continuous/intermittent/ only at dressing changes/none								
6. **PAIN (SEVERITY)** Patient's score (0–10)								
7. **WOUND MARGIN** a. colour b. oedematous								
8. **ERYTHEMA OF SURROUNDING SKIN** a. present b. maximum distance from wound (mm)								
9. **GENERAL CONDITION OF SURROUNDING SKIN** (e.g. dry eczema)								
10. **INFECTION** a. suspected b. wound swab sent c. confined (specify organism)								

WOUND ASSESSED BY:

Figure 15.5 Open wound assessment chart (reproduced by kind permission of Mosby International, from Morison MJ 2004 A framework for patient assessment and care planning. In: Morison MJ, Ovington LG, Wilkie K 2004 Chronic wound care: a problem-based approach. Mosby, London).

Box 15.2 Signs of clinical wound infection

- Localized pain
- Localized erythema
- Localized rise in skin temperature
- Local oedema
- Excess exudate
- Pus
- Offensive odour
- Pyrexia
- Bleeding
- Delayed healing

care products is useful, particularly if large areas require dressing, as in the case of an extensive venous leg ulcer.

Reflection and portfolio evidence

Find a copy of other wound assessment charts that may be in use in practice areas you have visited, or appear in the literature. Examples are provided by Benbow (2005) and Naylor (2004).

- Compare these other assessment tools with Morison's (2004) tool (see Fig. 15.5), and from your present experience and knowledge of wound care decide which tool would be the most valid to use and why. (Validity is the extent to which the tool measures what it is supposed to measure.)
- Test your chosen tool for reliability when two or more students observe the same wound, either in reality or using slides or computer simulation, and then compare any statements or scores for similarities and differences. (Reliability is the extent to which the tool measures consistently.)
- How would a tool help you in your decision making about wound management?
- Record your findings and learning in your portfolio.

Wound assessment charts can be useful tools when undertaking and recording the findings of wound assessments. Figure 15.5 shows an example of an open wound assessment chart developed by Morison (2004).

Facilitating wound healing

The general aim of wound management is to provide optimum conditions for facilitating natural wound healing as quickly and comfortably as possible with minimum

scarring. This includes identifying and addressing factors that may affect wound healing. These can be divided into three broad categories as follows:

- local factors relating to the wound environment (e.g. presence of necrotic tissue, oedema)
- general client factors (e.g. nutritional status, compliance with treatment)
- treatment – nursing and medical factors (e.g. radiotherapy, dressing choice).

Successful wound healing is dependent on the body's ability to heal. Wound care can only help to facilitate this process. Some wounds will not heal (for example inoperable fungating carcinoma), and here the aim of wound management is to contribute to an optimum quality of life for the client by containing wound odour and discharge, protecting the wound and controlling any pain.

The aims of local wound management are to provide an optimum environment to enable natural wound healing processes, to remove causes of delayed healing and to protect the wound from further damage (see Subject Knowledge). While moist healing has been accepted generally, in respect of wound care, the concept of wound-bed management for non-healing chronic wounds is a relatively new concept. As discussed previously (see Subject Knowledge), it has been recognized that non-healing chronic wounds require a different approach to wound healing, namely wound-bed preparation. As Collier (2002) identifies, wound-bed preparation requires removal of necrotic tissue/fibrinous tissue, control of oedema, achievement of a well vascularized wound bed, decrease in bacterial burden, minimization of wound exudate and correction of matrix abnormalities by, for example, the use of growth factors.

If a wound is necrotic, one of the first priorities is to remove the necrotic tissue. Devitalized tissue not only hinders healing and increases the risk of infection but also masks the extent of the injury (Benbow 2002). Removal of necrotic tissue can be achieved by mechanical, chemical, surgical (sharp) and biosurgical means (maggot/larval therapy), or by providing the right local conditions for autolysis to take place (see section on Annotated Further Reading: Falabella 2006).

Wound sites also need to be free of clinical infection. If a clinical wound infection is suspected (see Box 15.2) a wound swab should be taken before wound cleaning and sent for microscopy, culture and sensitivity. The use of topical antibiotics is rarely indicated because of the risk of contact sensitization and bacterial resistance. Rather, an appropriate systemic antibiotic should be prescribed (Dealey 2005). Chronic wounds in particular may be colonized by microorganisms that do not cause clinical infections and do not appear to affect wound healing.

Consideration should be given to whether the wound needs to be cleansed or redressed as unnecessary intervention delays wound healing. Wounds should be cleaned if there is superficial slough, pus, excessive exudate or visible debris such as grit or residue from previous dressings.

Reflection and portfolio evidence

Under the Subject Knowledge section you were given a list of conditions for optimum wound healing. Referring to this list, decide why unnecessary wound cleansing or redressing delays wound healing.

Reflect on the wound care activities you have observed during practice placement.

- How were the wounds cleaned and how often?
- What reasons were given for the choice of wound cleansing agent and the method of cleaning in each case?
- In wounds described as necrotic, what means were used to remove the necrotic tissue – mechanical, chemical, surgical, biosurgical or promoting autolysis? Why was the particular method chosen in each particular case you have seen?
- Record your findings in your portfolio.

Generally, if wounds require cleansing aseptically, they should be cleaned with warm (37 °C) sterile sodium chloride 0.9% solution, which is isotonic. Unlike antiseptics/antimicrobials, sodium chloride 0.9% solution does not have a toxic effect on skin tissue. Although antiseptics/antimicrobials may be used in specific circumstances, such as heavily contaminated wounds, it is necessary to weigh the benefits against the possible tissue damage they may cause. Despite these concerns, Benbow (2005) highlights that wounds with MRSA are often treated with such products, but there is little agreement about what constitutes the most effective practice. Preference should be given to irrigating wounds under moderate pressure (8 psi) rather than using cotton wool or gauze, which shed fibres into the wound, thereby delaying wound healing and providing a focus for infection. In addition, such mechanical cleansing can damage newly formed tissue.

The choice of dressing, if required, depends on a variety of factors. These include:

- the local conditions of the wound site and surrounding skin
- other requirements arising from the individual patient's needs, wishes and lifestyle
- cost-effectiveness and product availability.

Although it is not possible to determine the ideal characteristics of a wound dressing to suit all wounds, there are some features that the 'ideal' dressing should possess (Box 15.3).

Box 15.3 Features of an ideal dressing

Maintains a moist wound environment
Provides thermal insulation
Provides a barrier to microorganisms
Protects from trauma
Is non-toxic and non-allergenic
Is absorptive and removes excess exudate
Is sterile
Will not shed fibres into the wound
Atraumatic
Is flexible and conforming
Is comfortable
Controls odour
Is acceptable to the patient
Is easy to use
Requires infrequent dressing change
Is cost-effective
Has a reasonable shelf life and storage requirement
Is available

In many instances, a single dressing will not suffice. For example, a primary dressing may meet the requirements of the wound–dressing interface, but may not possess the absorptive qualities needed to contain exudate and a secondary absorbent dressing will need to be applied. Secondary dressings, including bandages, have the following functions:

- to protect and support the wound and surrounding skin
- to maintain the position of primary dressings
- to absorb moisture
- to control bleeding or oedema (as a result of pressure exerted by secondary dressings).

Vacuum assisted closure (VAC), or topical negative pressure (TNP), is a closed system comprising a foam sponge that fits into the wound. It is sealed by a semi-permeable film dressing and connected by tubing to a pump via a canister to collect wound exudate (Dealey 2005). TNP exerts a negative pressure on the wound, either continuously or intermittently, encouraging increased blood flow and faster granulation. With reference to a number of studies, Dealey (2005) highlights the following claimed benefits of TPN: reduction in tissue oedema, reduction of bacterial overload, management of chronic wound fluid, promotion of wound healing, improved take in skin grafts and cost-effectiveness. However, she does highlight the limited evidence regarding the efficacity of TNP, a concern echoed by Greenhalgh (2007). Dealey (2005), while acknowledging TPN is being used more widely, also cautions that it can be potentially harmful if inappropriately and inexpertly used.

In selecting a dressing the nurse needs to understand the properties, actions, indications and contraindications for the use of each dressing being considered, and match this information to the specific requirements of the patient and the wound (see Annotated Reading: Dealey 2005). The use of an algorithm and a dressing formulary will help nurses in decision making in this area of wound management.

Evidence-based practice

The World Union of Wound Healing Societies (2007), consisting of an international panel of experts, have produced a consensus document on *Wound Healing and the Role of Dressings*. Within the document, principles of best practice are discussed and myths regarding wound exudate are explored. It looks at what exudate is, what examining exudate may tell us, how to assess exudate and how to manage exudate – which includes information on dressing materials and indicated usage.

When undertaking wound care, it is essential that the nurse understands and adheres to the principles of asepsis to promote the prevention of cross-infection (see Ch. 5). If the client has several wounds that require redressing, the cleanest wounds should be dressed first.

There are occasions where wounds can be cleaned and dressed using a clean technique rather than an aseptic technique, depending on the outcomes of assessment (see Ch. 5). A clean technique adheres to the same principles of preventing cross-infection, but clean single-use gloves and/or safe-to-drink tap water are used rather than sterile alternatives. Following a review of five trials, Fernandez et al (2002) conclude that drinkable tap water may be as effective a wound cleanser as sterile water or sterile saline. These clean techniques are in more common use in caring for patients in the community. Gannon (2007), however, argues that for physiological reasons 0.9% saline should remain the cleansing solution of choice, unless contraindicated by the choice of dressing used. He points out that 0.9% saline is isotonic and does not impede wound healing, while water is hypotonic, which can cause cell oedema and rupture and increase the production of exudate.

Decision-making exercise

Mr Heron, a 60-year-old farmer, has a venous leg ulcer, which is shallow, clean, granulating and 5 cm × 5 cm. There is a moderate amount of exudate. He has no known allergies to specific dressing products. In the role of the community nurse:

- Select an appropriate dressing for the wound.
- Justify your choice in terms of promotion of wound healing, patient comfort and cost-effectiveness.
- Did you give consideration as to whether or not your choice of dressing would be available?
- Do you think you had enough information on which to base your decision? If not, what other information would you require before making a decision?

15.4 – WOUND MANAGEMENT ALGORITHMS AND FORMULARY

- Example of wound algorithm.
- Description and choice of dressing for four wound types.

EVALUATION OF THE EFFECTIVENESS OF WOUND MANAGEMENT

The evaluation of wound management should take place at two levels:

- An organization may wish to keep a record of specific wounds and evaluate the effectiveness of the measures taken to deal with and minimize the incidence of these wounds.
- At the level of individual wounds, an evaluation should be made each time the dressings are changed by observing and measuring to see if the wound is healing as expected.

Evaluating individual wounds is important for two reasons. First, as wound healing progresses and the characteristics of the wound change, different dressings may be required. Second, if there is no change or the wound has deteriorated, it is necessary to reflect on the possible factors responsible for delayed healing. The dressing choice may need to be revised or other treatment options considered. However, unless the wound has changed significantly, sufficient time must be given to allow the dressing to become effective before changing to another product. All members of the multidisciplinary team may need to be involved in the discussion and reappraisal of care. It is also important to evaluate patients' progress as a whole and to ascertain their views on the progress that they are making, giving consideration to their quality of life, so that areas of concern can be addressed.

Evidence-based practice

Vermeulen et al (2006) explored the level of agreement/disagreement between doctors ($n=79$) and nurses ($n=63$) when selecting dressings for open surgical wounds. Following assessment and agreement by an expert panel the subjects were asked to assess 18 photographs of wounds and decide on an appropriate dressing. They found a high level of disagreement between different doctors, different nurses and between the two professions, highlighting the importance of evidence-based practice and education in preparing professions to make appropriate choices.

MANAGEMENT OF ACUTE AND CHRONIC WOUNDS

Accidental wounds

An accidental wound is defined as an acute wound that has occurred as a result of an accident or a specific non-medical incident. They are sometimes referred to as traumatic wounds. Accidental wounds can range from minor cuts and abrasions to major wounds such as the loss of limb or crush injuries. Also included are burns, scalds, bites and stings.

In all emergency cases, it is necessary to assess the patient, and if possible to obtain a history of the wound. This includes the cause, circumstances, time of accident, estimate of blood loss and any other information relevant to the management of the patient. Psychological care of the patient – and any accompanying relatives or friends – is extremely important, as the suddenness of the situation can cause considerable distress and anxiety. It is also important to identify and address any pain the patient is experiencing.

The management of major accidental wounds is decided and directed by the accident and emergency medical officer. Rapid accurate assessment of the client's condition and underlying pathology is essential. Priority must be given to the re-establishment and maintenance of the airway, breathing and circulation and the control of bleeding before dealing with the wound itself. A head-to-toe examination must then be conducted to ensure that there are no other injuries that need to take priority over the management of the wound (Dealey 2005).

In the case of minor wounds, such as slight cuts and abrasions, an initial assessment of the patient is still necessary but attention can quickly be focused on wound care to minimize the risk of infection. It may be appropriate to offer health education or the patient may require a tetanus injection.

The cause of the wound will indicate likely damage and complications and will guide wound management decisions. Puncture wounds caused by stabbing have only a small entry site, but cut a deep track and may damage internal tissue and organs. As the wound penetrates deep into the body, the risk of infection is high. Abrasions can result in large tender areas where the superficial layers of skin have been removed. They often contain foreign particles such as grit, which can cause infection and tattooing if not removed effectively. If a large foreign body is embedded in the patient it must be removed in theatre as there is a risk of major haemorrhage when it is removed.

Accurate documentation is essential. In cases of criminal or civil prosecution or claims for industrial injury compensation, the patient's records may be used as evidence. Where a patient is a victim of a non-accidental injury that warrants police investigation, such as a stabbing or a road traffic accident, particular care must be taken with the patient's property, including clothing, as it may be required for further examination and used as evidence. Where child abuse is suspected, for example if a child appears to have cigarette burns on its buttocks, it is essential to follow the local hospital policy regarding the management and reporting of such cases, so that further action can be taken as appropriate. The nurse must use considerable tact when dealing with such situations.

Surgical wounds

Surgical wounds are classified as open or closed depending upon the reasons for surgery. Wounds healing by primary intention, using sutures, clips, staples or tape, will normally heal within 48 hours preventing ingress by bacteria (Dealey 2005) . The role of the nurse is to:

- prevent infection
- monitor the wound to detect the onset of any complications
- prevent trauma to the wound site
- promote nutritional and fluid intake.

Apart from using an aseptic technique to reduce the risk of a wound infection, nurses need to consider their own health: a nurse with a cold or sore throat will be a reservoir for infective organisms and should not be involved in wound care. Following surgery, wounds may be dressed with an island dressing which can be removed after 24–48 hours, or covered with a film dressing which is usually left *in situ* until the sutures are removed (Dealey 2005). The patient can resume normal hygiene activities, such as bathing, when wounds are dressed with film or hydrocolloid dressing (Bale & Jones 2006). Skin closing sutures pierce the skin and enter the subdermal layers and are therefore a potential route of entry for infection. Unless there is exudate, wound cleansing should not be undertaken, as the introduction of moisture to the sutures facilitates the passage of microorganisms by capillary action along the sutures into the subdermal layers. When removing sutures, the nurse must ensure that when the suture is cut and then drawn from the wound, the part of the suture that is above the surface of the skin is not allowed to pass beneath the surface of the skin. This prevents microorganisms from being drawn into the track left by the suture in the subdermal layers. If drainage tubes are used, they should be secured to prevent the shunting of the tubes in and out of the wound, thus reducing the risk of bacteria entering the drainage incision.

The wound should be assessed using a specific assessment tool for surgically closed wounds such as the tool developed by Morison (2004). The use of a clear dressing allows observation of the wound without removing the dressing, and so reduces the risk of contamination. In addition, the nurse must observe the drainage for colour and consistency and, in open drainage systems, odour.

To prevent trauma there should be no rubbing or pulling on the wound closures and drainage tubes. This can be achieved by applying a light dry dressing to the incision site. Wound drainage tubes should be secured and supported.

Surgical patients require an adequate fluid intake, and an increased calorie and protein intake to aid wound healing. Vitamins C, A, E, K, and B complex, and iron, zinc, manganese, copper and magnesium are also vital (see section on Further Annotated Reading: Burton 2006). The nurse should help the patient select appropriate food to meet these requirements. Liaison with a dietician is helpful in some instances. Assistance with feeding may be necessary.

Chronic wounds

The management of a patient with a chronic wound requires a different approach from those with an acute or surgical wound because of the longstanding nature of the problem and the prolonged healing time. The two most prevalent open chronic wounds are leg ulcers and pressure ulcers. In order to provide a framework for discussion, the management of pressure ulcers is used as an example. However, the principles of pressure ulcer management can be applied to any chronic wound.

The effects of the ulcer can be wide ranging, causing the patient to suffer not only physical, but also psychological, social and economic problems.

Pressure sores, bed sores, decubitus ulcers and pressure ulcers are some of the many terms used to describe the 'sores', and each has been criticized for its inaccuracy. They are not caused only by pressure and do not only occur in people who are in bed or lying down. No one term covers all the possible causes and situations in which sores can occur. For the purpose of discussion, the term pressure ulcer is used, as it is a widely used term recognized by all healthcare professionals.

Pressure ulcers are defined by Benbow (2005: 42) as 'areas of localized tissue damage that can extend to underlying structures such as muscle and bone. They are caused by excess pressure, shearing or friction'. It is the ischaemic changes in the tissues that cause the damage rather than the pressure itself. When direct pressure is exerted on the skin at a level greater than the mean capillary pressure of 25 mmHg, the capillaries are occluded and the blood supply to the tissues is restricted. This causes tissue ischaemia, and eventually, if the blood supply is not re-established, tissue necrosis. With shearing force the tissues are stretched to such an extent that capillaries rupture, resulting in a marked reduction in the amount of blood reaching the tissues and tissue necrosis.

Successful management of a pressure ulcer is important not only for the patient but for the financial health of the NHS (Table 15.1)

Assessment of the risk of developing pressure ulcers

Prevention is always better than a cure. There are several 'at risk' scales available to assist nurses in identifying those at risk of pressure ulcers in order that preventive care can be implemented. Waterlow (1985 and revised 2005) and Norton (Norton et al 1962) are examples of scales commonly used in the UK. Each has been critically appraised and found to be beneficial in some situations and to over or under-predict risk in others. No risk assessment tool has been able to identify all risk factors, therefore they should only be used as an aide-mémoire and should never replace clinical judgement. The RCN and NICE (2005: 27) highlight groups of people that are at risk of developing pressure ulcers:

those who are seriously ill, neurologically compromised i.e. individuals with spinal cord injuries, have impaired mobility or who are immobile (including those wearing a prosthesis, body brace or plaster cast), or who suffer from impaired nutrition, obesity, poor posture, or use equipment such as seating or beds which do not provide appropriate pressure relief. Older people and pregnant women are also at risk.

Table 15.1 Cost of healing pressure ulcers (Bennett et al 2004)

Grade (as EPUAP see Box 15.1)	Cost
1	£1064
2	£4402
3	£7313
4	£10 551

They do not specifically mention incontinence which is also acknowledged as a high risk factor (see Evolve 15.5 on risk assessment).

Preventive care can take many forms. The RCN (2001) gives recommendations on the use of pressure redistribution devices (e.g. overlays, cushions and alternating pressure mattresses); positioning (e.g. turns and redistribution of weight); seating; and education and training. They also specifically condemn the use of water filled gloves, synthetic sheepskins, genuine sheepskins and doughnut type devices as pressure relieving aids.

Once a pressure ulcer has developed the focus of care changes. Firstly, the ulcer needs to be assessed and graded and it is now recommended that the European Pressure Ulcer Advisory Panel (2003) classification is used across Europe (see Box 15.1).

---

evolve learning system

15.5 – PRESSURE ULCER RISK ASSESSMENT

- Website access to risk assessment tools.
- Exercise in comparing these tools.
- Commentary on evidence for choice of tools.

Assessment of a patient with a pressure ulcer

A thorough assessment of the patient can assist in the identification of both internal and external factors relating to the patient's condition and ability that may affect wound healing. The pressure ulcer assessment wheel (Fig. 15.6) incorporates many areas of patient assessment and some areas specific to the assessment of pressure ulcer, giving an overall assessment framework. Each of these is explained in turn as you progress around the wheel.

The 'inner wheel' highlights the many 'patient' factors that have an indirect effect on healing, namely:

- The importance of adequate 'oxygenation', 'nutrition' and 'hydration', which have been discussed previously (see Subject Knowledge).
- Anything that modifies the patient's ability or desire to move about ('mobility') may affect the wound.
- 'Pain' can prevent a patient from changing his or her position as often as required.
- 'Drugs' can have varying influences on healing, depending upon their effects – some drugs such as glucocorticosteroids may alter the texture of the skin, while others such as sedatives may reduce the patient's level of alertness, resulting in the associated problems of reduced movement and decreased awareness of risk.

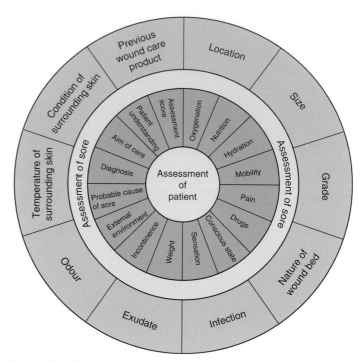

Figure 15.6 Pressure ulcer assessment wheel.

- Reduced 'consciousness' can lead to a patient being unable to identify the need to move, and can prevent him or her from doing so.
- Loss of 'sensation' can result in a patient being unaware of the position he or she is in and the need to change it.
- Extremes of weight, i.e. body mass index of above 30 or below 20, could compromise healing and increase the risk of further ulcer development.
- Faecal and urinary 'incontinence' can cause contamination of wound sites, excess moisture in the wound area and problems with adherence with certain dressings, particularly in relation to pressure ulcers on the buttocks, sacrum or hips.
- 'External environment' covers a large area relating to resources – the general environment (e.g. own home, hospital single room or multi-occupancy room, nursing or residential care) can affect the type of dressing or treatment available or possible, as can the amount of assistance the patient can expect from nursing staff, other carers and relatives or significant others.
- It is important to identify the 'probable cause of the ulcer' developing as this may influence the care required – if shearing force is suspected attention may be focused on handling and positioning patients to prevent further damage, but if direct pressure has caused the problem the main objective is to remove the pressure.
- The patient's 'diagnosis' can sometimes affect the wound healing – conditions such as diabetes mellitus, vascular disease, malignancy and anaemia can alter the cellular

environment and therefore interfere with the healing process.

- The 'aim of care' is not always apparent – for patients in the terminal stages of illness, it may not be possible to heal the pressure ulcer in the time the patient has left to live; in which case the aim of care may be to prevent the wound from deteriorating and to increase patient comfort, rather than to heal the ulcer.
- 'Patient understanding' of his or her condition and treatments and the patient's ability to comply with regimens may also affect the overall choice of treatment.
- A current assessment score using a risk calculator (see Evolve 15.5).

The 'outer ring' of the assessment wheel consists of the factors you should consider when dealing with the wound itself. These factors have been covered earlier. In addition to the points above, it is important to assess and manage the psychological impact of living with a chronic wound (see section on annotated further reading Hopkins et al 2006).

Any plan of care relating to pressure ulcer management needs to contain a core of information:

- an up-to-date assessment of the wound
- current at-risk assessment score and review dates
- cleansing solution to be used
- primary dressing requirements

- secondary dressing requirements – padding, bandaging
- method of carrying out dressing
- frequency of dressing changes
- referrals made and advice received
- associated factors – use of pressure relieving aids and mattresses, mobility programme and turning regimen
- patient and relative involvement
- patient and relative educational needs.

Pressure ulcers should not be seen as a nursing problem, but rather as a challenge to the full multidisciplinary team, in which each member has a role to play. The flowchart showing multidisciplinary involvement (Fig. 15.7) is not exhaustive, but serves to highlight the level of integration that may be required. Care should be implemented in accordance with the written patient care plan. It is advised that a limited number of nurses are involved in implementing the wound care. Continuity and consistency are important if the pressure ulcer is to be given the best chance of healing. Different nurses may use slightly different techniques; dressings may therefore be applied in a different manner. This can affect the rate and amount of wound healing; for instance, one nurse may pack a wound tighter than another. Continuity of care also helps evaluation, as the nurse becomes familiar with the wound and is better able to detect changes in its size, shape and general condition.

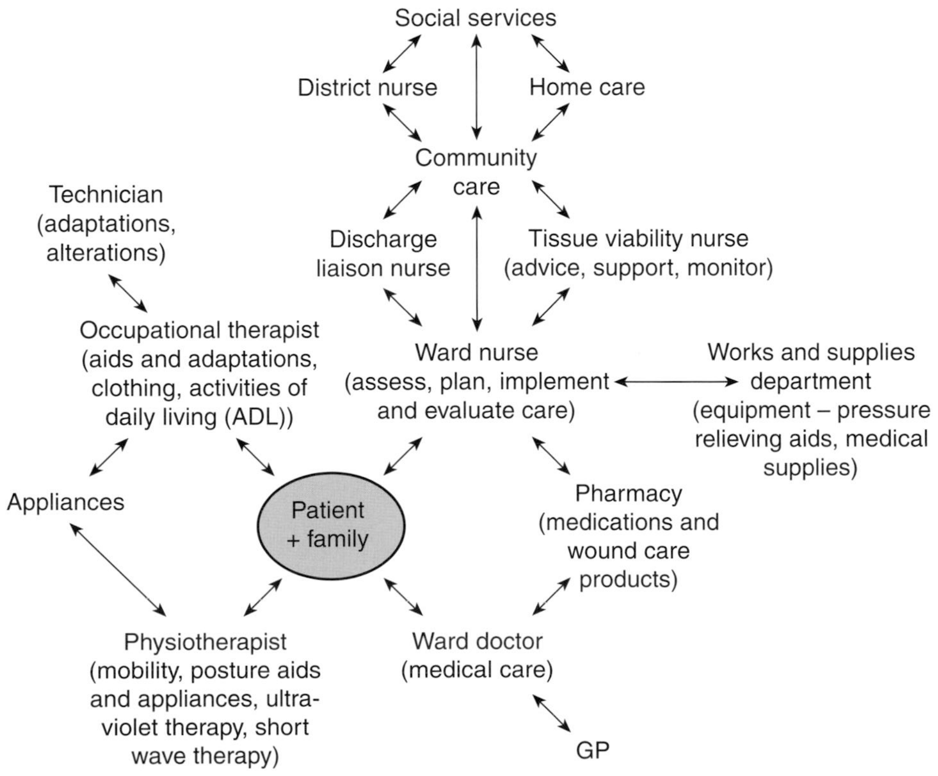

Figure 15.7 Multidisciplinary involvement in the management of pressure ulcers.

Decision-making exercise

Steven is 45 years old and suffers from cerebral palsy. He is cared for by his 67-year-old mother in a purpose-built ground floor flat and has two care assistants who attend him in the morning and at night to get him up and put him to bed. Steven attends a day centre 5 days a week. He is unable to walk and is confined to a wheelchair. He is difficult to feed and faecally incontinent. He has been catheterized for the past 2 years. During a visit to the day centre you notice a small broken area on his left buttock.

- Decide which factors you need to assess in order to plan the care Steven will require to heal the present ulcer.
- Draw a spider diagram showing which members of the multidisciplinary team can assist in the management of the present ulcer.
- Given the amount of support Steven already has, what other preventive measures may be necessary to prevent any further deterioration of Steven's skin?

If a pressure ulcer does not heal, further intervention through debridement and/or skin grafting is an option. Debridement helps remove non-viable tissue, control inflammation or infection, correct moisture imbalance and stimulate a non-advancing wound edge (Falabella 2006). Skin grafting has developed rapidly since the advent of genetic engineering. As well as the more established types of grafting, i.e. autografting (taking skin from one site to a second site on the same person), and pedicle or flap grafts, there are now many new techniques available. Collier (2006) describes a variety of innovations within tissue engineering to include the use of living dermal/epidermal cells or manufactured skin substitutes to replace damaged tissue. Although they have proven to be successful in some instances, the effectiveness is dependent on the status of the wound, patient condition and the clinical skills of the nurse undertaking the dressing procedure. Examples of tissue-engineered products are Dermagraft™, Intergra™ and Apligraf™

Wound care and technology

Basic technology such as photographing wounds to monitor healing has been used for many years. With the expansion of electronic information and communication technologies there are now opportunities for wider applications. Digital cameras, video recording and /or video conferencing could be used by nurses to obtain second opinions or treatment advice from nurses or medical staff working in other locations (see Evolve 15.6 for further information).

evolve learning system

15.6 – WOUND CARE AND TECHNOLOGY

- Technology to obtain treatment advice.
- Evidence of its effective use.
- Advantages and disadvantages.
- How to evaluate credibility of information on websites.

PROFESSIONAL AND ETHICAL KNOWLEDGE

This section focuses on professional and ethical issues that are relevant to the quality of care provision relating to skin integrity. The responsibility of the nurse to participate in organization wide strategies for promoting effective skin integrity as well as provide safe effective care, is explored.

Reflection and portfolio evidence

Reflect on the practice areas where you have worked in all fields of nursing.

- List examples of health promotion activities relating to skin integrity that you have observed.
- Reflect on the number of areas and occasions in which there was an opportunity to provide health promotion in relation to skin care and integrity.
- Record one incident where you took an active part in health promotion related to skin care and comment critically on what you learned through undertaking this activity.

PROMOTING SKIN HEALTH

The nurse has an important role to play in promoting health and there is considerable potential in all care settings to promote skin health. Health promotion activities can range from teaching parents the necessary skin care for their newborn babies to empowering individuals to manage their own chronic skin conditions, such as psoriasis and eczema.

The knowledge base provided in this chapter, along with a more in-depth understanding of health promotion (see Naidoo & Wills 2005), will enable the nurse to select the appropriate health promotion activity to assist specific individuals to achieve and maintain optimum skin health. To be effective it is essential that activities are planned, in order to achieve identified health goals. It is also important that the nurse recognizes individual limitations, and where necessary ensures that patients receive specific expert help. In addition, where longer-term interventions are needed and input from other healthcare professionals or agencies is required, as is often the case with chronic skin problems, consideration must be given to how continuity can be ensured. When planning health promotion for a group of individuals requiring healthcare services, for example patients with venous leg ulcers, the Department of Health's (2006) *Essence of Care: Benchmarks for Promoting Health* would provide a useful tool.

DEVELOPING SKIN CARE QUALITY SYSTEMS

There is considerable scope for nurses, along with other healthcare professionals, to be involved in the development and maintenance of quality systems of care relating to skin integrity. Examples of this include involvement in the development of standards of care, benchmarking, clinical guidelines and protocols, procedures, policies, integrated care pathways and auditing clinical practice (Birchall & Taylor 2003). Clinical guidelines and protocols promote quality standards and continuity of care by providing an agreed framework for decision making for the treatment and management of specific aspects of care. Integrated care pathways for the prevention of pressure ulcers and wound management are two examples relating to skin integrity in the development of quality systems of care. Recognition should be given to nationally produced guidelines as appropriate, for example the guidelines produced by the National Institute for Health and Clinical Excellence such as those for pressure ulcer management (NICE 2005).

Nurses also have a significant role in developing, undertaking and participating in audits of clinical practice. As an example which relates to skin integrity, hospitals often keep records of the incidence of pressure ulcers and will investigate what measures were taken to prevent the development of pressure ulcers and what care was given when pressure ulcers developed. Auditing may be undertaken to see if the agreed standards are being met for both prevention and care of pressure ulcers. The document *Essence of Care* (Department of Health 2003a, b) contains benchmarking tools related to eight fundamental aspects of care, one of which is pressure ulcers. These tools provide benchmarks of best practice against which nurses can measure the quality of practice in their own clinical areas.

IMPLICATIONS OF NURSE LED SKIN CARE

The role of the nurse in relation to skin integrity has developed greatly over the past 20 years. The Riverside Community Leg Ulcer Clinic was an innovation in its time (Moffatt & Oldroyd 1994), but such nurse-led clinics are now more commonplace. Collier & Radley (2005) set up a nurse-led complex wound clinic that allowed earlier discharge from hospital of patients with wounds that required prolonged specialist care. As well as providing care for patients

nurse-led services can provide advice and education to other nurses and clinicians. Due to increasing role development and the advancements in technology, it is necessary to explore the clinical, educational, professional and ethical implications for practice. Some of the more salient issues are discussed below.

Extended practice

With ever-growing technological development, nurses are taking on additional roles. As well as link nurses and clinical specialists there are now lead nurses and nurse consultants in tissue viability, dermatology, burns etc. who have a greater ability to carry out an extended range of wound care procedures and are often nurse prescribers. A higher level of skills and knowledge are necessary. The UK Central Council (1992) produced guidelines on the extended role of the nurse in its document *Scope of Professional Practice*. To date, there has been no corresponding publication from the Nursing and Midwifery Council (NMC) to guide extended practice, although clause 6 of its Code of Professional Conduct (Nursing and Midwifery Council 2008) does address professional knowledge and competence. The NMC have produced standards of proficiency for nurse and midwife prescribers (2005) and advice on complementary alternative therapies and homeopathy (2006) which could be relevant in wound management. The UK Central Council (1994) *Standards for Specialist Education and Practice*, which have been adopted by the NMC, differentiate between advanced practice and specialist practice. While stating that no standards will be set for advanced practice, they do give some guidance regarding the requirements of specialist practice.

Nurse prescribing

The Nurse Prescribers Formulary is published twice a year and contains details on items that can be prescribed by nurses who have been appropriately trained for this expanded role. Many wound dressings are included in this formulary giving community nurse prescribers the resources for total wound care management. Nurse prescribing has implication in terms of accountability and responsibility and has been shown to be beneficial to both patients, nurses and the NHS. Lowe & Hurst (2002) state that nurse prescribing is time saving, promotes continuity of care, increases patient concordance, gives an opportunity for health promotion, increases nurses' awareness of costs and prevents stock piling of dressings.

Community matrons

The NHS improvement plan (DH 2004) called for community matrons to be appointed to manage the care of patients with complex needs. They will have the authority to instigate care and support for patients and their carers and should prove beneficial for patients with complex wounds. This is a new clinical role, designed to prevent unplanned hospital admissions, improve quality of life and give patients and their families more choice in their care (Department of Health 2004). It is anticipated that 3000 community matrons will be employed by the NHS by 2008.

Record keeping

The Health Service Commissioner has highlighted inadequate record keeping in tissue viability as an issue in a number of related legal proceedings, professional misconduct cases and investigations (Culley 2001). Culley discusses the need for tissue viability nurses to produce accurate and effective records in all aspects of their expanding role. It can be argued that the same standard applies for any nurse who is involved in the management and record keeping of patients requiring care for skin integrity. Utilization of agreed evidence-based wound care assessment documentation, care pathways and protocols will facilitate this process. Effective clinical audits of record keeping will, as Culley (2001) suggests, monitor the effectiveness of the systems that are currently in place and inform improvements towards best practice. Record keeping is one of the *Essence of Care* (Department of Health 2003a) benchmarks and this document guides the nurse to identify best practice.

Consent

The Nursing and Midwifery Council (2008) stress the necessity of obtaining consent prior to giving any treatment or care. Although in many instances implied consent (Montgomery 1997) is adequate, it is also necessary to consider whether documented verbal or written consent may be required for some interventions. For example, should implied, verbal or written consent be obtained, and from whom, for larval treatment or allografting (replacing epidermal loss with genetically unrelated cells), particularly given the ethical considerations? The use of technology raises further issues of consent. Consent is also required for the taking of photographic and other digital images. The use of telemedicine means that information and images are subject to the Data Protection Act (1998). These issues need to be addressed to ensure that clear lines of accountability are drawn, that informed consent is obtained at an appropriate level and that clinical practice and documentation reflect professional, legal and ethically acceptable practice.

In any care setting nurses meet patients or clients with a variety of problems and needs relating to skin care. This chapter provides the knowledge and decision making skills that nurses need (within the limitations of their roles) to make informed decisions and provide appropriate, effective, evidence-based care for patients or clients and their families, in order that they might achieve and maintain optimum skin health. The importance of a holistic problem solving approach to care is stressed, as is the need for effective communication between healthcare professionals.

Decision-making exercise

Larval therapy involves the placement of live, sterile green-bottle larvae (maggots) on to a necrotic wound where they will digest the devitalized tissue and defaecate into the wound. The faecal material contains enzymes that are beneficial to wound healing. Having done their job the larvae are incinerated in the clinical waste.

- What information do you think a patient would require in order to give informed consent for the treatment to be used?
- Debate the legal and ethical requirements for informed consent and discuss the difficulties that may arise in providing this treatment for wound care.

PERSONAL AND REFLECTIVE KNOWLEDGE

PORTFOLIO ACTIVITIES

Reflection assists in making links between theory and practice, and helps to address the affective aspects of practice. In relation to affective aspects, reflection on observed practice, both in respect of others and one's self, as well as the response/reaction of the patient and significant others, enables you to consider the appropriateness of actions and alternative approaches to care, and to take forward new learning, as well as identifying areas for further development.

Reflection on wound management is often aided by keeping a diary of care that has been observed and practised. A wound management diary is available for printing in Evolve 15.7.

15.7 – WOUND MANAGEMENT EXERCISE

- Example of work-book to download for recording reflective learning on wound management.

CASE STUDIES IN NURSING PATIENTS WITH SKIN PROBLEMS

The following case studies will help you bring together the knowledge and decision-making skills required to address the needs of specific individuals with a variety of different skin problems.

Case study: Adult

Miss Green is 75 years old and lives alone in a one-bedroom ground floor flat. One morning, after the arrival of the district nurse, Miss Green slips on the kitchen mat and falls, sustaining a deep laceration to her head. The hot tea she is carrying splashes onto her arm causing a large but superficial burn.

- Decide what first aid treatment the district nurse should administer for the two skin injuries.
- On arrival at the accident and emergency department the doctor examines Miss Green and finds that during the fall she has sustained a fractured neck of femur. Miss Green subsequently requires a hip replacement. Decide what care Miss Green will require in respect of her hip wound for the first 10 postoperative days.

Case study: Child

Margaret and David MacDonnell take their 5-year-old son Robert on holiday to a well-known seaside resort. As it is an overcast day Margaret has not applied any sun protection to Robert. Robert spends the whole day in just a pair of trunks playing on the beach.

That evening Robert complains that his skin hurts and when David examines Robert he finds that his back is badly sunburnt.

- Decide what immediate measures should be taken to treat the effects of Robert's sunburn?
- Given the opportunity, how would you help Mr and Mrs MacDonnell ensure effective sun protection for Robert in the future?

Case study: Mental health

Josie is 28 years old and single. She is attending a day unit for the adult mentally ill for treatment of anxiety–depression. During the post lunch rest period Josie shouts for you to come to the female toilet where she says she requires your help. When you arrive you find that Josie has inflicted several superficial lacerations to her wrists and forearms using the broken handle of a teaspoon from her lunch tray.

- What immediate first aid measures are needed?
- Decide what measures the nurse will need to take to ensure that Josie receives appropriate wound care until her lacerations heal.
- Decide what actions the nurse should take to ensure appropriate reporting and recording of the incident and to minimize the risk of Josie repeating the behaviour.

Case study: Learning disabilities

Joseph is 40 years of age, has Down syndrome and lives in residential care. He has developed the habit of picking the skin on the back of his hand, which has resulted in a small but deep wound. Although the wound has been covered with a plaster, Joseph continues to pick at the wound site and the nurse thinks that the present dressing is inadequate.

- Decide what factors should be taken into account when choosing an appropriate dressing for Joseph?
- What nursing knowledge and skills would the nurse require to facilitate wound healing in Joseph's case?

SUMMARY

This chapter has focused on the knowledge and decision making needed to provide high-quality skin care for patients/clients and ourselves. It has included:

1. Information to understand the biological basis underpinning tissue viability, and also the psychological, social, cultural, environmental and economic factors involved.
2. An appreciation of the importance of conducting a thorough and appropriate assessment of the skin disorder/wound and of the patient as a whole, prior to the implementation of care.
3. Knowledge for the management of wounds/skin disorders based on current evidence-based protocols, care procedures and outcome measures to evaluate effective wound/skin care.
4. Health promotion strategies to encourage a healthy skin.
5. Acknowledgement of the vital role of specialist nurses and the multidisciplinary team in ensuring consistent

quality care especially for patients with chronic skin conditions/wounds.

6. Legal and ethical issues in skin care with particular reference to consent to treatment.

Annotated further reading and websites

Benbow M 2005 Managing infected wounds. Ch 9: Evidence-based wound management. Whurr Publishers, London, pp 95–114

This chapter explains the impact of infection on wound healing and discusses the assessment and management of different types of infected wounds.

Bethell E 2005 Wound care for patients with darkly pigmented skin. Nursing Standard 20:41–49

This article explores the main parameters for wound and skin assessment and discusses the differences that need to be acknowledged when nursing patients with darkly pigmented skin.

Burton F 2006 Best practice overview: surgical and trauma wounds. Wound Essentials 1:98–107

The author provides an overview of the nursing assessments and interventions that should be considered for patients with surgical or traumatic wounds.

Cullum N, Deeks J, Sheldon TA et al 2003 Beds, mattresses and cushions for pressure sore prevention and treatment (Cochrane Review). In: Cochrane Library, Issue 1. Update Software, Oxford

A review of 35 randomized controlled trials of the use of support surfaces for treatment and prevention of pressure ulcers. Although it is unable to determine the most effective surface it does provide a wide range of information on different support surfaces.

Dealey C 2005 Wound management products. Ch 4: The care of wounds: a guide for nurses. Blackwell Publishing, Oxford, pp 83–120

This chapter provides a comprehensive overview of wound management products.

Falabella AF 2006 Debridement and wound bed preparation. Dermatologic Therapy 19:317–325

This article discusses the important role of debridement in wound bed preparation and goes on to discuss the advantages and disadvantages of different types of debridement.

Vowden K, Vowden P 2003 Understanding exudate management and the role of exudate in the healing process. British Journal of Nursing 12: (20 Suppl.):4–13

This article discusses the role of wound exudate, highlights the differences between exudate in acute and chronic wounds and discusses strategies to manage wound exudate to facilitate wound healing.

http://science.uwe.ac.uk/research/
From the home page you can link to the Centre for Appearance Research (CAR). CAR was originally launched in 1988 under the title 'the Centre for Appearance and Disability Research' (CADR) and is part of the University of West England, Bristol. It conducts research into human appearance and disfigurement and provides a link to research articles and conferences.

http://www.epuap.org/
The European Pressure Ulcer Advisory Panel was formed in 1996 to provide guidance across the EU countries. The website contains information on the panel and guidelines for practice.

http://www.worldwidewounds.com/
This is the *Electronic Journal of Wound Management Practice* produced by the Surgical Materials Testing Laboratory, Bridgend, South Wales, in association with the Medical Education Partnership.

http://www.nice.org.uk
Home page for the National Institute for Health and Clinical Excellence (NICE). It provides links for both professionals and the public into a variety of pages that give guidance for best practice. Search wound derbridement.

http://www.eczema.org/
The National Eczema Society, founded in 1975, is dedicated to the needs of people with eczema, dermatitis and sensitive skin. A wide range of literature on skin conditions treatment and current research is provided on this website.

http://www.tvs.org.uk/
The Tissue Viability Society runs this useful website providing information for professionals, patients and carers. It contains some patient information leaflets that can be downloaded. Also provides information on forthcoming events and access to the *Journal of Tissue Viability*.

http://www.psoriasis-association.org.uk/index.html
The Psoriasis Association, which is a registered charity, runs this website providing information about psoriasis and treatments.

http://www.bad.org.uk/about
The British Association of Dermatologists is a long established association. On the website, information sheets about skin disease, general information about the skin, dermatology in the UK and current issues on skin disease are provided.

http://www.skin-camouflage.net/
The British Association of Skin Camouflage was formed in 1985. The website provides information on skin camouflage, promotes a positive change towards people with altered image, provides a network of trained camouflage practitioners and, through its magazine *The Cover*, provides up-to-date information on products and application techniques.

http://www.skincarecampaign.org
The Skin Care Campaign, established in 1992, and a subsidiary of the National Eczema Society, is an umbrella organization representing the interests of people in the UK with skin diseases. The website provides information about skin diseases and their treatment and initiatives to improve the health care of people with skin disease.

http://changingfaces.org.uk
Changing Faces is a national charity based in the UK, that supports and represents people with disfigurements. They provide information, including research articles. A new website for young people has also been developed called 'iface' http://iface.org.uk

http://www.ewma.org
The European Wound Management Association website provides access to their publications and conference details.

http://www.york.ac.uk/healthsciences/gsp/themes/woundcare/Wounds
This website give access to the Cochrane Wound Group and provides access to systematic reviews related to wound care.

http://www.wounds-uk.com
This website provides access to the *Wounds-UK* journal and links to many useful wound care sites.

References

Bale S, Jones V 2006 Wound care nursing: a patient-centred approach, 2nd edn. Elsevier, Edinburgh

Benbow M 2002 The skin. 2: Skin and wound assessment. Nursing Times 98:41–44

Benbow M 2005 Evidence-based wound management. Whurr, London

Bennett G, Dealey C, Posnett J 2004 The cost of pressure ulcers in the UK. Age and Ageing 33:230–235

Birchall L, Taylor S 2003 Surgical wound benchmark tool and best practice guidelines. British Journal of Nursing 12:1013–1014, 1016–1017, 1020–1023

Cancer Research UK 2005 Malignant melanoma factsheet. Available online: http://info.cancerresearchuk.org/images/pdfs/melanomafactsheet2005 (accessed 27 August 2008)

Cancer Research UK 2007 Stay safe. Available online: http://info.cancerresearchuk.org/healthyliving/sunsmart/staysafe/ (accessed 1 February 2008)

Calvin M 1998 Cutaneous wound repair. Wounds 10:12–32

Clarke A, Cooper C 2001 Psychosocial rehabilitation after disfiguring injury or disease: investigating the training needs of specialist nurses. Journal of Advanced Nursing 34:18–26

Collier M 2002 Wound-bed preparation. NTplus 98:55–57

Collier M 2006 The use of advanced biological and tissue-engineered wound products. Nursing Standard 21(7):68, 70, 72, 74–76

Collier M, Radley K 2005 The development of a nurse-led complex wound clinic. Nursing Standard 19:74–84

Culley F 2001 The tissue viability nurse and effective documentation. British Journal of Nursing 10(Suppl.):S30–S39

Data Protection Act 1998 Available online: http://www.opsi.gov.uk/Acts/Acts1998/ukpga_19980029_en_1 (accessed 1 February 2008)

Dealey C 2005 The care of wounds: a guide for nurses, 3rd edn. Blackwell Publishing, Oxford

Department of Health 2003a The essence of care: patient-focused benchmarks for clinical governance. Available online: http://www.dh.gov.uk/en/Publicationsandstatistics/Publications/PublicationsPolicyAndGuidance/DH_4005475 (accessed 1 February 2008)

Department of Health 2003b The essence of care: pressure ulcer risk assessment and prevention. HMSO, London

Department of Health 2004 The NHS improvement plan: putting people at the heart of public services. TSO, London

Department of Health 2006 Essence of care: benchmarks for promoting health. Available online: http://www.dh.gov.uk/en/Publicationsandstatistics/Publications/PublicationsPolicyAndGuidance/DH_075613 (accessed 1 February 2008)

Diffey BL 2002 Is daily use of sunscreens of benefit in the UK? British Journal of Dermatologists 146: 659–662

Diffey B 2007 Sunbeds, beauty and melanoma [Editorial]. British Journal of Dermatologists 157:215–216

European Management Association 2005 Cited by Moore Z, Cowman S 2007 Effective wound management: identifying criteria for infection. Nursing Standard 21:68, 70, 72, 74–76

European Pressure Ulcer Advisory Panel 2003 Pressure ulcer treatment guidelines. Available online: http://www.epuap.org/ (accessed 1 February 2008) and http://www.pressureulcerguidelines.org/ (accessed 19 August 2008)

Falabella AF 2006 Debridement and wound bed preparation. Dermatologic Therapy 19:317–325

Fernandez R, Griffiths R, Ussia C 2002 Water for wound cleansing. Cochrane Database of Systematic Reviews, Issue 4. Article no.: CD003861. DOI: 10.1002/14651858.CD003861

Gannon R 2007 Wound cleansing: sterile water or saline? NT 103:44–46

Greenhalgh DG 2007 Negative pressure therapy, a panacea or not [Editorial]? Wound Repair and Regeneration 15:433

Gross RD 2005 Psychology: the science of mind and behaviour, 5th edn. Hodder Arnold, London

Health Education Authority and BBC 2000 Sun Know How campaign. Available online: www.bbc.co.uk/weather/world/features/sun_know_how.shtml (accessed 1 February 2008)

Holloway S, Jones V 2005 The importance of skin care and assessment. British Journal of Nursing 14:1172–1176

Lowe L, Hurst R 2002 Nurse prescribing: the reality. In: Humphries JL, Green J (eds) Nurse prescribing, 2nd edn. Palgrave, London, ch 8

Ma W, Wlaschek M, Tantcheva-Poor I 2001 Chronological ageing and photoaging of the fibroblasts and the dermal connective tissue. Clinical and Experimental Dermatology 26:592–599

Mehta Products 2007 Bhoomibindi traditions. Available online: http://www.bhoomibindi.com/tradition_of_bindi.htm (accessed 1 February 2008)

Moffatt CJ, Oldroyd MI 1994 A pioneering service to the community: the Riverside community leg ulcer project. Professional Nurse 9:486, 488, 490, 492, 494, 497

Montague SE, Watson R, Herbert RA (eds) 2005 Physiology for nursing practice, 3rd edn. Elsevier, Edinburgh

Montgomery J 1997 Health care law. Oxford Polytechnic, Oxford

Moore Z, Cowman S 2007 Effective wound management: identifying criteria for infection. Nursing Standard 21:68, 70, 72, 74–76

Morison MJ 2004 A framework for patient assessment and care planning. In: Morison MJ, Ovington LG, Wilkie K 2004 Chronic wound care: a problem-based approach. Mosby, London, pp 46–66

Naidoo J, Wills J 2005 Public health and health promotion: developing practice, 2nd edn. Baillière Tindall, London

National Institute for Health and Clinical Excellence 2005 CG29 Pressure ulcer management: full guideline. Available online: http://www.nice.org.uk/Guidance/CG29 (accessed 29 January 2008)

National Institute for Health and Clinical Excellence 2006 Improving outcomes for people with skin tumours including melanoma. National Institute for Clinical Excellence, London. Available online: http://guidance.nice.org.uk/csgstim (accessed 1 February 2008)

Naylor W 2004 Wound management. In: Dougherty L, Lister SE (eds) The Royal Marsden Hospital manual of clinical nursing procedures, 6th edn. Blackwell Publishing, Oxford, pp 796–842

Norton D, McLaren R, Exton-Smith AN 1962. An investigation of geriatric nursing problems in hospitals. National Corporation for the Care of Older People, London

Nursing and Midwifery Council 2005 Standards of proficiency for nurse and midwife prescribers. NMC. London

Nursing and Midwifery Council 2006 Complementary alternative therapies and homeopathy (advice sheet). NMC. London

Nursing and Midwifery Council 2008 The Code: standards of conduct, performance and ethics for nurses and midwives. Nursing and Midwifery Council, London

Royal College of Nursing 2001 Pressure ulcer risk management and assessment. Royal College of Nursing, London

Royal College of Nursing and National Institute for Health and Clinical Excellence 2005 The management of pressure ulcers in primary and secondary care: a clinical practice guideline. Royal College of Nursing, London

Rumsey N, Clarke A, White P, Wyn-Williams M, Garlick W 2004 Altered body image: appearance-related concerns of people with disfigurement. Journal of Advance Nursing 48:443–453

Sator P-G, Schmidt JB, Hönigsmann H 2002 Objective assessment of photoageing effects using high-frequency ultrasound on

PUVA-treated psoriasis patients. British Journal of Dermatology 147:291–298

Thomas S 2003 Atraumatic dressings. World Wide Wounds. Available online: www.worldwidewounds.com/2003/january/Thomas/Atraumatic-Dressings.html (accessed 1 February 2008)

Tortora GJ, Grabowski SR 2003 Principles of anatomy and physiology, 10th edn. John Wiley, Chichester

UK Central Council 1992 The scope of professional practice. UK Central Council, London

UK Central Council 1994 Standards for specialist education and practice. UK Central Council, London

Vermeulen H, Ubbink D, Schreuder S, Lubbers M 2006 Inter-and intra-observer (dis)agreement among physicians and nurse: choice of dressings in surgical patients with open wounds. Wounds 18:286–293

Vowden K, Vowden P 2003 Understanding exudate management and the role of exudate in the healing process. British Journal of Nursing 12(20)(Suppl.):4–13

Waterlow J 2005 Pressure ulcer risk assessment and prevention: understanding the causes. Available online: www.judy-waterlow.co.uk/ (accessed 1 February 2008)

Westaby S (ed) 1985 Wound care. Heinemann, London

World Union of Wound Healing Societies 2007 Wound exudate and the role of dressings: a consensus document. Available online: http://www.wuwhs.org/datas/2_1/4/consensus_exudate_ENG_FINAL.pdf (accessed 1 February 2008)

Chapter 16

Sexuality

Steve Eastburn

INTRODUCTION

Sexuality is an essential element of people's lives and health. This chapter explores the nature of sexuality and how nurses can incorporate it in their day-to-day work. Nursing theory has acknowledged the significance of human sexuality, but it is an aspect of practice that some nurses have great difficulty with. This is probably due to two factors:

- firstly, sexuality is not easy to define
- secondly, it includes aspects of people's lives that usually remain private.

Sexuality is a delicate subject, surrounded by mystery and misunderstandings, and consequently can be avoided by nurses and clients. The aim of this chapter therefore is to explore the meanings of sexuality and identify its relevance for nursing practice.

OVERVIEW

Subject knowledge

The chapter begins by exploring definitions and meanings of sexuality. It includes an overview of the historical context and identifies some of the problems associated with understanding images of sexuality in the past. Masculinity, femininity and gender roles are then addressed, leading into an outline of the processes involved in the development of an individual's sexuality. This includes information on the male and female reproductive systems and the biological control of human sexual development and the human sexual response. It also includes psychosocial theory related to the development of sexual identity and gender roles.

Following this is an overview of sexual norms and a summary of key research on sexual behaviour in Britain. This ends with a consideration of the relationship between emotion and sexual behaviour.

Care delivery knowledge

Care delivery knowledge begins with an outline of sexuality as an aspect of nursing models and moves on to discuss the assessment of an individual's sexual health and sexuality related problems. It includes guidance on how to discuss sensitive issues with clients. To conclude this section, types of sexuality related problems are identified with appropriate nursing actions.

Professional and ethical knowledge

This section discusses the importance of nursing as a mainly female profession and identifies issues specific to the four branches of nursing. It includes an overview of legal issues and health policy related to sexuality.

Personal and reflective knowledge

This section comprises four case studies (p. 383), one for each branch of nursing. The case studies help to raise important issues for clinical practice and there are a number of questions to stimulate debate. You may like to read one of these before beginning this chapter, to use as a focus for reflection. After the case studies there are a number of exercises to help you develop your personal portfolio. The exercises encourage you to reflect on and learn from practice.

SUBJECT KNOWLEDGE

DEFINING SEXUALITY

Defining sexuality is not easy. Sexuality is a social construct, and open to change and interpretation. Consequently, complete and accurate definitions cannot exist as they are moulded by cultural norms. However, most address the following issues:

- sex
- sexual orientation
- gender and associated roles
- relationships
- self-image
- self-esteem
- human attraction
- love.

To understand sexuality it is essential to take into account its changing nature and the social and historical forces that shape it. Indeed, the World Health Organization (2002) offers the following as a working definition

Sexuality is a central aspect of being human throughout life and encompasses sex, gender identities and roles, sexual orientation, eroticism, pleasure, intimacy and reproduction. Sexuality is experienced and expressed in thoughts, fantasies, desires, beliefs, attitudes, values, behaviours, practices, roles and relationships. While sexuality can include all of these dimensions, not all of them are always experienced or expressed. Sexuality is influenced by the interaction of biological, psychological, social, economic, political, cultural, ethical, legal, historical, religious and spiritual factors.

(http://www.who.int/reproductive-health/gender/ sexual_health.html#2)

Note how the last part of this definition emphasizes the varying nature of sexuality and how the society in which we live has a massive impact on how sexuality is expressed.

Studies on the history of sexuality emphasize how people's attitudes and behaviour have changed (Foucault 1979). They are difficult to appreciate though, as comparisons of sexuality throughout the ages are based on today's norms. For example, a popular image of Roman life emphasizes overindulgence, particularly in sexual activity. Victorian times on the other hand are characterized by a repressed attitude towards sexuality, surrounded by taboos, and managed through strict social etiquette. More recently, possibly associated with the availability of effective contraception, the 1960s become notorious for 'free love' and liberated youth.

Although there may be some truth in these stereotypes they are generalizations and focus on sexual activity rather than a broader understanding of sexuality. In turn, they have inherent dangers. First, they may be inaccurate due to the passage of time and the tendency for some ideas to achieve mythological status. Secondly, they focus on certain social classes in history and ignore the behaviour and attitudes of most of the population. Finally there is an assumption that a person's sexuality develops during his or her 'formative' years and remains stable.

Focusing on recent history, understanding of sexuality based on stereotypes can influence the way we view older people. For example the 1930s and 1940s conjure up images of marriage for life, sexual faithfulness in the nuclear family, and sex as a taboo subject. Although more myth than reality, these images can influence the way a nurse cares for an older patient by making assumptions that people born in the 1930s and 40s acquired these norms and values, and even if they did, that they still hold the same norms and values today. Using these assumptions to guide practice then, a nurse may then not consider safer sex an appropriate topic to discuss with a 75-year-old person.

An important development in the recent history of sexuality though is the increasing acceptance of sexual activity as a valid topic for scientific study. This reflects more openness in society and the need to focus attention on human immunodeficiency virus (HIV) and acquired immune deficiency syndrome (AIDS).

MASCULINITY AND FEMININITY

Sexuality is a broad term reflecting what people do, say and feel, and particularly the way they interact. An accepted way of interpreting sexuality is by understanding masculinity and femininity, and the associated roles.

Descriptions of masculinity and femininity are associated with stereotypical images of males and females. These can be seen in films, cartoons and popular magazines and although they can be the butt of jokes, they can also be ideals or sources of aspiration. It could be argued that these stereotypes are outdated and that being masculine today encompasses the more feminine *caring* characteristics of the so-called 'new man' (although it could also be argued that the 'new man' is a myth and traditional gender differences and inequalities still exist). Similarly, the experience of being a woman has changed as many women take on paid employment, altering the traditional family life (Giddens 2005). Whatever the case, images of masculinity and femininity influence people in their day-to-day lives through their choice of jobs, the clothes they wear and the types of interests they develop.

Gender roles

The distinction between men's and women's roles in society can often be seen by the type of employment they take, and the social pressures influencing the decisions around their selection. From an early age children have ideas about what they would like to be when they 'grow up'. With responses like 'I want to be a train driver' or 'I want to be a nurse' you can guess with some confidence the gender of the child. Although children's aspirations differ from one society to the next, and from one generation to the other, boys' views of their future will clearly contrast with those of girls. Of course these childhood wishes are unlikely to come true for many, but nevertheless, adult roles are largely gender-specific and comply with general expectations. There are, of course, exceptions; but being exceptions, they tend to re-inforce the rule. For example, a female bricklayer and a male secretary will probably be seen as unusual, and may even acquire local celebrity status.

Gender role differences are also evident in leisure interests, household tasks and the relationships and interactions within a family. This can lead to gender associated disadvantage and in the 1970s Gove & Tudor (1972) found that marriage affected men's health more positively than women's (married men were healthier than single men whereas married women were less healthy than single women). Family structures, the nature of marriages and partnerships and employment patterns have changed significantly since the early 1970s though and evidence on the links between marital status and health is now less clear (Arber 1997).

Gender associated roles, particularly those arising from paid employment and within a family, enable people to express their sexuality to those around them and develop a positive self-image. Sometimes these roles are associated with immense pressures though, leading to role strain; i.e. the individual finds it difficult to wear too many hats. This is associated with role conflict which occurs when the demands arising from different roles become incompatible. For example, a woman can be a mother and be expected to make decisions regarding her children. She can also be a daughter and be expected to take advice from and listen to the wisdom of her parents. Such pressures can make the fulfilment of these roles difficult or impossible at times.

Reflection and portfolio evidence

Make a list of the different roles you currently take.

- Are there any competing pressures between these roles?
- How might these roles change in the future?
- What would happen if you suddenly had a big, unexpected demand from one of your role obligations?
- Devise a plan to balance between your obligations for each role with your available resources.

(You might find the time planning exercise in Ch. 9 on relaxation and stress useful here.)

DEVELOPMENT OF AN INDIVIDUAL'S SEXUALITY

The reproductive system

For the first few weeks after fertilization the embryonic internal and external genitalia for males and females are the same. At about the seventh week hormonal changes lead to sex differentiation and the male reproductive system develops under the influence of increased androgen levels.

In childhood, the greatest time of physical change related to sexuality occurs during puberty. These are controlled hormonally and in Western society the process usually begins at around 11–12 years of age for girls and 12–13 years of age for boys. It involves the development of fully functioning reproductive systems and the body changes that result in the characteristic adult male and female physiques (Fig. 16.1).

Adult male reproductive system (Fig. 16.2)

Testes

The testes have two functions:

- production of sperm
- secretion of testosterone.

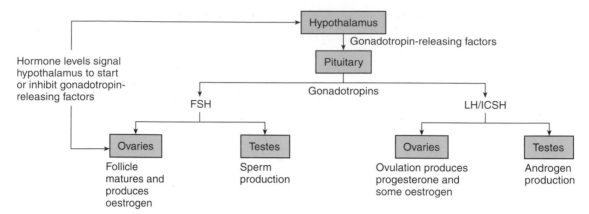

Figure 16.1 Hormonal control of sexual development. FSH, follicle-stimulating hormone; ICSH, interstitial-cell-stimulating hormone; LH, luteinizing hormone (after Offir 1982).

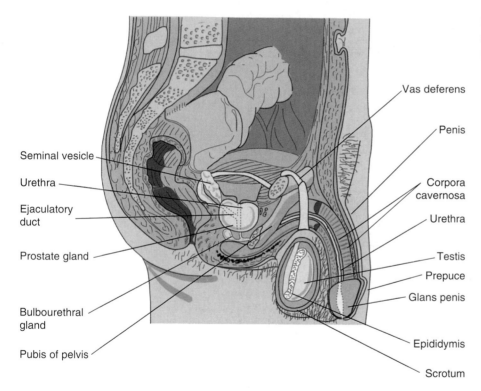

Figure 16.2 Anatomy of the male reproductive system (from Montague et al 2005, with kind permission of Elsevier).

The testes are made up of a fine network of convoluted seminiferous tubules. Under the influence of hormones, including testosterone and follicle-stimulating hormone, stem cells in the convoluted seminiferous tubules undergo a series of changes which results in the production of spermatozoa. These pass into the epididymis to mature before ejaculation. During ejaculation the sperm pass out of the tail of the epididymis into the vas deferens and ejaculatory duct where they mix with a fluid containing chemicals and nutrients secreted in the seminal vesicle, prostate gland and bulbourethral gland. This mixture is called semen

and its purpose is to allow the sperm to survive and move along the female reproductive tract.

Testosterone is a hormone secreted by the testes and is needed for spermatogenesis and the sex drive. It is also responsible for the development of the following male secondary sex characteristics:

- enlargement of the penis and testes
- enlargement of the larynx producing a deeper voice
- growth of facial hair and pubic hair
- increased sebaceous gland activity
- muscle development.

Penis

The penis contains three cylindrical masses of erectile tissue: two corpora cavernosa running along the top and sides, and a smaller corpus cavernosum on the underside, which contains the urethra. The glans penis at the end of the shaft of the penis is normally covered by a fold of skin, the prepuce or foreskin, which is sometimes removed surgically (circumcision). During sexual arousal the erectile tissue fills with blood and the penis enlarges and becomes firm.

Adult female reproductive system

Internal genitalia

The ovaries (Fig. 16.3) have two functions:

- production of ova
- secretion of progesterone and oestrogen.

Each ovary contains many oocytes. These are the cells that undergo a series of changes to develop into mature graafian follicles. Ovulation occurs when a follicle ruptures and releases an oocyte into the fallopian tube. This happens once a month during the menstrual cycle.

The hormone progesterone 'prepares' the woman's body for pregnancy. It increases the growth of the endometrium and breasts and influences cervical mucus production and uterine muscle activity. The hormone oestrogen influences oogenesis and follicle maturation, the onset of puberty and the development of female secondary sex characteristics, and the growth and maintenance of reproductive organs. Female secondary sex characteristics include:

- growth and development of breasts
- body hair, e.g. pubic hair
- changes in fat distribution to produce the female physique
- vaginal secretions.

The fallopian tubes extend from the uterus towards the ovaries and open into the peritoneal cavity with funnel-like projections. In reproduction, the oocyte moves into the first part of the fallopian tube and is fertilized in the ampulla partway along its length. Peristalsis and ciliated cells help the oocyte move to the uterus, which is a hollow, thick-walled muscular structure that assists in the implantation of the embryo, nurtures the developing foetus and moves the baby out through the vagina at birth.

The epithelial layer is the endometrium and this changes in thickness and structure, under hormonal control, during the menstrual cycle. The cervix is at the lower end of the uterus.

The vagina connects the cervix to the external genitalia. It expands during childbirth and intercourse and has an acidic environment to protect it from pathogenic organisms. It becomes lubricated during sexual arousal with secretions from the vestibular glands and the vaginal walls. The distal end of the vaginal orifice is partially occluded by the hymen, which usually ruptures during first intercourse, but it can also be ruptured by tampons or exercise.

External genitalia (Fig. 16.4)

The mons pubis is a fatty pad over the pubic bone. The labia majora are covered in skin and have many sebaceous glands and the labia minora meet at the anterior end at the

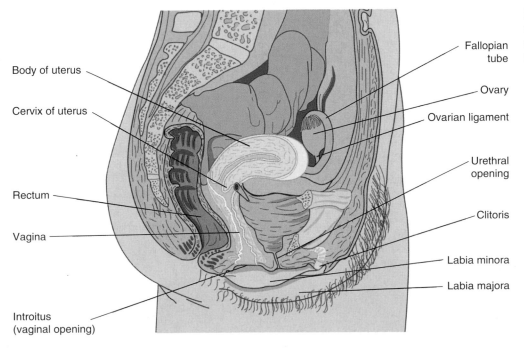

Figure 16.3 Anatomy of the female reproductive system (from Montague et al 2005, with kind permission of Elsevier).

Body of uterus

Cervix of uterus

Rectum

Vagina

Introitus (vaginal opening)

Fallopian tube

Ovary

Ovarian ligament

Urethral opening

Clitoris

Labia minora

Labia majora

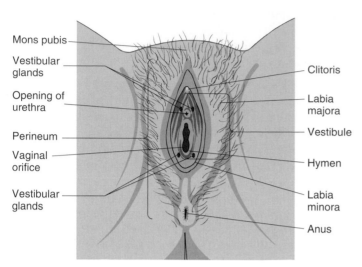

Figure 16.4 The female external genitalia (from Montague et al 2005, with kind permission of Elsevier).

clitoris. The clitoris is rich in nerve endings and plays an important part in the sexual response. The vestibular glands secrete a fluid which lubricates the vagina during sexual arousal.

The menstrual cycle

This is controlled by the level of circulating hormones (oestrogen, progesterone, follicle stimulating hormone and luteinizing hormone) but can also be influenced by emotional factors. It has three phases:

1. The proliferative phase: oestrogen causes cell proliferation in the uterus, the endometrium thickens and the cervical mucus becomes thinner and more profuse, which ends with ovulation.
2. The secretory phase: vascularity of the endometrium increases under the influence of progesterone and the cervical mucus thickens to block the cervical canal. Hormonal secretion from the corpus luteum declines if fertilization does not take place and the endometrium begins to degenerate.
3. The menstrual phase: the flow of blood and endometrial tissue, which lasts 3–6 days. Prostaglandins stimulate the uterus to contract and this causes the characteristic pain (dysmenorrhoea).

Premenstrual syndrome

Before the menstrual phase some women experience a range of symptoms. Pelvic congestion and overall body water retention can give a feeling of distension. Tiredness, irritability, depression and loss of concentration are common and the increase in body weight alongside these symptoms can initiate changes in body image and low self-esteem. The

reasons for these symptoms are unclear. Some theories suggest fluid retention is the cause, others that a deficiency of vitamin B_6, resulting from hormonal variations, affects brain functioning leading to mood changes.

The intensity of the premenstrual syndrome varies from individual to individual, but does not seem to be linked to the degree of hormonal change. Also, the significance and character of premenstrual changes have varied throughout history. This suggests that the premenstrual syndrome is influenced by social, psychological as well as biological factors (Obermeyer 2000).

Menopause

Some changes in the sexual response for women are associated with the menopause. Usually occurring between the ages of 45 and 55, it is the time when the ovaries cease to function and a woman's reproductive life ends. The reduced levels of oestrogen and progesterone are associated with a range of symptoms such as sweating, hot flushes, insomnia, depression, fatigue and headaches. Evidence to attribute these symptoms solely to hormonal changes is inconclusive though (Obermeyer 2000), as coming to terms with the end of a reproductive life plus other stressful life events commonly experienced at this age might also contribute. It is important to stress that the hormonal changes occurring during the menopause do not directly affect a woman's interest in sex. Oestrogen levels do not control sex drive nor do they affect a woman's ability to enjoy sex or have orgasms.

The 'mid-life crisis' in men

Men at this time of life often experience a slow decline in testosterone production. This results in less firm erections, less frequent ejaculations and a longer refractory period (see below). Men can also experience social and psychological pressures leading to a 'mid-life crisis' (Lachman 2004). However, in the same way that it is difficult to attribute menopause purely to biological factors, any changes in a man's sexual activity at this time of life cannot always be associated with decreasing androgen levels.

THE SEXUAL RESPONSE

The sexual response in men and women is controlled by complex interactions between the central nervous system, the peripheral nervous system, neurotransmitters, hormones and the circulatory system (Engenderhealth 2005). It has five stages:

1. Desire. We can respond to a variety of stimuli, including sight, sound, smell, touch and taste. Based on thoughts, feelings, and experiences, these create sexual desire.

2. Arousal. In men this results in penile erection, testicular elevation and flattening of the scrotal skin. In women it results in vaginal lubrication, clitoral enlargement, upper vaginal dilation, vaginal constriction of the lower third, uterine elevation and breast and nipple enlargement.
3. Plateau. In men this is associated with an increase in secretions from the urethral Cowper's glands and an increase in blood pressure, heart rate, respiratory rate and muscle tone. In women it is associated with retraction of the clitoris against the pubic bone and increases in blood pressure, heart rate, respiratory rate and muscle tone.
4. Orgasm. In men this is a rhythmical contraction of the perineal muscles, closure of the bladder neck and ejaculation. In women orgasm may be single or multiple and involves contractions of the perineal muscles, uterus and fallopian tubes. It is more common for women not to experience orgasm every time they engage in sexual activity than it is for men.
5. Resolution. This is when the physiological changes are reversed. There is also a refractory period, which is the resting time that must elapse before the next sexual response can be initiated (Masters & Johnson 1966).

The impact of age-related physiological changes on the sexual response

For men

Men may experience the following age-related changes:

- Arousal: erections may occur less frequently and more and longer direct stimulation of the penis is required to establish and maintain an erection.
- Plateau: may be prolonged and ejaculation more easily controlled.
- Orgasm: the number and force of contractions decrease, but the sensation may be equally satisfying.
- Resolution: the length of time between orgasm and the next possible erection increases.

For women

Reduced oestrogen levels result in thinning of the vaginal mucosa, replacement of breast tissue by fat and shrinking of the uterus. These may affect the sexual response in older women as follows:

- Arousal: longer direct clitoral stimulation may be required, the vaginal opening expands less and vaginal lubrication may be reduced to the extent that synthetic lubrication may be required.
- Plateau: sensation may alter due to a decrease in vasocongestion and a reduced tensing of the vagina.

- Orgasm: contractions may be fewer.
- Resolution: the clitoris loses its erection more rapidly, but the refractory period after orgasm does not seem to lengthen for women as it does for men.

Decision-making exercise

From the information on the effects of ageing on the sexual response:

- Can you see any physiological reasons why sexual activity might have to stop for older people?
- Can you see any physiological reasons why older people might not enjoy sexual activity?
- What implications do your answers have for nurses working with older people?

SEXUAL IDENTITY

A number of sociologists and psychologists have attempted to explain how people develop a sexual identity. There is agreement among many that relationships and interactions with those close to us play an important part. Others emphasize the biological factors and believe that our genetic make-up determines our sexual identity. The key theories are outlined below.

Freud's psychoanalytical theory

Freud's (1923) psychoanalytical theory offered an explanation of why boys and girls grow up differently, and it has since been developed by many psychologists. Freud focused on five stages of development. At each stage he identified the way in which individuals learn to balance the satisfaction of the 'libidinal' or pleasure drive of Id against those of the restrictive Ego and Superego.

Oral stage: 0–18 months of age

Newborn infants are unable to do little more than suck and drink and this satisfies the libidinal drive. During this stage of life only Id is present in the personality. Superego and Ego have not yet developed. Consequently the infant becomes frustrated if his demands are not met immediately.

Anal stage: 18 months to 3 years of age

During this period restrictions are placed upon the child; nourishment is no longer available on demand and potty training begins. This frustrates Id and results in temper tantrums. Eventually, Ego develops and the child exerts control over Id by using the potty. It is at this time that the libidinal drive passes to the anus and the child finds control of bowel movements pleasurable, both by expelling the contents and by retaining them.

Phallic stage: 3–5 years of age

During the first two stages of development the infant is unaware of gender differences. All children are seen as 'little males'. However, during the phallic stage the child becomes aware of its gender and discovers pleasure can be derived from either the penis or clitoris. The libidinal drive then focuses on this body area as the child derives satisfaction from playing with its sexual organ.

During this phase the child forms an incestuous desire for the parent of the opposite sex. In the male child this is called the Oedipus complex. Here the boy's love for his mother becomes very intense making him very jealous of anyone competing for her attention, including his father. However, he has noticed that girls and his mother do not have a penis. He suspects this is because they were castrated as a punishment when they were younger and he fears that if he continues the feelings he has for his mother then his father will castrate him also. To protect his penis he represses his feelings for his mother and identifies with his father. This way he retains both his penis and, by identifying with his father, he fulfils the desire for his mother.

In the female child a different process, the Electra complex, occurs. Initially the she is drawn towards her mother. She discovers, however, that unlike her father and boys, she does not possess a penis. She assumes she has been castrated, for which she blames her mother, and feels inferior to males, a phenomenon called 'penis envy'. Realizing she will not get a replacement penis, she replaces this desire with one for a baby, and she looks to her father to provide her with one. This brings problems though, as she will be in direct competition with her mother who she fears will reject her. To prevent this she internalizes the image of her mother as carer, so that her mother will continue to love her. This is the final part of the Electra complex, where the girl identifies again with her mother, and is called anaclytic identification.

The phallic stage is a very ambivalent time for a child of either gender and parental attitudes during this stage have profound ramifications on the child's development.

Latency stage: 5 years of age to puberty

Following the traumas of the phallic stage, this period is relatively quiet. Sexual interests are replaced by school, playtimes, sports and a range of new activities. The child also meets people from outside the family and makes new relationships.

Genital stage: puberty to adulthood

With the onset of puberty the individual experiences intense libidinal drives to engage in full sexual activity. The capacity for full physiological sexual responses has developed by this stage and in turn, individuals are able to experience themselves as complete sexual beings. At this stage boys lose their sexual attachment for their mother, and girls for their father, allowing them to make other sexual attachments. However, during this stage, the individual has to learn to express sexual energy in socially acceptable ways.

Despite criticisms, Freud's theory highlights the importance of relationships and interactions between children and the adults around them. The nature and quality of relationships during these formative years are significant in the development of an individual's sexuality. In certain settings nurses will work with people who have problems with their identity. An identity crisis in a patient, in particular in their sense of sexuality, is likely to have its origins in childhood development, and advanced nursing practice may involve exploration of an individual's relationships with their parents.

Neoanalytical theory

Some writers modified Freud's ideas, basing their explanations of gender identity on other experiences in early childhood. Chodorow (1992) emphasizes the importance of the early maternal bond that exists in all societies. Girls never completely break this bond and their identity incorporates a significant relational element. Boys on the other hand have to break this bond in order to develop a masculine identity characterized by independence, individuality and a rejection of the feminine. As a result, women require a close relationship in order to maintain their self-esteem, but men feel threatened by such close emotional attachments.

Chodorow's theory assumes a simplistic role of women as the main carer of children, especially in the early years, and has been criticized for failing to take into account other feelings, for example aggression and assertiveness. On the other hand it helps to make sense of some men's apparent inability to express their emotions.

Sociobiological theories

Sociobiologists use ideas from evolutionary biology to explain human behaviour and sexual identity. Birkhead (2000) argues sexual behaviour is influenced by the biological need to reproduce. People strive to be successful in reproduction so genetic information can be passed on to the next generation. Men have many sperm so it makes sense for men to use as many as they can. This has been given as an explanation for men being more promiscuous than women. On the other hand, women have relatively few ova, and their owners need to make sure that they are used carefully. It is in the interests of women therefore to be selective as to whom they choose as a mate. They need to make sure that their genes are amalgamated with others of a high quality.

This theory has implications for attitude development. Men should approve of casual sex and have many partners, whereas women should be less approving of casual sex and seek long-term commitment from few partners. Related to this is the explanation of men's jealousy and desire to control women's sexuality. Because a man provides for the mother and child he needs to make sure that he is rearing his own offspring and not someone else's. For this reason men would disapprove of their wives engaging in extramarital sex.

This sociobiological theory has its critics. Birkhead (2000) suggests that society is more complex than the picture painted here and sexual behaviour is more than purely reproductive. For example, the theory does not take into account the nature of sex and sexuality throughout an individual's lifespan. Also it attempts to legitimize inequalities between men and women by suggesting they are natural and normal; failing to explore the importance of socialization and the use of power in establishing and maintaining gender inequalities.

Social learning theory

This is concerned with how boys and girls learn their gender-related roles (Connell 2002). It does not see biology as particularly important in determining behaviour, but emphasizes the associations and interactions between children and others. This is, in the first place, the communication that takes place with parents. Behaviour consistent with gender is reinforced through rewards. So when parents and others react in a positive way towards a girl in a pretty dress playing with dolls and an urchin of a boy climbing trees, this behaviour is likely to be repeated.

Children learn their behaviour from significant role models, and these include parents, siblings, teachers and people in the media. This means that learning how to behave as a woman or a man is only partly influenced by parental upbringing. It is the influence of people and images from outside the family that explains why children differ from their parents. This theory is dynamic and takes account of an individual's changing nature and incorporates such things as trends and fashions. However, it tends to see people waiting to be moulded by the environment and those around them. In this sense, self-will, motivation and the ability to manipulate the environment are ignored.

Social learning theory attempts to explain how culture is learned; that is how individuals acquire certain patterns of beliefs, values, attitudes and norms. In turn, culture has a strong impact on sexuality and, of course, different cultures assign different meanings to sexuality. Some cultures emphasize equality between partners, including goals of mutual pleasure and psychological disclosure. Others believe that the exchange of pleasure, or communication of affection through sexual touching, plays no major role in the expression of sexuality (Monga & Lefebvre 1995). Some cultures permit premarital sex, while others condemn it. Culturally determined formal rituals can also play an important part in the development of a sexual identity, for example the circumcision of boys. Nurses therefore need an understanding of cultural differences so that they can give culture-specific care; within the bounds of what is legally and ethically acceptable (Jeffreys 2006).

NORMS

By learning from others and society, we acquire an understanding of what is 'normal'. However, this process may lead to prejudicial attitudes towards individuals or groups. Norms are socially acceptable behaviours that help to define what is 'right' in society. Nevertheless, society is made up of a number of sub-groups which may have different norms of sexual behaviour, and these are a potential source of conflict. For example the norms of sexual behaviour held by the youth culture could be very different from those held by parents or by professionals. There is a possibility that parents, teachers, doctors and nurses will see their own 'standards' as right and begin to impose them on those who they feel they are responsible for. For nurses working in the area of sexual health promotion with teenagers this creates an ethical problem. Should they try and persuade young teenagers not to have sex or should they accept this as a fact and offer advice on safer sex? The former might frighten the teenager off and prevent them using services or seeking help. The latter might expose the teenager to a range of physical and psychological risks.

There are also inequalities in the way that norms are applied to groups within society. Certain behaviours may be viewed as acceptable for men but not for women, or acceptable for adults but not for teenagers. Similarly attitudes towards a stable heterosexual couple may differ from that towards a stable homosexual couple.

Homosexuality

The idea of an open homosexual identity, where people attracted to others of the same gender have their own culture and lifestyle, is a relatively new phenomenon. Gay bars, newspapers, associations and holidays have not existed overtly for very long.

In the past, individuals were not labelled with a sexual identity that described them as either heterosexual or homosexual. In Roman times, for example, it formed part of a range of experiences for some people. In modern times, this may also be seen in people who have relationships with either gender or, occurring as a result of a situation, i.e. those in single-sex restrictive institutions such as prisons, monastic orders and boarding schools.

Bancroft (1989) describes the development of a gay culture through history, noting varying periods of acceptance and repression of homosexual activity. In the recent history of developed countries homosexuality has been characterized by rejection though. This was seen in public attitudes and inequalities within the legal frameworks of many countries. Minority groups are used as scapegoats for things going wrong in society, and commonly homosexuals have been perceived as a minority group responsible for many ills within society, from the downfall of the Greek empire to the spread of the HIV virus.

Hostility towards homosexuality may be denial that a mixed sexual identity can exist. Arguments based on the 'laws of nature' that are frequently used to justify this stance (i.e. 'Our bodies are not made for it') assume sexual activity is used solely for procreation; where homosexuality has no function. However, acceptance of this argument also excludes all non-procreational heterosexual activity.

The medical profession in the 19th century gave a different interpretation of homosexuality: a sickness for which treatments were developed. Although during the 20th century medicine's attitude towards homosexuality softened, the idea that it was something to treat remained and it was not until 1974 that the American Psychiatric Association removed homosexuality from its list of pathological diagnoses.

Female homosexuality is written about less frequently and has had a lower profile throughout history. This does not mean that women are less likely than men to be involved in homosexual activity, but is probably a reflection of the domination of women by men across a range of social institutions.

See the Evolve 16.1 web resource for a reflective exercise on sexual equality and a useful web link.

16.1 – EQUALITY

- Know the law as it relates to sexual equality.
- Reflect on the implications of equality in your practice.

SEXUAL BEHAVIOUR

Because of its sensitive nature, investigating sexual behaviour has been particularly challenging for researchers. For example, the National Survey on Sexual Behaviour in Britain (Wellings et al 1994) had a difficult start because the Department of Health withdrew its backing at the last minute and researchers had to find alternative support. The impetus for the work came from the need to find out more about the relationship between sexual practices and the spread of HIV and AIDS, but the political sensitivity of the subject meant that the researchers had problems in starting. This is very similar to the experiences of Kinsey in the USA (Kinsey et al 1948) and Lanval (1950) in Belgium, who both suffered in their attempts to discover more about sexual behaviour. Their research was condemned as pornographic and unworthy of academic attention. Despite these problems Kinsey persisted, and interviewed over 10 000 people on what sexual practices were common. It was apparent from the findings that the incidence of homosexuality, masturbation and premarital intercourse, and the active role of women in sexuality, differed from the social norms of the time, and this caused considerable political disquiet (Gagnon & Simon 2005).

Returning to Wellings et al (1994), who published one of the most extensive studies on sexual behaviour in Britain: as it focused on how the spread of HIV might be related to certain sexual practices it concentrated on issues like unprotected sex, numbers of partners and types of activities involving risks, although because of its quantitative nature it tells little about the meaning of sexual experiences to individuals. It does, however, give details of who does what with whom, at what age and how often, and relates these sorts of things to class and educational level. One major drawbacks was its failure to include people over 60 years of age. This perhaps reflects the commonly held view that 'older people don't do that sort of thing'.

See Evolve 16.2 for more information on this research.

16.2 – SEXUAL BEHAVIOUR

- Outline the findings of Wellings et al (1994) on sexual behaviour.
- Discuss contemporary heterosexual behaviour.
- Discuss contemporary homosexual behaviour.
- Understand sexual behaviour from a global perspective.

Evidence-based practice

A similar survey was carried out in the UK to try and help understand the trends in the incidence of sexually transmitted infections and teenage pregnancies. *The National Survey of Sexual Attitudes and Lifestyles* took place between 1999 and 2001 and was reported in three articles in *The Lancet* (Johnson et al 2001).

A sample of 4762 men and 6399 women aged between 16 and 44 were interviewed. The following is a selection of the findings:

- In the last 5 years the mean number of heterosexual partners was 3.8 for men and 2.4 for women.
- 4.3% of men reported paying for sex.
- 2.6% of respondents reported homosexual partnerships.
- Condom use has increased since 1990.
- There has been an increase in the number of sexual partners since 1990.
- The proportion of women reporting first intercourse before the age of 16 increased up to the mid-1990s and has now levelled off.
- A small minority of teenagers have unprotected first intercourse.
- Early motherhood is more strongly associated with educational level than family background.

Though similar to Wellings et al (1994), the National Survey of Sexual Attitudes and Lifestyles (Johnson et al 2001) was limited by only including people between 16 and 44. This excluded a small group of young teenagers and a very large group of people aged 45 and above. (See Evolve 16.3 material for more detailed findings.)

16.3 – SEXUAL BEHAVIOUR IN BRITAIN

- Outline the National Survey of Sexual Attitudes and Lifestyles (Johnson et al 2001).
- Compare the findings of Johnson et al (2001) with those of Wellings et al (1994).

Surveys on sexual behaviour are fraught with problems because of the sensitive nature of the topic. Findings from such surveys must be treated with caution because their accuracy and reliability may be influenced by individuals' honesty and openness in their responses. Nevertheless, this kind of research provides important information.

EMOTIONS AND SEXUAL ACTIVITY

Hart & Wellings (2002) believe that many medically oriented studies into sexual behaviour do not provide insight into the social and psychological factors involved. For example what is it that makes certain phenomena sexually arousing to some people but not to others, and how are desires and attractions explained?

The human sexual response is extremely complex. Emotions are central to these experiences and influence, and can be influenced by physical aspects of sexual activity. This is the psychosomatic circle of sex (Bancroft 2002).

Emotion can also have a negative effect on sexual performance, commonly shown by anxiety, which influences sexual responses through a number of mechanisms:

1. It excites the peripheral autonomic nervous system controlling physiological changes associated with sex. This affects the vasocongestion of genitals and orgasm, preventing these from occurring, slowing them down or speeding them up.
2. It can disrupt erotic stimuli. This is equivalent to having something on your mind, making it difficult to concentrate on anything else.
3. Anxiety and the sexual response become associated through past experiences, and the individual may subconsciously inhibit sexual responses to avoid anxiety, thereby reinforcing the initial anxiety.

Bancroft et al (2003) also investigated the relationship between mood and sexuality and found around 40% of people with depression experience a decreased sexual appetite. What is not easy to determine is the role sexual dysfunction has in creating depression in the first place (Werneke et al 2006). Also sexual problems and depression may be related to other underlying causes, for example biochemical or hormonal changes.

Decision-making exercise

List common life events for men and for women between the ages of 45 and 55.
How might these events affect people's intimate relationships with those close to them?
(The Evolve resource may prove helpful here.)

CARE DELIVERY KNOWLEDGE

This section focuses on the inclusion of sexuality in nursing models, communication issues as part of the assessment process, types of sexuality problems and frameworks for nursing actions.

NURSING THEORY

Some theorists explored the nature of health and nursing, and identified kinds of problems people experience that require nursing assistance. For example, Roper et al (2000) focus on the activities of living. Within this model 'expressing sexuality' is seen as an important activity that should be considered by nurses in all settings. This activity of living includes sexual activity, gender identity and relationship issues and the nurse's role is to help people express their sexuality despite the impact of their health condition. A useful application of these ideas, including a sections on expressing sexuality, can be found in Holland et al (2003).

Orem's (2001) model has self-care as its central concept to meet a range of needs that occur throughout life in both health and illness. One of the universal needs in this model is 'being normal' – a broad concept which includes reaching one's potential and living according to social norms and values. Although less specific than Roper et al (2000), Orem (2001) sees sexual activity and gender identity as important areas of concern for nurses because they are part of 'being normal'.

Other models of nursing are more process orientated and do not try to define the nature of human problems requiring help. They concentrate on the nature of the activity and what nurses do to help people. Peplau (1988), for example, focuses on the relationship between the nurse and the client. Using the client's perceptions, experiences and feelings, they identify clients' problems and consider methods of coping. This model therefore does not explicitly include sexuality as a relevant area of nursing concern. Implicit, though, is the importance of this aspect in people's lives and how there may be particular problems for some individuals.

ASSESSMENT OF SEXUALITY AND SEXUAL HEALTH

Reflection and portfolio evidence

During a clinical placement, make a point of looking at a written assessment of a client.

Use the definitions of sexual health above to help you answer the following questions:

- What aspects of sexual health/sexuality have been included in the written assessment?
- What aspects could have been included?
- How does the plan of care address any sexual health/ sexuality related issues?

DISCUSSING SEXUALITY WITH CLIENTS

Magnan et al (2006) found a high proportion of nurses believed it was their responsibility to give permission to clients to discuss problems related to sexual health by initiating these conversations. However, they also found that only a small proportion of nurses said they made time for this. In the care of older people in particular, sexual health issues were rarely addressed in nursing assessments (Bouman et al 2007). Despite nurses' reluctance there is evidence that clients want nurses to initiate such discussions (Higgins et al 2006); however, these findings suggest a dissonance between nurses' expressed beliefs and actions.

Attitudes and beliefs of health professionals can act as barriers to the discussion of sexual health issues. Gott et al (2004) found that healthcare professionals experienced particular difficulties discussing sexual health issues with patients of the opposite sex, patients from ethnic backgrounds different from their own, those who were older or who were homosexual. This suggests that nurses need to be aware of their own attitudes towards sexual health issues and how these attitudes might affect the way they see and care for patients.

Like many aspects of interpersonal activity there is no easy guide on how to manage conversations about sexuality. It has been argued that nurses face serious ethical issues by even considering that such conversations are theirs to be managed (Batcup & Thomas 1994). Take, for example, a client who has a health problem that the nurse feels could be seriously affecting his or her sexuality. If the client says nothing about the way he or she feels about him or herself, or does not admit to any such problem, does the nurse have a duty to dig deeper on the assumption that it may be the client's embarrassment that prevents him or her from telling the truth? If the nurse does this is the nurse in danger of setting the agenda and putting ideas into the client's mind? By asking specific questions the nurse can demonstrate to the client that it is legitimate to talk about issues related to sexuality or sexual activity. On the other hand, the questions could lead the client to consider aspects of life in detail, and begin to see 'new' problems. For example 'Does the pain affect your sex life?' implies that the client ought to have a sex life and suggests that a sex life might normally be affected by such pain. This type of question could lead the client along a line of discussion they had not previously considered. Sociologists have described this management of the conversation as a form of professional control, with the nurse exerting power over the client (Foucault 1973, Holmes & Byrne 2006).

Decision-making exercise

The questions that you ask during an assessment can contain implicit assumptions. Because of this, questions might be inappropriate or offensive to some patients.

Read the following statements and then answer the questions listed.

'I see from your records that your next of kin is your partner. Is she fit and well?'

'What method of contraception do you use?'

'Does the pain prevent you from having sexual intercourse?'

'Does this restlessness that you have at night in bed disturb your partner?'

- What are the possible assumptions in the questions?
- How might a client react if the assumptions are incorrect?
- How might this error of judgement affect your relationship with the client?

(See Evolve 16.4 for potential answers.)

16.4 – DISCUSSING SEXUALITY-RELATED ISSUES WITH PATIENTS

- Know how to discuss sexuality-related issues with patients.
- Be aware of assumptions nurses sometimes make in discussing sexuality with patients.

Language

One of the difficulties in conversations on delicate or sensitive subjects is deciphering the true meaning. Nurses sometimes need to take the lead and make sure that there is a mutual understanding. This involves exploration and clarification.

Reflection and portfolio evidence

Look at the following statements and identify the possible meanings for each.

'We no longer sleep together.'
'I can't stand her anywhere near me now.'
'I haven't had a relationship since it happened.'
'Since the operation I can't stand him to see my bits and pieces.'
'I'm not the man I used to be.'
'I got around a bit in my younger days.'
'The tablets have stopped me from getting it up.'

- Would you assume one particular meaning?
- How would you find out exactly what was meant?

Using the client's language and terminology may help the nurse and client feel at ease with some of these delicate subjects. However, there is still a danger that, despite using the same words, there is not a mutual understanding. The use of 'proper' or medical terms can also be misunderstood and can act as a barrier in the conversation. On the other hand, using slang or colloquial terms may be at odds with the perception of a professional nurse and can present as patronizing or condescending. The way to proceed is to be open with the client about the difficulties with terminology and to agree to use words you are comfortable with and ones that you both understand. Essential communication skills in assessing problems related to client's sexuality thus include:

- Using silence to allow the client to talk.
- Listening to what the client says and does not say, being aware of and sensitive to the way he or she expresses ideas, picking up clues and hints.

- Reflecting the client's ideas by repeating and paraphrasing their words.
- Clarifying the meaning behind statements, making sure that you both understand things in the same way.
- Interpreting the client's words to uncover the significance of events and explore the hidden feelings and meanings in the conversation.
- Focusing on certain topics as a way of encouraging and guiding clients to discuss areas of their concern.

Reflection and portfolio exercise

Some questions for initiating conversations on sexuality with clients might include:

- 'Has anything (e.g. a recent experience, illness, operation) affected your relationships with people close to you?'
- 'Tell me about your partnership/relationship/marriage.'
- 'How do you feel about yourself as a woman/man/ wife/ husband/ partner/mother/father?'
- 'Has your illness/operation/being in hospital changed the way you feel about yourself?'
- 'Has your illness/operation/being in hospital affected your sex life?'
- 'How are things between you and your partner?'
- 'Some of the tablets you are taking can affect aspects of your sex life. Have you noticed anything?'

In many areas, sexual behaviour and the risk of acquiring sexually transmitted infections will be the main focus of conversations. Knight (2004) gives some useful advice on how nurses can manage these situations.

- Explain to patients that it is essential to have a clear understanding of their sexual practices so that they can receive the best advice and support.
- Explain that the discussion is confidential.
- Negotiate with the patient what will be recorded in the patient notes.
- Avoid labelling terms such as 'gay', 'queer' and 'straight' unless the client introduces them.
- Do not make assumptions about sexual behaviour based on a patient's age, partnership status, disability or other characteristics.
- Ask specific questions about sexual behaviour in a direct and non-judgmental manner, for example:

  – Are you sexually active?
  – Do you have sex with men, women or both?
  – How many sexual partners do you have?
  – Do you use condoms for vaginal/anal intercourse?

POTENTIAL PROBLEMS RELATED TO CLIENTS' SEXUALITY

The way sexuality becomes part of an assessment depends upon the nature of the client's presenting health conditions. Sexuality can thus be an issue as:

- the client's primary reason for referral
- a problem secondary to another health condition
- a problem arising from difficulties coping with normal developmental changes.

Sexuality as a primary problem

Primary problems with sexuality include:

- difficulties with sexual activities or relationships
- unfulfilling sexual activity
- antisocial or inappropriate sexual behaviour
- fertility problems
- safer sex and contraceptive issues
- sexually transmitted infections.

These problems usually require the input of a specialist nurse. Sometimes, however, clients will raise these problems with generic nurses, for example practice nurses, health visitors or community psychiatric nurses, and it is therefore important to be aware of the specialist services available, e.g. sex therapists, psychosexual counsellors, fertility clinics and family planning clinics.

Sexuality problems secondary to other health conditions

Most nurses will encounter these types of problems as there are so many diseases, illnesses and health conditions that can affect an individual's sexuality. Because sexuality is a complex blend of physical, psychological and social factors, it is not always possible to identify a cause-and-effect relationship between illness and problem. For example a man with diabetes mellitus might have a low self-esteem. He might also have difficulties obtaining and maintaining an erection. It is difficult to judge just how the diabetes mellitus, the low self-esteem and the erectile dysfunction interrelate in terms of cause and effect. Physiological changes could cause the erectile dysfunction, which in turn could cause a low self-esteem. On the other hand the diagnosis of diabetes mellitus could induce feelings of poor self-worth, which in turn could generate erectile dysfunction. Table 16.1 lists the sexuality related problems that are sometimes associated with types of health conditions. The list is not exhaustive, but gives an indication of some of the problems to consider when working with clients.

Table 16.1 Sexuality related problems sometimes associated with certain types of health conditions

Type of health condition	Sexuality related problems
Musculoskeletal conditions	Sexual activity Body image Work and leisure activities Dressing and hygiene
Cardiovascular and respiratory conditions	Energy levels Breathing Body image Emotional state Male and female sexual response
Neurological conditions	Sensations Movement and coordination Male and female sexual response Libido
Endocrine and hormonal conditions	Body image Growth and development

Table 16.1—cont'd

Type of health condition	Sexuality related problems
	Libido Male and female sexual response Onset of puberty
Skin conditions	Body image Emotional state Sensations
Genitourinary conditions	Body image Choice of clothing Libido Male and female sexual response
Mental health problems	Body image Interpersonal relationships Libido Male and female sexual response Self-concept Work and leisure activities
Learning disabilities	Emotional state Relationship skills Self-concept Development of socially acceptable sexual behaviour Vulnerability to sexual abuse Work and leisure activities

Medications and sexual function

A number of medications have potential side-effects on sexual activity (Ford 2005) and some of these are listed in Table 16.2. Nurses assessing clients' problems need to be aware of these side-effects and provide this advice to clients to help them make fully informed decisions about the benefits and disadvantages of medications.

The list given in Table 16.2 is not exhaustive. It is possible that many clients taking prescribed medications experience side-effects that affect their sexuality and sexual activity. As well as this, alcohol and nicotine are known to contribute to erectile dysfunction. It is therefore important to find out about clients' medications and their use of leisure drugs.

Decision-making exercise

Think about a client with whom you have recently worked and who has been taking a range of prescribed medications. Identify the possible side-effects of these drugs on the patient's sexuality (you may wish to look in the current issue of the *British National Formulary* (British Medical Association and the Royal Pharmaceutical Society 2008) for this).

- Did the care staff know whether the patient was experiencing any of these side-effects?
- If not, why was this the case?
- Did the patient know about these possible side-effects?
- So that the patient could give proper consent to taking these medications, how much do you think he or she should have been told?

Table 16.2 Potential side-effects of medications on sexual activity

Type of medication	Drug	Side-effects on sexual activity
Diuretics (e.g. used for clients with heart failure)	Thiazides	Erectile dysfunction Decreased libido
	Spironolactone	Erectile dysfunction Decreased libido Gynaecomastia (enlargement of male breast)
Beta-blockers (e.g. used for clients with high blood pressure and clients with anxiety)		Erectile dysfunction
Sympatholytics (e.g. used for clients with high blood pressure)	Methyldopa	Erectile dysfunction Ejaculatory failure
	Prazosin	Erectile dysfunction Retrograde ejaculation in clients with benign prostatic enlargement
Antidepressants	Tricyclics and monoamine oxidase inhibitors	Erectile dysfunction Ejaculatory failure
Antipsychotics	Phenothiazines	Erectile dysfunction
Anxiolytics	Benzodiazepines	Erectile dysfunction
Cytotoxics		Amenorrhoea Decreased sperm count
Antihistamines		Decreased vaginal lubrication Erectile dysfunction
Glucocorticosteroids		Weight gain Changed fat distribution

Sexuality and normal developmental changes

People can experience difficulties in managing and coming to terms with normal developmental changes. Nurses have an important role in helping individuals to understand these changes and also in offering support and practical advice on how these changes can be managed. For example, issues such as menstruation, nocturnal emissions ('wet dreams'), masturbation, sexual relationships, safer sex, contraception, social roles and becoming an adult are surrounded by myth and taboo. By addressing these common phenomena, appropriately qualified school nurses can help children to understand the physical, psychological and social changes experienced during puberty and adolescence.

Other developmental changes require individuals to adapt and readjust. In many cases these changes have an impact on sexual identity and sexual activity. For example, the menopause can be associated with dryness of the vagina and women can experience problems coping with this physical change. Also around this time, children leave home and middle-aged adults might be involved in caring for ageing parents. As a result of decreasing androgen production in the late forties or early fifties, men experience less firm erections and an increased refractory period. At the same time men and women can be involved in important career decisions and planning retirement. These physical and social changes require psychological and behavioural adjustment. People having difficulties making the necessary adjustments can develop a low self-esteem and a negative body image. Again, these can have a direct impact on the quality of relationships, sexual identity and sexual activity.

NURSING ACTIONS

Clients present with a wide range of problems related to sexuality. Also, clients are individuals and their experiences of these problems will all be unique. Consequently, it is impossible to describe appropriate nursing actions in detail since a full assessment is required in order to plan care. Nevertheless there are guidelines to help nurses plan appropriate care. Annon (1974) describes levels of intervention using the P-LI-SS-IT model:

P – permission
LI – limited information
SS – specific suggestions
IT – intensive therapy.

Permission

This is when the nurse openly acknowledges to the client that sexuality is a legitimate issue for discussion. This means that the nurse must be seen to be willing to discuss sexuality, either by asking specific questions or by allowing and encouraging clients to raise the issue themselves. This says to the client that it is within the nurse's role to discuss sexuality and also that it is 'normal', usual and acceptable for clients to have concerns or problems related to their sexuality.

Limited information

This next stage requires the nurse to give explanations, facts or reasons about why the client might be having the sexuality problem. Obviously the nurse must have sufficient knowledge and experience to understand and interpret sexuality problems. Also this demands communication and teaching skills so that explanations can be understood and remembered. This level of intervention enables the client to make sense of the problems, and gives him or her the opportunity to consider ways of resolving or improving the situation. This stage might involve the nurse helping the client to correct any misconceptions or dispel any myths surrounding sexuality.

Specific suggestions

A client having difficulty resolving his or her own problems is likely to need specific guidance or advice. This means that the nurse must draw on research and previous experience to make practical, acceptable and realistic suggestions. The nurse must assess the client's abilities, knowledge and attitudes so that appropriate suggestions are made. Some suggestions could involve referral to other agencies. Therefore the nurse must be aware of the range of specialist services available, the nature of the services provided and the appropriate reasons for referral so that the client can decide how to proceed.

Intensive therapy

This level is usually beyond the skills of the generic nurse. Clients and partners can be involved in a programme of sessions to instruct, coach and demonstrate ways of overcoming the particular sexual problem. This could focus for example on relationship and communication difficulties between partners on alternative ways of 'pleasuring' or sexual expression between partners or on medical and surgical interventions to treat or improve the sexual response.

Taylor & Davis (2006) have developed Annon's original work into the 'EX – Plissit' model. This uses the same basic four stages of intervention but they emphasize the importance of permission giving as a core element of each of the stages. Also they suggest that nurses should continually reflect on their interactions with patients to help develop self awareness and challenge assumptions.

PROFESSIONAL AND ETHICAL KNOWLEDGE

This section examines the following aspects: nursing and gender, the medicalization of sexuality, information specific to the four branches of nursing, key legal issues related to nursing and clients' sexuality, and sexuality and health policy.

NURSING AND GENDER

Concepts of masculinity and femininity are especially important for nursing because the profession itself is associated very strongly with being female. This has implications for both men in nursing (Evans 2004) and women wanting to move into areas traditionally associated with masculine characteristics, e.g. management and leadership. In a broader context, feminine characteristics are used to explain the subservient role of nursing in the political hierarchy of healthcare professions (Versluysen 1980). Because nursing is viewed by many as a female profession, and women are often seen as subservient, nurses as a group command little political power (Salvage 1995, Maslin-Prothero & Masterson 2002). What is beginning to be touched upon here is the political nature of gender and sexuality. The descriptions of femininity and masculinity indicate the traditional views of the differences between men and women. These views are arguably not neutral because some characteristics are seen as more important for society and consequently attract higher social prestige and status. This is evident in the health service where medicine maintains power and prestige and is still seen as a male profession. Male nurses and female doctors as exceptions to these stereotypical images might be viewed with suspicion in some clinical areas. Also the day-to-day working relationships between doctors and nurses can be influenced by these gender politics (Stein et al 1990, Zelek & Phillips 2003).

Nurses must also be aware of the potential effects of their own gender on clients. Nursing often involves intimate activities where clients are required to expose their bodies and to be touched in sensitive, sometimes erogenous zones. This can result in embarrassing situations for the client and the nurse, and both can use a range of strategies to diffuse or cope with this embarrassment (Lawler 1991, Meerabeau 1999).

THE MEDICALIZATION OF SEXUALITY

A simple view of healthcare professions is that their role is to find solutions to health problems that exist in society. They use scientific methods to treat and care for people with all types of health problems. Some sociologists view professions in a very different way, and believe that rather than being objective scientists studying and finding treatments for health problems, they help to define and create 'new illnesses'. This process is known as 'medicalization' and has a long history, especially in the area of sexuality. Hart & Wellings (2002) describe the power the medical professions have had over sexual activity through their ability to define and give medical labels to aspects of human behaviour. In the 19th century, unacceptable behaviour such as masturbation was defined as a perversion and medicine helped to construct the list of adverse side-effects this behaviour could supposedly lead to. Similarly in the early 20th century homosexuality was seen by many as a 'condition' and treatment and cures were sought. More recently the medical professions have become very interested in sexual behaviour, in particular sexual pleasure and gratification. This medicalization of sex is evident in the way the pharmacological industry has invested massively in the research and production of drugs to enhance sexual performance. It might be argued that this emphasis on performance and sexual gratification raises expectations and helps to define what is normal and essential for health and well-being. Failure to reach these levels of gratification and performance have been defined as 'sexual dysfunctions' in need of 'treatment'. Hart & Wellings argue that this overly medical view of sex ignores the social and interpersonal dynamics of relationships.

INFORMATION SPECIFIC TO THE FOUR BRANCHES OF NURSING

Adult nursing

Staff working within this branch need to be aware of the relationship between sexuality and ageing. Degenerative changes associated with ageing can affect self-esteem, body image, sexual desire and sexual response. A decrease of circulating androgens lowers libido, and changes in neurological and vascular systems can affect sensation and response. These changes may not be important for some people, but many of these potential problems can be overcome by practical advice and medical intervention. Physiological changes do not in themselves prevent older people from having an active and pleasurable sex life and research suggests that sexual activity plays an important part in people's lives well into old age (Gott & Hinchcliffe 2003, Gott 2006, Bauer & McAuliffe 2007).

Many older people live alone and have few social contacts, thus reducing their chance of meeting a new partner. Also the attitudes that youth is beautiful and that older people should not be sexually active may force older people to believe that it is not right for them to have sexual desires. Comfort & Dial (1991) suggest that 'most of our aged stop having sex for reasons similar to those why they stop riding a bicycle: general infirmity, fear that it would expose them to ridicule, and for most, lack of a bicycle.' Furthermore, Read (2004) identified a number of physical and psychological factors that can affect an older adult's sexuality and sexual expression, for example incontinence, mobility, muscle tone, arthritis, skin condition and sensitivity, chronic illnesses such as arthritis and diabetes, social isolation, sense of unattractiveness, loneliness, grief and sense of mortality.

Learning disabilities nursing

A key concept to consider in caring for clients with learning disabilities is consent. If there are doubts about an individual's knowledge or level of understanding, then any relationships or sexual activities he or she is involved in could constitute abuse. This judgement of the ability to consent is difficult, but rests on a consideration of the individual's cognitive functioning and ability to assert his or her wishes in pressured situations (Murphy & O'Callaghan 2004). This has implications for nurses; in particular, how such a judgement is reached and how clients can be helped to gain the appropriate knowledge and skills. The Mental Capacity Act 2005 and the Code of Practice (Department for Constitutional Affairs 2007) have a significant impact on how a person's capacity to make decisions for themselves is assessed and determined. How this new policy will be applied to sexual relationships between people with learning disabilities is yet to be defined. However, one element of the assessment of capacity will address the person's understanding of sexual activity, sexual health and sexual health risks. Researchers are currently in the process of designing tools to help this assessment of sexual knowledge (Galea et al 2004, Lyden 2007).

A central issue in any assessment tool is deciding what is meant by appropriate knowledge and skills. For example, if a client expresses a desire to wear clothes normally worn by the opposite sex should this be discouraged or should nurses help the client to understand, promote and actively enjoy his or her chosen cross-dressing identity? On the one hand nurses might aim to encourage client decision making and choice, but on the other, aim to help clients develop attitudes and behaviour that allow for a degree of integration in the community. The difficulty in this case is that such an expression of sexuality may prevent what is usually understood as social integration. There may, however, be a cross-dressing community into which the client can integrate, but this may prove difficult because of the client's level of social skills or the stigma associated with learning disabilities. With regard to consent and choice nurses may have to consider whether it is appropriate for clients to make decisions about some aspects of their lives but not others. Like many other aspects of learning disabilities nursing there is a danger

that nurses might impose their own norms of sexuality, overtly or covertly, and restrict the client's potential. See the Evolve 16.5 resource for more information on this issue.

16.5 – NURSES SUPPORTING OR FACILITATING SEX FOR PATIENTS

- Understand the ethical issues involved in supporting or facilitating sex for patients.
- Understand the implications of this for the patient.
- Understand the implications of this for others.
- Apply this in a practical exercise.

Reflection and portfolio exercise

Ager & Little (1998) proposed the following rights for people with learning disabilities:

- The right to be informed about sexuality and its place in human life, at times and at a level that allows this area of human being and experience to be as positive as possible.
- The same right as everyone else to enjoy sexual activity. The concomitant right to remain celibate and to refrain from sexual activity of any kind.
- The right to contraceptive advice and services, both to avoid pregnancy and to avoid the risk of sexually transmitted infections.
- The same right as any other citizen to marry or form ongoing relationships.
- The same right to choose parenthood as that enjoyed by everyone else.
- The right not to be sexually abused and to be protected from sexual abuse.

How are these rights implemented in practice, in both learning disabilities and in other areas of care?

Children's nursing

Illness can intrude in the development of a child's sexuality. A variety of endocrine conditions as well as some chronic illnesses can directly affect growth and physiological development to the extent that puberty is delayed or absent. Similarly, chronic illness in childhood can influence exposure to the social and psychological experiences that seem to be important in the development of sexual identity. Sexual development in children is a complex process

(Bancroft 2003) and there seem to be a number of elements, for example:

- Role models in the child's immediate environment.
- Witnessing displays of affection between others (touch and language).
- Receiving comforting touch and praise that result in feelings of trust and security.
- Exploring one's own body and being allowed to gain pleasure from it (e.g. through masturbation).
- Learning that your body is your property and that others need your permission to touch it.
- Learning appropriate levels of privacy related to the body, in a way that prevents a feeling of guilt.
- Learning about other's needs for privacy.
- Having curiosity encouraged about gender and sexuality, receiving open and honest answers appropriate to the child's level of understanding.
- Having opportunities for play with peers of the same and of the opposite sex.
- Being free to participate in gender-based play.

Adolescence is characterized by experimentation, rebellion and risk taking behaviour. There are obvious risks in relation to unwanted pregnancies, sexually transmitted infections and emotional trauma during this stage of development; however, sexual development should include an understanding of rights, responsibilities and relationships as well as the mechanics of sexual activity. This has implications for nurses in many areas, particularly those in primary health care, school nursing, and health education and promotion (Treacy & Randle 2004, Haglund 2006).

The Royal College of Nursing (2001) raised the issue of child abuse in a hospital setting and produced guidelines for staff working in this potentially vulnerable situation. It recognized the range of types of abuse possible but focused on sexual abuse and how nurses may have allegations made against them by children and parents. The paper gives guidance on how staff can protect children from harm and protect themselves from false accusations. Men are particularly at risk of these accusations but the RCN says that all nurses need to be aware of this potential and take practical steps to avoid such situations.

Reflection and portfolio exercise

Imagine you are working on a children's ward.

What measures would you want to see in place to help prevent sexual abuse of the children on your ward?
What could make you suspect that a child on your ward was being sexually abused?
What would you do if you had this suspicion?

Check out the following websites on abuse for guidance

http://www.rcn.org.uk/__data/assets/pdf_file/0007/78532/001741.pdf
http://www.rcn.org.uk/__data/assets/pdf_file/0004/78583/002045.pdf
http://www.everychildmatters.gov.uk/_files/FD21D51F594298457CF64BE9CDF6F179.pdf

Mental health nursing

Mental health problems can impact on expressing sexuality and nurses are likely to be working with clients' unmet needs in this aspect of their lives (McCann 2000). The interrelationship between sexuality and mental health is complex. Low self-esteem and anxiety can intrude into personal relationships affecting libido and sexual function. This can become a vicious circle, with low self-esteem limiting sexual expression, which further reduces self-esteem. In this situation the client can feel out of control. In addition, the nurse needs to be aware of:

- The impact mental illness can have on personal relationships, in particular on the expression of intimacy within relationships (Wright et al 2007).
- The function of the psychiatric services in defining, monitoring and treating sexual deviance, and their social role in maintaining the stigmas surrounding certain sexual practices.
- The potential for therapeutic relationships between clients and professionals to develop into relationships involving inappropriate sexual expression.
- The balance required between the client's right to sexual expression and the need to protect vulnerable clients from exploitation – this will be an important issue for nursing and care staff working in homes for people with long-term serious mental health problems.
- The need for specifically designed sexual health education for people with mental health problems (Higgins & Barker 2006).
- The significant impact of commonly used neuroleptic medication on sexuality and sexual health (Higgins et al 2005, Stimmel & Gutierrez 2006) and how nurses regularly fail to address this issue with patients.

KEY LEGAL AND ETHICAL ISSUES

Sexuality is an important aspect of all branches of nursing. If nursing claims to be holistic in its outlook then it must take into account the links between health and all areas of people's lives. When people are unable to meet their own needs, nurses play an important role in assisting, guiding or advising.

In cases of extreme disability and dependence nurses may have to take over and act on the client's behalf, for example washing a client who is unconscious, or feeding a person with a severe learning disability. An ethical issue arises in the area of sexual need however. Earle (2001) raises the issue of facilitated sex and explains this as a continuum ranging from giving information to sexual surrogacy. Giving information to a client or creating a climate which allows for intimacy between client and partner may seem unproblematic whereas arranging paid-for sexual services or facilitated masturbation may raise legal and ethical dilemmas. Earle argues, though, that all levels of help on this continuum of facilitated sex could be seen as potentially problematic. Buying pornography for a client may be seen as acceptable by some professionals and not by others. Similarly escorting a client to a gay club to help him or her meet sexual partners may be interpreted as positive or negative depending on your perspective.

Reflection and portfolio evidence

Do you think it should be a nurse's role to help patients meet their sexual needs? Why?

What kind of help is appropriate / inappropriate?

If a patient wanted to pay for sex would you be willing to help them find a sex worker?

What are the legal and professional ramifications?

Read the following short article to see how this happened in practice: Parish C 2007 Hospice staff defend helping a 22-year-old to find a sex worker. Nursing Standard 21(22):8.

Sexuality is central to an individual's life, influencing thoughts, feelings and behaviours. Because of this, the relationship between the law and sexuality is wide ranging. It is beyond the scope of this chapter to cover legal aspects of sexuality in detail; however, it is important to be aware of the areas of law that might need to be considered by nurses across a range of settings. These include laws related to: sex discrimination, families, child care, reproduction, abortion, sexual deviance, sexual abuse, rape, indecency, consent, confidentiality, privacy. This is not exhaustive and for a more detailed introduction to

these areas see Dimond (2005). Two recent developments in legislation related to sexuality are the Sexual Offences Act 2003 and the Civil Partnership Act 2004. The Sexual Offences Act 2003 attempts to clarify what constitutes a sexual offence and it brings together under one umbrella some old and diverse laws on sexual offences. The Civil Partnership Act 2004 enables same sex couples to register their partnerships. The first couples did this on 21 December 2005. The act gives same sex couples the same legal and financial rights (tax, pension, etc.) as heterosexual married couples.

POLICY AND SEXUALITY

Sexual health has become an important issue for policy makers over the last decade. The Department of Health (2002) published the National Strategy for Sexual Health and HIV with the following aims:

- to reduce the transmission of HIV and sexually transmitted infections (STIs)
- to reduce the prevalence of undiagnosed HIV and STIs
- to reduce unintended pregnancy rates
- to improve health and social care of people living with HIV
- to reduce the stigma associated with HIV and STIs.

A criticism of these aims might be that they are disease focused and tend to ignore many other aspects of sexuality and positive sexual health. The Royal College of Nursing produced a guidance document, *Sexuality and Sexual Health in Nursing Practice* (Royal College of Nursing 2000). While it incorporates a disease focus, it does emphasize a broader nature of sexual health and suggests how sexuality can become part of clinical work. The report acknowledges difficulties nurses may have in discussing sexuality based problems with clients but goes some way in breaking down barriers and stigma.

Improving sexual health is priority D in the Department of Health (2004, 2005) policy *Choosing Health: Making Healthier Choices Easier*. This focuses mainly on teenage pregnancy and sexually transmitted infections but sets an agenda for improving services. Similarly the National Institute for Health and Clinical Excellence (2007) produced guidance on the prevention of sexually transmitted infections and the reduction of teenage pregnancies.

PERSONAL AND REFLECTIVE KNOWLEDGE

This final section now finishes with four case studies based on clients with sexuality related problems. There are a number of questions after each case study to help you consider the issues. After these are a number of exercises to help you reflect on your practice and develop your portfolio evidence.

CASE STUDIES RELATING TO SEXUALITY

Case study: Adult

Mrs Ellis is a resident in a private nursing home. She is 75 years old and has been a widow for 10 years. Despite having severe osteoarthritis in her knees and hips she sees herself as relatively fit. She is mentally alert and enjoys mixing with other residents, especially during meal times and organized social events. She has early signs of heart failure, which prevents her from having surgery for her arthritis and also makes her feel tired and out of sorts at times. She requires assistance with dressing, personal hygiene and going to the toilet, but is able to move around the home independently in her wheelchair. She has made a close association with a man in the home and they spend time together most afternoons.

- How might Mrs Ellis's age and disability affect the way she sees herself as a woman?
- What would your reaction be if you were Mrs Ellis's primary nurse and she said she would like to develop the relationship with her friend into a sexual one?
- What are the potential problems with confidentiality and what should Mrs Ellis's primary nurse do to maintain confidentiality?

Case study: Learning disabilities

John Brown is 26 years of age and has a moderate learning disability. He lives at home with his parents and visits a day centre every day where he participates in a social skills training programme, which is partly organized by a community nurse. The nurse discovers from the day centre staff that John regularly visits a local public toilet to engage in homosexual activities. This emerged at a day centre group meeting when another of the service users, who openly admits to visiting the same toilets, said he had seen John there.

John is usually withdrawn and initiates little conversation or interaction with people at the day centre. He has a close relationship with the nurse, but is reluctant to talk about his sexual activities with anyone. John is not used to making decisions in his life and has everything organized for him by his parents. Generally the staff see John as an inoffensive young man who creates no fuss in the day centre because on the whole he does as he is told.

- Supposing the claim about John's sexual behaviour is true, should the nurse be concerned? Why or why not?

- Do you think the nurse should do anything and if so, what?
- How do you think John's parents might react if they discovered what he was doing?
- Do you think John's parents have a right to know?

Case study: Child

Susan Jones is 15 years old and has cystic fibrosis. This is a hereditary condition affecting a number of body systems. The respiratory system produces large amounts of thick, sticky sputum, breathlessness can be particularly disabling, and the illness is likely to lead to a premature death. Susan needs oxygen therapy much of the time and requires regular physiotherapy to keep her chest clear. Like other children with this condition, Susan's physical development has been retarded and she is short for her age and underweight.

Susan lives at home with her parents and 12-year-old sister. She has missed a lot of school over the last year and although a couple of friends visit on occasions she has lost touch with her peer group. Her parents are very caring and worry about her repeated chest infections. They believe that the infections flare up after Susan has had friends around and as a result they discourage too many visitors.

- How might Susan's ill health have affected her self-concept?
- Adolescence is a crucial time for the development of a sexual identity. What important aspects of adolescence might Susan have missed out on?
- How could a community nurse promote the development of Susan's sexual identity?

Case study: Mental health

David Anderson is a 35-year-old single man who lives alone in his new four-bedroom detached house on the outskirts of a large city. He has been admitted to an acute admission ward in a psychiatric hospital suffering from severe depression. He has recently split up from his partner of 6 months and the advertising business he owns is struggling, to the extent that he is considering laying off staff. His career has been all-consuming and David has never been one for 'getting married and settling down'. He has had a number of short-term relationships over the last 10 years and he explains the breakdown of his recent relationship as mainly his fault. He has not been interested in sex and 'found it difficult to perform these days'.

- How might recent events be contributing to the way David feels about himself?
- Describe the possible relationship between David's lifestyle and his sexual difficulties.
- As David's primary nurse what could you do to help him regain his ability to express his sexuality?

SUMMARY

This chapter has focused on developing knowledge and insight into human sexuality and the implications for practice. It has included:

1. Defining sexuality and examining how the concept has evolved to become integrated into self-concept and within society.
2. Expression of sexuality was examined in gender identification and development.
3. Examining the human sexual response and sexual behaviour throughout the lifespan.
4. The implications for practice were considered, beginning with an examination of approaches for discussing and assessing sexuality with clients.
5. To be comfortable in assessing clients, however, nurses need to be comfortable with their own sexuality. Consequently, exercises were included to help to raise self-awareness.
6. Potential areas of difficulty that clients might experience were highlighted and some actions that nurses could use to help to address them were suggested, particularly by incorporating the use of Annon's (1974) P-LI-SS-IT model.
7. The implication of nursing being predominantly a female profession was considered. Nursing practice often involves intimate activities and the juxtaposition of delivering care with the potential effects of gender was also discussed.
8. Finally, in a brief overview of contemporary policy, the *National Strategy for Sexual Health and HIV* (Department of Health 2002) and *Sexuality and Sexual Health in Nursing Practice* (Royal College of Nursing 2000) were highlighted. Although they were criticized for being disease focused, it was recognized that sexuality is, at last, being addressed by policy makers. This has been added to by the policy on making healthier choices (Department of Health 2004, 2005) and NICE guidelines (2007).

Annotated further reading and websites

Gott M 2005 Sexuality, sexual health, and ageing (rethinking ageing). Open University Press, Maidenhead

This book integrates theoretical insights into sexuality, sexual health and ageing, with research findings from studies conducted with older people and the professionals that work with them.

Heath H, White I 2001 The challenge of sexuality in health care. Blackwell, Oxford

A comprehensive overview of issues in sexuality and health care. It describes the normal processes and issues that arise at different stages of a person's life connected with sexuality. It goes on to discuss sexuality in relation to illness, disfigurement, physical and mental disability.

Wells D (ed) 2000 Caring for sexuality in health and illness. Churchill Livingstone, Edinburgh

An introduction to the theory and practice of psychosexual care. It focuses on the role of the healthcare professional in promoting sexual health and includes exercises to help reflect on practice.

http://www.sexualityandu.ca
This Canadian website is a useful source of information on sexuality education including topics such as sexually transmitted infections, contraception and lifestyle choices. It has sections for health professionals, parents, teachers, adults and teenagers.

http://www.sexualhealth.com
This site provides a range of information on and links to sexuality education, counselling and therapy.

http://www.bbc.co.uk/health/sex/
This site covers a number of factsheets and articles on sex and sexual health. It has particularly good links to UK organizations related to sexuality.

http://www.engenderhealth.org
This site covers men's and women's health. It has a worldwide perspective and includes a selection of online courses and professional material for people wanting to learn about sexuality.

http://www.equality.salford.ac.uk/legislation/sexlaw.php
This site provides a valuable overview of legislation related to sexuality and sexual health.

http://www.dh.gov.uk/en/Policyandguidance/
Healthandsocialcaretopics/Sexualhealth/index.htm
This is the Department of Health policy and guidance site for sexual health services. It provides useful links to a range of other sites related to sexual health.

http://www.directgov.gov.uk/en/HealthAndWellBeing/DG_4002934
This is a government site with a focus on sexual health.

http://www.mind.org.uk/NR/rdonlyres/4E259C31-6E41-4522-8A45-741E331CB61E/1044/SummaryfindingsofLGBreport.pdf
A report based on research carried out in 2003 on the mental health and well being of gay men, lesbians and bisexuals. It makes important recommendations for mental health services.

http://www.gro.gov.uk/gro/content/civilpartnerships/
The General Register Office guidelines on civil partnerships.

http://www.stonewall.org.uk/information_bank/partnership/
civil_partnership_act/default.asp
This site is by Stonewall and it provides a detailed explanation of civil partnerships.

http://www.opsi.gov.uk/acts/acts2004/ukpga_20040033_en_1
The Civil Partnership Act 2004.

http://www.opsi.gov.uk/ACTS/acts2003/20030042.htm
The Sexual Offences Act 2003.

http://www.homeoffice.gov.uk/documents/sex-offence-protect-learning-dis
This Home Office booklet is written for people under 16 with a learning disability and explains how they can protect themselves from sexual abuse.

http://www.homeoffice.gov.uk/documents/adults-safe-fr-sex-harm-leaflet
This Home Office booklet sets out the main aspects of the Sexual Offences Act 2003 designed to protect adults.

http://www.opsi.gov.uk/si/si2007/uksi_20071263_en_1
The Equality Act (Sexual Orientation) Regulations 2007.

http://www.dh.gov.uk/en/Policyandguidance/
Equalityandhumanrights/Sexualorientationandgenderidentity/index.
htm
The Department of Health's policy and guidance on sexual orientation
and gender identity. This contains links to many reports on anti-
discriminatory practice and ways to promote equality for lesbian, gay,
bisexual and transgender (LBGT) people in health and social care, both
as service users and as employees.

References

Ager J, Little J 1998 Sexual health for people with learning disabilities. Nursing Standard 13(2):34–39

Annon J S 1974 The behavioural treatment of sexual problems. Enabling Systems, Honolulu

Arber S 1997 Comparing inequalities in women's and men's health: Britain in the 1990s. Social Science and Medicine (44)6:773–787

Bancroft J 1989 Human sexuality and its problems. Churchill Livingstone, Edinburgh

Bancroft J 2002 Biological factors in human sexuality. Journal of Sex Research 39(1):15–21

Bancroft J 2003 Sexual development in children. Indiana University Press, Indiana

Bancroft J, Janssen E, Strong D, Carnes L, Vukadinovic Z, Scott Long J 2003 The relation between mood and sexuality in heterosexual men. Archives of Sexual Behavior 32(3):217–230

Batcup D, Thomas B 1994 Mixing the genders, an ethical dilemma: how nursing theory has dealt with sexuality and gender. Nursing Ethics 1(1):43–52

Bauer M, McAuliffe L 2007 Sexuality, health care and the older person: an overview of the literature. International Journal of Older People Nursing 2:63–68

Birkhead TR 2000 Promiscuity. Faber and Faber, London

Bouman WP, Arcelus J, Benbow SM 2007 Nottingham Study of Sexuality and Ageing (NoSSA II). Attitudes of care staff regarding sexuality and residents: a study in residential and nursing homes. Sexual and Relationship Therapy 22(1):45–61

British Medical Association and the Royal Pharmaceutical Society 2008 British National Formulary 55. British Medical Association, London

Chodorow N 1992 Feminism and psychoanalytical theory. Yale University Press, New Haven

Comfort A, Dial L 1991 Sexuality and aging: an overview. Clinical Geriatric Medicine 7(1):1–7

Connell RW 2002 Gender. Polity Press, London

Department for Constitutional Affairs 2007 Mental Capacity Act 2005 Code of Practice. TSO, London. Available online: http://www.dca.gov.uk/legal-policy/mental-capacity/mca-cp.pdf (accessed 21 August 2008)

Department of Health 2002 The national strategy for sexual health and HIV. HMSO, London

Department of Health 2004 Choosing health: making healthier choices easier. HMSO, London

Department of Health 2005 Delivering choosing health: making healthier choices easier. HMSO, London

Dimond B 2005 Legal aspects of nursing, 4th edn. Pearson Education, Harlow

Earle S 2001 Disability, facilitated sex and the role of the nurse. Journal of Advanced Nursing 36(3):433–440

Engenderhealth 2005 Sexual response and sexual practices. Available online: http://www.engenderhealth.org/res/onc/sexuality/response/pg2.html (accessed 20 August 2008)

Evans J 2004 Men nurses: a historical and feminist perspective. Journal of Advanced Nursing 47(3):321–328

Ford A 2005 Medicines and sexual function: introduction. Proceedings of the Western Pharmacology Society 48:164

Foucault M 1973 The birth of the clinic. Tavistock, London

Foucault M 1979 The history of sexuality, vol. 1. An introduction. Allen Lane, London

Freud S 1923 The ego and the id. Hogarth Press, London

Gagnon JH, Simon W 2005 Sexual conduct: the social sources of human sexuality. Aldine, Chicago

Galea J, Butler J, Iacono T, Leighton D 2004 The assessment of sexual knowledge in people with intellectual disability. Journal of Intellectual and Developmental Disability 29(4):350–365

Giddens A 2005 Sociology. Blackwell, Oxford

Gott M 2006 Sexual health and the new ageing. Age and Aging 35(2):106–107

Gott M, Hinchcliff S 2003 How important is sex in later life? The views of older people. Social Science and Medicine 56(8):1617–1628

Gott M, Galena E, Hinchliff S, Elford H 2004 'Opening a can of worms': GP and practice nurse barriers to talking about sexual health in primary care. Family Practice 21(5):528–536

Gove WR, Tudor JF 1972 Adult sex roles and mental illness. American Journal of Sociology 78:812–835

Haglund K 2006 Recommendations for sexuality education for early adolescents. Journal of Obstetric, Gynecologic, and Neonatal Nursing 35(3):369–375

Hart G, Wellings K 2002 Sexual behaviour and its medicalisation: in sickness and in health. British Medical Journal 324:896–900

Higgins A, Barker P 2006 Sexual health education for people with mental health problems: what can we learn from the literature? Journal of Psychiatric and Mental Health Nursing 13(6):687–697

Higgins A, Barker P, Begley CM 2005 Neuroleptic medication and sexuality: the forgotten aspect of education and care. Journal of Psychiatric and Mental Health Nursing 12:439–446

Higgins A, Barker P, Begley CM 2006 Sexuality: the challenge to espoused holistic care. International Journal of Nursing Practice 12(6):345–351

Holland K, Jenkins J, Solomon J, Whittam S 2003 Applying the Roper Logan and Tierney model in practice. Churchill Livingstone, Edinburgh

Holmes D, O'Byrne P 2006 The art of public health nursing: using confession technè in the sexual health domain. Journal of Advanced Nursing. 56(4):430–437

Jeffreys MR 2006 Teaching cultural competence in nursing and health care. Springer, New York

Johnson MA, Mercer CH, Erens B 2001 Sexual behaviour in Britain: partnerships, practices, and HIV risk behaviours. Lancet 358:1835–1854

Kinsey AC, Pomeroy WB, Martin CE 1948 Sexual behaviour in the human male. Saunders, Philadelphia

Knight D 2004 Health care screening for men who have sex with men. American Family Physician 69(9):2149–2158

Lachman M 2004 Development in midlife. Annual Review of Psychology 55(1):305–331

Lanval M 1950 An inquiry into the intimate lives of women. Cadillac, New York

Lawler J 1991 Behind the screens. Nursing: somology and the problem of the body. Churchill Livingstone, Edinburgh

Lyden M 2007 Assessment of sexual consent capacity. Sexuality and Disability 25(1):3–20

McCann J 2000 The expression of sexuality in people with psychosis: breaking taboos. Journal of Advanced Nursing 32:132–138

Magnan MA, Reynolds KE, Galvin EA 2006 Barriers to addressing patient sexuality in nursing practice. Dermatology Nursing 18(5):448–454

Maslin-Prothero S, Masterson A 2002 Power, politics, and nursing in the United Kingdom. Policy, Politics, and Nursing Practice 3(2):108–117

Masters W, Johnson V 1966 Human sexual response. Churchill, London

Meerabeau L 1999 The management of embarrassment and sexuality in health care. Journal of Advanced Nursing 29(6):1507–1513

Mental Capacity Act 2005 (Chapter 9) Stationery Office, London. Available online: **http://www.england-legislation.hmso.gov.uk/acts/acts2005/ukpga_20050009_en_1** (accessed 20 August 2008)

Monga TN, Lefebvre KA 1995 Sexuality: an overview. Physical Medicine and Rehabilitation: State of the Art Reviews 9(2):299–311

Montague SE, Watson R, Herbert RA (eds) 2005 Physiology for nursing practice, 3rd edn. Elsevier, Edinburgh

Murphy GH, O'Callaghan A 2004 Capacity of adults with intellectual disabilities to consent to sexual relationships. Psychological Medicine 34:1347–1357

National Institute of Health and Clinical Excellence (NICE) 2007 Preventing sexually transmitted infections and reducing under 18 conceptions. Available online: http://guidance.nice.org.uk/PHI3 (accessed 20 August 2008)

Obermeyer CM 2000 Menopause across cultures: a review of the evidence. Menopause 7(3):184–192

Orem D 2001 Nursing: concepts of practice, 6th edn. Mosby, London

Peplau H 1988 Interpersonal relations in nursing. Macmillan, London

Read J 2004 Health factors that inhibit sexual activity in elderly people. British Medical Journal 329:559–561

Royal College of Nursing 2000 Sexuality and sexual health in nursing practice. Royal College of Nursing, London

Royal College of Nursing 2001 Protection of nurses working with children and young people. Royal College of Nursing, London

Roper N, Logan W, Tierney A 2000 The Roper–Logan–Tierney model of nursing: based on activities of living. Churchill Livingstone, Edinburgh

Salvage J 1995 The politics of nursing. Heinemann, London

Stein L, Watts D, Howell T 1990 The doctor–nurse game revisited. New England Journal of Medicine 322(8):546–549

Stimmel L, Gutierrez MA 2006 Sexual dysfunction and psychotropic medications. CNS Spectrums 11(8 Suppl. 9):24–30

Taylor B, Davis S 2006 Using the extended PLISSIT model to address sexual healthcare needs. Nursing Standard 21(11):35–40. Available online: **http://nursingstandard.rcnpublishing.co.uk/resources/archive/GetArticleById.asp?ArticleId=6382** (accessed 21 August 2008)

Treacy V, Randle J 2004 Breaking sexuality taboos. Paediatric Nursing 16(2):19–22

Versluysen MC 1980 Old wives' tales? Women healers in English history. In: Davies C (ed) Rewriting nursing history. Croom Helm, London, pp 175–199

Wellings K, Field J, Johnson A M et al 1994 Sexual behaviour in Britain: the national survey of sexual attitudes and lifestyles. Penguin, Harmondsworth

Wellings K, Nanchahal K, Macdowall W et al 2001 Sexual behaviour in Britain: early heterosexual experience. Lancet 358:1843–1850

Werneke U, Northey S, Bhugra D 2006 Anti depressants and sexual dysfunction. Acta Psychiatrica Scandinavica 114(6):384–397

World Health Organization 2002 Gender and reproductive rights. Available online: http://www.who.int/reproductive-health/gender/sexual_health.html#2 (accessed 20 August 2008)

Wright ER, Wright DE, Perry BL, Foote-Ardah CE 2007 Stigma and the sexual isolation of people with serious mental illness. Social Problems 54(1):78–98

Zelek B, Phillips SP 2003 Gender and power: nurses and doctors in Canada. International Journal for Equity in Health 2(1):1–5

Chapter 17

Confusion

Jan Dewing

INTRODUCTION

There is a difference between the everyday experience and understanding of confusion (for example missing the point or being suddenly caught out and feeling a sense of embarrassment) and confusion in the context of health care. Here, confusion is fundamentally a lack of orientation with respect to time, place and/or self. It is generally marked by poor attention and thinking, which leads to difficulties in comprehension, loss of short-term memory and usually, irritability alternating with drowsiness. Having confusion often means the person does not or cannot act as others would expect them to in any given context or situation. It is vital to appreciate that the lived experience of what it is really like for the person is one where they can feel bewildered, perplexed and unable to self-orientate and it is others around the person who appear to be saying and doing unusual things.

Further, acute confusion or delirium is a clinical sign or more accurately a syndrome (a collection of symptoms) which generally occurs suddenly as an impairment in a person's mental state secondary to a medical condition or as a consequence of some medical treatment. Healthcare practitioners must be knowledgeable about confusion, particularly acute confusion, its possible underlying causes, what it is like to be confused and how to respond to the person and their families or carers in a way that is both compassionate and therapeutic. Confusion can also be seen to be present on a longer term basis, often as part of a neurological condition (for example head trauma or dementia) and again nurses need to have an overall appreciation of the causes and particularly how to respond to the person who is confused in the best way to support their health and overall best interests.

Figures for the rates of delirium vary according to which patient group or setting is being discussed. Delirium occurs in about 15–20 % of all general admissions to hospital (Meagher 2001). There is an increase with age: 0.4% in those over 18 years of age, 1.1% in those over 55, 13.6% in those over 85 years (Burns et al 2004). The incidence is higher in older people and for those with a pre-existing cognitive impairment and prevalence is higher in people with malignancy and HIV. Despite this relatively frequent occurrence, delirium remains under-diagnosed and often poorly managed, with up to 60% of cases being missed or diagnosed at late stage (Meagher 2001). Furthermore, patients with delirium have longer hospital stays by two to three times the usual length, a higher frequency of complications, e.g. infections and pressure sores, and increased mortality rates. Older people also have an increased risk of requiring long-term institutional care following an episode of delirium. Dementia usually affects older people and becomes more common with increasing age. Sometime after the age of 65 about 1 in 20 people develop dementia and this level rises until about 1 in 5 people over the age of 80 have dementia. Although still rare, dementia can affect younger people.

OVERVIEW

This chapter explores a selection of contemporary evidence around what is known about confusion, the various causes of confusion and strategies to help people who are confused.

Subject knowledge

In this section of the chapter, the physiological factors that may lead to individuals becoming confused are identified. This is followed by an exploration of the psychological and environmental factors that also may lead to and/or worsen the experience of confusion.

Care delivery knowledge

In this section, the assessment and care planning of people who are experiencing acute and longer term confusion is considered. The area of risk assessment is also considered.

Professional and ethical knowledge

In the Professional and Ethical Knowledge section, values and beliefs about confusion and attitudes towards people who experience confusion are considered. Increasing numbers of older people receive health care, and although this group of people are at greater risk of developing acute confusion, it does not follow that all older people will do so. Consequently, within this section there is a short discussion on ageism and discrimination. Capacity and consent are central concerns for professional practice in any context and this is considered next. This is followed by a more detailed look at confusion in older people, specifically the sort of confusion that can exist as part of dementia. Working with families and carers and involving them in care of the person who is confused can be a helpful strategy; however, the provision of information and support for the family and carers is essential if they are to have as positive an experience of care as is possible.

Personal and reflective knowledge

Finally, the Personal and Reflective Knowledge section summarizes the main points of the chapter to help you to consolidate your knowledge. You will find some reflective cues you can work with to help you identify your values and beliefs about caring for people who experience confusion. On pages 402–403 there are four scenarios, one relating to each of the branch programmes, and you might find it helpful to read through the relevant scenario before you start the chapter and use it as a focus for reflection while reading. These scenarios are followed by activities that you can use to develop your learning portfolio. You may also find it helpful to undertake one or more of the following suggestions to support the way you are organizing your learning.

SUBJECT KNOWLEDGE

PHYSIOLOGICAL

As a term used within health and social care, confusion has been somewhat of a 'cover all' and is often used inappropriately without a formal assessment. Its vernacular usage describes people experiencing a low level of disorientation or a minor change in their mental state. However, it is also used to mean an acute confusion, confusional state or delirium, which is a life-threatening condition requiring specific medical and nursing interventions for the underlying cause(s) (Eriksdotter Jönhagen 2002). The term 'delirium' is favoured by the international medical community, although in the UK it is not often so referred to by healthcare practitioners, especially nurses. Thus it is vital to clarify what is being talked about – confusion in a non-specific general sense or acute confusion/delirium – and to appreciate that acute confusion is the same as delirium. Additionally, nurses must appreciate that the label of confusion is simply a way of summarizing a syndrome with a collection of symptoms. These symptoms indicate that some other processes are occurring that require systematic medical assessment and diagnosis.

TYPES OF CONFUSION

When talking about confusion, it is helpful to ascertain if the person is confused in regard to place, person and/or time. Confusion is generally classified as short-term or long-term. Short-term or acute confusion (delirium) has a sudden onset, is reversible and involves no significant destruction of brain cells. It can occur in individuals regardless of age. People with extensive life threatening injuries can be at risk of experiencing an acute state of confusion (Pisani et al 2006). In older people almost any severe physical illness can bring about confusion. However, younger people and children can also develop acute confusion through various causes, including epilepsy (especially following a seizure), hyperpyrexia, post electro-convulsive therapy and poisoning. Delirium is also common in the last weeks of life, occurring in up to 44% of people with advanced cancer and in up to 88% of people with a terminal illness in the last days of life (Keeley 2007).

In contrast, long-term or chronic confusion occurs due to the effects of a continuing acute confusion/delirium or to degenerative and often progressive changes in the brain. The main underlying cause of this type of confusion is dementia. Dementia is a term used to cover numerous types of disease processes which tend to be slow in onset, are usually irreversible and involve substantial destruction of brain cells to the extent of interfering with social and personal functioning. The most frequently occurring dementias are Alzheimer's disease, Lewy body dementia and vascular dementia.

PHYSIOLOGICAL FACTORS

There are six major physiological factors that can lead to the development of confusion:

- infections
- endocrine disturbance
- electrolyte imbalance
- poisoning
- trauma
- dementia.

Infection

Any infection which causes a fever can lead to confusion or delirium. Infections arise due to pathogens invading the body systems, commonly via the urinary or respiratory tracts, although there are many other possible entry sites for infections. Additionally, some infections, such as a chest infection, may cause hypoxia, preventing adequate oxygenated blood reaching the brain and worsening the confusion. Pathogens may also be transported from the primary site of infection via the circulatory system to infect the nervous system directly, again worsening the confusion. The problem of hospital acquired infections must also be considered, especially with people who are already vulnerable to infection.

Endocrine disturbance

Disorders of the endocrine system can interfere with the operation of the nervous system resulting in confusion. For example, a malfunction of the thyroid gland can lead to hypothyroidism, one of the symptoms of which can be

confusion (El-Kaissi et al 2005). Similarly, if diabetes mellitus has not been stabilized, or if food has not been taken after the administration of insulin, hypoglycaemia and associated confusion can develop.

Electrolyte imbalance

The main cause of electrolyte imbalance is a sodium depletion. Sodium is an important element in maintaining osmotic stability within body tissues. In cases of chronic renal failure, congestive heart disease, cirrhosis of the liver, inappropriate intake of water or secretion of antidiuretic hormone, the resulting sodium deficiency leads to the electrolyte abnormality of hyponatraemia, often shown by tiredness and confusion. Although not as common, it can be induced iatrogenically (i.e. induced as a consequence of medical interventions, often polypharmacy), particularly in older people who are prescribed diuretics. Diuretics can cause excessive sodium to be excreted. In turn, this leads to electrolyte disturbances which then results in confusion.

Electrolyte imbalance is often seen towards the end of life where multiple organ failure sets in (Keeley 2007). Furthermore, the habitual use of laxatives, a common practice by some people with eating disorders and older people, can lead to problems of hydration, electrolyte imbalance and eventual confusion (Kumar et al 2007). Electrolyte disturbances can also result from an inadequate intake of food and drink, i.e. malnutrition. In addition, malnutrition can result in the body lacking the vitamins thiamine and B_{12}. The deficiency of these leads to changes in mental health observed by characteristics such as forgetfulness, depression, irritability and confusion. Factors such as infections, vitamin deficiencies and electrolyte imbalances can mimic some of the signs of dementia. This is one of the reasons why, when a person is being assessed for a dementia, a full blood screen is taken.

Reflection and portfolio evidence

Drawing on your experience to date and/or on your next clinical placement consider the following:

- How do you feel about caring for someone who is acutely confused – and what has influenced these feelings?
- What factors have you encountered that have caused a delirium in a patient you have helped nurse?
- What blood test is undertaken to determine whether someone has an electrolyte imbalance?
- How do you know if diuretics are working effectively?
- How would you establish if someone was malnourished?

Poisoning

In addition to environmental toxins, poisons that cause confusion include alcohol and drugs. The misuse and abuse of alcohol or drugs which was once considered a problem only among the young is now becoming a growing problem among people of all age groups, including older people. The misuse of alcohol or other substances is a common cause of physical and mental health problems, especially in older men. Older adults are particularly vulnerable to the mental and physical effects of these substances because the changes that happen through ageing that mean these poisons cannot be metabolized rapidly by the liver as they can with a younger healthy person (McLoughlin & Farrell 1997).

Alcohol

Intoxication with alcohol can lead to short-term confusion and, sometimes, memory lapses associated with brain damage. In turn, this can result in physical, psychological and social problems. In the long term, prolonged excessive consumption of alcohol can cause vitamin B_{12} deficiency, leading to irreversible damage to the brain, and the development of Korsakoff syndrome, of which chronic confusion is one of the main features.

Drugs

Drug-related confusion may result from:

- an overdose; either accidental or intentional
- the drug's cumulative effect
- an interaction between different drugs
- underlying predisposing factors such as the person's reaction to the drug(s).

According to the National Institute of Drug Abuse (2007), confusion can result from the misuse and abuse of many of the most common recreational and hard drugs. In addition, confusion can be induced by certain neuroleptic drugs and compound analgesics. In addition, some stimulants and sedatives can also lead to disorientation with time, place or person if they are stopped suddenly, particularly in people who have abused illicit drugs or alcohol.

Ghodse (1995) noted that a wide range of psychoactive drugs can impair an individual's general awareness and ability to concentrate. In particular, lysergic acid diethylamide (LSD or acid) results in altered perception and confusion. The illicit use of 3,4-methylenedioxymethamphetamine (MDMA, better known as ecstasy) has always been a public concern. MDMA, banned in the UK since 1971 as a class A drug, has been popularized as a recreational drug among contemporary youth culture arising from the mistaken belief that it has relatively harmless properties. MDMA inhibits the reuptake of serotonin leading to an accumulation of excessive amounts of the neurotransmitter within the neural

synapses. This gives the euphoric feelings associated with taking the drug. Excessive serotonin also raises the body temperature, which can result in dehydration, inappropriate blood clotting, convulsions and coma (Jones & Owens 1996). Following publicity of this fact, many users attempted to compensate for the dehydration by drinking copious amounts of water. Day (1996) found that some users of MDMA drank so much water that they severely disturbed their electrolyte balance. In the long term, exposure to MDMA damages the neuroreceptors and reduces the secretion of serotonin (Kish et al 2000), which is associated with depression, memory impairment and, subsequently, confusion.

For multiple reasons, older people are more likely to be prescribed medication for new conditions and to continue with existing long-term medication. Occasionally, due to the side-effects of the drugs, or due to the interaction of a combination of drugs, confusion in the form of an iatrogenic dementia can develop (Strickland et al 1999).

Decision–making exercise

To celebrate a milestone birthday, Jeremy Banko, with a group of his friends, went out drinking and then on to a night club. After he collapsed on the dance floor, he was taken to the nearest accident and emergency department. The paramedics established from his friends that Jeremy took some ecstasy tablets approximately 45 minutes prior to collapsing. During the assessment the nurse observed and documented that Jeremy was alternately very talkative and very quiet, hypotensive, tachycardic, pyrexial and he appeared to be dehydrated; he was also showing signs of agitation resulting in verbal aggressive behaviour and was overly responsive to being touched.

- How do you feel about what Jeremy allegedly did and what are the likely consequences for the way you would care for him?
- What immediate nursing actions would be taken to stabilize Jeremy's physiological condition?
- What medical interventions may be made to limit the effects of the drug?
- How would the nursing and medical actions be affected by Jeremy's mental state?
- How might Jeremy be supported to enjoy safer nights out with his friends and take more responsibility for his health?

Trauma

Physical damage to the brain can result in confusion (Engel & Romano 2004). The nature of the confusion is governed by the part of the brain affected and the extent of the injury. If the injury is minor and reversible then it is likely that the confusion will reverse as the trauma subsides. For example, confusion arising from concussion reduces as the concussion resolves. On the other hand, if the confusion arises from a major trauma that has caused permanent damage to the brain, complete recovery is unlikely. Agitation, restlessness, and aggression arising from confusion are frequently found in the early stages of recovery from traumatic brain injury. These behavioural symptoms can slow down or disrupt patient care and impede rehabilitation efforts (Levy et al 2005). In severe cases of traumatic head injury, residual confusion may persist and may need careful management and in particular avoiding triggers that induce agitation, restlessness, and aggression.

Dementia

Alzheimer's disease

Alzheimer's disease is presently the commonest type of dementia in the developed world. However, it is becoming clearer that there are many variations of Alzheimer's and that we no longer think of it as one type only. Ultimately, in Alzheimer's disease(s), the cerebral cortex can be seen to atrophy. This means that there is shrinkage of the brain in the areas that are responsible for cognitive and intellectual functioning. It occurs as the result of several processes from the build up of amyloid plaques and neurofibrillary tangles. These plaques are found outside of the neurons and impair their function.

The neurofibrillary tangles are composed of a protein called tau protein. Tau proteins play a crucial role in the structure of the neuron. In people with Alzheimer's tau proteins cause abnormality through overactive enzymes resulting in the formation of neurofibrillary tangles which in turn cause the death of the cells. In Alzheimer's disease the number of tangles becomes so large that they interfere with the functioning of the brain. See the Evolve presentations for further details on types of dementia, more information on the medical diagnosis of delirium and dementia and what nurses need to know.

evolve

17.1 – PEOPLE'S EXPERIENCES WITH ACUTE CONFUSION/ DELIRIUM AND DEMENTIA

- Understand what it might feel like to experience acute confusion/delirium.
- Know how to address the concerns of families/carers.
- Understand what it might feel like to experience dementia.

It has generally been thought that the signs found in people with dementia reflect the widespread and progressive deterioration of function in the cortex and extending into sensorimotor cortical areas as well. Consequently, Alzheimer's disease is characterized by progressive mental and functional deterioration. This results in changes to people's:

- memory
- language
- cognitive abilities (e.g. concentration, problem solving, sequencing of tasks, way finding)
- personality
- mood
- emotions
- physical health.

However, it is now known that some of the consequences seen in people with dementia are not entirely due to physiological changes associated with dementia but more to do with how others treat the person with dementia and negative effects from the environment. Kitwood (1997: 49–53) captures this very well proposing the following 'equation' to explain' what we see in dementia:

$$1 D = P + B + H + NI + SP$$

P = Personality, which includes coping styles and defences against anxiety

B = Biography, and responses to the changes in circumstances associated with later life

H = Health status, including the acuity of the senses

NI = Neurological impairment, separated into its location, type and intensity

SP = Social psychology (relationships between people) which constitutes the fabric of everyday life

Thus D, which = dementia, can be viewed as the product of a complex interaction between the five elements of the above equation.

Vascular dementia

In the developed world, vascular disease is thought to be the second most common cause of dementia. Vascular disease is at least partially preventable and treatable, so increasing awareness of the association of managing blood pressure for example, may decrease the incidence of dementia in the longer term. Vascular dementia may progress in stages; each stage can consist of some deterioration with the possibility of a period of partial recovery. This type of dementia can also be called Multi-Infarct Dementia and its features include:

- Sudden difficulty or in comprehension when doing routine tasks
- Confusion
- Irritability or aggression
- Balance and co-ordination difficulties
- Absence of speech or changes in speech
- Drowsiness or sleepiness
- Occasionally people may have convulsions or seizures. These might only happen once or may continue to be a problem for the person intermittently and may signal the beginning of another phase of deterioration.

Lewy body dementia

Another form of dementia that is being more frequently diagnosed is Lewy Body dementia and is said to be a variant of

Alzheimer's. Lewy bodies are tiny, spherical protein deposits found in nerve cells in the brain. Their presence disrupts the brain's normal functioning, specifically interrupting the action of important chemical messengers, including acetylcholine and dopamine. The onset of Lewy Body can be very similar to that of Alzheimer's. Early symptoms include changes to:

- Language
- Memory
- Ability to judge space and distance
- Slowness of movement
- Stiffness and tremor
- States of confusion – which may vary in degree from day to day
- Hallucination – (auditory or visual)
- Parkinsonian symptoms – such as tremors or jerkiness
- Delusions – can be quite common
- Depression – can be quite common.

In a few cases, the person experiences changes in their heart rate and blood pressure to the extent it may result in unsteady balance/fainting. Abilities and mood can change very quickly, and might fluctuate. This can make life very puzzling for the family and/or carer.

Pick's disease

Pick's Disease, also referred to as frontal lobe dementia, usually begins in younger people (aged 40 to 65 years) and can have many similarities to that of Alzheimer's. Early symptoms are alterations in the personality and may consist of some of the following:

- Lack of inhibition (may behave in inappropriate ways, e.g. anti-social/aggressive)
- Loss of judgment
- Some loss of language
- Some loss of memory
- Difficulty recognizing ordinary objects
- Obsessional (repeating) behaviour
- Overeating (especially sweet things)
- Putting objects (other than food) into their mouth
- Inappropriate emotions e.g. crying, laughing, grimaces and gesturing
- Often unable to recognize people close to them.

Other dementias

About 10% of people with Parkinson's Disease also develop dementia. Other less common forms of dementia include: Huntington's Disease; Aids Related Dementia; Creutzfeldt-Jakob Disease (C.J.D.) and Korsakoff's Disease or Alcohol related dementia. People with Down's Syndrome and other learning disabilities as they are living longer, are developing dementia at increased rates. It is said that up to 40% of people with Downs will develop a dementia if they live to the age of 60 (Arshad et al 2001). The term 'younger onset dementia' is used to describe any form of dementia diagnosed in people under the age of sixty-five. Although most dementias affect people who are over this age, occasionally younger people in their 30s, 40s and 50s are diagnosed with dementia.

Another model of physiological causes of confusion is shown in Evolve presentation 17.2.

17.2 – DIAGNOSIS OF ACUTE CONFUSION/DELIRIUM AND DEMENTIA

- Describe how delirium is diagnosed.
- Differentiate between delirium, functional psychosis and dementia.
- Construct a definition of dementia.
- List the most frequently occurring types of dementia.

PSYCHOSOCIAL FACTORS

PSYCHOLOGICAL CAUSES OF CONFUSION

Confusion can arise from a number of psychological factors and may be due either to already existing predisposing factors within the person or to precipitating factors (Inouye 1999). It is vital to appreciate that psychological factors always have some contribution to make to delirium, in terms of how the person is able to keep away or minimize the effects of changes in their mental state or in terms of how they respond to the effects of delirium (MacLeod 2006). Functional disorders that give rise to perceptual dysfunctions, such as delusions or hallucinations, can also lead to confusion as the person's sense of reality changes and they experience and react to a reality that is not shared by others around them.

Psychological symptoms of depression are common in patients with delirium. Up to 40% of patients referred to mental health services with suspected depressive illness have delirium (Meagher 2001). Distinguishing delirium from depression is particularly important since in addition to delaying appropriate treatment, many antidepressants have marked anticholinergic activity and if given to a individuals with acute confusion, can worsen the confusion/delirium. It is necessary to keep in mind that a person can develop an acute confusion or delirium on top of an existing dementia. Whatever psychological factors are involved in the causation of delirium, a delirium presents significant distress which in turn has further psychological impact. A structured approach to recognizing, assessing and managing delirium and compassionately supporting the person through their experience is therefore essential.

THE EXPERIENCE OF DELIRIUM

Acute confusion or delirium is not simply a clinical sign or a syndrome. For those experiencing delirium it is a lived experience – and possibly a fearful one (Fagerberg & Eriksdotter Jönhagen 2002). Additionally, it is one where most people retain and recall their experience, like vivid but strange dreams, and this may have implications for subsequent psychological care (Fleminger 2002). Given the way in which the person can present during a delirium in regards to their varying grasp of reality, this is easy to lose sight of (Burns et al 2004).

Schofield (2007) describes the experience of delirium as being either hyperactive or hypoactive.

With the hyperactive experience, the person can experience changes from misperception that result in them being:

- restless
- excitable
- on guard – suspicious
- wanting to be continuously on the move
- searching
- shouting
- resistive
- experiencing visual hallucinations.

With a hypoactive experience you will find that the person becomes less active both physically and psychologically. Consequently the person can be:

- less alert
- slower in responses and speech
- apathetic
- sleepy and harder to rouse
- indifferent to what is going on around them.

The few accounts of experiences of delirium in the literature indicate that many people experience a mix of both of the above (Schofield 2007, Sörensen Duppils & Wikblad 2007).

THE EXPERIENCE OF DEMENTIA

There have for many years been accounts written by families and carers about the person with dementia. Echoing this, much of the research was also carried out with families and carers as it was thought that people with dementia could not contribute and indeed did not have anything useful to contribute. Until the last 10 years there has been little written by people with dementia themselves. However, there are now more accounts being written by people with dementia about their experiences of living with dementia. The writing takes on various forms such as narrative, poetry and factual accounts of receiving treatment and care. People with dementia are also sharing their experiences through paintings and other creative forms of expression. These expressions often provide very candid and personal descriptions of experiences, thoughts and feelings.

To 'hear' more from people with dementia visit http://www.dasninternational.org/presentations.php

Being given a diagnosis of dementia can lead to a range of emotions and responses including depression and anger. However, it can also lead people to clarify what is important to them in their life and to make plans for their future. It is vital that nurses, whatever their own values and beliefs about dementia, are able to care for and support people with dementia to live as meaningful and as free a life as possible, regardless of the effects of dementia. Thus 'cognitive' rehabilitation is important in the earlier stages of dementia. As the dementia progresses and people need more care, the emphasis should again be on nursing contributing to the person living as full and actively meaningful a life as possible, until palliative and end of life care is needed.

ENVIRONMENTAL INFLUENCES ON CONFUSION

A variety of environmental factors can contribute to and exacerbate confusion. They include:

- excessive and prolonged noise and/or light
- lack of personal space
- prolonged poor lighting
- distortion of light and darkness
- a lack of familiar people along with too many unfamiliar people
- unfamiliar routine and the busyness of the routine.

Some people experience an increase in their symptoms around dusk when natural lighting changes in their environment. This is sometimes referred to as sundown syndrome or sundowning (Dewing 2000, Sörensen Duppils & Wikblad 2007). As well as changes in light causing problems, noise, particularly excessive noise, is highly 'toxic' to people with confusion (Schofield & Dewing 2001). Marshall (2001) contends noise is as disabling to people with confusion as stairs are to people who use wheelchairs.

A familiar environment is particularly important in the care of all people experiencing delirium (Simon et al 1997) and those living with a dementia. Most people function adequately in their own or their usual environment, but will deteriorate rapidly if moved to a new unfamiliar environment. This is because the nature of the syndrome and disease makes their intellectual functioning less effective, combined with the effects of an unfamiliar environment that creates more demands on the person than they have the competence for. Indeed this excess challenge can mean people lose preserved abilities at an accelerated rate, even temporarily. This, in dementia, is sometimes referred to as 'excess disability' and in part it explains why a person changes their competence from one setting to another within a short time scale.

Attention to reducing the 'strangeness' of the immediate environment should consequently form a core part of any care planning. It also plays a role in a therapy known as reality orientation therapy – a strategy that can be used to help some individuals who are confused. However, it should be noted that after a certain point in the dementia process reality orientation can bring people more distress than benefits. The layout of wards, units and the home, including hallways, doorways and exits, directional signing, signing of spaces and places (e.g. toilets and dining areas) and the design and décor of an area can all be modified or adapted to better suit the needs of people with confusion. People with dementia need similar clear and uncluttered environments; however, they should also be sensorily stimulating and promote interest (learning), pleasure and fun.

Reflection and portfolio evidence

Drawing on your experience of a particular care setting where you have nursed someone who has experienced acute confusion or dementia, reflect on:

- How you feel the environment influenced the person's competence?
- What did you do to make the immediate bed-side area (or the area where care was being offered) less strange for the person?
- What else do you feel you could have done?
- Looking more broadly at that setting, what changes could have been made to make the place feel less strange?

See Evolve presentation 17.1, which looks at delirium and dementia from the perspective of people who have it or are living through it.

CARE DELIVERY KNOWLEDGE

NURSING ASSESSMENT OF PEOPLE EXPERIENCING ACUTE CONFUSION/DELIRIUM

It must be remembered that confusion per se is a symptom of an underlying pathological condition rather than a condition in its own right. Where an acute confusion is suspected, the purpose of assessment is to identify and rapidly treat the condition causing the confusion (Wills & Dewing 2001). The individual who is confused will probably have difficulty in comprehending what is said to them and in communicating back, so it is essential that the assessor has good interpersonal skills. This is facilitated by achieving a calm and focused presence, a clear yet gentle approach and the use of active listening and observation skills. Three major areas should form the focus of assessment: physiological, psychological and environmental. If any assessments have been carried out, you should familiarize yourself with these as it may avoid duplication of questions for the patient and/or family.

Physiological and psychological nursing assessment

This part of the assessment is to consider how the underlying physiological factors that may be contributing to the confusion affect the person physically and from this to establish what care is needed to support the person until they are self-caring again. It begins by observing the person to see how they look, for example for signs of illness, discomfort, distress, pallor or flushing of the skin. In particular, observing the condition of the skin will indicate the level of hydration and nutritional state while cyanosis may indicate a poorly oxygenated blood supply to the brain. It is often possible to establish if the person is hyper- or hypoactive from their appearance and facial expressions.

Establishing a relationship will assist with the assessment process. The individual's ability to communicate and comprehend should be also determined as this can give indications of the responsiveness level and any fluctuations in concentration. It may be that aids to communication such as spectacles or a hearing aid are needed, especially for older people. If so, it should be verified that these are worn correctly and are effective, as sensory deficits may add to the person's experience of confusion.

An assessment model will act as a guide as to how to progress with the assessment. For example, in older persons' services there is likely to be a single assessment process in place, which is specific about assessment (Department of Health 2004). Regardless of what model is being used, the nurse needs to gain consent from the person (or their parent/legally authorized representative) to begin any assessment. As part of the assessment, the nurse will record the vital signs of temperature, pulse, respiration and blood pressure. It is important to keep in mind that what you are doing may appear suspicious to the person who is acutely or chronically confused as it may not make sense or it may look like something else that the person has negative feelings about. To help address this possibility, explaining what you are doing and the reasoning behind it is important; as is doing the assessment at a pace that the person can cope with.

To give greater rigour to the assessment, there are a number of ways that a delirium can be identified. Subject to the person's intellectual ability, asking them to count backwards from 20 through to 1 is a simple test for delirium. The person with delirium is generally unable to achieve this without loss of attention. In some situations the onset of delirium is rapid, e.g. in young children following anaesthesia (Funk et al 2007), and assessment will likewise need to be rapid. In more controlled situations and with adults, several screening tools can be used to detect delirium, although they can be time consuming to use for the nurse, exhausting for the person who is confused.

The confusion assessment method (Inouye et al 1990) is a widely used assessment tool. It takes about 5–10 minutes to use (Box 17.1). However, it should be noted that it does

Box 17.1 The Confusion Assessment Method Instrument (adapted from Inouye et al 1990)

1. [Acute Onset] Is there evidence of an acute change in mental status from the patient's baseline?

2A. [Inattention] Did the patient have difficulty focusing attention, for example, being easily distractible, or having difficulty keeping track of what was being said?

2B. (If present or abnormal) Did this behaviour fluctuate during the interview, that is, tend to come and go or increase and decrease in severity?

3. [Disorganized thinking] Was the patient's thinking disorganized or incoherent, such as rambling or irrelevant conversation, unclear or illogical flow of ideas, or unpredictable switching from subject to subject?

4. [Altered level of consciousness] Overall, how would you rate this patient's level of consciousness? (Alert [normal]; Vigilant [hyperalert, overly sensitive to environmental stimuli, startled very easily]; Lethargic [drowsy, easily aroused]; Stupor [difficult to arouse]; Coma; [unrousable]; Uncertain)

5. [Disorientation] Was the patient disoriented at any time during the interview, such as thinking that he or she was somewhere other than the hospital, using the wrong bed, or misjudging the time of day?

6. [Memory impairment] Did the patient demonstrate any memory problems during the interview, such as inability to remember events in the hospital or difficulty remembering instructions?

7. [Perceptual disturbances] Did the patient have any evidence of perceptual disturbances, for example, hallucinations, illusions or misinterpretations (such as thinking something was moving when it was not)?

8A. [Psychomotor agitation] At any time during the interview did the patient have an unusually increased level of motor activity such as restlessness, picking at bedclothes, tapping fingers or making frequent sudden changes of position?

8B. [Psychomotor retardation] At any time during the interview did the patient have an unusually decreased level of motor activity such as sluggishness, staring into space, staying in one position for a long time or moving very slowly?

9. [Altered sleep–wake cycle] Did the patient have evidence of disturbance of the sleep–wake cycle, such as excessive daytime sleepiness with insomnia at night?

From http://www.hartfordign.org/publications/trythis/issue13.pdf

not give an indication of the severity of delirium. The nine cues offer the nurse a structure for assessing delirium.

There are no specific tools for use with children or adults with learning disabilities. With children, the nurse would assess the child using knowledge about developmental stages in particular considering their cognitive milestones, while bearing in mind that many children show indications of developmental 'regression' during periods of stress, anxiety and when separated from their families.

Reflection and portfolio evidence

Based on your reading so far, describe how you would go about assessing a person (choose from either a child, young adult with learning disabilities or an older person with a mild dementia) who is said to have an acute confusion. In your notes make sure you identify the key principles underpinning how you would approach and relate with the person as well as what you would do.

NURSING ASSESSMENT OF PEOPLE EXPERIENCING LONGER TERM CONFUSION

Assessing for dementia is a complex matter. The assessment usually takes place over several weeks and sometimes months. Diagnosis, although complex in the early stages, is best begun earlier rather than later. It is important that nurses contribute to the education of people that getting a proper diagnosis of dementia is essential to:

- Rule out other conditions that may have symptoms similar to dementia and that may be treatable. These include depression, chest and urinary infections, severe constipation, vitamin and thyroid deficiencies and brain tumours.
- Rule out other possible causes of confusion, such as poor sight or hearing, emotional changes and upsets, such as moving or bereavement, or the side-effects of certain drugs or a combination of drugs.
- Get access to advice, information and support from social services, voluntary agencies and support groups.
- Allow the person with dementia to plan and make advance arrangements for the future.
- Enable access to certain drugs – particularly if Alzheimer's disease is diagnosed.

The assessment will usually include a general physical examination and a number of tests, such as blood and urine tests, to identify physical conditions that may be causing the confusion. A series of questions designed to test thinking and memory will also be used and in most cases, where a dementia is suspected, the person will be referred to a specialist for a detailed memory assessment. This may take place in the home, in outpatients, in a day hospital over several weeks or, very occasionally, as a hospital inpatient. In the specialist assessment, the person being diagnosed may undergo a series of detailed and standardized cognitive and psychological tests and a brain scan. It is now becoming more usual that once the diagnosis has been reached it is shared directly with the person whom it concerns. There are more community services (such as support groups and counselling) available to support people and their families once a diagnosis has been shared.

Environmental assessment

It is important to include environmental factors in any assessment as confusion worsens in unfamiliar surroundings (Dewing 2001). For example, when patients are admitted to a ward/unit staffed with unfamiliar people their state of health may deteriorate with a consequent loss of sleep and increased distress. Therefore, when assessing patients in a new environment it must also be considered whether they can function to their fullest abilities in their usual surroundings (Clare 2003). In dementia, the person can sometimes appear more disabled then the degree of their condition would indicate. This is referred to as excess disability (Sabat 1994) and is generally caused by the person being in an unfamiliar environment and where the people in that environment act in such a way that the person with dementia is not able to fully understand what they are doing or what their intention is.

It is helpful to look at the environment and its impact from the patient's perspective. Noise and light are two factors that significantly impact on sensory input and can worsen confusion, both during the day and at night. Both excessive and low levels of sensory input can be detrimental. The number of different staff a person encounters is also a key factor. Signage and orientation cues are also key factors in helping a person work out where they are and what is going on. As a minimum, the person should be able to find their way to the toilet and back to their bed area/room again. The more inadequate the environment is, the more the nurse will need to repeatedly intervene to help the person feel orientated and safe in the environment.

RISK ASSESSMENT

Risk assessment can apply to assessment of the risk of acquiring acute confusion or the risk of there being serious adverse consequences of a confusion once it is acquired. There are numerous systematic reviews that indicate the risk level of acquiring an acute confusion in particular circumstances (e.g. with cardiac and non-cardiac surgery; major elective surgery; hospitalized older people; people with alcohol withdrawal syndrome; post transplantation; and terminal illness). These reviews usually summarize the most likely adverse effects of acquiring an acute confusion and their consequences, and by using this information, Inouye (1999) argues, delirium is preventable in about one third of people.

In addition to the findings reported in the reviews though, other factors influence how nurses assess risk: for example, nurses' own values and beliefs about risk; their level of skill and nursing expertise; the organization's overall approach to risk management; and national policy to risk and accident/incident prevention. There is a growing tendency to prevent all risk in vulnerable patients, in an effort to avoid accidents and incidents. However, the drive to prevent risk must be balanced with the person's human rights, for example to walk and move around freely and decline care. Sometimes excess attention to preventing risk can actually increase restlessness and agitation, and may lead to aggressive expression and behaviours. This makes the lived experience worse for the individual and makes caring for the person more demanding than it needs to be.

PLANNING NURSING CARE FOR PEOPLE WHO ARE CONFUSED

It is now known that multiple interventions are necessary for effective nursing care of the person with confusion/delirium or the person with a dementia. With an acute confusion, this includes an compassionate approach and communication, environmental modifications, multiprofessional team working and rapid, specific interventions to eliminate the known causes (Milisen et al 2005, Schofield 2007). Indeed, Milisen et al (2005) reduced the severity and duration of acute confusion in patients with hip fractures by implementing an education programme for nurses that addressed assessment and administration of analgesia on a regular basis. Similarly, Meagher (2001) identifies six key interventions in terms of environmental and general supportive measures:

- Education of all staff and families about delirium.
- Correcting sensory impairments.
- Providing a safer environment free of clutter.
- Providing an environment with appropriate stimulation and removing/preventing excessive noise.
- Ensuring warmth and nutrition needs are met.
- Use of reality orientation techniques.
- Use of clocks and calendars.

Whatever the intervention, it is necessary to communicate both compassionately, clearly and concisely. Carers should expect to give repeated verbal reminders of the day, time, location and identity of key individuals, such as members of the team and relatives. Avoiding the use of medical jargon and abbreviations and discussion of a confused person in their presence is helpful because such talk could contribute to suspicious and even paranoid thoughts. Where English is not the person's first language then the services of an interpreter will need to be used. The fewer staff that come in contact with the person the better, thus ensuring consistency. Involving family members with care giving can assist in helping the person feel more secure. However, family members and carers may feel uncertain about what to do.

To implement the above research within a plan of care requires simplification of the environment and giving the person as much space as possible. Ensuring that lighting is adequate during the day is important, and, in addition, provide an indirect 40–60 W light at night time. This is best angled towards the ground as this will help to reduce mis-perception. Controlling and ideally preventing sources of excess noise (such as that produced by staff, equipment and visitors) is vital. Provide clear signposts and cues for the person, including a clock, a calendar, a note from the family saying that they know where the person is and when they will be returning, identifying the room or bed area, and a chart with the day's schedule. Having a few familiar objects by the bedside or in the room can be help-ful. Some literature suggests that using the radio and TV can help orientate the person, but other literature suggests avoiding TV and radio as it can lead to sensory overload and worsen confusion. If it is used, then it should not be left on for long periods.

It is possible that the person will be suspicious about receiving care and at times even resistive. Thus introduc-ing different aspects of nursing care slowly can help. It is often necessary to break up care interventions into smal-ler activities rather than expecting to carry out multiple interventions in one episode. The person should be encour-aged to maintain their activity levels and to walk around if this is what they would usually do. Between activity and nursing care, they may need to have a period of sleep. At times, it may be necessary to discuss with other patients any concerns they may have about what the person is doing and their own safety.

Much of what has just been said about planning care for people with acute confusion can also apply for people with dementia. In the earlier stages of dementia, the person is usually able to adjust to a new environment with environ-mental cues and support from people around them. As the dementia progresses the person needs more help to make sense of new places. Nurses tend to adopt a reality orienta-tion approach to working with people who have dementia. This can be helpful up until the point where the person moves completely beyond recognition of place and also moves beyond living in chronological time. In this case the principles of validation therapy are more suited to working in a harmonious way with people who have dementia. Both of these approaches will be outlined now.

Reality orientation

Confusion is usually evident when there are signs of disor-ientation of time, place and person, or any one or more of these three. These cause difficulties for the person regard-ing perception of self, others, the environment and the relationships between them. Reality orientation attempts to address this by using a variety of cues, stimuli and tips to help remember time, place and names. Continued use of reality orientation reduces the need for the person to ask staff/carers the time or the date or the location of places, such as the toilet or bedroom, and it decreases the chance that the person will be labelled confused or disorientated. Holden & Woods (1982) claim it also helps to maintain a safe environment, and promotes a sense of security, dig-nity, independence and self-esteem. There are two main ways of offering reality orientation:

- Intensive group sessions (often as part of a memory sup-port group offered to people with early dementia)
- Ongoing 24-hour reality orientation relying on the use of cues, signs and colours placed at strategic points around the ward/unit or in the person's house. For example, the person may have a colour coded bed area, the toilet may have a clear picture of a toilet on the door, and the living area may have a large clock, a calendar and weather description in a prominent area. Thus adapting the envi-ronment is a part of reality orientation.

If cognitive deterioration is temporary or not so advanced, it may slow the pace of deterioration and it often improves the patient's mental state. Critics of reality orientation argue that it distresses people if expectations are not achieved. It is also criticized for its repetitive nature. Reality orientation is unlikely to help people living with severe dementia.

In practice, reality orientation confronts the individual with facts (such as the day, date, names and news). For example, a nurse may say:

Nurse: 'Hello Mr Smith. My name is Asha.'
Mr Smith: 'Asha . . . who are you? Er, do I know you?'
Nurse: 'I am Asha, the nurse who is looking after you this evening.' [uses hands to show her uniform and name badge at the same time]
Mr Smith: 'Oh yes, . . . I'm in hospital.'

Notice that the use of the nurse's name alone was an insufficient cue for Mr Smith. The nurse repeats the greeting and use of cues every time she meets the patient throughout the shift and encourages or reminds others to do similarly. Each correct response is given positive reinforcement. It is important not to react negatively should an incorrect response be given and to support the person until they can achieve a sense of orientation with people, place and time. The use of reality orientation should be used only to support orientation and not to test the person or to expose deficits. The nurse must be patient in repeating the same cues many times and avoid saying things such as 'What did I just tell you' or 'Do you not remember what I said to you last time?'

Cognitive stimulation therapy (CST) is one specific structured form of reality orientation for people with dementia. It has been developed from the findings of two

Cochrane reviews (Woods et al 2005). This reality orientation therapy incorporates aspects of several psychological therapies, found through scientific trials to improve cognition and behaviour, and generally takes place several times a week in a group session led by a therapist.

Validation therapy

Once a person moves beyond a certain stage in dementia, they become mostly unable to respond to reality orientation. Thus, reality orientation methods should not be used as it is most likely going to lead to frustration and distress. The distress may lead to the person responding and behaving in ways that nurses then find challenging – which then presents a new set of nursing care difficulties. Feil (1982) developed validation therapy as an alternative to the distress she saw as a result of the inappropriate use of reality orientation. Like 24-hour reality orientation, it is an ongoing process. However, unlike reality orientation, it seeks to identify the underlying cause and emotion(s) attached to what the person is saying or doing. To do this, the nurse must not allow any factual errors to interrupt the meaningful dialogue on topics of interest to the individual. The nurse needs to accept the lived reality of person at that time and place. It is hypothesized that the content of 'confused' talk reflects the emotional meaning of past events that are being triggered by the current place or situation. For example, worrying about getting home in time to meet the children from school may reflect that parenting was a time of reward and security or even anxiety. The response to the disorientation is directed at exploring what things were like for that person, and how this relates to how they are feeling now. It is suggested that even the most confused behaviour has some meaning for that person.

Therefore, when a person aged 80 years says something like: 'My father is waiting for me, I must go home,' the nurse does not confront the patient with reality by replying 'Your father is not waiting for you' or even 'Your father is dead and . . .'.

Instead the nurse thinks why the person might need their father, what the father represents to this person and what emotions are attached to this need or want. The nurse's response is focused on the possible emotions.

Nurse: 'You look concerned. It sounds serious wanting your father. Would you like to talk to me?' Or 'Do you miss him badly?'

It remains to be demonstrated how effective validation therapy is. A recent Cochrane Review found insufficient evidence (from the few randomized trials that exist) to allow any conclusion about the efficacy of validation therapy for people with dementia or cognitive impairment (Neal & Barton Wright 2003).

Evolve presentations 17.3 and 17.4 offer more information on the nursing assessment and management of the person with a delirium or dementia.

17.3 – NURSING ASSESSMENT AND MANAGEMENT OF DELIRIUM

- Explore a model for establishing diagnosis.
- Describe the fundamental care needs of a person with delirium.
- Appraise the nursing interventions for the management of delirium.

17.4 – NURSING ASSESSMENT AND MANAGEMENT OF DEMENTIA

- Outline the assessment process for dementia.
- Give examples of the fundamental care needs of patients with dementia.

Decision-making exercise

Mr Navraj Singh, a retired accountant, is admitted to an acute medical ward. He is known to be dehydrated and have a chest infection. Soon after admission, and while waiting for a medical assessment, he becomes increasingly restless. The ward cleaner reports that he has seen Mr Singh stacking up chairs and other pieces of furniture on his bed. When you approach Mr Singh, he tells you that the floor is dirty and he is worried about the things he can see on the floor, although he does not elaborate on what these 'things' are. You can see he has poured the contents of his water jug on the floor, along with numerous tissues and the newspaper. He says he wants his wife immediately and is beginning to look and call out for her. The other patients in the four bedded area and their visitors seem to be watching him.

- How would you assess the situation?
- What skills would you need to draw on when interacting with Mr Singh?
- What are the priorities for Mr Singh's care?
- How would you prepare Mrs Singh when she arrives to visit her husband?

Policy background

Following publication of *A First Class Service: Quality in the New NHS* (Department of Health 1998), a number of national standards were set and are being implemented via the National Service Frameworks (NSF) for Mental Health (Department of Health 1999b), Older People (Department of Health 2001) and Long Term Conditions (Department of Health 2005). The NSFs are key tools for delivering the government's health and social care strategy. There is also a forthcoming national strategy on dementia care that will be significant in shaping the design and delivery of care.

People covered by these three NSFs are said to be the most intensive users of the most expensive services. Further, the numbers are increasing due to factors such as an ageing population, health inequalities and certain lifestyle choices that people make. All these groups of people are not just high users of primary and specific acute services but also social care and community services and often of urgent and emergency care. The Department of Health contends that there are huge benefits to the population and financial savings if health and social care communities invest in effective interventions and management. Key themes in the NSFs are about independent living for as long as possible, care planned around the needs and choices of the individual, easier, timely access to services and joint working across all agencies and disciplines involved.

Whenever possible, the plan of care should be made with the cooperation of all involved in the care, for example informal carers, relatives and members of the multidisciplinary team (Department of Health 2000, 2002) and, most importantly, the person with confusion. However, with a severely confused person, this may be beyond their ability at some points in time (see section on capacity and consent later in this chapter). Plans must also incorporate strategies to assist carers to cope with the needs of the person who is confused, particularly if they have a dementia. Over a period of time, this is likely to include providing information about the pattern of the illness, promoting involvement in the care process, providing information about benefits, accessing support agencies, coordinating health and social care services and how to comment and/or complain.

SUPPORTING FAMILIES AND CARERS

Informal carers comprise families, friends and neighbours. At the present time around 6 million people in Great Britain have some informal caring responsibilities (Department of Health 1999a). Around half of these are within the working age range of 45–65 years, with the majority of the remainder being over the age of 65 (Department of Health 2002). However, some informal carers are of school age (Department of Health 1999a). With adequate support, informal carers can continue to maintain a reasonable level of well-being and social contact. In most areas of the country, support for informal carers may take the form of a mixture of practical help and support provided by health and social services, charitable or voluntary agencies as well as family, friends and neighbours. With devolution though, each part of the UK is moving towards different provisions for carers. More information on individual rights for carers can be obtained from www.carersuk.org. Additionally, the provision of free nursing and personal care differs across the UK and many carers and families find negotiating the referral and assessment systems in health and social care stressful and some say there is an inequity across the UK.

Informal carers play an important part in meeting the needs of those with acute and longer term illness, extreme frailty and disabilities. They are often placed or find themselves under great strain through caring responsibilities combined with the broader consequences of being a carer (financial hardship; social isolation; perceived lack of support). Some informal carers become ill themselves as a result of the stress of caring for their relative (Hunt 2003). For some carers, particularly those caring for people with dementia, sleep is often disturbed, which impacts adversely on health and coping resilience. In practical terms it is a matter of concern when carers experience high distress levels since they become more likely to either provide less quality of care or eventually to stop caring. Unsupported, informal carers can actually worsen their caring and quality of life by generating extreme distress for themselves and the person they are caring for (Lo & Brown 2000). Extremes of stress prevent the carer from being able to adapt to new situations and even from appreciating the healthy aspects of the person they are caring for. At its worst, neglect or abuse may take place (Action on Elder Abuse 2007,http://www.elderabuse.org.uk) so knowing what the signs of abuse are is very important.

Much of the distress associated with caring can be avoided, however, if carers are provided with adequate support (Mitchell 2000). Many carers tend to feel inadequate or guilty at accepting community support and services and many carers also have feelings of concern about quality of care and services their relative may receive. Nurses can contribute towards promoting the health and well-being of carers by reinforcing that accepting community support is a positive action to take and that the carer will still be valued as a key part of a caring team.

Opinions vary about if and how the presence of family members influences the experience of confusion for the person with an acute confusion/delirium. Conn & Lieff (2001) and Segatore & Adams (2001) suggested that families should be encouraged to stay with the person who is experiencing confusion as their presence had positive effects. However, Andersson et al (2003) found that their presence might, in some circumstances, worsen the confusion. The presence of relatives during an acute confusional state is remembered by the confused person (McCurren & Nones Cronin, 2003) where relatives are often perceived as being a rescuer or someone who will make everything clear or even better.

Unusual talk and behaviour from a person who is confused might be experienced as frightening and distressing for many relatives (Milisen et al 1998, Conn & Lieff 2001). Eriksdotter & Jönhagen (2002) argue it is important for nurses to inform families about the symptoms of confusion. Making families aware of the symptoms and that they are likely to be short term can help families adjust for the period of time that the symptoms are present. Helping families use effective interventions can also provide the family with a structure to work with so they feel they are 'doing their best'.

As far as dementia is concerned, the government and care provider organizations (such as NHS and primary care trusts) claim they have made huge efforts in providing an improved range of support options for carers and yet it seems that carers' own organizations still feel that support for carers is inadequate. Within contemporary society, the care of dependent and older frail people often relies on the contribution made by families and informal carers and it is thus hard for the state to repay in real terms all the care that is given by families and friends. Although the Carers and Disabled Children Act 2000 states that carers are entitled to an assessment, it is important that carers are also included within any care plan as it cannot be assumed that they will automatically carry on caring. An admission to hospital or into any care service can often mean a crisis in caring has occurred and thus it becomes a point where decisions might be made about alternative arrangements for care. Within mental health services, carers are seen as an integral part of the National Service Framework for Mental Health (Department of Health 1999b) and the Revised Care Programme Approach (Department of Health 2000). Unfortunately, this was not extended to the National Service Framework for Older People, which only requires the patient to be directly involved in care planning (Department of Health 2001).

The document *Caring about Carers* (Department of Health 1999a) emphasizes the government's commitment to supporting the approximately 6 million carers within the UK, by enabling flexible work patterns and helping carers take a break without losing their employment. The Carers (Equal Opportunities) Act 2004 which came into force in England and in Wales in 2005 gives carers rights to information. For example, Section 1 of the Act places a duty on local authorities to inform carers of their right to a carer's assessment and ensures that work, life-long learning and leisure are considered when a carer is assessed. Section 2 of the Act means that when a carer's assessment is completed, it must take into account whether the carer works or wishes to work, any learning or courses the carer is taking or wishes to take, and any other leisure activities the carer undertakes or wishes to undertake. In an effort to ensure joined up planning, the Act also gives local authorities new powers to gain the help of housing, health, education and other local authorities in providing support to carers. Section 3 states that if the local authority requests another authority to plan services, that authority must give that request due consideration. Further, the Working and Families Act 2006 extends the right of carers to have flexible provision for work. It remains to be seen if this is enough legislation or even if legislation can be responsive to carers' needs.

Evidence-based practice

Many carers now have access to the Internet, either from within their own home, from a local library or through Internet cafes and support groups. There are many useful resources available on the Internet that the practitioner, or increasingly carers, can access; they include:

- Age Concern (http://www.ageconcern.org.uk/)
- Alzheimer's Association (http://www.alz.org/) and Alzheimer Scotland (http://www.alzscot.org/)
- Crossroads (http://www.crossroads.org.uk/English/carers.htm#how)
- Help the Aged (http://www.helptheaged.org.uk/)
- Saga (http://www.saga.co.uk/)
- Princess Royal's Trust for Carers (see sections on young carers) (http://www.carers.org/)
- http://www.mecopp.org.uk/ provides a variety of services to black and minority ethnic carers and communities locally, regionally and nationally in Scotland.

These websites are some of the ones that have been around for some time. The Evolve presentations list other websites that may be useful to you. It is always worthwhile keeping up to date with these and other related sites as they offer useful insights into the implementation of policy, information that you can use with families and carers and for getting a deeper appreciation of carers' and families' lived experiences.

Reflection and portfolio evidence

Amaka is caring for her mother full time. Amaka has given up her job to care for her mother and also has two teenage children studying for exams, to care for. They live in the family home in a busy central city street. Amaka's mother has advanced dementia. She goes to an Afro-Caribbean day centre twice a week. Amaka feels she manages to care for her mother well during the day. Recently, her mother has started getting out of bed at night looking for the toilet. However, if Amaka does not get up in time, her mother seems to end up walking downstairs and often tries to get out of the house through the front door. Amaka is now feeling very tired with her sleep being regularly disrupted and exams coming up soon.

- How might the children be affected by having their grandmother living with them?
- What financial problems might Amaka and her family experience?
- How can looking after her mother affect Amaka's health and well-being?
- What interventions might be suggested to help Amaka's mother find her way to the toilet at night and to prevent her leaving the house?

PROFESSIONAL AND ETHICAL KNOWLEDGE

NEGATIVE ATTITUDES TOWARDS PEOPLE WHO ARE CONFUSED

Negative attitudes can range from thinking that people who are confused are funny or entertaining because of their disorientated talk and behaviours or they are difficult to nurse because of the altered behaviour, memory impairment and resistiveness to care and treatment. Rogers & Gibson (2002) found that nurses felt that caring for acutely confused patients increased their workload, threatened their safety, affected their self-esteem and created mental conflicts about what was the best way to care for the person. Where there is any passive acceptance of confusion as being 'expected' or that it is an inevitable characteristic of a particular condition, disorder or experience, complacency can be fostered as can a less than compassionate approach to caring for the person. This can lead to low self-esteem, dependence and isolation and further confusion. It is therefore important to nurture a shared view within teams that confusion, as in acute confusion/delirium, is a medical emergency and should be responded to as such (unless it emerges at the end of life, although even in this situation it is still possible to alleviate symptoms). It is impossible to overemphasize the importance of a comprehensive medical and nursing assessment to help identify the cause(s) of the confusion and endeavour to promote a realistic programme of care or management. In order to improve the probablity of care being accepted by the person who is confused, the nurse needs to establish a trusting relationship and demonstrate skills in being both technically competent and compassionate. Promoting a relationship with a person who is confused, either acutely confused or with a dementia, can be challenging and the nurse must be prepared to work with the person who might have challenging behaviours. To establish an effective helping relationship, the fundamentals of promoting respect, privacy and dignity for the person, whatever their altered cognitive state, is core to nursing practice.

ATTITUDES TOWARDS OLDER PEOPLE

There is an interrelationship between personal and professional values (Dewing 2007). All nurses bring their personal values and beliefs with them into their work in some way. Values form part of what is sometimes referred to as personal or tacit knowledge, therefore they need active reflection to see how they influence ways of working in health care. Given working with older people often produces situations where values and beliefs can be core to decision making, care planning and care delivery, it seems reasonable to argue that nurses need to reflect on their values and beliefs about ageing and older persons. Developing critical insight is an essential skill in nursing as this helps to set personal standards to work along with professionally required standards laid down to nurses by the Nursing and Midwifery Council.

A central value, to be examined when choosing to work with older people, is ageism. Ageism is pervasive in Western cultures and affects all age groups, but is directed mainly at older people (Heath 1999: 12). Ageism, often referred to as age discrimination, exists in many areas of life such as consumerism, design, crime, media, civic and voluntary life and politics. Fundamentally, ageism is an abuse of human rights, which causes personal suffering and hardship and cultural and economic problems. It was reported in *Adding Life to Years* (Department of Health 2002) that although 17% of older people felt that they had received an inferior service to younger people, evidence to substantiate these claims was not found. The report cautions, however, that because no evidence was found, it does not follow that ageism is absent from the National Health Service. Indeed, Age Concern found that within contemporary society, ageism remains a major problem, particularly in health care (Age Concern 2006).

Stereotypes, myths and ageism are reinforced in a society that values the younger generations more than the older generations. As part of ageism, the phenomenon of stereotyping can occur. In stereotyping, all older people are 'lumped together' into a generally negative portrayal. This includes older people (or the 'elderly') being seen as being frail, cantankerous or confused. The National Service Framework for Older People (Department of Health 2001) has as its first standard the theme of preventing ageism in health care. However, the new law on age discrimination which came into force in England in October 2006 only covers the areas of employment, training and education; it does not provide protection against age related discrimination in health and social care services.

CAPACITY AND CONSENT

Increasingly issues of capacity and informed consent may be raised in relation to the treatment of delirium. Urgent interventions needed to prevent serious deterioration or death, or in the interests of a patient's safety, are deemed to be covered by common law in the United Kingdom. Although opinions differ, most agree that (a) if medical colleagues would deem a treatment appropriate and (b) if reasonable people would want the treatment themselves, then it can be given if urgently necessary. Mental capacity legislation is now in effect across Scotland, England and Wales and must be addressed alongside common law.

The Mental Capacity Act 2005 which came into effect in England and Wales during 2007 affects everyone aged 16 years and over and provides a statutory framework to empower and protect people who may not be able to make some decisions for themselves, for example, people with dementia, learning disabilities, mental health problems, stroke or brain injuries, or for any other reason. It provides clear guidelines for carers and professionals about who can take decisions in which situations. At its heart, the Act states that everyone should be treated as able to make their own decisions until it is properly shown that they cannot. It also aims to enable people to make their own decisions for as long as they are capable of doing so, even where those decisions might go against what professionals would feel were best or 'right' in any particular situation. A person's capacity to make a decision will be established at the time that a decision needs to be made (i.e. it is situational). A lack of capacity could be present because of a severe learning disability, dementia, mental health problems, a brain injury, a stroke or unconsciousness due to an anaesthetic or a sudden accident. However, it must no longer be assumed that capacity is lacking simply due to a diagnosis or condition. There is also a new criminal offence of neglect or ill-treatment of a person who lacks capacity.

The Act also sets out to protect people who lose the capacity to make their own decisions. It will allow the person, while they are still able, to appoint someone (for example a trusted relative or friend) to make decisions on their behalf once they lose the ability to do so. This will mean they can make decisions on the person's health and personal welfare. (Previously, the law only covered decision making for financial matters.) It will ensure that decisions made by others, on the person's behalf, are in their best overall interests and wherever possible will be based on the person's known wishes and preferences. To assist this, the Act provides a checklist of things that decision makers must work through. It also introduces a code of practice for healthcare workers, including nurses, who support people who have lost the capacity to make their own decisions.

PERSONAL AND REFLECTIVE KNOWLEDGE

APPLYING THE KNOWLEDGE IN THIS CHAPTER TO ALL BRANCHES OF NURSING

You can develop the section of your portfolio on working with people who are experiencing short term or longer term confusion by collecting summarized and synthesized information or evidence gathered from multiple aspects of your work (activities and projects you have been involved in as well as day-to-day practice), clinical supervision, research, websites, journal articles and written reflections. Remember that accounts by patients/users can also count as evidence.

To complete your portfolio you need to provide *synthesized* evidence of insight into personal and professional growth (Stuart 1998). (Descriptive reflection alone is not sufficient.) This is achieved by summarizing from a number of reflections on how your (1) feelings, (2) values and beliefs, (3) knowledge and skills have developed over time, again using structured reflection on your own or alongside mentorship and/or clinical supervision where necessary to assist this process.

Examples that you could include within your portfolio are:

- Evidence of any activity, project and papers/articles that you used when working with a person who was confused or their families/carers showing how you drew on theory to inform your practice and how effective this was.
- Summaries from your reflections of caring with a person with confusion – setting out what you have learned, what you now do differently and what you still need to develop and how this will be achieved.
- Identifying your level/experience/personal ability in caring for a person with confusion and supporting their family/carer.

- Identifying the transferable skills you have developed when caring for people who are confused, that you can use in future practice.

CASE STUDIES ON THE CARE OF PEOPLE EXPERIENCING CONFUSION

Four scenarios now follow, one from each branch of nursing. You should work through the relevant one for you and respond to the questions to help you consolidate the knowledge you have gained from this chapter. Reading through the others might also be of interest to you.

Case study: Mental health

George Ferguson has been referred to the community mental health team. George, a retired local policeman, has lived in the same house since his marriage to Ida 58 years ago. A year ago Ida died and since that time there has been a progressive deterioration in George's behaviour. He has lost a significant amount of weight, and more recently he has been found by neighbours 'wandering' around his village. Neighbours are very supportive. Recently he has taken to sleeping during the day and leaving his house, with the doors open, at night. His neighbours find him very forgetful and generally disorganized. One neighbour contacted the GP after smelling smoke coming from the house and finding a pan of beans burnt out on the gas ring of the cooker.

- What are the possible causes for George's current problems?
- What might George feel his problems or needs are?
- What information should the community psychiatric nurse obtain in the assessment and why?

- What support and community services might be available to help George to remain at home for as long as possible?
- On what basis would a decision be made that George might require admission to a nursing home?

Case study: Adult

Frank Hecker, originally from Austria, is a 58-year-old retired dentist. He is admitted to the accident and emergency department after being found in a collapsed state in the street. He smells strongly of alcohol, is very restless and at times agitated, and appears disorientated of time, date and place. He is also tearful and verbally aggressive towards staff. When you are attending to him he keeps mistaking you for one of his friends and calls you 'Anya'. You notice in your assessment that his chest sounds congested, and you can see and feel his extremities are cyanosed. You also think that you can smell acetone on his breath as well as the smell of alcohol.

- What are the possible reasons for Frank's behaviour?
- What immediate actions should be taken by nursing and medical staff?
- How will you explain to Frank what is happening to him?

Case study: Child

Kimberley Kingston, aged 8 years, was cycling when she hit the kerb and fell off her bike, hitting her head on the ground as she landed. She is reported to have lost consciousness briefly and was brought into the accident and emergency department. A skull X-ray shows no sign of a fracture, but she is to be kept in hospital overnight for observation. Kimberley is frightened and does not appear to know where she is or why she is there. She has no recollection of the accident.

- Why has Kimberley's confusion arisen?
- What immediate actions should be taken to help reduce Kimberley's confusion?
- How long would you expect Kimberley's confusion to last?
- How will you explain to the parents and younger sister what is happening and what support might they need?

Case study: Learning disabilities

Pravin Dutt, a 34-year-old man, acquired brain damage at birth. Since the death of his mother 9 years ago he has been living in a group bungalow with live-in carers. Using the continued support from his carers Pravin has coped well with day-to-day activities of living. He has also benefited from an active behaviour modification programme.

Recent changes in management and organization at the home with new staff arriving and a new resident have resulted in Pravin becoming much more dependent upon others, in particular with elimination, and he has developed faecal incontinence. His GP felt he might be depressed and prescribed a course of an antidepressant medication. This has been followed by changes in his mental state manifesting as disorientation of time, date and place, restlessness and challenging behaviour.

- Identify the most probable causes for Pravin's change in behaviour.
- What actions should the carers take to relieve Pravin's distress?
- What actions could be taken to minimize Pravin's faecal incontinence?
- What are the likely outcomes of the nursing actions taken and when would you expect them to be achieved by?

SUMMARY

This chapter has explored how physiological, psychological and environmental factors can lead to the development of confusion. The main points stressed are as follows:

1. An acute confusion/delirium is symptomatic of an underlying pathology and the focus of the initial nursing assessment must be to help identify the cause and establish what symptoms the person who is confused needs nursing interventions for.
2. Acute confusion, while a medical emergency, is generally treatable.
3. Long-term confusion, specifically associated with dementia, is usually as a result of an untreatable organic pathology and only amenable to symptomatic medical management, although there is much that nursing can offer to support the person maintain their quality of life for as long as possible.
4. Although older people are the most likely to experience both acute and longer term confusion, there are many stereotyped views on both confusion and older people (especially those living with dementia). Thus, it is important to be aware of these in order to give appropriate and compassionate care.
5. No matter how confused a person appears the fundamentals of privacy, dignity, respect and consent are still central aspects of nursing care.
6. Various strategies from assessment and care planning can help the person and their families/carers while they are experiencing confusion. Central to nursing interventions is providing the best environment possible in which the person is nursed.

7. It is important to remember that the use of medication with neuroleptic effects is rarely recommended.

Annotated further reading and websites

Irving K, Foreman M 2006 Delirium, nursing practice and the future. International Journal of Older People Nursing 1:121–127

Neville S 2006 Delirium and older people: repositioning nursing care. International Journal of Older People Nursing 1:113–120

Bryden C 2005 Dancing with dementia. Jessica Kingsley, London
Written by a woman living with dementia, this book offers a detailed and helpful account of one person's journey with dementia, both the desperation and joy of life with a condition that reduces cognitive abilities and ultimately will end her life.

Wilkinson H, Kerr D, Cunningham C, Rae C 2004 Home for good? Preparing to support people with a learning disability living in residential settings when they develop dementia. Final Report. Joseph Rowntree Foundation, York

Wilkinson H, Kerr D 2004 Top tips: fact sheet for caring for people with learning disability and dementia. Joseph Rowntree Foundation, York
Both the above are available from the Joseph Rowntree Foundation – www.jrf.org.uk

Kerr D 2007 Understanding learning disability and dementia: developing effective interventions. Jessica Kingsley, London

This book covers all the essential issues in supporting a person with a learning disability when they develop dementia. It provides essential knowledge for anyone involved in the provision of services, assessment of need and direct care and support for people with a learning disability who also have a dementia.

Buijssen H 2005 The simplicity of dementia: a guide for families and carers. Jessica Kingsley, London

This book offers an introduction for relatives, carers and professionals looking after or training to work with people with dementia. The book sets out and draws on two 'laws of dementia'. The author explains the causes of communication problems, mood disturbances and 'deviant' behaviours, with particular emphasis on how these are experienced by the person with dementia. The book contains numerous case examples.

http://www.alzheimers.org.uk
This is the Alzheimer's Society website. It is an excellent, comprehensive website that contains resources for practitioners, carers and people living with dementia, not only of Alzheimer disease but also for people who have acquired CJD. The library section also contains an excellent resource of downloadable papers for professional use.

http://www.alzscot.org/pages/carer.htm
This is the Alzheimer Scotland website, which also contains useful resources.

http://www.direct.gov.uk/en/CaringForSomeone/DG_071391
A comprehensive website for carers.

References

Action on Elder Abuse 2007 Available online: http://www.elderabuse.org.uk (accessed 8 December 2007)

Age Concern 2006 Ageism: a benchmark of public attitudes in Britain. Available online: http://www.ageconcern.org.uk/AgeConcern/Documents/Ageism_Report.pdf (accessed 23 August 2008)

Andersson EM, HallbergIR, Edberg AK 2003 Nurses' experiences of the encounter with elderly patients in acute confusional state in orthopaedic care. International Journal of Nursing Studies 40:437–448

Arshad P, Sridharan B, Brown R 2001 Treatment for Alzheimer's disease in people with learning disabilities: NICE guidance. British Journal of Psychiatry 179:74

Burns A, Gallagley A, Byrne J 2004 Delirium. Journal of Neurological Neurosurgery and Psychiatry 75(3):362–367

Clare L 2003 Cognitive training and cognitive rehabilitation for people with early-stage dementia. Reviews in Clinical Gerontology 13:75–83

Conn DK, Lieff S 2001 Diagnosing and managing delirium in the elderly. Canadian Family Physician 47:101–108

Day M 1996 The bitterest pill: the drug ecstasy. Nursing Times 92 (7):4–20

Department of Health 1998 A first class service: quality in the new NHS. HMSO, London

Department of Health 1999a Caring about carers: a national strategy for carers. HMSO, London

Department of Health 1999b National service framework (mental health). HMSO, London

Department of Health 2000 Effective care co-ordination in mental health services: modernizing the care programme approach. HMSO, London

Department of Health 2001 National service framework for older people. HMSO, London

Department of Health 2002 Adding life to years: report of the expert group on healthcare of older people. HMSO, London

Department of Health 2004 Single assessment process for older people. HMSO, London

Department of Health 2005 National service framework for long term conditions. HMSO, London

Dewing J 2000 Sundowning: is it a syndrome or not? A literature review. Journal of Dementia Care 8(6):34–37

Dewing J 2001 Care for older people with a dementia in acute hospital settings. Nursing Older People Journal 13(3):18–20

Dewing J 2007 Values underpinning help, support and care. In: Neno R, Aveyard B, Heath H (eds) Older people and mental health nursing: a handbook of care. Blackwell, Oxford, pp 40–51

El-Kaissi S, Kotowicz MA, Berk M, Wall JR 2005 Acute delirium in the setting of primary hypothyroidism: the role of thyroid hormone replacement therapy. Thyroid 15(9):1099–1101

Engel GL, Romano J 2004 Delirium: a syndrome of cerebral insufficiency. Neuropsychiatry Clinical Neurosciences Journal 16:526–538

Eriksdotter Jönhagen M 2002 Delirium in the elderly. Dementia 2:2–7

Fagerberg I, Eriksdotter Jönhagen M 2002 Temporary confusion: a fearful experience. Journal of Psychiatric and Mental Health Nursing 9:339–346

Feil N 1982 Validation: the Feil method. Edward Feil Productions, Cleveland

Fleminger S 2002 Remembering delirium. British Journal of Psychiatry 180:4–5

Funk W, Hollnberger H, Geroldinger J 2007 Physostigmine and anaesthesia emergence delirium in preschool children: a randomized blinded trial. European Journal of Anaesthesiology 25(1):37–42

Ghodse H 1995 Drugs and addictive behaviour: a guide to treatment. Blackwell Science, Oxford

Heath H 1999 Perspectives on ageing and older people. In: Heath H, Schofield I (eds) Healthy ageing: nursing older people. Mosby, London, pp 3–20

Holden UP, Woods RT 1982 Reality orientation: psychological approaches to the 'confused' elderly. Churchill Livingstone, Edinburgh

Hunt CK 2003 Concepts in caregiver research. Journal of Nursing Scholarship 35(1):27–32

Inouye SK 1999 Predisposing and precipitating factors for delirium in hospitalised older patients. Dementia and Geriatric Cognitive Disorders 10:393–400

Inouye S, van Dyck C, Alessi C, Balkin S, Siegal A, Horwitz R 1990 Clarifying confusion: the confusion assessment method. Annals of Internal Medicine 113(12):941–948

Jones C, Owens D 1996 The recreational drug user in the intensive care unit: a review. Intensive and Critical Care Nursing 12(3):126–130

Keeley P 2007 Delirium at the end of life. British Medical Journal. Available online: http://clinicalevidence.bmj.com/ceweb/conditions/spc/2405/2405_background.jsp (accessed 6 December 2007)

Kish SJ, Furukwa Y, Ang L et al 2000 Striatal serotonin is depleted in brain of a human MDMA (ecstasy) user. Neurology 55(2):294–296

Kitwood T 1997 Dementia reconsidered: the person comes first. Open University Press, Buckingham

Kumar V, Yoselevitz S, Gambert SR 2007 Laxative use and abuse in the older adult. Clinical Geriatrics 5(5):38–45

Levy M, Berson A, Cook T et al 2005 Treatment of agitation following traumatic brain injury: a review of the literature. Neurorehabilitation 20(4):279–306

Lo R, Brown R 2000 Caring for family carers and people with dementia. International Journal of Psychiatric Nursing Research 6(2):684–694

MacLeod AD 2006 Delirium: the clinical concept. Palliative and Supportive Care 4:305–312

McCurren C, Nones Cronin S 2003 Delirium: elders tell their stories and guide nursing practice. Medical Surgical Nursing 12(5):318–323

McLoughlin D, Farrell M 1997 Substance misuse in the elderly. In: Norman IJ, Redfern SJ (eds) Mental health care for elderly people. Churchill Livingstone, Edinburgh, pp 205–221

Marshall M 2001 Care settings and the care environment. In: Cantley C (ed) A handbook of dementia care. Open University Press, Buckingham

Meagher DJ 2001 Delirium: optimising management. British Medical Journal 322(7279):144–149

Milisen K, Foreman MD, Godderis J, Abraham IL, Broos PL 1998 Delirium in the hospitalized elderly: nursing assessment and management. Nursing Clinics of North America 33(3):417–439

Milisen K, Lemiengre J, Braes T, Foreman MD 2005 Multicomponent intervention strategies for managing delirium in hospitalized older people: systematic review. Journal of Advanced Nursing 52(1):79–90

Mitchell E 2000 Managing carer stress: an evaluation of a stress management programme for carers of people with dementia. British Journal of Occupational Therapy 63(4):179–184

Neal M, Barton Wright P 2003 Validation therapy for dementia. Cochrane Database of Systematic Reviews 2007, Issue 4

NHS and Community Care Act 1990 HMSO, London

National Institute of Drug Abuse 2007 Commonly abused drugs. National Institute of Health, New York

Pisani M A, Araujo K L B, Van Ness P H, Zhang Y, Ely E W, Inouye S K 2006 A research algorithm to improve detection of delirium in the intensive care unit. Critical Care 10(4). Available online: http://ccforum.com/content/10/4/R121 (accessed 6 December 2007)

Rogers AC, Gibson CH 2002 Experiences of orthopaedic nurses caring for elderly patients with acute confusion. Journal of Orthopaedic Nursing 6(1):9–17

Sabat S 1994 Excess disability and malignant social psychology: a case study of Alzheimer's disease. Journal of Community and Applied Social Psychology 4:157–166

Schofield I 2007 Delirium. In: Neno R, Aveyard B, Heath H (eds) Older people and mental health: a handbook of care. Blackwell, Oxford, pp 168–181

Schofield I, Dewing J 2001 The nursing contribution to the acute care of older people with a delirium in acute settings. Nursing Older People Journal 13(1):21–25

Segatore M, Adams D 2001 Managing delirium and agitation in elderly hospitalized orthopaedic patients: part 2 – interventions. Orthopaedic Nursing 20(2):61–73

Simon L, Jewell N, Brokel J 1997 Management of acute delirium in hospitalized elderly: a process improvement project. Geriatric Nursing 18:150–154

Sörensen Duppils G, Winbald K 2007 Patients' experiences of being delirious. Journal of Clinical Nursing 16(5):810–818

Strickland TL, Longobardi P, Gray GE 1999 Health issues of minority elderly: dementia in minority elderly. Clinical Geriatrics 7(11):83–93

Stuart GM 1998 Therapeutic nurse–patient relationship. In: Stuart GM, Laraia MT (eds) Principles and practice of psychiatric nursing. Mosby, St Louis, pp 17–53

Wills T, Dewing J 2001 Supporting older people with acute confusion: the contribution of mental health nurses. Nursing Older People Journal 13(1):17–19

Woods B, Spector AE, Prendergast L, Orrell M 2005 Cognitive stimulation to improve cognitive functioning in people with dementia. (Protocol) Cochrane Database of Systematic Reviews, Issue 4

Chapter 18

Continence

Alison Kelley and Anita Counsell

KEY ISSUES

SUBJECT KNOWLEDGE
- Definition of continence and incontinence
- Biology of the urinary system
- The process of defaecation
- Different types of incontinence and their causes
- Effects of the ageing process on continence
- Psychological and environmental causes of incontinence
- Behavioural problems caused by or causing incontinence
- The stigma of incontinence

CARE DELIVERY KNOWLEDGE
- Nursing assessment of urinary and faecal incontinence
- Ways of promoting urinary and faecal continence
- Aids and appliances used to manage incontinence

PROFESSIONAL AND ETHICAL KNOWLEDGE
- The effect of national policies on the Continence Advisory Service
- Education for continence promotion
- Quality assurance of continence care
- The rights of clients to quality continence care

PERSONAL AND REFLECTIVE KNOWLEDGE
- Empathy with the incontinent client
- Consolidation of knowledge through case studies

INTRODUCTION

People have the right to be continent whenever that is achievable. When true continence is not achievable, people have the right to the highest standards of continence care and incontinence management.

Urinary incontinence is a worldwide problem. A prevalence of 32% was found in the UK and over 30% in four European countries (Hunskar et al 2002). *Good Practice in Continence Services* (Department of Health 2000) suggests that urinary incontinence may, in the general population, be as high as 1 in 10 to 1 in 5 women over 65 years and 1 in 14 to 1 in 10 males over 65 years, and this may rise to 1 in 2 in homes caring for the infirm elderly. The Children's NSF (Department of Health 2004 section 10:17, p. 32) states 'there are at least 500,000 children who suffer from nocturnal enuresis and a significant number with daytime wetting and faecal incontinence'.

The presence of symptoms of leaking urine have an impact on the quality of life and pyschological well-being of an individual (Shaw 2001), and bowel problems remain a taboo topic in western societies (Norton 2005). However, incontinence is a treatable condition, where provision of appropriate physiological and psychological intervention can help a client achieve continence. Education of the general public to dispel negative and misguided attitudes is of prime importance.

This chapter aims to explain the reasons elimination problems occur and to introduce you to the knowledge and skills you will need to assess clients with continence difficulties and to plan their care. It also discusses the impact of national policies to ensure this care is of a high standard.

OVERVIEW

Subject knowledge

This section covers the normal anatomy and physiology of micturition and defaecation, how continence is gained, and then describes how alterations from the normal can give rise to incontinence. It explores how continence is affected when ability to cope with activities of daily living change, and examines how society and its attitudes can affect elimination behaviour.

Care delivery knowledge

This section outlines the skills needed to assess clients' problems, ways of promoting continence, how to manage incontinence and additional treatments that can be offered by referring clients to the continence advisor and the multidisciplinary team.

Professional and ethical knowledge

Policy issues around promoting and managing continence are highlighted. The responsibilities of the continence advisor, the nurse and the multidisciplinary team, and the vision for integrated services are outlined. Educational needs and ethical issues of continence care are discussed.

Personal and reflective knowledge

The aim of the exercises is to help you use the knowledge gained and develop them for your portfolio.

On pages 434–435 there are four case studies, each one relating to one of the branch programmes. You may find it helpful to read one of them before you start the chapter and use it as a focus for your reflections while reading as part of your portfolio development.

SUBJECT KNOWLEDGE

BIOLOGICAL

Continence is a skill gained when a person learns to recognize the need to pass urine and/or bowel motion, has the ability to reach an acceptable place to void, is able to hold on until they reach there and is able to void/eliminate effectively on reaching that place (Getliffe & Dolman 2007).

The first section examines the physiological mechanism used to achieve continence and then how it may fail and cause urinary and faecal incontinence. Other types of physiological failures that can cause problems with elimination are also considered.

ANATOMY AND PHYSIOLOGY OF THE LOWER URINARY TRACT

The urinary system consists of two kidneys, two ureters, a bladder and a urethra. Urine is made in the kidneys when the blood is filtrated to remove waste products and keep water and electrolytes balanced in the body. Antidiuretic hormone (ADH) will decrease urine production, and will normally rise at night to decrease the amount of urine produced. Urine passes down the ureters from the kidneys. It is important that it does not reflux back to the kidneys,

causing renal damage. This is prevented by; the angle at which the ureters enter the bladder; peristalsis in the ureters causing urine to flow towards the bladder; and the narrowing along the ureter.

To understand continence fully it is important to know about the organs involved in storage and evacuation (bladder and urethra) and how they relate to the lower bowel and the male and female reproductive organs (Fig. 18.1).

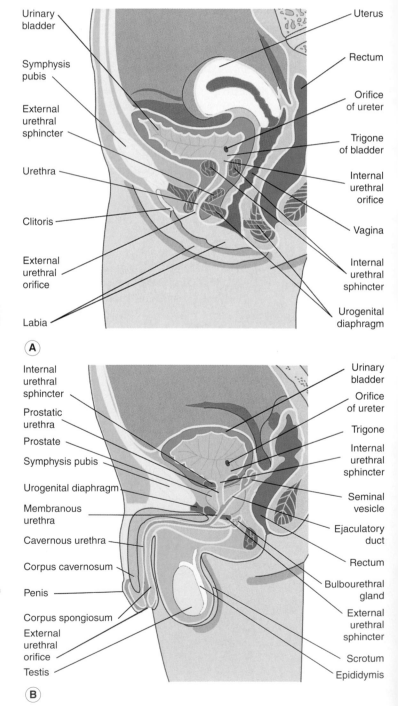

Figure 18.1 Anatomy of the urinary system.

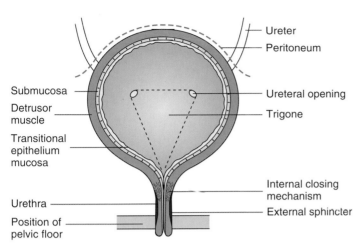

Figure 18.2 Cross-section of (female) urinary bladder (after Cheater 1992b).

The bladder is made of four layers of tissue:

- an inner layer of transitional epithelium
- a connective tissue layer
- smooth muscle
- an outer coating covering the upper surface, the peritoneum (Fig. 18.2).

The epithelial layer has the ability to stretch and it also produces mucus to protect the tissues from the acidity of the urine. The smooth muscle is known as the detrusor muscle and is made up of layers of longitudinal and circular muscle to allow it to both stretch and contract. Stretch receptors monitor the fullness of the bladder and are found throughout this muscle, but are concentrated in the sensitive trigone, a triangular area between the ureters and the urethra. Urine enters the bladder through the ureters and leaves through the urethra (see Fig. 18.2) (Getliffe & Dolman 2007).

The urethra is a tube running from the bladder and is 3–5 cm long in the female and 18–22 cm long in the male. It has a thick mucosal lining containing mucus-producing cells, and is folded to enhance the watertight seal of the bladder. At the bladder neck the smooth muscle passes from the bladder to the urethra, forming the internal closing mechanism. This is more distinct in men than women, being found just above the prostate gland (Fig. 18.3). (Getliffe & Dolman 2007).

The external sphincter is made of voluntary muscle and in men it is a separate ring just below the prostate gland. This allows the sphincters to work independently so during ejaculation the bladder is closed but the urethra can be open. In women the internal closing mechanism is less distinct and the external sphincter surrounds this. It is also sensitive to oestrogen levels. These factors may give rise to an incompetent sphincter (discussed later in the chapter).

The pelvic floor is a muscular sling supporting the abdominal organs. It is pierced by the rectum posteriorly and the vagina and urethra anteriorly. It is very important in continence, contracting to maintain urinary and faecal continence, but relaxing to allow expulsion of urine and faeces (Emmanuel 2004). The bladder and the proximal urethra sit well supported above the pelvic floor, a position needed to maintain continence (see Fig. 18.2).

Decision-making exercise

The coordination of bladder emptying is controlled by nerve pathways. Damage to these pathways can upset their balance and cause incontinence.

- How will damage in the following areas affect the micturition process?
  - the frontal lobe of the brain
  - the midbrain or pons
  - the cervical spine
  - the lumbar spine
  - the sacrum
  - the nerves forming the spinal reflex arc.
- Compare your answers with the problems described in the following discussion of altered physiology.
- As you gain nursing experience, list the conditions caused by damage to the central nervous system or spinal cord and look at the patient's subsequent continence.

The bladder is controlled by both the somatic and the autonomic nervous system, which allows it to store urine and expel it at a suitable time. The parasympathetic system innervates the detrusor muscle of the bladder, allowing the bladder to relax during its filling phase while the sphincters remain closed. It allows filling up to approximately 300 mL without registering changes of pressure. This is known as compliance. Once this volume is reached the sensory parasympathetic nerves transmit impulses to the sacral area of the spinal cord (S2–S4). A spinal reflex arc is completed allowing impulses to pass back to the bladder through the parasympathetic motor nerves, causing the muscle to contract and the sphincter to open, resulting in micturition (Fig. 18.4).

The voluntary control works in an inhibitory manner: sensory impulses are sent through the pudendal nerve to the cortical micturition centre in the frontal lobe of the brain saying bladder is full. Inhibitory impulses are passed back to the sacrum to prevent the sacral reflex arc initiating micturition. When the individual is ready to pass urine, the inhibition is lifted (see Fig. 18.4). These voluntary nerve pathways pass through the pons in the brainstem and it is thought that this area ensures that the sphincters' opening and the bladder's contraction are coordinated (Fader & Craggs 2003). The reflex arc action occurs in babies, and the inhibitory process begins to develop in infants from the age of 18 months as the central nervous system matures.

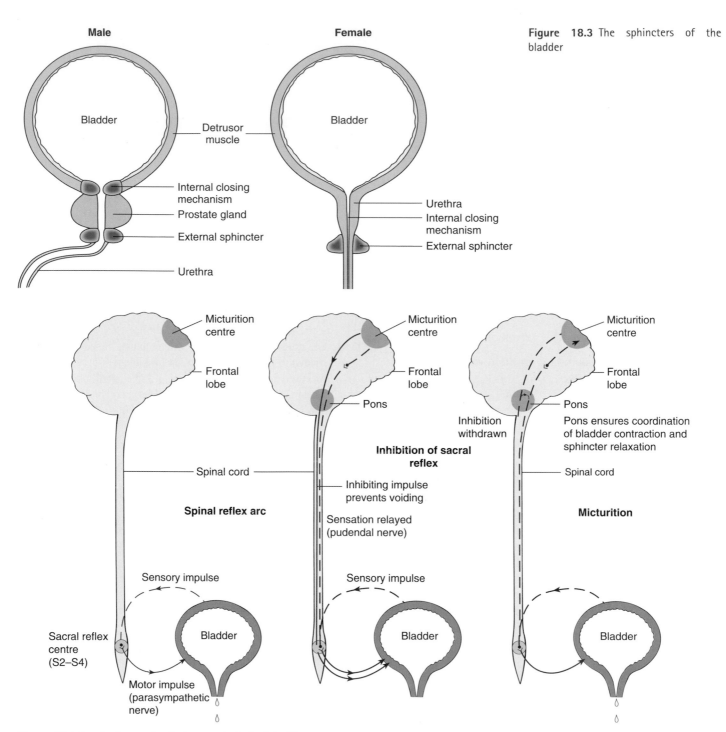

Figure 18.3 The sphincters of the bladder

Figure 18.4 Involuntary and voluntary control of micturition.

ALTERED PHYSIOLOGY OF THE LOWER URINARY TRACT

Three main types of incontinence result from an alteration of the normal physiology described above. These are:

- stress incontinence
- overactive bladder
- voiding difficulties.

The conditions will be discussed separately so that you can understand the different symptoms of each type. This is important when you assess patients as some clients may have more than one condition causing their continence difficulties.

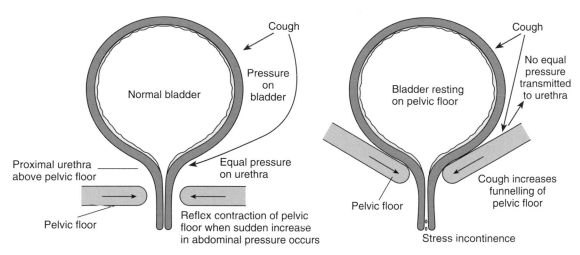

Figure 18.5 Diagram showing the relationship between the bladder and the pelvic floor for continence, and how a lax pelvic floor causes stress incontinence.

Stress incontinence

Stress incontinence is more common than diabetes or asthma (Bishop 2005). It is defined as an involuntary loss of urine during increase in intra-abdominal pressure caused by laughing, sneezing or lifting. It occurs during the filling phase of the bladder causing leakage of urine. When the bladder is held in the correct position by the pelvic floor the inner closing mechanism and the external sphincter of the bladder prevent leakage (Fig. 18.5). If the pelvic floor is weak the bladder prolapses downwards and there is no compensatory pressure helping to counteract the pressure on the bladder and leakage may occur (see Fig. 18.5); this is made worse if the urethral closing mechanism is also weak, for example when oestrogen levels are low (Dolman 2007). Table 18.1 lists the common causes of stress incontinence.

Overactive bladder

Overactive bladder is characterized by involuntary bladder contractions during its filling phase and produces symptoms of urgency, frequency, urge incontinence, nocturia and nocturnal enuresis (see Table 18.2 for definitions of terms) (Wein et al 2002). The inhibition impulse from the cortical micturition centre of the cortex is not sufficient to prevent the sacral reflex action occurring, so the bladder starts to contract and voiding begins. This may be due to damage to the central nervous system, for example a cerebrovascular accident (stroke), tumours, spinal cord injuries or malfunction of the conduction of the nerve impulses, as seen in multiple sclerosis (MS) and Parkinsonism. Local bladder factors may be responsible for causing spasm that overrides cortical inhibition, for example caffeine (Bryant

Table 18.1 Common causes of stress incontinence

Mechanism	Cause	Reference
Weakness of pelvic floor muscles (due to muscle or nerve damage)	Pregnancy	Eason et al (2004)
	Childbirth Trauma during childbirth (vaginal delivery)	
	Forceps delivery	Klein et al (1997)
	Obesity	
Increased abdominal pressure	Chronic cough Prolonged lifting of heavy weights Childbirth	
Oestrogen deficiency (oestrogen receptors are found in pelvic floor, bladder and bladder neck, thus there is good muscle tone in the presence of oestrogen)	Pregnancy Last part of menstrual cycle Menopause	Dolman (2007)

et al 2002), urinary tract infections, concentrated urine or external factors such as prostatic enlargement or constipation. Overactive bladder may occur in the absence of any detectable pathology (Fig. 18.6) (Getliffe & Dolman 2007).

Voiding difficulties

There are two reasons for voiding difficulties and each is described in the following section.

Table 18.2 Definitions of terms used in connection with incontinence

Urgency	The need to pass urine in a great hurry
Sensory urgency	Urgency in the absence of unstable bladder contractions; the bladder is hypersensitive
Frequency	Visiting the toilet to pass urine more often than is acceptable to the patient; this usually means more than seven times during the day and more than once at night
Urge incontinence	While experiencing urgency the patient may not be able to get to the toilet in time and is therefore incontinent
Reflex incontinence	Urine loss due to detrusor hyperreflexia (or involuntary urethral relaxation) when there is aneuropathic absence of sensation
Hesitancy	Difficulty in initiating voiding
Dribbling	Dribbling of urine after voiding, due to pooling of urine in the urethra between internal and external sphincter
Nocturnal enuresis	Bed-wetting while asleep
Passive incontinence	Wetting at rest without any coincident activity or sensation
Dysuria	Pain or burning while actually passing urine
Haematuria	Blood in the urine

Bladder outflow obstruction

This condition can occur when the outlet to the bladder becomes obstructed (Fig 18.7). The most common cause in males is prostatic enlargement. It is estimated that approximately 2.5 million men in the UK may have symptoms of this type of obstruction (Brown & Das 2002). The condition may also occur in both males and females with urethral narrowing or stricture, and more rarely with urethral cancers and stones.

Symptoms of this problem could include bladder filling problems, such as frequency and urgency of micturition, and bladder voiding symptoms, such as hesitancy, poor stream and varying degrees of retention of urine. Urinary tract infection and longer term damage to the upper renal tract and detrusor muscle of the bladder may occur.

Detrusor hypoactivity (atonic bladder)

In some cases, if the detrusor muscle of the bladder fails to contract fully it will not completely empty and the bladder will retain urine (Fig 18.8). To some degree, these symptoms may mimic those of outflow obstruction, such as

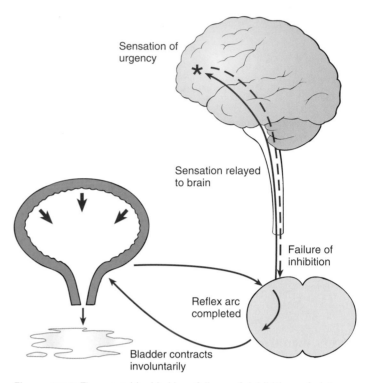

Figure 18.6 The unstable bladder: failure of inhibition of detrusor contraction (reproduced with kind permission of Coloplast Ltd).

repeated urinary tract infection. Where bladder sensation is present, the patient will know their bladder is not empty and experience frequency and urgency of micturition.

The causes of this condition may be due to muscle weakness seen more commonly in elderly clients (Norton 2005). They include underlying neuropathy such as stroke (Brittain et al 1998) and peripheral neuropathy in diabetes. Spinal cord damage may also be a contributory

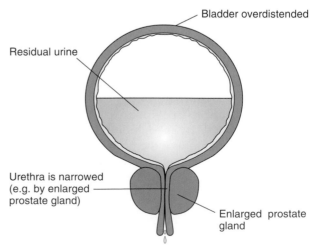

Figure 18.7 Obstruction with overflow incontinence (reproduced with kind permission of Coloplast Ltd).

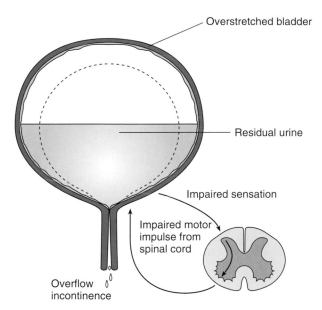

Figure 18.8 The underactive detrusor (reproduced with kind permission of Coloplast Ltd).

factor either as a result of trauma or disease. Approximately 1 in 10 patients suffering with multiple sclerosis exhibit this type of voiding dysfunction (Kobashi & Leach 1999). Also clients with multiple sclerosis or stroke may experience a condition termed detrusor sphincter dyssynergia. Here the detrusor muscle does contract but the sphincter fails to relax leading to a non-emptying bladder.

If the nervous control is completely damaged, as seen in some children with spina bifida, the bladder cannot empty at all and this is known as atonic bladder.

Influences on bladder function

There are other influences on the normal functioning bladder that may cause incontinence: these are fluid intake, urinary tract infection, drugs and constipation. The last two will be discussed later.

Many clients will cut down their fluid intake mistakenly believing it will reduce their incontinence. Concentrated urine will encourage bladder spasm and thus cause urgency and frequency (Getliff & Dolman 2007). This problem is also found in young children especially when starting school, unless encouraged to drink. They may drink minimal amounts, which may cause some girls to exhibit daytime wetting and may also be a factor in children who wet the bed (Butler et al 2005). The opposite problem sometimes occur in clients with learning disabilities who drink excessive amounts of water and produce large volumes of urine, causing frequency. Urinary tract infection will also cause bladder spasm giving urgency and frequency and may exacerbate urinary problems.

ANATOMY AND PHYSIOLOGY OF THE LOWER BOWEL

'Faecal incontinence is the most embarrassing, socially unacceptable and demoralizing of symptoms' (Irvine 1996: 226). Looking after a person with faecal incontinence is poorly tolerated by carers and frequently leads to the discontinuation of community care. Faecal incontinence is not as widespread as urinary incontinence. The Department of Health (2000) estimates a prevalence of faecal incontinence of 1% among total population of adults, rising to 17% in the very elderly.

The large intestine consists of the caecum and colon and terminates with the rectum and anal canal. It receives 600 mL of chyme from the small intestine daily and reduces it to 150–200 mL of faeces by reabsorbing water from the chyme as it travels through the colon. Faeces are stored in the rectum and eliminated though the anal canal (Norton & Chelvanayagam 2004). The rectum has a mucosal lining (i.e. columnar epithelial), which produces mucus to lubricate the passage of stool. The anal canal has a squamous epithelial lining, which is dry and very sensitive and can distinguish between flatus and stool, allowing flatulence to escape to relieve gaseous distension, but retaining faeces. The muscle layer of the rectum is smooth involuntary muscle and contains specialized stretch receptors, which monitor the fullness of the rectum. In the anal canal the smooth involuntary muscle thickens to form the internal sphincter, which is surrounded by a layer of voluntary muscle, the anal sphincter (Fig. 18.9) (Emmanuel 2004). Vascular projections (anal cushions) are found in the anus; these help to reduce feacal leaking and may give rise to haemorrhoids (Barrett 2002).

Faeces formed by the large bowel enter the rectum by a series of peristaltic movements known as the gastrocolic reflex, which is stimulated by physical activity and ingestion of food (Emmanuel 2004). Once 150 mL or more of

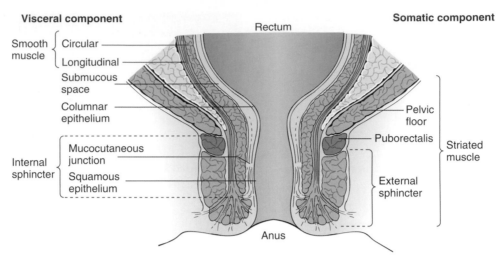

Figure 18.9 Section through the lower rectum and anus (from Bendall 1989).

stool is in the rectum, the individual gets a feeling of fullness and impending defaecation and the internal anal sphincter relaxes and allows the stool to enter the anal canal. If defaecation is not convenient, the external sphincter remains closed and the faeces return to the rectum (Edwards et al 2003). However, if it is appropriate, the external sphincter relaxes and defaecation occurs. This is most efficiently achieved in a squatting position as pressure from the abdominal muscles will cause the external and internal anal sphincters to relax, the pelvic floor will drop down to form a funnel, and the bowel will empty easily (Horton 2004).

The nervous control is a reflex action involving the myenteric plexus and stimulated by a full rectum. The internal anal sphincter is controlled by the autonomic nervous system and the external sphincter is controlled by the somatic nervous system (pudendal nerve).

If the defaecation mechanism is working properly the individual should be able to pass 150–200 mL of formed but soft stool regularly. However, the frequency of defaecation varies between individuals, ranging from three times a day to once in three days (Emmanuel 2004). The consistency of the stool may show individual differences; these can be assessed using the Bristol Stool Scale, 3 and 4 on this scale being considered to be preferable (Fig. 18.10).

The pelvic floor is responsible for keeping the rectum in the correct position. The muscle of the pelvic floor, which anchors the rectum to the pubis (i.e. the puborectalis), is of great importance in maintaining faecal continence. The puborectalis maintains an angle of 60–105 ° between the rectum and the anal canal. This angle acts as a flap valve, which closes when abdominal pressures rise, for example due to sneezing or lifting, preventing leakage through the canal (Fig. 18.11). During defaecation the pelvic floor

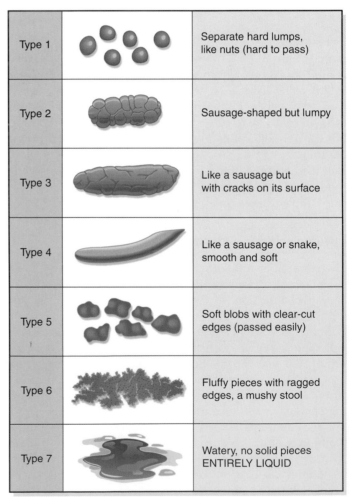

Type 1		Separate hard lumps, like nuts (hard to pass)
Type 2		Sausage-shaped but lumpy
Type 3		Like a sausage but with cracks on its surface
Type 4		Like a sausage or snake, smooth and soft
Type 5		Soft blobs with clear-cut edges (passed easily)
Type 6		Fluffy pieces with ragged edges, a mushy stool
Type 7		Watery, no solid pieces ENTIRELY LIQUID

Figure 18.10 The Bristol Stool Scale (reproduced with kind permission of Norgine Ltd).

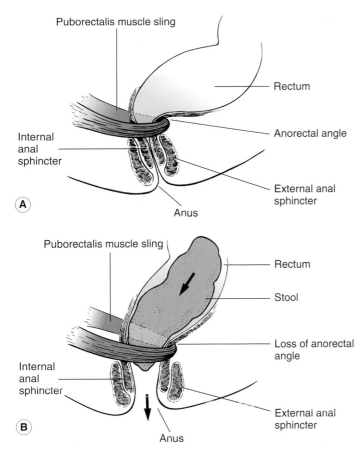

Figure 18.11 Faecal continence and the anorectal angle.

relaxes increasing this angle allowing easy passing of stool (see Fig. 18.11). The nerve supply of the pelvic floor is innervated by the same nerve as the external sphincter, the pudendal nerve. This nerve synapses with the autonomic system at S2–S4 (Edwards et al 2003).

ALTERED PHYSIOLOGY OF THE LOWER BOWEL

Faecal incontinence is defined as involuntary and/or inappropriate passing of liquid or solid stool. Norton & Chelvanayagam (2004) classify the causes of faecal incontinence under the following headings:

- anal sphincter or pelvic floor damage
- gut motility/stool consistency
- anorectal pathology (e.g. haemorrhoids, anal fistula, rectal prolapse)
- neurological disease
- secondary to degenerative neurological disease
- impaction with overflow
- lifestyle (discussed in management of constipation).

Anal sphincter or pelvic floor damage and/or anorectal pathology

Faecal incontinence may occur when abdominal pressure increases for example when sneezing or lifting (see Fig. 18.11). It may be due to the following: damage of the anal sphincters, the pudendal nerve, weakness of the pelvic floor, (the puborectalis muscle) and increase of the anorectal angle (Norton & Chelvanayagam 2004). Damage to the internal or external anal sphincters (or both) due to forceps delivery or perineal tears during childbirth are often responsible for faecal incontinence in younger women (Porrett 2006). If the external sphincter is damaged, women may experience urgency, while damage to the internal sphincter may cause faecal seeping. Reduced muscle tone and nerve degeneration cause anorectal abnormality (Harari 2004).

Gut motility/stool consistency

A bad attack of diarrhoea may cause faecal incontinence, especially in those who are very ill, bed bound or have mobility problems. This may be due to infection or gastro-intestinal disease. Severe and prolonged attacks of diarrhoea should have a medical referral as should rectal bleeding (Norton & Chelvanayagam 2004).

Neurological causes

Neurogenic bowel refers to constipation or faecal incontinence that occurs in patients with major neurological disease or injury, for example stroke or multiple sclerosis (Wiesel & Bell 2004). Spinal cord injury also leads to bowel dysfunction of varying types depending on the level and the degree of neurological completeness of the lesion (Ash 2005). The differences in the areas and seriousness of the neurological damage mean that management of this group must be individualized as there is a fine line between relieving constipation and causing faecal incontinence.

Secondary to degenerative neurological disease

Elderly patients with dementia may be faecally incontinent due to decreased intellectual function, loss of social awareness and neurological sensation and an inability to control their bowels (Norton & Chelvanayagam 2004).

Faecal impaction

Constipation affects up to 27% of the population of the Western world (Lembo & Camilleri 2003). Faecal impaction can be the result of chronic constipation (Table 18.3) and may give rise to faecal incontinence of either solid or liquid stool (Norton & Chelvanayagam 2004). The latter is seepage from above the obstruction, and slime as a result of

Table 18.3 Causes of constipation

Mechanism	Causes
Insufficient material in the bowel	Lack of fibre in the diet Poor fluid intake
Abnormal neurological control	Spinal or nerve injury affecting autonomic nervous system Hirschsprung disease (a condition where there is an absence of nerves in the wall of bowel) Psychological factors, by an inhibitory effect on autonomic innervation (Dykes et al 2001)
Obstruction	Tumours Diverticular disease Haemorrhoids Congenital abnormalities
Pregnancy	High progesterone levels causing decrease in motility of the gastrointestinal tract
Metabolic causes	Diabetes mellitus Hypothyroidism Dehydration
Drugs	Aluminium (antacids) Anticholinergics Diuretics Iron Analgesia opiates Verapamil
Laxative abuse	Overuse of laxatives can cause damage to the nerves in the colon, resulting in atonic bowel
Environmental	Anything preventing defaecation, e.g. lack of privacy, dirty toilets, insufficient toilets
Immobility	Lack of exercise means the bowel itself is less active. The client may have difficulty reaching the toilet

bacterial breaking down hard faeces and extra mucus. It is foul smelling and known as spurious diarrhoea. Thompson et al (1999) defined constipation as demonstrating two of the following symptoms: straining at stool; lumpy hard stools; sensation of incomplete emptying; and fewer than two bowel movements a week (ROME II criteria).

Faecal impaction may not always be due to large amounts of small hard stool but large amounts of soft faeces, when the client may be unable to completely empty from their bowel despite regular bowel movement. This can also cause faecal incontinence. The term 'faecal loading' may be the best term for this type of bowel problem (Barrett 2002). Impaction is often found in the frail elderly who may have impaired rectal sensation and thus do not initiate defaecation effectively (Harari 2002).

GENERAL ALTERED PHYSIOLOGY CAUSING CONTINENCE PROBLEMS

Returning to the original definition of continence, we can see that physiological changes in other systems of the body can affect the continence state of the client. For example when identifying the place for elimination the client needs to be orientated. Clients with dementia, confusion or disorientation may become incontinent simply because they are unable to locate the toilet (Eustice 2007). Finding the correct receptacle may also be a problem: the demented patient may confuse washbasins with urinals. To locate a toilet, a person needs to be able to follow a signed route, which can be difficult in dim corridors or if the person is blind or partially sighted. The sign also needs to be recognizable, because notices in small print or the modern stylized pictures may not be obvious to the disorientated. A sign only saying 'toilets' is also unsuitable, causing discomfort to people who fear sharing facilities with the opposite sex. People may have to ask for the toilet, which can be embarrassing for some, but very difficult for clients with communication problems due to physical illness (e.g. stroke) or mental illness (e.g. depression).

The ability to reach the toilet is essential and clients with problems like stiff joints or poor balance can find this difficult. In addition this effort may tire them, resulting in an incontinent episode before they reach the toilet. Obstacles en route such as stairs, narrow passages, sharp corners, loose mats and heavy doors can also hamper the journey. Memory loss causes problems as the client may forget what their goal is after setting out to go to the toilet and wander around until it is too late (Stokes 2002). On reaching the toilet itself the client needs dexterity to remove clothing before eliminating; inappropriate clothing may slow the client so much that they may begin to void or defaecate too soon. To complete the toileting sequence a person must be able to squat, or for men have the stability to stand to urinate, and this may cause problems for the disabled. This type of incontinence is often known as functional incontinence (see Evolve 18.1).

evolve
learning system

18.1 – FUNCTIONAL INCONTINENCE

- Identify the causes of functional incontinence.
- Describe the types of patients that may have this type of incontinence.
- List ideas of how to manage these problems.
- Recognize aids to support continence.

Ageing

Any of the general physiological factors discussed above can be a problem for the elderly, but they are not inevitable.

The ageing process may affect continence in many other ways and the following factors should be considered

- Circulatory changes and kidney deterioration mean that urine production is less efficient; this results in larger amounts of urine being produced during the night – 35% of the 24-hour volume as opposed to 20% in younger adults (Weiss & Blaivas 2000).
- Hormonal change in the amount of oestrogen circulating in a woman's body decreases. As a result, the soft convoluted tissue of the vagina and urethra become less elastic with less pronounced folds, resulting in the loss of the watertight seal in the urethra. This deficiency also causes the pelvic floor muscle tone to become lax, and may lead to stress incontinence (Cardosa et al 2000).
- The elderly man has a tendency towards prostatic enlargement and therefore overflow incontinence.
- There is a deterioration of detrusor contractility (Pfisterer et al 2006). The bladder may not empty completely so that a residual volume builds up in the bladder.
- Deterioration of nerves occurs so that the sensation of bladder fullness becomes less acute, and the older person will feel the urge to urinate when the bladder is 90% full, and not 50%, as in the younger person. There is also a tendency towards an overactive bladder in the elderly due to neural changes (Pfisterer et al 2006).
- The immunological system becomes less efficient thus increasing the incidence of infections. This, coupled with a residual volume of urine in the bladder, increases the likelihood of urinary tract infections. Raz et al (2000) list infections as one of the factors that can cause transient incontinence in the elderly.

In summary, often continence difficulties in the elderly are multifactorial; for example, nocturia may be due to less efficient urine production, decreased antidiuretic hormone, bladder storage problems and sleep related issues (Wein et al 2002).

PSYCHOSOCIAL

DEVELOPMENT OF CONTROL

To acquire continence the child needs to develop physically, mentally and socially. During the first 18 months of life bladder emptying is purely a reflex action. The bladder is stable and empties completely, and Yeung et al (1995) found there is cerebral arousal during emptying. During the first 3 years of life the bladder capacity increases and the frequency of voiding decreases (Jansson et al 2000). Eventually the child then becomes aware of the urge sensation of passing urine and wanting to defaecate, associating this with feeling wet or soiled. The ability to control the bladder and anal sphincters and also the pelvic floor is

developed. The sequence of developing control of elimination is normally bowel control when asleep, followed by the child being clean during the day, then the child gaining urinary continence during the day and finally becoming dry at night. There are a number of essential skills the child needs to develop before they are ready for toilet training (Schum et al 2002); gross motor skills of sitting and walking, the fine motor skills involved in dressing and undressing, and communication skills to alert their parent or carer that they need to go to the toilet are essential (Harris 2004). For children with special needs, this signal may be a nonverbal cue or a type of behaviour.

All these factors must be mastered to make 'potty training' successful. When the child has developed these diverse skills and is interested in using the toilet, they are ready for toilet training. Time should be given by the parent or carer to help the child get used to the potty or toilet, giving praise and encouragement when the child is successful. Toilet training takes time and accidents can occur, especially if the child is engrossed in play. This may upset the child and the parent.

Physical problems (illness) and emotional worries (parents' divorce, starting school, etc.) may prolong toilet training, or even cause a child already trained to regress and start wetting again.

Nocturnal enuresis can be defined as involuntary voiding during sleep (Butler 2000). Children who have never been dry at night are classed as having primary nocturnal enuresis, whereas those who have been previously dry for 6 months or more are classed as having secondary nocturnal enuresis. Butler et al (2001) suggest that 15–22% of boys and 7–15% of girls wet the bed regularly at the age of 7 years.

Reflection and portfolio evidence

Schum et al (2002) identified 27 skills a child needed to develop for toilet training to be successful.

- List the skills you need to go to the toilet.
- Relate these to a child's developmental steps.
- Work out what the child needs to be doing to be 'toilet ready'.
- When working with a health visitor or school nurse you may be able to assess children's developmental steps and relate it to their toilet readiness.
- Record your learning in your portfolio.

It is thought that bed-wetting may be multifactorial (Enuresis Resource and Information Centre 2002), arising from the three following conditions, known as the 'Three Systems Approach':

- Lack of antidiuretic hormone production at night resulting in high night-time urine production (Medel et al 1998).

- Bladder (detrusor) instability which causes bladder spasm and a low bladder capacity which will need emptying at night.
- Lack of arousal from sleep; being unable to wake from sleep when the bladder is full (Neveus et al 1999).

BEHAVIOURAL FACTORS

Incontinence in an individual cannot always be explained by physical factors alone. The emotional and mental state of the individual, along with his or her attitude, will also have a bearing on the problem. In children, regression may occur when a sibling is born, giving secondary nocturnal enuresis. Encopresis is defined as the passage of normal stool in socially inappropriate places and is found in children with emotional and behavioural problems who need psychological support as part of the child treatment (West & Steinhart 2003).

In an adult the beginning of continence problems can sometimes be traced to emotional traumas, for example bereavement, rejection or moving to a new place (Stokes 2002). Many people become incontinent on admission to residential care or soon after, and this may be related to the loss of independence and personal responsibility and a decreasing sense of self-worth. Duggan et al (2000) found clear evidence that urinary incontinence causes depressive symptoms in older clients.

Continence is an acquired habit, and the motivation to be continent can be diminished in the apathetic or confused elderly person; for example, if a toilet is cold, unpleasant or a distance away, the call to micturate or defaecate may be ignored. Confused or demented people are very dependent upon familiar stimuli in order to maintain their activities (Stokes 2002). Most people have a lifetime of conditioned reflexes to pass urine while seated with no clothing over the genital areas on a toilet in privacy and with the sensation of a full bladder. If an individual is taken to the toilet or sat in a chair with a bare bottom on an underpad, confused messages are given as to where and when to pass urine.

Reflection and portfolio evidence

Think of the different public toilets you have visited, both pleasant and unpleasant.

- List what makes these toilets acceptable or unacceptable to you.
- During your allocations look at the patient toilet; is it up to your personal standards?
- Reflect on how an ill or frail person must feel using this toilet and how you may improve it if necessary.
- Record your findings in your portfolio.

STIGMA AND INCONTINENCE

Incontinence can be viewed as a great social stigma. Embarrassment and shame may prevent people reporting their problems with maintaining continence to a health professional (Duggan et al 2000). There are many myths, for example having children causes incontinence, and incontinence is an inevitable part of ageing. Acceptance of these myths may prevent clients, especially women, asking for help (Duggan et al 2001).

Expectation that some sectors of society will be incontinent – e.g. the elderly, people with learning difficulties and women who have had children – encourages passive acceptance of the condition. This is compounded by attitudes of some staff in the caring professions who, for example, accept incontinence as the norm for an elderly person within a nursing home environment (Nazarko 2000).

People often cope by adapting their lifestyle to hide their incontinence by reducing their social activities and not playing sport. Outings by bus or car can be an ordeal because of worrying about being able to get to a toilet when needed, and staying overnight with friends can be out of the question in case of wetting beds or furniture. The guilt, shame, frustration and feelings of the hopelessness of a situation that does not seem to have a solution can cause isolation in all those with continence difficulties. Duggan et al (2000) found patients with urinary incontinence reported loneliness as a major problem, particularly in younger patients.

Butler (2002) looked at the impact of nocturnal enuresis on children and suggested that older children with this condition may exhibit psychological symptoms including low self-esteem and behavioural problems; however, if the bed wetting is treated successfully, no long-term effects were apparent.

Wilkinson (2001) found that Pakistani women with these problems had low self-esteem and had feelings of being unclean and sinful. Muslim women found the worst consequence was that it prevented them praying.

This shame can affect the individual's sexuality and relationship with those closest to them (Roe et al 1999). There is a high correlation with impotence, and it has been shown that stress incontinence is associated with sexual dysfunction among middle-aged women. The feeling of being unclean or smelly, and perhaps wearing incontinent aids, will hamper a person's self-image and question their sexual attractiveness. Sexual activity is regarded as a private and personal matter and like incontinence is also taboo. Discussing this dual problem needs to be conducted with delicacy. It is important to remember that clients who have to rely on pads or catheters may still wish to have a sex life, and if these are causing problems, help and counselling should be sought from a specialist.

Reflection and portfolio evidence

- How do you feel when you are changing a baby?
- How do you feel when you are changing an elderly person's wet and soiled bed?
- Are your feelings different; if so why?
- List the things that would cause you concern if you were incontinent?
- With your reflections in mind, list ways that you may be able to support people who have problems with continence.

CARE DELIVERY KNOWLEDGE

ASSESSMENT OF URINARY INCONTINENCE

Care pathways are vehicles for planning patient focused care. Accurate assessment of the individual with incontinence is essential to ensure that the reason for incontinence is found so a pathway with suitable interventions for the specific problems is identified (Brown et al 2006). The NICE guidelines for urinary incontinence (2006: 32) provide a good example of a care pathway for the management of urinary incontinence in women. Ideally the assessment will be multidisciplinary, involving doctors, nurses, physiotherapists and occupational therapists (NICE 2006).

When assessing and caring for a client with elimination difficulties nurses need to understand how the client and carer feel, and also to be aware of their own feelings towards the situation, so that negative attitudes are not transferred from the assessor to the client. The environment should be private and provide a relaxed atmosphere. The assessment should not be rushed and mutually understood terminology should be used. A holistic assessment should include the influencing and functional factors of incontinence as well as the urinary symptoms and specific physical examination (see Table 18.4).

Assessment of urinary problems

The assessment should cover:

- urinary symptoms
- baseline chart
- urinalysis
- post-void residual volume
- vaginal examination
- rectal examination.

Urinary symptoms

It is important to gain the client's perspective in order to determine the severity of the problem. Wetting a

Table 18.4 Components of a holistic assessment of a client presenting with incontinence

Mobility	Difficulty in walking to or sitting on the toilet
Dexterity	Problems with opening doors or removing clothing
Communication	Problems with sight or hearing, speaking
Diet and fluids	Amount and type of fluid drunk, type of diet especially the amount of fibre eaten (see Ch. 8, 'Nutrition')
Elimination	The client's view of the problem, constipation history
Sleep	Tiredness may indicate lack of sleep due to nocturia
Psychological	Memory loss, confusion making finding the toilet difficult, behaviour associated with wanting to pass urine, any anxiety or depression caused by the incontinence
Environmental	Information about the toilet facilities at the client's home, location of toilet, up or down stairs, height of toilet, handwashing facilities, privacy
Recreational	To what extent has the problem affected their lives, socially, at work, their family, sexual relationships
Past medical history	Neurological, urological, and gynaecological problems. In women, details of menstrual cycle/menopause, obstetric history: number of children, weight of babies, type of delivery, were forceps used. In men, prostate history

teaspoonful a day into a panty liner may not seem much, but to certain individuals this loss of control can be devastating, both psychologically and socially.

Assessing the bladder symptoms and questioning should establish what type of urinary symptoms the client has. Firstly, an overall picture is needed, for example:

- How often do you pass urine? (frequency)
- How long can you hold following the desire to pass urine? (urgency)
- Do you wet before you reach the toilet? (urge incontinence)
- Is it painful to pass urine? (dysuria)
- Do you wake at night to pass urine? (nocturia)
- Do you strain to pass urine?
- Do you have to wait to start? (hesitancy)
- Do you gush or dribble? (poor stream)
- Does your bladder empty without warning? (decreased sensation)
- Do you leak when you cough or laugh? (stress incontinence)

BLADDER CHART
showing stress incontinence
Week commencing: 05/04/03   Name: A. Smith

> Please tick in the **plain** column each time you pass urine

> Please tick in the **shaded** column each time you are wet

Special instructions : Chart for 1 week. Please measure the amount of urine passed.
Please state if wet on exertion with an E, e.g. getting out of bed, coughing, laughing, lifting, etc.

	Monday		Tuesday		Wednesday		Thursday		Friday		Saturday		Sunday	
Midnight													150	✓E
1 a.m.														
2														
3														
4														
5														
6														
7	550	✓E	500	✓E			500	✓E	550					
8					600	✓E								
9										✓E				
10		✓E	300				250	✓E	300		600	✓E	500	✓E
11	300				300									
Noon								✓E				✓E	200	✓E
1 p.m.			350	✓E	200				300		300			
2					350					✓E			300	
3	300													
4		✓E			200			✓E			300	✓E		✓E
5			300				✓E	300						✓E
6					200				300				350	
7		✓E		✓E				✓E				✓E		
8	450						300				450		200	
9									150	✓E				✓E
10	200		450	✓E	300	✓E	150	✓E				✓E		
11									300	✓E	200		250	✓E
Totals	5	4	5	4	6	4	6	5		4	5		7	7

BLADDER CHART
showing possible overactive bladder
Week commencing: 05/04/03 Name: A. Smith

> Please tick in the **plain** column each time you pass urine

> Please tick in the **shaded** column each time you are wet

Special instructions: Chart for 5 days. Please measure the amount of urine passed.

	Monday		Tuesday		Wednesday		Thursday		Friday		Saturday		Sunday	
Midnight	50		50		50									
1 a.m.							100		50					
2	100				50									
3			50						50					
4					50		100							
5			100						50					
6	300	✓												
7	100		100	✓	200	✓	150		200	✓				
8			50		50		50	✓						
9	100								50					
10	50	✓	50		100		50		50	✓				
11	50				50	✓	50	✓						
Noon			100	✓			50		30	✓				
1 p.m.	50		80						50					
2	40		100		30	✓	100		100					
3	30	✓	40	✓			30	✓						
4														
5	100	✓	60		100		50		30	✓				
6	50		30	✓	50		30	✓	40	✓				
7														
8			100		50	✓	100		60					
9	100	✓			50				50	✓				
10	60		100	✓			150							
11					50		50	✓	100					
Totals	14	5	13	5		4	14	5	14	6				

Figure 18.12 Example of charts.

Charting (bladder diary/bladder chart)

To confirm the urinary symptoms, a chart should be filled in, usually by the patient or a carer (Fig. 18.12). The chart should be completed over a minimum of 3 days (Groutz et al 2000). It is the most useful nursing tool in assessing incontinence as part of a baseline assessment and a record of progress during treatment (NICE 2006). A well-kept chart will show times of voiding and episodes of incontinence. If the bladder capacity is needed the volume of urine is also recorded. The fluid intake may also need monitoring if the nurse needs to assess whether the client is drinking enough and has a balanced input and output (see Evolve 18.2).

evolve
learning system

18.2 – BASELINE CHARTS AND BLADDER DIARIES

- Diagnose the type of continence problems.
- Motivate patients.
- Plan bladder retraining.
- Provide a detailed toilet regime for demented patients and those with learning disabilities.

Urinalysis

A specimen of urine should be taken for testing. The presence of protein or blood will indicate infection and a specimen should be sent to microbiology for culture and sensitivity. If the urine testing sticks are able to identify nitrites then the presence of infection is 90% certain; if no nitrites are present there is no infection (NICE 2006).

Residual volume

A post-void residual volume of urine should be determined on initial assessment using an ultrasound scanner (Goode et al 2000) or by intermittent catheterization. Symptoms of a client with an increased residual volume may mimic the symptoms of detrusor muscle instability. If there is a residual volume and inappropriate treatment is commenced, e.g. drug therapy for bladder spasm, this may cause the volume to become greater and eventually cause hydronephrosis and severe kidney damage.

Physical examination

A nursing assessment should include a physical examination of the client, but the nurse must remember that the patient may find this embarrassing. The perineal area should be examined for signs of infection, prolapse, vaginitis and urethritis. A vaginal examination may need to be done by an experienced nurse if stress incontinence is suspected. The strength of the pelvic floor can be assessed and the ability of the client to identify her pelvic floor muscles (NICE 2006). A digital examination of the rectum may be necessary to diagnose if a man has prostate enlargement; again this should only be done by a nurse specialist or a doctor (Royal College of Nursing 2004).

PROMOTING URINARY CONTINENCE

General nursing interventions

Information

If the client understands their problem the reasons for the treatments will be clear and their compliance and motivation should improve.

Fluid intake

Ensuring suitable fluid intake is important for a healthy bladder. This should be around 1500 mL a day for an adult (Archibald 2006). Abrams & Klevmar (1996) suggest this is dependent on weight, e.g. a client weighing 57 kg (9 stone) needs 6 mugs of fluid (1750 mL) while a client of 68 kg (11 stone) needs 7–8 mugs (2200 mL). This ensures the bladder is fully filled and the urine is not concentrated. Drinks that cause bladder spasm, e.g. alcohol or caffeine, should be avoided (Bryant et al 2002). This intervention is particularly important for clients with an overactive bladder, and improvements in the clients' symptoms are often seen

following this simple treatment. Cranberry juice is often encouraged as it may prevent urinary tract infection (Howell & Foxman 2002) (see Evolve 18.3).

> **18.3 – THE CRANBERRY JUICE DEBATE**
>
> - List the actions of cranberry juice (CJ).
> - Describe the evidence for preventing UTI.
> - Discuss evidence for reducing episodes of infection.
> - Summarize its use in clinical practice.

Prevention of constipation

Pressure on the bladder and urethra will cause differing urinary problems, for example bladder spasm due to irritation caused by a rectum filled with hard stool.

Evidence-based practice

Stress incontinence is often associated with both elderly women and women having undergone childbirth; however it may occur at any age. It can be common for young female athletes to experience loss of urine during sporting activities. Carls (2007) conducted a small survey into this problem using females taking part in high impact sports from high schools and colleges in Illinois and also explored the knowledge they had about the condition.

171 questionaires were distributed and 86 were returned. Despite the poor response rate the results raised some significant findings. 28% of the athletes reported small amounts of stress incontinence during sports activities. Some felt this had a negative effect on their social activities and had even given up their sports, and many had not told anyone of their condition. 91% were unaware that pelvic floor exercises could help to prevent the condition. This evidence demonstrates the importance of primary health education in continence promotion of everyone regardless of age.

Specific nursing interventions

Stress incontinence

Following accurate assessment and diagnosis of this condition, the first line of treatment should be pelvic floor muscle training (PFMT) lasting at least 3 months (NICE 2006). Modification of an exercise programme should be on an individual basis with regular follow-up (Bo 2004). Motivated women with no obvious vaginal prolapse experiencing mild to moderate stress incontinence have a good success rate using this treatment modality (NICE 2006).

PFMT can also be used effectively in men, especially after surgery such as radical prostatectomy (Dorey 2007).

Longer term compliance and motivation are important factors for successful outcomes of PFMT. Biofeedback to promote the awareness of movement of the pelvic floor can be useful. This will be visual, electronic or mechanical (Thakar & Stanton 2000). With little or no pelvic floor movement, a course of electro muscle stimulation could be considered. Usually using either a vaginal or rectal probe, electrical impulses are directed into the pelvic floor muscle which will produce a muscle contraction that may lead to strengthening of the pelvic floor (Barroso et al 2004).

When first line PFMT fails, secondary treatment options should be considered. These may include medication such as duloxetine (Yentreve). This drug acts on the sympathetic nervous system, causing sphincter contraction during the filling phase of the bladder (Smith et al 2006). Other drug treatments could include topical oestrogen in menopausal and post-menopausal women. Oestrogen may increase the activity of alpha receptors in the bladder, so allowing the sphincters to work more effectively, although research to support this is inconclusive (Cardosa et al 2000).

Surgery may also be a second line option.

Reflection and portfolio evidence

This exercise for your own private work is physical, rather than the reflection in most such exercises.

Using the anatomy and physiology information discussed earlier, locate the pelvic floor.

- Identify the pelvic floor muscles around the anus by imagining you are holding back flatulence. You should be able to use these muscles without clenching your buttocks, sitting, lying, or standing, in fact anywhere.
- Repeat the previous action by imagining you need to pass urine, but you are in an inappropriate place: feel the muscles that inhibit this action.
- A typical regimen used for continence promotion could be to tighten the muscles around the vagina and anal sphincter, hold for a count of 5–10, then slowly release; repeat four times regularly throughout the day. This exercise is for 'slow twitch' (support) muscles of the pelvic floor. Fast tightenings (tighten and release immediately) are also needed to exercise the 'fast twitch' muscles.

Bayliss (1996:137–139) gives a detailed explanation of these exercises.

Overactive bladder

Conservative treatments for this condition will always start with fluid modification, particularly caffeine reduction (Bryant et al 2002). First line treatment should be bladder training lasting at least 6 weeks (NICE 2006). Bladder training is based on the principal of suppressing an urge to micturate, gradually building up the time between voids (Anders 1999). Prompted or timed voiding where specific times for voiding are set, may be useful for confused clients (Eustice et al 2006). This is explained in Evolve 18.2.

If bladder training is ineffective, drug therapy may be appropriate (Table 18.5). This therapy will usually be in the form of an antimuscarinic preparation. Antimuscarinics block muscarinic receptors of the parasympathetic nervous

Table 18.5 Drug treatment for incontinence

Drug	Dose	Side-effects
For detrusor instability *Anticholinergic (antagonizes the parasympathetic action decreasing bladder spasm)* (NB Antispasmodics should not be given to client with or a history of narrow angle glaucoma)		
Oxybutynin (Cystrin, Ditropan)	2.5–5.0 mg bd–tds Start with minimum dose for the elderly For children 5 years and above 2.5 mg bd	Dry mouth with foul taste Constipation
Slow release oxybutynin (Lyrinal XL)	Start with 5 mg daily, increase 5 mg per week up to 30 mg daily	Less dry mouth
Oxybutynin patch (Kentera)	Each patch delivers 3.9 mg or 15 mg daily	Side-effects lessened
Tolterodine (Detrusitol)	2 mg bd, 1 mg in liver failure	More bladder specific anticholinergic Similar side-effects, less dry mouth
Trospium chlorine (Regurin)	20 mg bd	As above (Does not travel across blood–brain barrier)

Table 18.5—cont'd

Drug	Dose	Side-effects
Solifenacin (Vesicare)	5–10 mg daily	As above
Anticholinergic and calcium antagonist (prevents the uptake of calcium by muscle thus reducing muscle spasm)		
Propiverine (Detrunorm)	15–30 mg bd or tds low dose for the elderly	As oxybutynin
For nocturnal enuresis *Synthetic antidiuretic hormone*		
Desmotabs	200–400 mg nocte	Do not use if client has water retention
For stress incontinence *Reuptake inhibitors (acts on the sympathetic nervous system, causing sphincter contraction during the filling phase of the bladder)*		
Duloxetin (Yentreve)	40 mg bd	Nausea, vomiting Contraindicated in: Hepatic impairment Pregnancy Breastfeeding
Oestrogens (increase the receptability of alpha receptor especially the urethral sphincter)		
Oestradial		Urethritis – use topical cream
For outflow incontinence *Alpha blockers (block action of noradrenaline (norepinephrine) to relax smooth muscle in the prostatic urethra)*		
Tamsulosin	0.4 mg daily	Minimal as drug is prostate specific
5 Alpha reductase inhibitors (androgen deprivation, shrinks benign hyperplastic tissue of prostate)		
Finasteride	5 mg daily	Decreased libido

system in the bladder, so reducing bladder sensation and contractibility (Haab & Castro-Diaz 2005). Recent treatment guidelines do not provide robust evidence to demonstrate significant differences in efficacy between various antimuscarinics (NICE 2006).

Evidence-based practice

Kay and Granville(2005) reviewed literature on the effect of antimuscarinic agents in managing overactive bladder in elderly patients. Side-effects of these drugs include constipation, blurred vision and a dry mouth but of more concern is the possibility of central nervous system dysfunction including cognitive impairment. Antimuscarinics block neurotransmitter binding sites to reduce the parasympathetic effect on the detrusor muscle. There are five muscarinic receptors subtypes (M1–M5) through the body; M2 and M3 predominate in the detrusor muscle. The literature reviewed showed that age increases the permeability of the blood-brain barrier to albumen, and that some of these drugs are more likely to cross the blood–brain barrier and bind with M1 receptors. It is this that gives rise to drowsiness and the adverse effects of cognitive impairment. When selecting therapies for overactive bladder, the health care professional must be aware of the effects these drugs may have on the elderly and prescribe accordingly.

Voiding difficulties

Although outflow obstruction and detrusor hypotrophy show similar symptoms, the underlying causes will eventually need different approaches to treatment.

Outflow obstruction

Treatment options for this condition will either be conservative, medical therapy or surgical intervention. Conservative treatment will involve enrolling the patient onto a 'watchful waiting' programme. Medical treatment will usually be a drug that acts on the alpha receptors in the prostate and bladder neck, or in the case of prostate cancer, will usually be a hormone manipulating drug or anti-androgen.

The obstruction may cause acute urinary retention, the treatment of which is surgery, a prostatectomy, or an indwelling catheter if the patient is unfit for surgery (Heath & Watson 2003).

Detrusor hypotrophy (atonic bladder)

Residual urine is defined as 'the volume of urine left in the bladder immediately following completion of voiding' (Abrams et al 2005). A residual over 100 mL could be significant and should be treated. These treatments could include external bladder stimulation (Dasgupta et al 1997), double voiding (Rigby 2005) or catheterization.

Intermittent catheterization has long been considered an effective and safe method of emptying the bladder (Choong & Emberton 2000). Newer treatments such as sacral nerve stimulation are also becoming more popular (Jonas et al 2001).

Nursing interventions for confused elderly and children

As well as planning the promotion of continence, intervention using specific plans is also needed for those unable to cope with treatments, such as the confused or demented, or the client with learning disabilities. Ways of helping the child with nocturnal enuresis are also important.

Toileting programmes

Toileting programmes help where incontinence is related to the behaviour of the client, or for those who cannot ask to be taken to the toilet. It is useless to toilet a patient every 2 hours without having a prior knowledge of their voiding habits. For example, a client may require the toilet more often in the morning if he/she has taken diuretic tablets and less during the rest of the day when the effect has worn off. Charting is a very good method of ensuring the correct toileting pattern is found and toileting is carried out at the necessary times. The individual needs to be encouraged to go to the toilet to pass urine either at the same time as they passed urine on the previous days or when they were incontinent of urine. Ostaskiewicz et al (2005) shows some evidence that these regimens are effective. Rigid regimens, e.g. everyone is toileted after meals, are best reserved for those people, usually the very demented, for whom all efforts at retraining have failed and where incontinence is intractable. In the demented patient or clients with learning disabilities, communication may be the biggest problem.

Nocturnal enuresis

Children with nocturnal enuresis should be assessed holistically and individually by the multidisciplinary team, so that if there are physical problems they can be referred on as appropriate. As this problem may be multifactorial, a thorough assessment of urinary symptoms is needed including a baseline chart showing fluid input as well as

Table 18.6 The 'Three Systems': signs and symptoms and treatment of choice

Signs	Symptoms	Treatment of choice
Nocturnal : polyuria due to lack of ADH (vasopressin)	Wet soon after sleeping Large wet patches Dilute urine Sleep through wetting Dry if wake to go to the toilet	Desmopressin • can be used long term • best response with older children with primary enuresis (Butler 2002) • needs structural withdrawal using reward charts
Low bladder capacity and bladder instability	Urgency Frequent small voids during day Varying sizes of wet patches Wet more than once a night Wake during or immediately after voiding	Encourage regular intake (6–7 cups a day) avoiding fizzy drinks and caffeine (Enuresis Resource and Information Centre 2002) Regular voiding through the day (6–7 times) Avoid delaying going to the toilet Medication: oxybutynin (Neveus 2001) Relax
Inability to rouse from sleep	Sleep through wetting Difficult to wake even in response to loud noises	Alarms (sensor placed in child's pyjamas or on the bed; this is attached to an alarm and will make a noise when urine wets the sensor) (Butler et al 2001)

urinary output, bladder capacity, number and type of wet episodes and urinalysis. From this information, the cause of the problem can be diagnosed and treated (Table 18.6). Throughout all treatments regular reviews should take place to monitor progress and praise for improvement (Enuresis Resource and Information Centre 2002). A positive attitude from the parents is essential to prevent negative feeling being transferred to the child.

℮volve
learning system

18.4 – NOCTURNAL ENURESIS

- Outline information that should be given to parents.
- List simple treatments for nocturnal enuresis.
- Explain the treatments for nocturnal enuresis.
- Alarm treatment.
- Medications used for nocturnal enuresis.
- Discuss research on the efficacy of these treatments.

Learning difficulties may delay continence but should not be a barrier to acquiring these skills (Harris 2004). Toilet training should start at a time when a child is starting to cooperate with simple instructions. Other milestones also need to be assessed to confirm the child is 'toilet ready' such as the child's mobility and dexterity and ability to know if he or she is 'wet' (Price & Butler 2001).

Individual learning programmes can be introduced using the principles of behaviour modification. The programme must be tailored to the client; it needs to be broken into a series of smaller skills with suitable rewards identified for successfully achieving the skill (Smith & Smith 2003).

ASSESSMENT OF FAECAL INCONTINENCE

This assessment will follow a similar pattern to that discussed for urinary incontinence, especially the questions relating to mobility, environment, dexterity, psychological factors, fluid intake and diet. Those areas that differ are discussed below.

Main complaint

The following key issues are important:

- Discover what terms are used for defaecation, and the client's understanding of diarrhoea and constipation. People vary enormously in what they consider a normal bowel action, in terms of both frequency and consistency (Edwards et al 2003).
- The client's normal defaecation pattern should be noted: the frequency of passing stool, at what time of day and if there are any associated habits (e.g. reading the newspaper, smoking a cigarette).
- The client's perspective of the problem.

Defaecation history

This needs to include the following:

- Using the Bristol stool scale (see Fig. 18.10), ask the patient to identify which is their type and consistency of stool.
- Amount?
- Ease of passing stool?
- Is there rectal sensation of the need to defaecate?
- Is there need to strain, or pain on passing faeces?
- Has the client noted any differences in the stool such as a change in colour or consistency or in the normal eliminating pattern? (A black stool indicates gastrointestinal bleeding, pale stool indicates biliary problems, excess pus or mucus indicates inflammation, for example ulcerative colitis or Crohn disease, altered bowel function may be due to a tumour.)

Faecal incontinence history

This needs to include the following:

- Description of how bad the incontinence is (staining, light soiling, liquid stool, etc.).
- How often the incontinence occurs.
- Whether the client is aware that it is happening.
- Whether the incontinence is due to urgency and not being able to reach the toilet in time.
- Any foods that may cause constipation, diarrhoea, wind or stomach cramps.

Medication history

A list of the client's drugs should be made as they may be responsible for constipation or diarrhoea. For example opiates taken for pain will cause constipation. Record any drugs taken for a bowel problem such as laxatives; note whether there is any laxative abuse as the colon may have become resistant to their effect or even atonic (Metcalf 2007).

Physical examination

The perineum should be observed for signs of prolapse or haemorrhoids. A digital rectal examination (DRE), by an experienced nurse, will show if the rectum is empty or full of hard, soft or loose stool (Royal College of Nursing 2004). DRE should not be undertaken in children if it can be avoided.

The commonest cause of soiling in children is constipation with faecal loading, leading to overflow (Bracey 2002). A similar in-depth assessment needs to be performed, especially in respect of the diet, but the causes may be more complex including psychological problems and difficulties within the family.

There are specific symptoms that warrant a medical referral for investigation; these are rectal bleeding, change in bowel pattern, sudden loss of weight and abdominal pain (Vance 2004).

MANAGEMENT OF FAECAL INCONTINENCE

The treatment will be discussed in the order of the causes shown in Subject Knowledge section (altered physiology of the lower bowel).

Anal sphincter or pelvic floor damage

Restoring the anorectal angle to improve continence can be a more difficult problem, and surgery may be needed. Strengthening of the puborectalis and thus the anal sphincters can be done by pelvic floor exercises concentrating on the anal area (Edwards et al 2003). Electrical stimulation can also help (Norton & Chelvanayagam 2004).

Gut motility/stool consistency

Many types of diarrhoea need medical intervention, e.g. antibiotics for serious infectious diarrhoea, specific treatments for ulcerative colitis or bowel cancers. Chronic diarrhoea may need to be managed by using drugs (Metcalf 2007). Other important nursing care is essential for these patients; replacing fluid lost, and care for skin in the anal area. The latter is done with careful cleansing; often, using wet wipes instead of ordinary toilet paper prevents leaving faecal matter on the skin (Metcalf 2007).

Anorectal pathology

If the problem is due to haemorrhoids, anal fistula or rectal prolapse, medical referral for treatment is needed.

Neurological disease

When caring for patients with neurological problems, interventions depend on the type of nerve damage and nervous disorder. Treatments can range from drug therapy to manual evacuation. The specific care for spinal injuries is expanded on in Evolve 18.5.

18.5 – SPINAL INJURY BOWEL DYSFUNCTION

- List the different types of bowel dysfunction experienced by patients with spinal injury.
- Describe the symptoms these types of bowel dysfunctions cause.
- Outline the most suitable bowel programme for each type of bowel dysfunction.

Secondary to degenerative neurological disease

A structured approach is needed for the demented client; a programme can be constructed using the individual's bowel pattern as a base and then checking, prompting and encouraging the patient to follow what is normal for them (Stokes 2002).

Impaction with overflow

If the incontinence is due to impaction of faeces, the aim of treatment is twofold: firstly, to clear the rectum and colon; secondly, to avoid constipation and keep the rectum empty (Edwards et al 2003).

If the impaction is due to hard faeces, the rectum should be emptied from below by giving daily enemas, either phosphate or micro-enemas. Softener laxatives (Table 18.7) may be prescribed to treat the impaction from above. If the

impaction is soft then any softening agent will give very loose stools and exacerbate the incontinence, so a micro-enema should be used with a stimulant laxative if necessary. If the impaction is great, manual evacuation may be suggested, as a last resort (Royal College of Nursing 2004). In cases of severe cognitive impairment invasive treatments may be inappropriate (NICE 2007). There are serious risks associated with manual evacuation, for example stimulation of the vagus nerve causing dysrhythmias, and perforation of the colonic wall (Royal College of Nursing 2004). Polyethylene glycol (Movicol) is the only oral laxative recommended for the treatment of faecal impaction (Kyle 2006) and may eventually reduce the need for invasive treatments. Movicol can safely be used in children and toddlers and is very effective (Loening-Bauke 2005).

Lifestyle

Simple improvement to a client's lifestyle may be enough to keep the bowel empty, to include good dietary habits and an intake of sufficient roughage. Edwards et al (2003) recommend 30 g fibre daily and a good fluid intake, e.g. 2000 mL per day. Bracey (2002) suggests that a child's fibre intake should be equal to age + 5 in grams and the fluid intake is calculated by weight as follows:

- 1–3 years: 95 mL per kg
- 4–6 years: 85 mL per kg
- 7–10 years: 75 mL per kg
- 11–14 years: 55 mL per kg.

Too much bran should not be eaten without a good fluid intake as this may increase faecal loading in the elderly. An increase in exercise should be encouraged. If these lifestyle changes are unsuccessful, then a suitable laxative may be needed (see Table 18.7).

Reflection and portfolio evidence

Many frail and elderly patients are at risk of constipation as they do not feel like eating and drinking.

- List the foods that contain fibre.
- Look at the menu cards on the wards and identify which contain high amounts of fibre.
- Will these meals tempt these ill patients?
- Think of ways you can introduce more fibre into your patient's diet.
- Your patients should drink 8–10 glasses of fluid a day.
- Think of ways you can help the patient to reach this target.

Discuss these ideas with your mentor and the dietician and reflect on this problem in your portfolio.

Table 18.7 Drug therapy for faecal incontinence: (a) in treating constipation and (b) in treating diarrhoea

Name	Dose	Starts working after	Action	Side-effects and contraindications
(a) Constipation treatments				
Osmotic laxative				
Lactulose	10–15 mL bd children 5–10 years 5 g bd	Up to 2 days	It attracts water as it passes through the gut, softening the stool	Nausea and vomiting and problems with flatus
Fletchers' phosphate enema	1 × 128 mL enema	30 minutes	Increases water content causing rectal distension which stimulates motility	Local irritation; avoid long-term use; contraindicated in Hirschsprung disease
Micro-enemas (sodium citrate), e.g. Micolette, Micralax, Relaxit		30 minutes	Allows water to penetrate and soften the stool thus stimulating defaecation	Local irritation; avoid long-term use; contraindicated in inflammatory bowel disease
Movicol	1–3 sachets daily 8 sachets in 1 litre daily for faecal impaction		Isotonic laxative which does not lose water if client is dehydrated	Abdominal distension and nausea; caution in pregnancy, women breastfeeding, cardiac patients, intestinal obstruction; licensed for children over 5 years (Ungar 2000)
Stool softeners				
Arachis oil retention enema	Single dose enema		Covers the stool with a hydrophobic coat softening the stool and retaining water; the colon is also lubricated	Made from peanuts; be careful in clients with nut allergy
Stimulant laxative				
Senna	2–4 tablets nightly, children over 6 years half adult dose	24 hours plus	Increases rectal motility, i.e. increases peristalsis	Abdominal cramps; may colour the urine red; do not use in intestinal obstruction
Dantron (Co-danthramer)	1–2 capsules nightly or suspension 5–10 mL at night	6–12 hours	As above	Abdominal cramps; may colour the urine red; may cause cancer thus only use in elderly, or the terminally ill
Docusate sodium	Up to 5 × 100 mg capsules daily in divided doses	24 hours plus	Changes the surface tension of the stool allowing water to enter and soften it; this also has a stimulant effect	Abdominal cramps; do not use over a long period of time, or in intestinal obstruction
Bisacodyl tablets	10 mg nightly	10–12 hours	Increases rectal motility	Abdominal discomfort; avoid prolonged use; do not take at the same time as antacids
Bisacodyl suppositories	10 mg in the morning	20–60 minutes	As above	As above
Fletchers' Enemette (docusate)	5 mL	20–30 minutes	As above	As above
Picolax (sodium picosulphate)	10 mg sachet	3 hours	As above	Do not use in gastrointestinal obstruction on congestive cardiac failure
Bulking agents				
Bran		Up to 4 days	Attracts water, increasing faecal mass and thus stimulating peristasis	Flatulence, abdominal distension, intestinal obstruction; adequate fluids are essential

Continued

Table 18.7—cont'd

Name	Dose	Starts working after	Action	Side-effects and contraindications
Ispaghula husk, e.g. Fybogel	1 sachet bd	As above	As above	As above
Regulan	1 sachet 1–3 times a day, for children over 6 years 1/2 to 1 level 5 mL spoon	As above	As above	As above
(b) Antidiarrhoeal agents				
Codeine phosphate	15–30 mg tds-qds		Stimulates opium receptors to decrease the gastrointestinal transit time	Short-term use only; may produce morphine-like dependence; not recommended for children
Loperamide	2 mg capsules after each loose stool, up to 8 mg max		Synthetic opiate inhibits relaxation of the anal sphincter thus retaining liquid stool	Short-term use only. Do not use in liver disease, inflammatory disease, and children under 12 years

For both urinary and faecal incontinence it must be remembered that very simple actions like being near to a toilet, a suitably placed commode, or an adapted bedpan or bottle, and clothes that are easily removed can promote continence in clients where the problem is functional.

> **Evidence-based practice**
>
> Beloosesky et al (2003) queried the safety of using sodium phosphate laxatives as bowel preparation for elderly patients undergoing rectal procedures. He studied 36 patients over 65 who had bowel cleansing for colonoscopy using this medication. It was demonstrated that serious electrolyte abnormality (hypokalemia) may occur. Davies (2004) also looked at this problem in a literature review and suggested phosphate enemas, for similar reasons, were inappropriate for elderly and frail patients, those with cardiac problems or electrolyte imbalance, paralytic illeus, colonic obstructure and patients who had just had surgery. She suggested that glycerine suppositories, bisacodyl suppositories, micro enema polyethylene glycol (Movicol) were suitable alternatives.

GENERAL MANAGEMENT OF INCONTINENCE

There are clients who, despite all efforts to regain continence, never achieve it and clients who are too ill or frail to benefit from or indeed manage the treatment programmes recommended. The aim of management should be to ensure that the client keeps their dignity and self-esteem and is socially acceptable by using pads, sheaths or catheters. Aids must prevent leakage of urine, faeces or any smell, be discreet under clothing and be comfortable to wear.

Absorbent products

These fall into three designs:

- pads placed on the bed or chair
- pads built into the gusset of normal style pants
- body worn pads, all in one or fitted with pants (Fig. 18.13).

All these products may be disposable or reusable (Nazarko 2002).

Disposable underpads or bedpads are possibly one of the least effective and most misused of all items. Disposable pads were designed to protect chairs and beds, and well-applied body worn pads render these redundant (see Evolve 18.6).

18.6 – PADS AND PANTS

- List types of pads.
- Describe the construction of a disposable pad.
- Assess for the correct choice of pad.
- Know how to fit pads correctly.
- Outline skin care for patients using disposable pants.

Sheaths

External sheaths may be a useful alternative for men as a management method for intractable urinary incontinence. Sheaths are made of latex or silicone materials and are held in place by an adhesive interior. They can then be attached to a urinary drainage bag and would usually need to be changed once every 24 hours. However, many men will

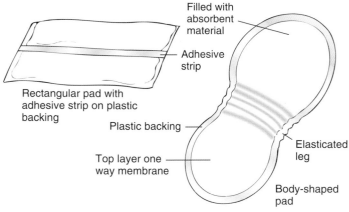

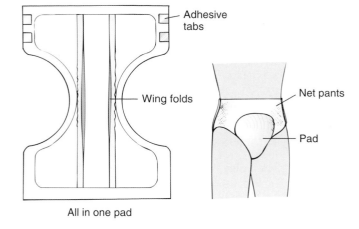

Figure 18.13 Types of disposable body worn pads.

use a sheath on an intermittent basis only. A comprehensive assessment should include accurate sizing, skin integrity and ease of application of the sheath (Fader et al 2001). Sheaths may not be suitable if penile retraction is present, or if the underlying cause of the incontinence is a urinary tract infection or chronic retention of urine.

Catheters

A catheter is a hollow tube used for draining urine. Two types of catheter are used in practice: intermittent and indwelling. An intermittent catheter is a simple plastic tube with inlet holes at the tip and no balloon (a Nélaton catheter). An indwelling catheter is a more flexible tube with a balloon to hold it in place and another lumen to allow the balloon to be inflated (a Foley catheter).

Intermittent catheters

The biggest single advance in the management of neurogenic voiding difficulties has been the introduction of intermittent catheterization. The catheter is introduced periodically into the bladder to remove residual volumes greater than 100 mL in clients experiencing problems of overflow incontinence or recurrent urinary tract infection (Getliffe & Fader 2007). Intermittent catheterization is used in all areas of nursing where patients have problems with residual volumes of urine, for example people with spinal injury or peripheral neuropathy, children with spina bifida, the elderly with hypotonic bladder tendencies and postoperatively.

The frequency of intermittent catheterization will depend on the size of the residual volume of urine found in the bladder. The client with an atonic bladder may need to be catheterized four to six times a day. If the problem is due to a hypoactive detrusor muscle, the client will still be voiding and the residual volume may build up slowly. Catheterization may only be needed two or three times a

week just to ensure the detrusor muscle is not over-stretched making it more lax. Bladder volume equals void plus residual volume and should not be more than 500 mL (Getliffe & Fader 2007). Many clients self-catheterize and for this they need good dexterity, motivation and understanding of the procedure; if they are unable to do it, a carer can be taught, as long as the patient and carer find this acceptable (see Evolve 18.7).

18.7 – TEACHING INTERMITTENT CATHETERIZATION

- Describe types of intermittent catheters.
- Outline areas needed to be included in a teaching programme.
- Provide an example of information given to patients who are going to intermittently catheterize at home.

Evidence-based practice

Pillona et al (2005) investigated how valuable intermittent catheterization was to patients over 70, with a post voidal residual volume of more than 50% of their bladder capacity, in comparison to indwelling catheters. It was a small study of 21 patients who had differing bladder problems including acontractile bladder, underactive detrusor and detrusor sphincter dysynergia. All suffered from urinary tract infection (UTI), six complained of incontinence and four were unable to void. 12 clients were taught to self catheterize and the others were catheterized by carers.

Pilona et al (2007) found that while intermittently catheterizing, no patient had a urinary tract infection; those who were incontinent regained continence and their bladder function partially returned. 18 participants reported a much improved quality of life.

Continued

Indwelling catheters

Indwelling (or Foley) catheters may be used for a client with chronic incontinence after all alternative methods of management have been unsuccessful or are inappropriate.

Catheter management

Long-term indwelling catheters can have serious complications; one of the main ones is the risk of catheter associated infection, with care being focused on its prevention. It is important to ensure a correct type and size of catheter and that a suitable drainage bag system is chosen (Fig. 18.14). The drainage bags can be free-standing or body worn. The latter is usually attached to the leg; however, recently a bag has been designed to fit round the waist – the 'belly bag'; these are particularly suitable for wheelchair bound clients. Catheter valves can also be used; the valve is inserted into the end of the catheter and allows bladder filling and intermittent drainage without interrupting the closed system. The length of time a catheter will be *in situ* will determine the most appropriate catheter material, i.e. either latex or Teflon-coated latex for short-term catheterization (up to 4 weeks), and silicone or hydrogel-coated for long-term catheterization (12 weeks) (Getliffe & Fader 2007). There is some evidence that silver-alloy coated catheters help to reduce risk of catheter associated infection for up to 21 days (Johnson & Kuskowskil 2006).

Catheters come in two lengths: 25 cm for women and 45 cm for men, and with differing diameters, which are measured in Charrières (ch) (0.3 mm = 1 ch). Size 10–12 ch should be used for female clients, 12–14 ch for males and 6–10 ch for children. The smallest catheter possible should be used as one that is too large can cause bladder irritability, occlude urethral glands and cause ulceration of the bladder or urethra or strictures (Getliffe & Fader 2007). The catheter is held in place by a catheter balloon; due to the drainage eyelet's position above the balloon a small residual volume will collect in the bladder. The inflated balloon will sit next to the sensitive trigone and may cause irritation and bladder spasm; thus a small 10 mL balloon is used for most adults (Getliffe & Fader 2007). A 30 mL balloon should only be used following bladder surgery to minimize bleeding

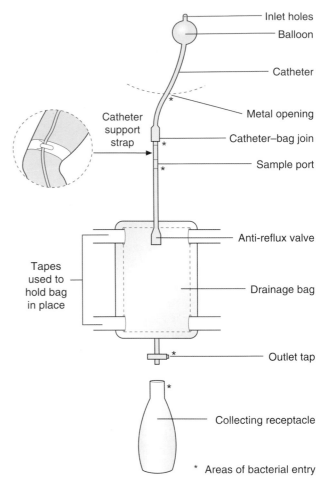

Figure 18.14 Closed urinary drainage system.

(Heath & Watson 2003) The natural defences against urinary tract infection include the tightly closed folds of the urethra and the bladder's flushing action caused by regular emptying. The invasive nature of catheterization compromises these defences and infection may be a consequence (Getliffe & Fader 2007). The ways in which catheter-associated infection occurs and means of preventing it are shown in Table 18.8.

A major complication in up to 50% of clients with long-term catheters is encrustation (Getliffe & Fader 2007). This forms when urine becomes infected with bacteria and forms a biofilm. Urease-producing microorganisms, e.g. *Proteus mirabilis* or *Staphylococcus aureus*, work on urine to split urea and release ammonia; this in solution makes the urine alkaline and encourages mineral salts to precipitate, encrusting the surface of the catheter (Getliffe & Fader 2007). Catheter maintenance solutions may be of benefit for these patients (Table 18.9); however, identifying when the catheter blocks and planning catheter changes accordingly may be the best answer (Getliffe & Fader 2007).

Table 18.8 Some complications of catheterization

Problem	Cause	Action	Reference
Catheter associated infection	Microorganisms introduced by:		
	(a) poor catheterization technique	Improve aseptic technique	DH 2001c
	(b) migration between urethra and catheter	Daily meatal cleansing using clean water	Getliffe 2003
	(c) migration within the closed system by:		
	• break in closed system	Use specimen port to take specimens Empty bag when two-thirds full Change drainage bag every 7 days	Getliffe & Fader 2007
	• poor emptying technique	Wash hands before and after emptying and use clean gloves Empty into disposable receptacle or receptacle that is used for an individual client and can be hot washed	Getliffe & Fader 2007
	(d) poor fluid intake	Increase to 1500 to 2000 mL a day Introduce cranberry juice as a prevention of urinary tract infection	Howell & Foxman 2002
Catheter not draining urine	Kink in tubing	Check tubing and reposition as necessary	
	Drainage bag positioned above bladder	Reposition drainage bag below the bladder	
	Drainage bag too full	Empty regularly as per procedure	
	Inadequate fluid intake	Increase to approx. 10 drinks per day	Getliffe & Fader 2007
	Constipation	Clear constipation (see text)	
	Encrustation/blocked catheter	See below	
Urine bypassing catheter			
(a) While catheter is still draining	Detrusor spasm due to:		
	• too large a catheter	Recatheterization with smaller catheter	Getliffe & Fader2007
	• too large a balloon	Recatheterization with smaller balloon	
	• concentrated urine	Increase fluid intake	
		Anticholinergic medication	
		Bladder washouts not recommended	
(b) When there is no drainage from the catheter	Debris	Intermittent bladder washouts	Rew 1996
	Encrustation	Change catheter and observe tip for encrustation. If this is an ongoing problem planned catheter changes should be adopted	Getliffe 1994

Table 18.9 Catheter maintenance solutions (Rew 1996)

Solution	Content	Action
Suby G (pH 4)	3.23% citric acid + magnesium oxide (to decrease tissue irritation)	Reduces encrustation; helps dissolve existing mineral deposits to keep the catheter patent for longer
Solution R (pH 2)	6% citric acid solution + magnesium carbonate	Aims to dissolve encrustation
Mandelic acid (pH2)	Acidic solution	Aims at inhibiting growth of urease producers
Saline	Antiseptic solution	For removing debris and clots only

Reflection and portfolio evidence

Sometimes patients are discharged from hospital with little information about their catheter, making ordering difficult for the district nurse. If a client has a long-term catheter and is admitted to hospital similar information is also needed. More worryingly, it sometimes happens that there are clients who have a catheter and the nurse cannot find the reason for it being put in originally. It is then a decision making issue as to whether the catheter should be removed or not.

In your practice placement, check the care plans of your catheterized patients and see what information has been documented.

- Can you see clearly when the catheter is due out, to be changed or to be evaluated?
- Find out the type of catheter: its material, size, length, and its balloon size.
- Find out which drainage system is being used.
- Do you understand the rationale for the client's catheterization?
- Obtain a company name, batch number, expiry date so that you can lodge a complaint if there is a problem with the patient's catheter.
- Write up your experiences with critical commentary and add to your portfolio.

PROFESSIONAL AND ETHICAL KNOWLEDGE

This part of the chapter will give an outline of recent national policies, how they impinge on continence care and the way the future service will become integrated. This should allow you to identify the role that nurses will have as part of a multidisciplinary framework to care for clients with elimination problems.

PROVIDING A CONTINENCE ADVISORY SERVICE

Continence advisors emerged as specialist providers of continence care in the early 1970s. At that point services were patchy, and there was no universal job description for this type of specialist (Rhodes 1995). As a result, many continence advisors' roles were focused on coping with the problem rather than on promoting continence. This certainly changed over the years and an important document, *Agenda for Action on Continence Services* (Sanderson 1991), began the emphasis on the need for integration of continence services. Further reviews and reports by the Royal College of Physicians (1995) and Anthony (1998) highlighted disparity in services and education of service providers.

These reviews led to a working party being formed to produce the document *Good Practice in Continence Services* (Department of Health 2000). This document set out national guidelines on how continence services should be delivered, highlighting the need for multidisciplinary assessment and management of the problem. These guidelines were then echoed for the first time in mandatory documentation, *The National Service Framework for Older People* (Department of Health 2001a). This document set the requirement that service providers should establish integrated continence services for older people by April 2004. Other national service frameworks (NSF) such as the NSF for children (Department of Health 2004), the NSF for diabetes (Department of Health 2003) and the NSF for long term conditions (Department of Health 2005), all provided support and momentum for striving to improve continence care nationally.

In the same year as the *National Service Framework for Older People* was published, the document *Essence of Care* (Department of Health 2001b) was produced. This outlined a benchmarking programme for patient care, identifying eight areas of concern. One area highlighted was care of the client with bladder and bowel problems. This document provided an audit tool for all multidisciplinary team members to use to benchmark their services locally and compare them to other services outside their organization. Other national audit tools such as the National Audit of Continence Care for Older People (Royal College of Physicians 2005) enabled continence care providers to audit their services in a similar way.

In 2006, the first clinical guidelines for the treatment of urinary incontinence were published. *The Management of Urinary Incontinence in Women* (NICE 2006) set out a framework for the evidence-based recommendations for assessment and treatment of this condition. As a result, uniformity throughout the health service should be achieved with regards to this treatment, as clear, definitive treatment algorithms have been produced. NICE (2007) has also produced guidelines for faecal incontinence.

Evidence-based practice

Dingwall & McLafferty (2006) conducted a study to explore nurses' perceptions about whether urinary continence is promoted for older people in acute medical and health care of the elderly wards in Scotland. The work was conducted across hospitals including a teaching hospital and three rehabilitation areas and included both trained and untrained staff. The information was obtained using focus groups and semi-structured interviews.

The results suggest that nurses continue to use containment strategies despite being aware of the detrimental effect that long-term catheters may have on the elderly patient. This was reported to be due to personal preference, lack of valid and reliable continence assessment tools to use in planning good quality care, poor documentation in acute areas giving little or no information around the reason for catheterization. Finally, the nurses seemed unaware of the presence of the continence nurse specialist and their advisory role. This showed there is still much work to be done to ensure the elderly receive good evidence-based care.

EDUCATION FOR CONTINENCE PROMOTION

Good Practice in Continence Services (Department of Health 2000) sets out clearly the need for all nurses and healthcare professionals involved with clients with bladder and bowel dysfunction to identify, assess and treat these clients effectively. Prior to this, work by Cheater (1992a) and Palmer (1995) has shown that good quality care for these clients is hampered by lack of knowledge. Laycock (1995) found that an average of 9.4 hours was devoted to continence in pre-registration nursing programmes and much of this was in a clinical setting. *Essence of Care* (Department of Health 2001b) highlights the need for education for assessors and planners of continence care and also support and education for carers of people with continence problems. As a result, recommendations that service providers not only deliver in-service training but also work with higher education institutions to provide valid educational programmes to both pre and post-registered nurses are in place. Higher education institutes now offer degree programmes and postgraduate modules within this speciality.

Decision-making exercise

The first factor to be benchmarked for the section 'Continence and bladder and bowel care' of *Essence of Care* (Department of Health 2001b: 98) reads 'Assessment of individual patient'. And the benchmark of best practice reads:

Patients' positive response to the trigger questions always leads to an offer of an initial bladder and bowel continence assessment which, if accepted by the patient, is completed

With this in mind, what assessment is given to clients, of all ages, with continence problems on the ward or in the community?

- Find out what assessment tools are used on the wards and in the community.
- Are the assessments adapted for the specific groups found in that clinical area.
- Is the tool detailed enough to make a nursing diagnosis of the problem and plan suitable care.
- Assess the client using the tool.

QUALITY ASSURANCE OF CONTINENCE CARE

The *Good Practice in Continence Services* guidelines (Department of Health 2000) suggests targets for all areas of health and the use of performance indicators and audits to monitor progress. This process sits within a clinical governance programme and with reforms in the NHS this governance is mandatory in healthcare trusts. *Essence of Care* (Department of Health 2001b) addresses many quality issues associated with the delivery of a continence service, and does set out clear performance standards and targets. Although these mechanisms are in place, recent reports from the Royal College of Physicians (2005) suggest that there is still much to be done about the quality of assessment and treatment of clients with urinary and faecal incontinence, and the progression towards an integration of continence services. Government White Papers such as *Our Health, Our Care, Our Say* (Department of Health 2006) demand transparent quality assurance processes from the NHS, as much of this paper promotes and supports patient experience and choice. Many continence advisory services will be 'marketed' to users and quality assurance will be an important part of this process.

ETHICAL CONSIDERATIONS

Some areas of continence assessment and care give rise to ethical dilemmas for the nurse. *Essence of Care* (Department of Health 2001b) states that clients have a right to clear explanation of their treatment and full information about available products, and the right to participate fully in the discussions of care. Vinsnes et al (2001) found the care that nurses give patients is at odds with their underpinning knowledge, e.g. pressures on a busy ward may mean an indwelling catheter instead of regular intermittent catheterization is used to save time, or the client who needs a different type of pad or appliance that is not usually supplied by the organization, may cause difficulties. Nurses have a professional responsibility to seek out best practice guidelines and protocols (Dingwall & McLafferty 2006).

Another area of concern is digital rectal examination and manual evacuation, with many nurses confused about the professional and legal aspects of digital rectal examination and manual evacuation of faeces (Royal College of Nursing 2004). The intimate and invasive nature of these procedures make nurses worry that they may be accused of abuse. Recent cases of professional misconduct where inappropriate digital rectal examination and manual evacuations were used with frail elderly people has increased this dilemma (Willis 2000). In the past these skills had to be learned on the job with

experience (Willis 2000). The Royal College of Nursing (2004) guidelines consider there is a need for these procedures in certain cases, but that they must be carried out by a competent practitioner who has the knowledge to judge the appropriateness of their action. It is recommended that employers also have procedures in place that will guide and support their employees in this practice. Nurses need a suitable rationale for using the procedures and to have received instruction and training in performing the technique. Most importantly there needs to be consent of the client to permit the procedure; consent can only be given when the client is in full knowledge of the facts. This will still cause dilemmas in caring for the demented clients who may need this procedure.

Digital rectal examination and manual evacuation are not the only invasive and embarrassing interventions needed to care for a client with continence problems. Vaginal examination and urodynamics investigations are also invasive and compromise the client's dignity, so the same principles of good practice should be followed.

PERSONAL AND REFLECTIVE KNOWLEDGE

Reflective and decision-making exercises have been provided throughout the chapter. By completing these exercises and also keeping a reflective journal of your practice learning, you will build up your knowledge base and expertise and develop empathy with the incontinent client.

CASE STUDIES IN THE MANAGEMENT OF INCONTINENCE

In this final part of the chapter, case studies are presented with related decision making questions in order for you to consolidate the knowledge you have gained from this chapter and your experiences in the practice setting.

Case study: Adult

Sally Taylor is a 32-year-old woman who gave birth to her first child 3 months ago. She is a single parent living in a rural community and is generally fit and well. She has recently visited her GP as she is finding it more difficult to walk, lift her shopping and bend down without leaking urine. She has always had to rush to the toilet, but this leakage coupled with an increased frequency in how often she has to pass urine has become a problem.

- Using the assessment tool described in the chapter try and identify Sally's urinary problems.
- A frequency volume chart showed that Sally had cut down on her oral fluids, only having 4 drinks a day, usually tea or diet cola.

- A vaginal examination carried out by the GP did not reveal anything unusual apart from a weak pelvic floor.
- What may be the causes of Sally's urinary symptoms and what advice would you give?
- Evolve will give you Sally's assessment and base line chart and possible treatments so you can compare your answers.

Case study: Learning disabilities

Susan is a 26-year-old woman with moderate learning difficulties. She lives in a supervised bungalow and goes out to work each day to a local hotel where she cleans. She is taken there by bus. At the bungalow she is able to make her bed and help in the kitchen making simple meals under supervision.

Susan has had no continence problems since she came to the bungalow 6 years ago, but over the last 6 months she has started to wet once she has got to work.

- List all the reasons you can think of for Susan wetting at work and what assessments you could carry out with her.
- When a baseline chart was completed by the home staff, it showed a good fluid intake of 10 cups of fluid a day but the urinary output was high. What reasons can you give for this pattern? (*Clue:* the staff only charted the drinks they gave Susan).

Case study: Mental health

Ted Woodman is 78 and was widowed 3 months ago. He has two children who are married with children but they live far away from their father. Although they ring him regularly they are unable to visit. He has been neglecting himself and now appears unkempt and has lost weight. His sons have contacted the GP who has diagnosed him as having depression. He has prescribed antidepressants and referred him to the community psychiatric nurse. He finds Mr Woodman is very depressed and has only been eating crisps and sausage rolls and drinks tea when he can be bothered to make it. Recently he has been becoming more confused and is refusing to wash, and his underwear is soiled. Today he feels nauseous and is complaining of 'tummy pains'.

- What could be the cause of Mr Woodman's nausea and pain?
- Do you think they could be due to continence difficulties?
- Could a holistic continence assessment highlight the causes of Mr Woodman's problem?
- What interventions do you suggest?
- Are there any ethical issues that may make the treatment and care of Mr Woodman difficult?

Case study: Child

Beth is 8 years old and lives with her mother and two sisters, (Amelia 4 and Alice 9) in a three bedroom detached house on a new estate. Mum and Dad split up 6 months ago. Beth goes to the local primary school and appears to be doing well in her studies. Mum is a dental nurse and has gone back to work full time so Beth and her sisters go to a child minder before and after school.

Beth wets the bed about 4 nights a week. It is usually once a night but she tends to soak the bed. Mum has hoped that she will grow out of it as her ex-husband was also a bed wetter when he was young. Beth is a Brownie and wants to go to the Brownie sleepover so Mum will need to address the problem and approaches the school nurse for help.

- What issues physical, psychological and social, may contribute to Beth's problems?
- What areas of Beth's holistic assessment will be important to diagnose her problem? (use the three systems approach from the Text)
- What interventions can you suggest?
- What advice and support can you give to Mum?
- Evolve will give you Beth's assessment and base line chart and possible treatments so you can compare your answers.

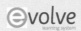

18. 8 – CASE STUDY SUPPORT
• Hints and information to help complete the case studies.

SUMMARY

In order to be an effective decision maker in relation to continence care you need knowledge and skills in continence promotion and the management of incontinence. This chapter has included:

1. An outline of the normal and altered anatomy and physiology of related organs.
2. Information on the psychosocial pressures and the many causes of urinary and faecal incontinence in all age groups.
3. A comprehesive overview of assessment of urinary and faecal incontinence.
4. Information on promotion of continence and management of incontinence.
5. An outline of current national guidelines on continence care.
6. A review of ethical issues related to continence care

Annotated further reading and websites

Cardoza L, Staskin D, Kirby M 2000 Urinary incontinence in primary care. ISIS Medical Media, Oxford

A reference guide covering reasons for incontinence, investigations that are performed, clear interventions for these clients along with tips for care and some coping strategies. It has good clear pictures and diagrams to illustrate key points.

Getliffe K, Dolman P 2007 Promoting continence, 2nd edn. Baillière Tindall, London

This is a very informative book. A full discussion on catheters and their drainage systems is found in Chapter 9. An in-depth chapter on the elimination problems of the elderly and clients with neurological disabilities is in chapter 6; chapter 5 (Mainly children: childhood enuresis and encopresis) is useful for child branch students; and chapter 10 is useful for nurses from the Learning Disabilities branch.

Norton C, Chelvanayagam S 2005 Bowel continence nursing. Beaconsfield Publishers, Beaconsfield

This book covers all types of lower bowel dysfunction. Nursing assessment, investigations and interventions are discussed in depth. The anatomy and physiology chapter (2) is clear and has helpful diagram. And the psychosocial aspects chapter (5) is useful.

http://www.stmarkshospital.org.uk
St Mark's Hospital website giving practical advice for clients and information for professionals.

http://www.eric.org.uk
Site of the Enuresis Resource and Information Centre, where parents and clients can get information on day time wetting, bed-wetting, soiling and constipation. Questions and expert answers displayed.

http://www.continence-foundation.org.uk/
For people with bladder and bowel problems. The Continence Foundation gives information about causes, symptoms, treatments and products. Useful information for professionals.

http://www.aca.uk.com
The Association for Continence Advisors for advice and education for professionals.

http://www.incontact.org
For patient support and information on bladder and bowel problems.

References

Abrams P, Klevmar K 1996 Frequency volume charts: an indispensable part of lower urinary tract assessment. Scandinavian Journal of Urology and Nephrology 179(Suppl.):47–53

Abrams P, Cardozo L, Khoury S, Wein A 2005 Incontinence. Health Publication, Paris, vol 1

Anders K 1999 Bladder retraining. Professional Nurse 14(5):14–16

Anthony B 1998 Provision of continence supplies by NHS trusts. Middlesex University, London

Archibald C 2006 Promoting hydration in patients with dementia in health care settings. Nursing Standard 20(44):49–52

Ash D 2005 Sustaining safe and acceptable practice in spinal cord injured patients. Nursing Standard 20(8):55–64

Barrett J 2002 Pathophysiology of constipation and faecal incontinence in older people. In: Potter J, Norton C, Cottenden A (eds) 2002 Bowel care in older people: research and practice. Royal College of Physicians, London

Barroso J, Ramos J, Martins-Costa S et al 2004 Transvaginal electrical stimulation in the treatment of urinary incontinence. British Journal of Urology International 93(3):319–323

Bayliss V 1996 Female urinary incontinence. In: Norton C (ed) Nursing for continence, 2nd edn. Beaconsfield Press, Beaconsfield, pp 123–152

Beloosesky Y, Grinblat J, Weiss A, Grosman B, Gafter U, Chagnac A 2003 Electrolyte disorders following oral sodium phosphate administration for bowel cleansing in the elderly. Archives of Internal Medicine 163(7):803–808

Bishop M 2005 A wee problem. Nursing Standard 20(12):20–21

Bo K 2004 Pelvic floor muscle training is effective in treatment of female stress urinary incontinence, but how does it work? International Urogynaecology Journal 15(2):76–84

Bracey J 2002 Solving children's soiling problems. Churchill Livingstone, Edinburgh

Brown C, Das G 2002 Assessment, diagnosis and management of lower urinary tract symptoms in men. Journal of Clinical Practice 56 (8):591–603

Brown J, Bradley C, Subak L et al 2006 The sensitivity and specificity of a simple test to distinguish between urge and stress incontinence. American College of Physicians 144:715–723

Bryant C, Dowell C, Fairbrother G 2002 Caffeine reduction education to improve urinary symptoms. British Journal of Nursing 11(8):560–565

Butler R 2000 A fresh approach to understanding childhood nocturnal enuresis. Urology News 4(8):29–32

Butler R 2002 The impact of nocturnal enuresis on the child. Nurse2Nurse 02(10):27–28

Butler R, Holland P, Robinson J 2001 An examination of structural withdrawal programme to prevent relapse in nocturnal enuresis. Journal of Urology 166:2463–2466

Butler R, Golding J, Heron J, ALSPAC Study Team 2005 Nocturnal enuresis : a survey of parental coping strategies at 7{1/2} years. Child Care, Health and Development 31(6):659–667

Carls C 2007 The prevalence of stress urinary incontinence in high school and college-age female athletes in the Midwest: implications for education and prevention. Urological Nursing 27(1):21–24

Cardosa L, Staskin D, Kirby M 2000 Urinary incontinence in primary care. ISIS Medical Media, Oxford

Cheater FM 1992a Nurses' education, preparation and knowledge concerning continence promotion. Journal of Advanced Nursing 17:328–338

Cheater FM 1992b The aetiology of urinary incontinence. In: Roe B (ed) Clinical nursing practice: the promotion and management of continence. Prentice-Hall, Hemel Hempstead, pp 20–40

Choong S, Emberton M 2000 Acute urinary retention. British Journal of Urology International 85(2):186–201

Dasgupta P, Haslam C, Goodwin R, Fowler C 1997 The 'Queen Square bladder stimulator': a device for assisting emptying of the neurogenic bladder. British Journal of Urology 80(2):234–237

Davies C 2004 The use of phosphate enemas in the treatment of constipation. Nursing Times 100(18):32–35

Department of Health 2000 Good practice in continence services. HMSO, London

Department of Health 2001a National service framework for older people. HMSO, London

Department of Health 2001b Essence of care: patient focused benchmarking for healthcare professionals. HMSO, London

Department of Health 2001c Guidelines for preventing infections associated with the insertion of short term indwelling urethral catheters in acute care. Journal of Hospital Infection 47(Suppl.):39–46

Department of Health 2003 The diabetes national service framework. HMSO, London

Department of Health 2004 National service framework for children, young people and maternity services. HMSO, London

Department of Health 2005 Long term (neurological) conditions national service framework. HMSO, London

Department of Health 2006 Our health, our care, our say. HMSO, London

Dingwall L, McLafferty E 2006 Nurses' perceptions of indwelling urinary catheters in older people. Nursing Standard 21(14):35–42

Diokno AC 2003 Incidence and prevalence of stress urinary incontinence. Proceedings 3(8E):824–828

Dolman M 2007 Mainly women. In: Getliffe K, Dolman P (eds) Promoting continence, 3rd edn. Baillière Tindall, London, pp 185–227

Dorey G 2007 Why men need to perform pelvic floor exercises. Continence Journal, Nursing Times 103(19):40–43

Duggan E, Cohan S, Bland D, Preisser J, Suggs P, McGann P 2000 The association of depressive symptoms and urinary incontinence amongst older adults. American Geriatric Society 48(4):413–416

Duggen E, Roberts C, Cohan S et al 2001 Why older community dwellers do not discuss urinary incontinence with their primary health physicians. American Geriatric Society 49(4):462–465

Dykes S, Smilgin Humphreys S, Bass C 2001 Chronic idiopathic constipation :a psychological enquiry. European Journal of Gastroenterology and Hepatology 13(1):39–44

Eason E, Labrecque M, Marcoux S 2004 Effects of carrying a pregnancy and a method of delivery on urinary incontinence: a prospective cohort study. BMC Pregnancy and Childbirth 4(1):4

Edwards C, Dolman M, Horton N 2003 Down, down and away: an overview of adult constipation and faecal incontinence. In: Getliffe K, Dolman P (eds) Promoting continence, 2nd edn. Baillière Tindall, London, pp 185–227

Emmanuel A 2004 The physiology of defaecation and continence. In: Norton C, Chelvanayagam S (eds) 2004 Bowel continence nursing. Beaconsfield Publishers, Beaconsfield

Enuresis Resource and Information Centre 2002 Bed-wetting: treating the underlying problem. Ferring, London

Eustice S 2007 Frail elderly. In: Getliffe K, Dolman P (eds) Promoting continence, 3rd edn. Baillière Tindall, London, p 137

Eustice S, Roe P, Paterson J 2006 Prompted voiding for the management of urinary incontinence in adults. Cochrane Lbrary (4) CDOO213

Fader M, Petterson L, Deans R et al 2001 Sheaths for urinary incontinence: a randomised crossover trial. British Journal of Urology International 88(4):367–372

Fader M, Craggs M 2003 Continence problems and neurological disability. In: Getliffe K, Dolman P (eds) Promoting continence, 2nd edn. Baillière Tindall, London, pp 259–303

Getliffe K 1994 The characteristics and management of patients with recurrent blockage of long-term urinary catheters. Journal of Advanced Nursing 20:140–145

Getliffe K 2003 Catheters and catheterization. In: Getliffe K, Dolman P (eds) Promoting continence, 2nd edn. Baillière Tindall, London, pp 259–303

Getliffe K, Dolman M 2007 Assessing bladder function. In: Getliffe K, Dolman M (eds) Promoting continence, 3rd edn. Ballière Tindall, London, pp 21–53

Getliffe K, Fader M 2007 Catheters and containment products. In: Getliffe K, Dolman P (eds) Promoting continence, 3rd edn. Baillière Tindall, London, pp 259–308

Goode P, Locher J, Bryant R 2000 Measurement of residual urine with portable transabdominal bladder ultrasound scanner and urethral catheterisation. International Urogynecology Journal and Pelvic Floor Dysfunction 11(5):296–300

Groutz A, Blavas J, Chaikin D 2000 Non-invasive outcome measures of urinary incontinence and lower urinary tract symptoms: a multicenter study of micturition diary and pad tests. Journal of Urology 164(3/1):678–701

Haab F, Castro-Diaz D 2005 Persistence with antimuscarinic therapy in patients with overactive bladder. International Journal of Clinical Practice 59(8):931–937

Harari D 2002 Epidemiology and risk factors for bowel problems in older people. In: Potter J, Norton C, Cottenden A (eds) 2002 Bowel care in older people : research and practice. Royal College of Physicians, London

Harari D 2004 Bowel care in old age. In: Norton C, Chelvanayagam S (eds) 2004 Bowel continence nursing. Beaconsfield Publishers, Beaconsfield

Harris A 2004 Toilet training children with learning difficulties : what the literature tells us. British Journal of Nursing 13(13):771–776

Heath T, Watson R 2003 Mostly male. In: Getliffe K, Dolman P (eds) Promoting continence, 2nd edn. Baillière Tindall, London, pp 259–303

Horton N 2004 Behavioural and biofeedback therapy for evacuation disorders. In: Norton C, Chelvanayagam S (eds) 2004 Bowel continence nursing. Beaconsfield Publishers, Beaconsfield

Howell A, Foxman B 2002 Cranberry juice and adhesion of antibiotic-resistant uropathogens. JAMA 287(23):3082–3083

Hunskaar S, Lose G, Sykes D, Voss L 2004 Prevalence of stress urinary incontinence in women in 4 European countries. BJU International 93:324–330

Irvine L 1996 Faecal incontinence. In: Norton C (ed) Nursing for continence, 2nd edn. Beaconsfield Press, Beaconsfield, pp 226–254

Johnson J, Kuskowskil M 2006 Systematic review: antimicrobial urinary catheters to prevent catheter-associated infection in hospitalisation patients. Annals of Internal Medicine 144(2):116–126

Jansson V, Hanson M, Hanson E, Hellstrom A, Sille U 2000 Voiding patterns in healthy children 0–3 years old. Journal of Urology 134:2050–2054

Jonas U, Fowler C, Chancellor M et al 2001 Efficacy of sacral nerve stimulation for urinary retention: results 18 months after implantation. Journal of Urology 165(1):15–19

Kay G, Granville L 2005 Antimuscarine agents : implications and concerns in the management of overactive bladder in the elderly. Clinical Therapeutics 27(1):127–138

Klein M, Janssen P, Macwilliam L 1997 Determinants of vaginal–perineal integrity and pelvic floor functioning in childbirth. American Journal of Obstetrics and Gyneacology 176:403–410

Kobashi K, Leach G 1999 Bladder dysfunction in multiple sclerosis. Neuro-rehabilitation and Neural Repair 13(2):117–123

Kyle G 2006 Assessment and treatment of older patients with constipation. Nursing Standard 21(8):41–46

Laycock J 1995 Must do better: survey of continence education in schools of nursing, medicine, physiotherapy and GP training. Nursing Times 91(7):64

Lembo A, Camilleri M 2003 Chronic constipation. New England Journal of Medicine 349(14):1360–1368

Loening-Baucke V 2005 Prevalence symptoms and outcomes of constipation in infants and toddlers. Journal of Pediatrics 140 (3):359–367

Medel R, Dieguez S, Brindo M et al 1998 Monosymptomatic primary enuresis: differences between patients responding or not responding to oral desmopressin. British Journal of Urology 81:46–49

Metcalf D 2007 Chronic diarrhoea: investigation treatment and nursing care. Nursing Standard 21(21):48–56

National Institute for Health and Clinical Excellence 2006 Guidelines for the management of urinary incontinence in women. National Institute for Clinical Excellence, London

National Institute for Health and Clinical Excellence 2007 Faecal incontinence: the management of faecal incontinence in adults. National Institute for Clinical Excellence, London

Nazarko L 2000 How age affects fluid intake. Nursing Times 96(31):8–10

Nazarko L 2002 Educational needs of nurses working in nursing homes. Blackwell Science, Oxford, p 133

Neveus T 2001 Oxybutynin, desmopressin and enuresis. Journal of Urology 166:1459–2462

Neveus T, Lackgren G, Tuverno T et al 1999 Osmoregulation and desmopressin: pharmcokinetics in enuretic children. Paediatrics 103:65–70

Norton C, Chelvanayagam S 2004 The causes of faecal incontinence. In: Norton C, Chelvanayagam S (eds) 2004 Bowel continence nursing. Beaconsfield Publishers, Beaconsfield

Norton C 2005 Eliminating. In: Redfern S, Ross F (eds) Nursing older people. Churchill Livingstone, London, pp 395–412

Ostaskiewicz J, Roe B, Johnson L 2005 Effects of timed voiding for the management of urinary incontinence in adults: a systematic review. Journal of Advanced Nursing 52(4):420–431

Palmer M 1995 Nurses' knowledge and beliefs about continence interventions in long-term care. Journal of Advanced Nursing 21:1065–1072

Pfisterer M, Grifiths D, Schaefer W, Resnick N 2006 The effect of age on the lower urinary function, a study in women. American Geriatric Society 54(3):405–412

Pillona S, Krhut J, Mair D, Maderbacher H, Kessler T 2005 Intermittent catheterisation in older people: a valuable alternative to indwelling catheters? Age and Ageing 34:57–60

Porrett T 2006 Understanding pelvic floor dysfunction and its relevance to colorectal nursing. Gastrointestinal Nursing 4(3):20–26

Price K, Butler U 2001 Bladder and bowel management in children with disabilities. Current Paediatrics 11:143–148

Raz R, GennesinY, Wasser J 2000 Recurrent urinary tract infection in post menopausal women. Clinical Infectious Diseases 30(1):152–156

Rew M 1996 Use of catheter maintenance solutions for long-term catheters. British Journal of Nursing 8(11):10–13

Rhodes P 1995 The postal survey of continence advisors in England and Wales. Journal of Advanced Nursing 21:286–294

Rigby D 2005 Underactive bladder syndrome. Nursing Standard 19 (35):57–64

Roe B, Doll H, Wilson K 1999 Help seeking behaviour and health and social service utilisation by people suffering from urinary incontinence. International Journal of Nursing Studies 36(3):245–253

Royal College of Nursing 2004 Digital rectal examination and manual removal of faeces: guidance for nurses. Royal College of Nursing, London

Royal College of Physicians 1995 Incontinence causes and management and provision of services. Royal College of Physicians, London

Royal College of Physicians 2005 The national audit of continence care for older people. Royal College of Physicians, London

Sanderson J 1991 Agenda for action on continence services. Department of Health, London

Schum T, Kolb T, McAuliffe T, Simms M, Underhill R, Lewis M 2002 Sequential acquisition of toilet training skills: a descriptive study of gender and age differences in normal children. Pediatrics 109 (3):48–54

Shaw C 2001 A review of the psychosocial predictors of help seeking behaviours and impact of life in people with urinary incontinence. Journal of Clinical Nursing 10(1):15–24

Smith P, Smith L 2003 Continence training in intellectual disability. In: Getliffe K, Dolman P (eds) Promoting continence, 2nd edn. Baillière Tindall, London, pp 303–337

Smith PP, McCrery RJ, Appell RA 2006 Current trends I the evaluation and management of female urinary incontinence. Canadian Medical Association Journal 175(10):1233–1240

Stokes G 2002 Psychological approaches to bowel care in older people with dementia. In: Potter J, Norton C, Cottenden A (eds) 2002 Bowel care in older people: research and practice. Royal College of Physicians, London

Thakar R, Stanton S 2000 Regular review: management of urinary incontinence in women. British Medical Journal 321(7272):1326–1331

Thompson W, Longstreth G, Drossman D, Heaton K, Irvine E, Muller-Lissner S 1999 Functional bowel disorders and functional abdominal pain. Gut 45(Suppl. 2):43–47

Ungar A 2000 Movicol: its treatment of constipation and faecal incontinence. Hospital Medicine 61(11):37–40

Vance M 2004 Rectal bleeding: when to refer in. In: Norton C, Chelvanayagam S (eds) 2004 Bowel continence nursing. Beaconsfield Publishers, Beaconsfield

Wein A, Lose G, Fonda D 2002 Nocturia in men, women and the elderly, a practical approach. British Journal of Urology International 90 (Suppl. 3):28–31

Weiss J, Blaivas J 2000 Nocturia. Journal of Urology 163(1):5–11

West A, Stienhardt K 2003 Containing anxiety in the management of constipation. Archives of Disease in Childhood 88:1038

Wiesel P, Bell S 2004 Bowel dysfunction : assessment and management in the neurological patient. In: Norton C, Chelvanayagam S (eds) 2004 Bowel continence nursing. Beaconsfield Publishers, Beaconsfield

Wilkinson K 2001 Pakistani women's perceptions and experiences of incontinence. Nursing Standard 16(5):33–39

Willis J 2000 Bowel management and consent. Nursing Times 96(6):6–7

Vinsnes A, Harkless G, Haltback J, Hunskarr S 2001 Healthcare personnel's attitudes towards patients with urinary incontinence. Journal of Clinical Nursing 10(4):455–461

Yeung L, Godley H, Ho C et al 1995 Some new insights into bladder function in infancy. British Journal of Urology 76(2):235–240

Chapter 19

Rehabilitation and recovery

Janet H. Barker and Brenda Rush

KEY ISSUES

SUBJECT KNOWLEDGE
- The social and political context of rehabilitation
- Social roles
- Sick role
- Labelling and stigma
- Altered body image
- Loss and grieving
- Motivation
- Management of change
- Teams and leadership

CARE DELIVERY KNOWLEDGE
- Assessment in rehabilitation
- Goal setting
- The nurse as an educator or facilitator of change

PROFESSIONAL AND ETHICAL KNOWLEDGE
- Impact of health and social policy on the provision of care
- Social exclusion
- Inter-professional working
- Ethical considerations

PERSONAL AND REFLECTIVE KNOWLEDGE
- Rehabilitation in professional practice

INTRODUCTION

There has been a shift from custodial care to rehabilitation in a variety of contexts ranging from the care of the elderly to children's disorders and from physical disorders to enduring mental illness. Indeed, health policy over a decade and a half ago, in the form of *The Health of the Nation* (Department of Health 1991a), identified rehabilitation as a key area in the strategy for health. The long-term conditions National Services Framework (NSF) (Department of Health 2005) reiterates this commitment to rehabilitation and the provision of services to meet the needs of people requiring such interventions. Rehabilitation can be seen as an area of central importance to healthcare delivery.

Various definitions of rehabilitation are available, but Wade's (2005: 814) is comprehensive, proposing rehabilitation is:

an educational, problem-solving process that focuses on activity limitations and aims to optimize patient social participation and well being, and so reduce stress on care/family

The word 'process' in the above definition suggests an activity that moves forward through a series of actions aimed at achieving an identified result.

Rehabilitation is associated with the notion of recovery but the two do not mean the same thing. Rehabilitation focuses on the helping process whereas 'recovery' focuses on the experience of the person who is trying to overcome a particular disability. A psychologist, service user and writer, Patricia Deegan, described recovery from mental health problems in terms of regaining a sense of self and a sense of purpose 'within and beyond the limits of the disability' (Deegan 1988: 11). The notion of 'recovery' from mental illness developed from service users themselves and Deegan's work has influenced contemporary thinking about mental health care by health care professionals and policy makers. For example, one of the *Ten Essential Shared Capabilities* for mental health practice (Hope 2004: 3) is 'promoting recovery':

Working in partnership to provide care and treatment that enables service users and carers to tackle mental health problems with hope and optimism and to work towards a valued life-style within and beyond the limits of any mental health problem.

The Chief Nursing Officer's review of mental health nursing (Department of Health 2006: 17) similarly advocates a 'recovery approach' which stresses the need for optimism by nurses, where recovery does not necessarily mean a full return to previous functioning, or a cure, but rather the instillation of hope about the possibility of positive change in an individual.

Recovery is also relevant to people with physical disabilities. For example, the woman whose life has involved playing tennis, running and skiing will have to revise her sense of self as an active 'sporty person' if she becomes incapacitated through severe arthritis or a serious road traffic accident. However, with support and positive attitudes from healthcare professionals, the effects of an illness can be minimized so that they interfere with a person's lifestyle as little as possible. Rehabilitation then can promote recovery. Repper & Perkins (2003) discuss the notion of recovery and rehabilitation in mental health nursing, although their ideas are transferable to other branches. They note the importance of giving hope and the importance of a supportive nurse–patient relationship. Allvin et al (2007: 557) define recovery from a postoperative perspective as:

an energy-requiring process of returning to normality and wholeness as defined by comparative standards, achieved by regaining control over physical, psychological, social and habitual functions, which results in returning to preoperative levels of independence/dependence in activities of daily living and an optimum level of psychological well-being.

This definition reminds us that recovery can be a difficult process, encompassing many aspects of a person's life which will need to be considered by the rehabilitation nurse.

As will be discussed later in this chapter, it is suggested that the role of nurses in the process of rehabilitation is often poorly defined (Kvigne et al 2005). However, Jinks & Hope (2000) indicate nurses are the 'glue' within the multidisciplinary team, acting as coordinators of care and providing a holistic overview. It is argued by Low (2003) that in acting as coordinators of care, nurses fulfil one of the most central roles within the rehabilitation process. The Royal College of Nursing (2007a: 9) suggest that 'the role of the nurse is to be there, offer personal support and practice expertise but always to enable the person to follow their own path'.

Blanche-Spelich et al (2004) propose that the process of rehabilitation knows no boundaries, being equally relevant to individuals with a range of health problems/illnesses/disabilities across all ages, ethnic and social groups.

Rehabilitation activities are undertaken in a range of settings, from acute inpatient care to day and community settings. As such, rehabilitation can been seen as an aspect of every nurse's practice and warrants close consideration.

OVERVIEW

This chapter addresses factors that influence the process of rehabilitation and recovery. Numerous terms are used to describe people who are recipients of care. In this chapter the terms patient, client and service user are used interchangeably to represent this group.

As identified above, recovery is a concept associated with rehabilitation in mental health; however, it can readily be applied to other branches of nursing. Therefore, wherever recovery is pertinent to discussions in this chapter it will be included.

Within contemporary service delivery, user and carer involvement is fundamental to successful rehabilitation programmes and you will also see this reflected throughout this chapter.

The chapter is divided into four main parts.

Subject knowledge

The first section, Subject Knowledge, develops the scope of rehabilitation. Rehabilitation is undertaken in a wide range of settings and it would be impossible to address all care groups here. However, the social, psychological and health policy aspects are common and have great relevance to all forms of rehabilitation and for this reason form a large component of this section.

Care delivery knowledge

The second section of the chapter, Care Delivery Knowledge, examines the roles of service users, carers and nurses in rehabilitation. The use of decision-making exercises and suggestions for portfolio work will help you to develop an understanding of the issues that underpin the associated nursing care.

Professional and ethical knowledge

The third section of the chapter, Professional and Ethical Knowledge, focuses on three main issues: the impact of health policy, the nurse's role in interprofessional working and ethical issues in rehabilitation.

Personal and reflective knowledge

Finally, in Personal and Reflective Knowledge, the main points of the chapter are revisited both through the use of case studies and in providing suggestions for portfolio evidence. You may find it helpful to read one of the case studies on page 456 before you start the chapter and use it as a focus for your reflections while reading.

SUBJECT KNOWLEDGE

As identified above, rehabilitation is undertaken in a wide range of settings and it would be impossible to address all care groups here. However, the social, psychological and health policy aspects are common and have great relevance to all forms of rehabilitation and for this reason form a large component of this section.

THE SOCIAL AND POLITICAL CONTEXT OF REHABILITATION

The underpinning social and health policy context has great relevance to all forms of rehabilitation. Consequently it is important for nurses to first understand these issues, with the RCN (2007b) stating that an understanding of such issues is essential if the nurse is to fulfil their role in advocating for changes to care delivery and management services for patients.

Social policy relates to central and local government activities associated with the provision of services related to health, education, housing and social services, including social security and income support. It addresses questions concerning how much welfare the state should provide and how this is to be funded. Health policy, as one aspect of this, is of particular interest to those involved in the delivery of care. Scott (2001) argues that the overlapping of health policy with nursing policy requires nurses to have an understanding of how one impacts on the other and the implication of this for care delivery.

Developed countries are viewed as having a mixed economy of welfare made up of:

- state sector
- private sector
- voluntary sector
- informal carers.

Recently in the UK there has been an emphasis on involving patients and the public in developing health and social services and delivering. The way in which this involvement has developed can be understood from the prevailing political and social climate. Barnes et al (2000) identify three models of user involvement, which show different emphases over time. These are, the 'consumerist' approaches during the 1980s and early 1990s; the 'democratic model' in the mid-1990s and the 'stakeholder model', representing approaches in the early 21st century.

The consumerist model

In the political context of the 1980s and 1990s the emphasis on introducing an internal market (Department of Health 1989) in health care led to the view that patients should be viewed as customers or consumers of health services. The Conservative governments between 1979 and 1997 emphasized the responsibility of individuals to maintain their own health. Indeed, the first reference to the public as customers of health services appeared in *Patients First* (Department of Health and Social Security 1979). This consumerist approach was reflected by a change in the roles of service providers who were concerned to improve the efficiency and effectiveness of services to patients.

The early 1990s saw a number of policies that developed the consumerist model. For example, the NHS and Community Care Act (Department of Health 1990) required local authorities to consult with service users and carers, then, in 1991, the *Patients' Charter* (Department of Health 1991b) established a framework for patient entitlements. The involvement of the 'consumers' was acknowledged in *Local Voices* (Department of Health 1992), which recommended community involvement to help in the planning and monitoring of services in the NHS.

The democratic model

In contrast to the consumerist approach, the democratic model is associated with service users who challenged the inequalities in power between service providers and consumers (Beresford & Croft 1993). This can be most clearly seen in the rise of the user movement in the UK when groups of mental health service users were established to argue against what they saw as an unfair distribution of power in favour of the professions. The democratic model is about more than having a voice in health and social care services. It is concerned with how citizens are treated and regarded, based around a belief that everyone should have a greater say and more control over state funded institutions which influence the lives of the population.

Closely associated with the democratic model is the notion of 'empowerment'. Empowerment has been described as a process and an outcome (Ryles 1999). As a process, the empowerment of patients by health professionals is considered possible if professionals relinquish their own power, but as Masterson & Owen (2006) argue, social change is needed to allow new-found power to be exerted. So, at the level of care delivery empowerment can be understood as the nurse maximizing the patient's independence and minimizing dependency. At a political–social level, it can be seen through policies which enable individuals to influence the development and delivery of healthcare services. When considering the outcomes of empowerment, it appears that the concept is more easily understood by its absence. For example, Gibson (1991) identified powerlessness, helplessness, hopelessness, oppression, loss of control over one's life and dependency as indications of a lack of empowerment.

The stakeholder model

With political changes from the late 1990s during the period of the New Labour government, Barnes et al (2000) argue that consumerism and empowerment have evolved into the stakeholder model. This position suggests that public services are best planned and delivered when the views of key parties, including those of service users, professionals, the general public and government, are actively sought and taken into account. The idea of 'partnership' is emphasized rather than the empowerment of one group. Under a stakeholder model, service users' and carers' views and knowledge are accepted as equally important to those of other stakeholders and they are therefore regarded as 'partners'. So the goal of this model is to ensure that users' and carers' voices are heard and their views have influence. Inequalities in power between the different parties are accepted as the reality, rather than being open to challenge. In the stakeholder model, service users and carers will usually be invited to participate on the terms set out by policy makers and professionals.

The stakeholder model has been espoused in a series of Labour government reports since 1997, which have emphasized the need to involve patients and the public in decision making about health and social care (for example Department of Health 1997, 2000, 2001c). These culminated in the Health and Social Care Act (Great Britain 2001), which placed a duty in law on the NHS to make arrangements to involve and consult patients and the public in decisions about health services and can be seen in various consultation groups such as Patient Advice and Liaison Services (PALS), Local Involvement Networks (LINks) and Patient and Public Involvement Forums (PPI Forums).

See Evolve 19.1 for more information on patient and public involvement.

SOCIAL ROLES

The social and political context explains how a society views rehabilitation. To explore what it actually means for individuals requires an understanding of how individuals interact within society. It is suggested that individuals and society interact through taking various social roles. This provides a sense of purpose and belonging for all individuals within society and allows the individual to develop a concept of self. A loss of social role can occur following illness or disability or as a result of the often prolonged process of rehabilitation. Therefore as Wade (2005) proposes, a significant aspect of rehabilitation is enabling individuals to maintain and/or resume as far as possible their social roles and is central to planning rehabilitation programmes.

Social roles are associated with the individual's status within his or her society. Status encompasses such things as:

- gender (e.g. male or female)
- occupation (e.g. nurse, farm worker, tailor)
- family relationships (e.g. daughter, brother, parent).

Status is also culturally defined and may be either:

- fixed or ascribed (e.g. gender or ethnicity), or
- achieved (e.g. marital status or class).

For each status there are identifiable expected and acceptable ways of behaving. These are known as 'norms'. The group of norms attached to a particular status is a 'role'. Therefore each status is accompanied by a role, which shapes and directs social behaviour. Individuals then perform this role in relation to one another (Table 19.1). This enables individuals to interact with each other, predict how others will behave and have a clear idea of what is expected in terms of their own role. For example, in the interaction between nurse and client, each knows what is expected of them and how the other should respond. Both nurse and client can then concentrate on the situation they are in without being inhibited by other aspects of their lives.

When someone becomes ill they may not be able to fulfil their normal roles and this affects their perceived status and self-esteem. For example, if a woman experiences a

19.1 – PATIENT AND PUBLIC INVOLVEMENT

- Be familiar with government legislation and recommendations on public involvement in strategic decisions on health care.
- Be familiar with government legislation and recommendations on patients' rights to involvement in their own care in partnership with health professionals.

Table 19.1 Role of the nurse

Status	Nurse
Norms	Knowledge of illness Cares for people Gentle and kind
Role	Wears a uniform Practical Busy

stroke that affects her ability to do domestic activities, she may feel that this affects her role as a provider of care for her husband. This may have an impact on the way the husband and wife interact and their expectations of each other.

The above discussion presents social roles and obligations as clearly identified and explicit concepts. However, roles can be seen as fluid and changeable.

An alternative way of thinking about roles is seeing them as having generally defined aspects but certain elements within them being subject to individual negotiation. For example it can be said that there is no script as to how a student nurse should behave; rather this is negotiated between students and their teachers, placement supervisors and clients. This negotiation occurs in relation to an individual's understanding of the role and their beliefs.

Evidence-based practice

Men are perceived as being socialized into a particular gender role and as such this has implications for the ways in which they view health and their response to disease. White & Johnson (2005) conducted in-depth interviews with men admitted to hospital with chest pain. They found that all the men delayed seeking help and tried to explain their symptoms as common everyday problems such as wind or heartburn. It is suggested this is in part due to the 'macho' ideal present within Western society and the socialization of men into roles that promote the image of men as strong, productive, fit and healthy. Delaying initial treatment of acute chest pain can have serious implications for treatment and outcomes and the eventual impact on men's general well-being.

The sick role

Parsons (1951) argued that in times of illness, Western societies allow individuals to take a sick role. This means that individuals are not expected to contribute economically to society during the time of their sickness and are not subject to any moral blame for their illness. However, they are expected to comply with treatment and do all in their power to work with the professionals to aid their recovery (see Table 19.2 for rights and obligations of the sick role). The social exchange in Parsons' theory means that compliance with treatment and trying to get well again allows the sufferer to experience a form of no fault–no blame agreement in the eyes of society.

The implication of sick role theory for individuals is that they are expected to accept, rather than to challenge care decisions made by professionals which results in an imbalance in power between professional experts and patients. Unlike the stakeholder model mentioned earlier, in this

Table 19.2 The sick role (after Parsons 1951)

Right or obligation	Provisos
Two rights	
The sick person is exempt from performing his or her usual social role	This exemption is relative to the severity of the illness It must be legitimized by others – often the doctor is the legitimizing agent
The sick person is not responsible for his or her illness	The person is not expected to 'pull themselves together' As he or she is exempt from responsibility, there is an expectation of 'being taken care of'
Two obligations	
The sick person must get better as soon as possible	Being ill is unacceptable and the person must be motivated to get well
The sick person must seek medical advice and comply with the treatment prescribed	Help must be sought from a competent and acceptable source in relation to the severity of the illness

situation there is little or no acceptance of a partnership approach here. The view is that patients need to be given information to help them to understand that they are sick and that their cooperation is an essential element in the recovery process. To involve them in their care makes good sense, particularly in the light of research evidence that such involvement helps to promote compliance, user satisfaction and effective treatment (Anthony & Crawford 2000).

Reflection and portfolio evidence

Think of a client in whose care you have recently been involved during a clinical placement.

- Identify the various roles that individuals may have.
- How might their illness or disability affect these roles?
- How could the nurse help the client adjust to the new role demands in the short term?
- What long-term role adjustments might this client have to make?
- On your last practice placement, did the clients meet Parsons' (1951) criteria for the sick role (see Table 19.2)?
- If they did, how?
- Have you ever taken the sick role?

LABELLING AND STIGMA

Becoming ill can be viewed as deviant and the sick role offers a way of describing how behaviour is regulated. An alternative way of viewing this is through labelling theory. This offers an interactionist view of society and an explanation as to how a client's role is negotiated and maintained.

Lemert (1951) suggested two forms of deviation: primary and secondary. Primary deviation is any act that an individual may engage in before being publicly labelled as deviant. These acts are seen as relatively unimportant as they have little impact on an individual's self-concept. What is important is society's response to the individual. Public recognition and labelling of deviant behaviour coupled with the consequences of such identification produces a response from the individual. This response is the secondary deviation. Society's reaction to the individual assigns a new role and status, which has an effect on how an individual sees themselves and their behaviour. The move from primary deviance to secondary deviance happens when an individual labelled as deviant by others accepts the 'new' social status and role.

Williams (1987) discusses deviance in relation to a medical diagnosis. Secondary deviation occurs where the diagnosis is accepted and associated with a negative social status. As a result of illness or surgery, labels such as diabetic, schizophrenic or amputee may be applied. Therefore the labelled individual is marked as different from the rest of society and may invoke negative social reactions. 'Stigma' is the term applied to such responses.

The seminal work on stigma was produced by Goffman (1963), who identified various sources and attributes associated with this phenomenon (Table 19.3). The negative social responses to conditions that attract stigmas are related to feelings such as fear or disgust that are attached to certain labels and the attribution of stereotypical traits to individuals. Therefore, people in wheelchairs are often viewed as both mentally and physically disabled, while someone with a mental illness is considered to be potentially violent.

Sayce (2000) suggests that the concept of 'stigma' is not always useful as it focuses on the individual. 'Stigma' literally means a mark of disgrace or shame and can be seen to focus on what is wrong with the person. Thus it does not provide any foundation for challenging prejudice or improving rights for people with a disability. Rather, the focus needs to be on those who do the stigmatizing and act unfairly towards the person. In this way discriminatory practices can be highlighted and collectively acted upon.

Reflection and portfolio evidence

On your last clinical placement:

- What diagnostic labels were attached to clients?
- What effect did the diagnostic label have on the client? – the client's family? – the care team?
- How can the nurse minimize the negative effects of stigma attached to diagnostic labels?

Stigmatized ideas are culturally determined; that is they are based on society's norms and values, which are learned early in life, and they are reinforced through everyday conversations and the media. Individuals with stigmatizing illnesses may be viewed as socially inferior and may also be subject to discrimination and socially disadvantaged. The imposing of such social disfavour may result in poor self-concept and identity. Goffman (1963) suggests that the stigmatized individual may adopt various responses when interacting with a non-stigmatized individual (Table 19.4).

Table 19.3 Sources and attributes of stigma (after Goffman 1963)

Sources	Abominations of the body	Physical disabilities
		Mental illness, sexual deviance
	Blemishes of character	Race, nation, religion
	Tribal stigmas	
Attributes	Discreditable	Those that are not visible or known and are therefore only potentially stigmatizing such as epilepsy, acquired immunodeficiency syndrome (AIDS), diabetes mellitus
	Discrediting	Known, visible and provoking a reaction in others, for example facial disablement or deformities, symptoms of mental illness

Table 19.4 Responses to stigma (after Goffman 1963)

Passing	Tries to conceal attribute and pass as normal (e.g. an individual not disclosing a history of mental illness to an employer)
Covering	Tries to reduce the significance of the condition (e.g. attempts to resume 'normal behaviour')
Withdrawal	Opts out of social interaction with 'normal' people (e.g. all social activities involve others with a similar disorder)

Finlay (2005) highlights how the labels nurses attach to patients have implications for the care received. Often patients are labelled as 'good' when they are seen as compliant, uncomplaining and get better; bad when viewed as less cooperative and demanding of time. However, the use of such labels is subjective. What is seen as demanding by one person may be viewed as looking for support and reassurance by another.

ALTERED BODY IMAGE

Many stigmatizing illnesses have an impact on the way an individual perceives his or her body and therefore his or her body image. Body image affects the social, spiritual, physical and psychological aspects of well-being, and as such, an understanding is vital to the provision of care (Walker et al 2006).

Price (1990) suggests that body image has an impact on the process of rehabilitation, having consequences for and affecting the client's well-being. He identifies three components to body image:

- how individuals perceive and feel about their bodies (body reality)
- how the body responds to commands (body presentation)
- how the first two components compare with an internal standard (body ideal).

Throughout life there is an attempt to achieve and maintain a balance between the three elements (Table 19.5). Thus body image depends not only on the individual's response to his or her own body, but also upon the appearance, attitude and responses of others. This is important for nurses to remember when delivering care, as their own responses may have a great impact on how clients perceive themselves.

In considering Price's (1990) work, Walker et al (2006) identify that body image and self-image are interconnected, self-image being central to an individual's confidence, motivation and sense of achievement. It is a product of an individual's personality, being moulded by socialization, and represents an assessment of self-worth. When the three elements of body image are in a state of equilibrium, meeting both personal and social expectations and therefore enabling a successful presentation of self, there is a corresponding positive self-image. If, however, changes occur that result in an alteration of one or more of the body image components, a negative self-image may follow (Fig. 19.1).

Personal responses to altered body image will be influenced by a variety of factors, including:

- visibility
- associated shame or guilt
- significance for the future – work, social life, personal
- support during transition
- personal coping strategies.

Newell (2002) suggests that nurses have a role helping patients to deal with the distress associated with altered body image. There are three areas in which the nurse can take an active role

1. Public health – promoting public awareness of the issues faced by people who are subject to stigmatisation due to disfigurement.
2. Advisory role – preparing individuals who undergo procedures that may result in changes to their body image or disfigurement.
3. Providing specific interventions or referring to experts where necessary.

Table 19.5 Components of body image (after Price 1990)

Reality	As it really is: tall/short, fat/thin, dark/fair Norm for race and relative to wider social group Not a constant state, dependent upon age and physical changes
Presentation	Dress and fashion Control of functions, movement and pose How others receive us
Ideal	How a body should look and act (culturally determined and includes size, proportion, odours and smells) Personal norm for personal space Body reliability, which may be unrealistic Applied not only to self, but to those around us

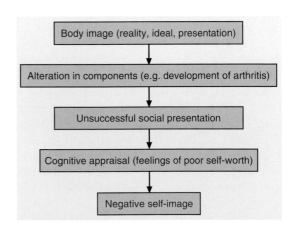

Figure 19.1 Impact of body image on self-image.

LOSS AND GRIEVING

Decision-making exercise

Gareth Pearce, aged 23, is developing his career as a professional footballer. He played for a third division team when he was spotted by a scout for a premier league team, who subsequently signed him on. He appeared to have a promising career ahead of him. However, in his fourth match in the first team, as a result of a bad tackle, Gareth finds himself in the accident and emergency department with a fractured left tibia and fibula. He is accompanied by his wife and young son. The orthopaedic surgeon informs Gareth that he will not be playing football again for the rest of the season and that the fracture is so severe that at this stage he is uncertain whether Gareth will be able to play football again.

- What losses might Gareth and his family experience as a result of the accident and during his hospitalization?
- What responses or behaviour could this evoke?
- How might a knowledge of the grief reaction help the nurse to support Gareth and his family over the immediate crisis?

(For further information on the grief reaction see Ch. 13, 'End of life care'.)

Grief is usually associated with death and dying, but it also occurs during other times of loss. Costello (1995) suggests that grief is the feelings that are evoked through the loss of something valued, and, as observed by McGrath (2004), there are many potential and actual losses experienced by people who have or are recovering from health threatening events. These losses relate to things such as lifestyle changes, altered physical or psychological functioning and loss of body parts. Such experiences can result in a severe emotional stress response (see Ch. 9, 'Stress, relaxation and rest'). It can also invoke the grieving process.

In her work with terminally ill people and their families, Dunne (2005) provides an overview of the various ways in which people deal with grief and cites the classic work of Kubler Ross (1975) in which it is identified that people who face death experience a number of emotional responses (Table 19.6). She suggests that not all individuals will go through all these stages, that some may never reach acceptance, and that individuals may move to and fro between the stages. Although this process is viewed in terms of the individual's impending 'loss' through their own death, it can also be applied to losses experienced from illness and disability.

Table 19.6 Stages of grief (after Kubler Ross 1975)

Stage of grief	Features
Denial	Feeling that 'This can't be true', emotions are not expressed and the person tries to continue as if nothing has happened
Anger	Following acknowledgement of the reality an individual may express anger; this may be directed at themselves, friends, family, carers, God, everyone or everything in general
Bargaining	The person seeks to avoid the inevitable by proposing 'bargains' such as becoming a good person or going to church regularly if only they are allowed to live longer or have less pain; these 'bargains' are made privately or silently
Anger, depression	As the individual begins to feel that bargaining is futile they may lapse into depression or revert to their anger, questioning 'Why me?' For the person to feel this way there has to be a certain element of acceptance
True acceptance	Or resignation to their fate

Evidence-based practice

Lohne & Severinsson (2005) investigated patients' experiences of hope and suffering following spinal cord injury. Two main themes emerged.

- 'Vicious circle' – here people talked of feelings of loss, loneliness and dependency on others as they progressed through a cycle of good and bad days. They alternated between an acceptance of what had happened to them and the limitations this imposed and a belief that things would improve.
- Longing – every patient expressed a longing to return to their former life, leading to a constant comparison between who they were before the injury and who they had become.

All expressed the need for someone to talk to about their suffering and longing. Lohne & Severinsson suggest that nurses are ideally placed to provide patients with this type of support and therapeutic engagement.

MOTIVATION

Motivation is an important factor in the process of rehabilitation. Motivated behaviour is described by Gross (2005) as being purposeful and goal directed. When a client's physical ability is present, but motivation is lacking, rehabilitation can become a frustrating experience for those providing care – both for health professionals and informal carers.

Resnick (2002) identifies the understanding of motivation to be essential if the nurse is to facilitate an individual's rehabilitation and suggests that theories related to self-efficacy, such as in the work of Bandura (1977), provide both an explanation of motivation and a framework for promoting patient activity.

Self-efficacy relates to the confidence an individual has in their ability to achieve identified goals and is seen as a strong predictor of an individual's likelihood of overcoming barriers to success (Sherwood & Jeffery, 2000). Bandura (1977) suggests that cognitive processes play a central role in whether individuals are able to adopt and maintain new patterns of behaviour. Albery & Munafo (2008) state that self-efficacy is central to individuals' behaviour in relation to striving to achieve goals and their response to the illness they are experiencing.

Self-efficacy is based in social learning theory in which it is suggested that individuals' ideas about themselves are developed and learned over time. It involves four processes:

1. Performance of behaviours.
2. Observing others' behaviours (modelling).
3. Feedback on own behaviour from valued sources.
4. Interpretation of the experience of performing the activities.

Through these processes, over time, an individual learns what is appropriate behaviour though their own activities, their internal experience of these, and through feedback from and observation of others. Self-efficacy develops through this process and relates to an individual's beliefs as to whether they are able to perform activities/behaviours in an appropriate way. Individuals evaluate their behaviour against self-imposed standards/expectations. If the individual believes s/he will not be able to perform to the appropriate standard, s/he is likely to avoid the activity. Within rehabilitation, involvement in planned care activities is dependent on the individual's perception of their ability to perform well. For example, if following an amputation an individual believes s/he is capable of learning to walk appropriately with a prosthesis, then s/he is more likely to participate in the rehabilitation process.

Resnick (2002) asserts that self-efficacy has been proved to be a significant factor in the recovery of older adults and recommends the use of scales (such as the Self-Efficacy for Functional Activities Scale; Resnick 2002) to measure patients' confidence in their abilities to do certain things. This then allows nurses to identify what, if any, interventions are needed to strengthen individuals' self-efficacy.

MANAGEMENT OF CHANGE

Altered health status may necessitate lifestyle changes to reduce risk factors associated with particular disorders. Rehabilitation therefore involves developing skills, attitudes and norms in individuals to enable optimum well-being to be realized. For example, someone with hypertension may be asked to stop smoking, lose weight, take up an exercise routine and reduce their level of stress. As Karner et al (2005) identify, such lifestyle change can have a major impact on the likely prognosis and health outcomes for an individual. Such a regimen involves major lifestyle changes, an increased knowledge relating to diet and exercise and the development of alternative coping skills.

To facilitate change the nurse must adopt the role of 'change agent'; someone who creates an environment conducive to change, overcomes resistance to change, understands how to encourage acceptance of the need for change, generates ideas and implements and evaluates the process.

TEAMS AND LEADERSHIP

A rehabilitation programme requires the involvement of a variety of health and social care professionals to help to return the client to their optimum level of functioning. In turn, multidisciplinary involvement requires a coordinated approach to ensure that the needs of the client are addressed. This is best achieved through teamwork.

A team is a group of people working together; it is more than an aggregate of individuals, but rather what Huczynski & Buchanan (2001) describe as a psychological group, where individual members of the team have a sense of collective identity and interact in a significant way. A multidisciplinary team is usually considered to be a formal group, created by an organization to achieve specific goals related to identified tasks. However Huczynski & Buchanan suggest that for a group to become a team there is a need to develop certain positive characteristics such as 'cooperation, coordination and cohesion' (p. 301).

In groups, a hierarchy develops with a leader at the top. In formal groups, such as teams, this leader is either appointed formally or becomes the person with the highest status. Leadership is concerned with guiding, directing and influencing others towards an identified goal or result. In a formally appointed leader, control is based upon power and the leader is able to exert power to influence the group. This is not the same for all leaders, however, and styles of leadership can vary (Table 19.7).

The ability of the leader to influence others in the group relates to the power structure within the group, which may stem from a variety of sources. The way in which communication occurs within a group will thus vary according to the group structure and the style of leadership. With an

Table 19.7 Leadership styles and their characteristics

Autocratic	Defensive, restrictive, fearing, obedience, punishment, reward, threat, constant surveillance
Democratic	Open, accepting, trusting, recognition, satisfaction, self-discipline, challenge
Laissez faire	Permissive, abdicating, indifferent, self-direction, differences, ultraliberal, equality

autocratic leadership communication tends to go in one direction – from the leader to the other members. Conversely, the democratic style encourages multi-directional communication that flows between group members and the leader. Communication within a group with laissez-faire leadership only occurs when the leader is asked to provide information. These different styles of leadership and communication structures become appropriate to use depending upon the particular situation.

CARE DELIVERY KNOWLEDGE

As identified at the beginning of this chapter, rehabilitation is a problem-solving process, being cyclical in nature and therefore requiring the use of a systematic approach, such as the nursing process, to facilitate the assessment, planning, implementation and evaluation of care. Systematic approaches to care such as these are well documented elsewhere, but issues related to assessment and goal setting warrant closer consideration within the rehabilitation setting.

ASSESSMENT IN REHABILITATION

Assessment is often described as the first stage of the nursing process. This suggests that it is a one-off activity that only occurs within the nursing domain. Such an assumption is inappropriate, however, particularly in rehabilitation. Pryor & Smith (2002) propose that assessment within rehabilitation is continuous with nurses gathering and interpreting information at every stage of the process. Central to all assessment is service user and carer involvement.

Nazarko (2001) proclaims assessment is a 'crucial' aspect of rehabilitation. The process of rehabilitation requires an assessment of multiple factors in an effort to ensure an individual's needs and abilities are fully identified. This allows for rehabilitation to be ability-led and therefore reflect the needs of the individual. Wing (1983: 55) suggests that:

the value of assessment is to determine the severity and the chronicity of disablement and its main causes, to discover what talents might be developed, to lay down a plan of

rehabilitation, to allocate the appropriate professional help to the client and relatives, and to monitor progress and update the plan as necessary.

Although Wing was writing some 25 years ago, this assertion still holds true today. It is only through rigorous assessment that an appropriate rehabilitation programme can be developed. Within such a programme reassessment to monitor progress is essential. One-off assessment only tells how an individual functions at a particular time. Ongoing assessment allows identification of changes in the client's status.

Assessment is also essential to provide a baseline from which to identify an individual's level of recovery and rehabilitation success. This should include identification of an individual's capabilities before their current illness to provide a true picture of what is achievable. Frequently the client's family and friends will be involved in the assessment, providing that this does not compromise confidentiality, as this information is helpful to identify the client's previous levels of social, cognitive and practical skills.

Assessment requires the collection of data based on:

- direct observation
- interviews
- assessment tools.

The National Service Framework for Older People (Department of Health 2001a) advocates a multidisciplinary assessment using shared documentation. However, the focus of observations and interviews and the types of assessment tools used are usually determined by the individual's illness or disorder. For example, Harrison (2005) suggests that in cardiac rehabilitation a strong emphasis should be placed on psychological assessment in relation to depression and anxiety. Identification of psychological distress and provision of appropriate interventions are seen as important predictors of long-term outcomes.

Although particular illnesses or disorders may require a specific type of assessment, the basic principles of data collection and assessment skills remain the same.

Reflection and portfolio evidence

Think of a client you have recently been involved in caring for.

- What data would you need to develop a rehabilitation programme?
- Who would be involved in the assessment process?
- How would the data be collected?
- Identify specific assessment tools to aid the process.

The development of a trusting relationship is central to assessment. Without such a relationship with both client and their families/carers, the gathering of relevant information becomes difficult, if not impossible. To facilitate this, good communication skills are essential and those factors that promote and act as barriers to communication must be considered (see further discussion of communication in Ch. 1).

Evidence-based practice

Twelve projects funded by the Department of Health (Farrell 2004) and using a variety of research methods provide evidence on the value of patient and public involvement. The findings of the studies reveal that patient satisfaction increases through involvement in care, with a reduction in anxiety and increased positive health effects. Involving patients in their care as equal partners means that a better nurse–patient relationship is developed and there is also greater satisfaction for nurses. Good communication skills are essential to facilitate involvement. Information giving is an important part of this, so that patients can make informed choices about their care. The right information should be given at the right time in the right way, in the right environment. With a nurse's busy workload, it is not always easy, since time and a private place needs to be found for discussion. Nevertheless, it is vital that patients and/or their carers are helped to feel they are having a say about the care received.

GOAL SETTING

Holliday & Ballinger (2007) propose goal setting as a 'core skill' for those working in rehabilitation. Goals facilitate communication between health professionals, clients and carers. They also have a motivational aspect, giving a sense of direction, and when achieved, increasing self-esteem and feelings of satisfaction.

There are two types of goals: long-term and short-term. The overall goal of a rehabilitation programme may be to restore an individual to a certain level of functioning. This is a long-term goal. Rehabilitation is often a lengthy undertaking and the daily grind of working towards a too distant goal is demoralizing and demodulating. Consequently, to maintain a sense of progress, there is a need to identify smaller goals that are attainable in a shorter space of time. Short-term goals also provide the means of evaluating the rehabilitation programme. This is essential both from the clients' perspective – to enable clients to see their own improvement – and from the formal and informal carers' view to determine whether the care they are giving is appropriate.

Goals set the desired outcomes or objectives that identify the direction of care. Thus, the rehabilitation process can stand or fall on the quality and relevance of the goals that are set. Goal setting is not without its problems and these include determining appropriate target times and levels of achievement. When identifying goals it must be remembered that what is important to the nurse or carer may not be so to the client, therefore mutual goal setting is essential. To this end, it is useful to remember the findings of Lewinter & Mikkelsen (1995). They interviewed individuals who had undergone rehabilitation following a stroke. Generally, the physical retraining aspects of the rehabilitation programmes were evaluated well. However, they found that the care programmes failed to address psychological and social needs, in particular counselling and group support. Individuals were also critical of the lack of sexual counselling (a topic that staff avoided – there is more information on this in Chapter 16, 'Sexuality') and cognitive training. If a goal is viewed by anyone involved in the rehabilitation process as irrelevant, the motivation to achieve the goal will be lacking and difficulties will arise (see Table 19.8 for those behaviours associated with resistance to change), whereas goals that are too complex will act as a disincentive if they are beyond the client's ability. Therefore there is a strong need for discussion, negotiation, and at times compromise, between all involved.

Goals also need to be set in order of priority. Different members of the multidisciplinary team may have conflicting views about what is essential for the rehabilitation of an individual and the priority each goal should take. Additionally, what is a priority to the team may not be so for the client. However, if the priorities of goal setting are not universally agreed between the client, his/her carer

---

Table 19.8 Common resistance to change behaviours (after Vaughan & Pillmoor 1989, by kind permission)

Lip service	Individuals listen to suggestions, agree while change agent is present, but do not undertake proposed action or behaviour in their absence
Aggression	Person displays aggressive behaviour, which results in them not having to face or undertake the change
Destruction	In an attempt to reduce feelings of anxiety individuals may demonstrate destructive behaviour (e.g. a family member may encourage the client not to adhere to a diet when trying to lose weight or to have a cigarette when attempting to give up smoking)
Lack of continuity	Individuals may find excuses not to do certain things – 'I'm too busy today to do my exercises'; the excuses increase until the proposed change

and the team, there may be a resistance to change and the rehabilitation plan may well be undermined. It is essential therefore that all individuals communicate effectively and openly in setting and prioritizing goals.

> **Evidence-based practice**
>
> Bloom et al (2006) found that goal priorities significantly differed between rehabilitation team members and patients with multiple sclerosis. In a study of an inpatient rehabilitation setting, 27 patients and the clinical team, in separate groups, were asked to rate pre-identified goals as to their significance to the rehabilitation process. The patients placed greater emphasis on goals related to areas such as health, mobility and daily activities. They also found that the patients had higher expectations of achievement of their goals than the health professionals.

Goals should express what is to be accomplished rather than describing what is to be done to or by the individual. They should also be phrased in a positive manner, identifying clearly the outcome to be achieved, for example 'Be able to make a cup of tea unaided' rather that an unclear goal such as 'Reduce dependency upon others'. This approach puts the process in a positive framework and clearly states what is expected as opposed to identifying what is not wanted. If this is combined with writing goals in behavioural terms, i.e. stating what is to be observed if the goal is achieved and when it is expected to be achieved by (Table 19.9), then goals become what Dougherty & Lister (2004) identify as appropriate; that they are understood clearly by both patients and health professionals and that they are realistic, achievable and easy to evaluate.

Table 19.9 All behavioural goals must contain the five elements listed here with examples

Behavioural goal	Evelyn is becoming mobile following a hip replacement and will be able to walk for 30 m using a walking frame without sitting down twice daily for 5 days
1. Who will demonstrate behaviour?	Evelyn
2. What will he or she do?	Walk 30 m
3. Under what conditions?	Using her walking frame
4. To what standard?	Without sitting down
5. Expected time or interval by which?	Twice a day for 5 days

> **Evidence-based practice**
>
> It is known that less than 20% of patients maintain programmes for cardiac rehabilitation. Paquet et al (2005) explored the experience of patients with cardiac disease in the 3 month period following hospitalization in an attempt to understand the issues involved in non-maintenance of programmes of care. They found that many patients were reluctant to make lifestyle changes because they felt that it was they who were in the best position to identify their needs. The goals that had been set they viewed as an outside pressure rather than a personal objective. Paquet et al suggest that for rehabilitation programmes to be successful it is therefore essential to take account of the patient's preferences and goals.

THE NURSE AS AN EDUCATOR OR FACILITATOR OF CHANGE

The RCN (2007b) identify education as a key aspect of the nurse's role in rehabilitation, and an integral part of this is teaching about health promotion and self-care. This includes identification of the risk factors associated with certain illnesses or disorders and helping clients to make changes to reduce these by adopting a healthier lifestyle. This aspect of rehabilitation helps to reduce the dependency of an individual on others and encourages the client to take responsibility for his or her own well-being. Individuals must accept such responsibilities if they are to become more than passive consumers of care. However Croghan (2005) identifies that not all people are at the point where they are able to make lifestyle changes and it is important to assess the client's 'readiness' and motivation to change. She suggests the use of Prochaska & DiClemente's (1983) transactional model of behaviour change (see Box 19.1) in assessing readiness. In assessing motivation and readiness for changes in lifestyle the nurse is then able to identify approaches that will help the individual and tailor plans to fit their needs.

> **Box 19.1** Transtheoretical model (Prochaska and DiClemente, 1983)
>
> Pre-contemplation – not considering change
> Contemplation – is aware of need to change
> Action planning – actively planning approaches to making changes
> Implementation – attempts are made to change
> Maintenance – change is achieved and individual tries not to relapse

Evidence-based practice

Ostir et al (2002) investigated the impact of premorbid emotional health on the recovery of functional ability in people who had experienced a stroke, heart attack or hip fractures. They found that those who had depressive symptoms prior to the disabling event were less likely to recover functional ability than those who had positive emotional health. It is suggested that depressive symptoms reduce the individual's motivation to maintain rehabilitation regimes and are related to poor lifestyles – inactivity, poor nutrition, smoking, lack of social interaction, increased feelings of helplessness and hopelessness. To address these it is therefore recommended that recovery programmes should include:

- An understanding of the patient's physical capabilities and the knowledge to maintain a reasonable level of fitness.
- An awareness of the adverse effects of smoking, obesity, poor diet, lack of exercise and stress.
- An appreciation of the benefits of a healthier way of life.
- An ability to identify individual risk factors and take measures to modify them.

Evidence-based practice

Karner et al (2005) considered how individuals respond following myocardial infarction to proposed lifestyle changes such as losing weight or giving up smoking, and what factors might facilitate or constrain people making required changes. Four main factors were found that have an influence on whether on not patients made health related lifestyle changes. These were identified as incentives:

- Somatic – related to how individuals experience body signals that individuals perceived as related to health improvement or illness.
- Social/practical – includes levels of social support, work and environment factors.
- Cognitive – incorporates knowledge, understanding and beliefs of the issues and lifestyles.
- Affective – involves the emotional response to the illness and lifestyle changes, including levels of self-esteem and will power.

PROFESSIONAL AND ETHICAL KNOWLEDGE

IMPACT OF HEALTH AND SOCIAL POLICY ON THE PROVISION OF CARE

The Department of Health has published a number of National Service Frameworks which are long-term strategies for improving specific areas of care. All of the NSFs emphasize the need for health professionals, service users and carers to work together. These documents provide guidance on good practice with the aims of providing good quality care.

The Long-term (Neurological) Conditions NSF was established in March 2005 with the aim of helping people with these conditions achieve independent living and have care planned around their needs and choices. The NSF provides a strategy for health and social services working together with local agencies such as providers of housing, transport, education, employment, transport, benefits and pensions. It is expected that a systematic approach to care will be taken through the implementation of integrated patient pathways.

This builds on the *NHS Plan* (Department of Health 2000), which introduced the idea of 'intermediate care'. It was envisaged that a new form of services would be developed to reduce the pressure placed on acute services by those with sub-acute and longer term/rehabilitation needs.

Intermediate care is also a major tenet of the National Service Framework for Older People (Department of Health 2001b). It is proposed that intermediate care can improve recovery rates and increase patient satisfaction, while at the same time reducing costs incurred through inappropriate admissions to NHS services (such as acute units) and private sector facilities (nursing/residential homes). Units specializing in rehabilitation are viewed as enabling people to regain physical functioning at a faster pace and promoting early discharge enabling people to stay in their own homes for longer. Although much that has been written regarding intermediate care relates to physical disorders, such models may also be of benefit in the mental health setting.

The Department of Health (2001b) identified three issues central to the successful implementation of these services:

- consultation with service users and carers
- mapping of local need
- development of care pathways.

Nurses are seen to play a large role in the development of intermediate care, with a number of nurse-led units being planned.

The success of a rehabilitation programme depends upon the availability of support and resources in the individual's own home. Where resources are limited it is essential that needs are prioritized to ensure that the individual receives the optimum level of care available. However, Nazarko (2001) suggests that intermediate care models are based on the premise that care in the community is in place and able to meet the demands placed on it by the new initiatives. This she proposes, is not so, and may result in rehabilitation services failing to meeting the demands placed on them.

SOCIAL EXCLUSION

Social exclusion is said to affect a wide range of social groups – low income families, those in care, ex-prisoners, ethnic minorities, those with mental health problems, people with disabilities and older people (Social Exclusion Unit 2001). These groups are often at risk of falling into poverty, discriminated against in the job market and prevented from participating in normal social activities due to lack of mobility either as a result of their disability, age or lack of money to enable use of transport. Such discrimination often leads to poor morale, loneliness and depression. The costs of social exclusion to the individual are:

- financial
- poor access to services
- stress
- poor health
- lack of hope.

The Social Exclusion Unit (2001: 51) sees poor health and disability as one of the 'key causes of social exclusion' and proposes a number of initiatives aimed at addressing inequalities in health and supporting those with long term health needs and/or disabilities. These include focusing health services to ensure those in most need receive appropriate care interventions and ensuring that patients are involved in health care decisions relating to such interventions.

WHY INVOLVE SERVICE USERS?

The notion of the 'expert patient' has been promoted by the Department of Health's Expert Patients Programme (Department of Health 2001c) which states that patients with a long-term illness should be given the confidence, skills and knowledge to manage their condition and be more in control of their lives. If patients are 'experts' in their own illness and ways of managing it, and there is evidence that people do find ways of coping with their problems (Faulkner & Layzell 2000), it can be seen that they have a right to expect health professionals to take account of their views. The focus on 'rights' reflects the democratic model discussed above, and was encompassed in Shields's (1985) ideas on the reasons why service users' views should be sought on their care. Shields argued that since in a democracy public services are accountable to citizens, they have a right to participate. Given that nurses are accountable to the public on qualification, it is argued that service users have a right to have their views heard by professionals.

When people go into hospital or receive care in the community, they are likely to feel vulnerable and out of control of the situation in which they find themselves. For this reason Frisby (2001) suggests that there is a moral imperative to involve service users because of the inequalities in power characteristics of the nurse–patient relationship. In addition, service users and carers can be a resource for nurses. By finding out what service users can do for themselves or how they have coped with their difficulties previously, nurses can learn alternative approaches and simultaneously save time that might have been taken up with trying interventions that are not helpful to the patient.

In the modern NHS, satisfaction surveys and the involvement of service users, patients and carers in the development of National Service Frameworks (see Department of Health website www.dh.gov.uk) are accepted on a point of principle. The purpose of involvement under an illness model is to help the professionals and planners to understand more about the needs and experiences of users, in order to enable them to be more effective in their work of devising treatment regimens which are acceptable to service users and patients themselves. However, adoption of an illness model may have the effect of downplaying the effects of environment and social disadvantage (Sayce 2000). An alternative approach is the disability inclusion model.

DISABILITY INCLUSION MODEL

A recent view of people who have endured mental distress, driven by the mental health service user movement, is the 'disability inclusion model' (Sayce 2000: 129) or 'social inclusion and recovery model' (Repper & Perkins 2003). This approach aims to break down the stigma and discrimination of people with a psychiatric diagnosis. The values of social inclusion have been adopted by the review of mental health nursing (Department of Health 2006) and Sayce (2000) has argued that this model neither removes responsibility from users as in an illness model, nor blames them for being mentally ill. The disability inclusion model puts responsibility upon service users to object to discrimination wherever it occurs and is associated with the recovery movement, which encourages users to take stock and set new life paths. Recovery in this sense means recovering a valued sense of self and a life that is meaningful to the individual, rather than necessarily the recovery from symptoms. According to the review of mental health nursing (Department of Health 2006):

> The recovery approach is based around a number of principles that stress the importance of: working in partnership with service users (and/or carers) to identify realistic life goals and enabling them to achieve them; stressing the value of social inclusion . . . stressing the need for professionals to be optimistic about the possibility of positive individual change.
>
> (Department of Health 2006: 17)

The disability inclusion model is about finding ways of leading an individually fulfilling life and encouraging nurses and other health professionals to focus on service users' strengths, while at the same time making allowances for their disabilities, in the same way as you would expect facilities for physically disabled people to be provided. In this sense, recovery does not depend on illness-based services, which can be seen as creating dependence and isolation. Instead: 'Recovery is totally dependent on civil rights and opportunities for inclusion ... [beliefs] based on valuing people who are different and not just those who fit in' (Sayce 2000: 132).

This view is most closely aligned to the 'democratic' model of involvement discussed earlier. Politically, the disability inclusion model is supported by the Disability Discrimination Act (Great Britain) 2005, and organizations that advocate inclusion for people with mental health problems such as the Sainsbury Centre for Mental Health. At the level of service delivery a disability inclusion model reminds nurses that service users have rights and responsibilities and reminds service users that they have the backing of the law to assert these. However, a view that a person experiencing health problems is 'disabled' will not in itself promote involvement. It is clear that the need for an Act of parliament was due to negative public attitudes and discrimination endured by people with physical or mental disabilities. So in addition, it is essential that service users must be perceived as 'experts' in respect of their experiences as health care recipients. Evolve 19.2 has more information on the Act.

19.2 – THE DISABILITY DISCRIMINATION ACT (DDA) 1995

- Know the aims and provisions of the Act.

INTERPROFESSIONAL WORKING

Gibbons et al (2002) identify that the involvement of different professional groups in the rehabilitation process could result in an uncoordinated approach. There are many barriers to interprofessional working – professional jealousies, role boundary confusion, attitudes of one profession towards another and unrealistic expectations of others. If interprofessional working is to be effective there is a need to address such issues. However Xyrichis & Lowton (2008), in a comprehensive review of literature, identified two main issues that affect the effectiveness of interprofessional teams, the team structure and the team process. Within the team structure, the team premises are seen to have an impact of the integration of member in teams – if all members are not based on the same site, some members may be less integrated into the team than others. Smaller teams are identified as working more effectively than large teams. Leadership is seen as an important issue: if good leadership is lacking poor decision making occurs.

In terms of team processes, Xyrichis & Lowton (2008) identify that regular team meetings are central to innovation, effective working and interprofessional communication. The setting of clear goals shared by all members has a significant effect on the effectiveness of the team as these were seen as clearly identifying individuals' and disciplines' roles and responsibilities. Finally, auditing of team processes is seen as essential, providing feedback on team effectiveness and performance.

Most literature relating to the nurse's role within the rehabilitation team suggests that the nurse has a vital part to play in interprofessional working. As mentioned earlier, nurses are seen as the glue which holds the diverse aspects of care together (Jinks & Hope 2000) and their coordination role is a key aspect of care provision in the rehabilitation process (Low 2003). Low also identifies that no other health professional has such close and continuous contact with patients. This contact provides nurses with a unique view of patients' needs and responses to care, while at the same time providing consistency and stability for the patient and their family. The RCN (2007b) suggest the nurse's role in ensuring continuity of care also enables the building of relationships with patient and carers which may facilitate more active involvement in the rehabilitation process.

Long et al (2002) identify six interlinking roles for nurses in the rehabilitation setting:

- assessment – identifying actual and potential problems
- coordination and communication
- technical and physical care
- therapy integration and therapy carry on – ensuring the environment is conducive and treatment regimens maintained
- emotional support
- involving the family.

Long et al (2002) suggest there may be a tension for nurses between their traditional role of 'caring' which is often seen as 'doing for' the patient and 'rehabilitation therapy' which demands a standing back and encouraging independence. However, Pryor & Smith (2002) found that nurses in the rehabilitation setting put teaching and coaxing central to their role and identified seven domains (listed below), which represent the 'how' and the 'what' of specialist practice in this area.

- Rehabilitative approach – facilitating recovery, focusing on abilities rather than disabilities. Requires a range of interpersonal skills to enable development of therapeutic relationships/environment; assessment, setting of appropriate goals; ability to 'see the big picture'.
- Teaching and coaching – every interaction seen as an opportunity to teach/develop patient independence/self-care.

- Observation, assessment and interpretation – activities associated with getting to know the patient and developing an appropriate plan of care.
- Therapeutic interventions – involves both nursing based and collaborative interprofessional working approaches.
- Managing situations – anticipating changing needs and responding to the rapidly changing nature of the patient and family experiences holistically.
- Management, advocacy and coordination – acting as coordinator of care at an individual and ward level.
- Monitoring and quality assurance – ensuring care is evidence based and quality assured.

The RCN (2007b) identify that nurses have eight areas of influence in the rehabilitation setting (see Box 19.2).

It should not be forgotten that there are 6 million people providing unpaid care for family or friends with physical or mental health problems and disabilities (Carers UK 2007). Caring for someone close is not something that people plan for and yet most people will find themselves doing this for a short or long period at some time in their lives. In a survey of almost 3000 carers, asking them to identify their priorities, one in five carers wanted recognition from professionals. This suggests that the involvement of carers in decision-making about services or professional care is essential. It is important to remember that while carers give so much to others, they can also suffer ill health, poverty and discrimination themselves. Caring can be very stressful and when a loved one needs to receive health services the carer might feel guilty about not having been able to cope with the situation themselves or feel that the professional care the person is receiving is not as good as the individual care they have been providing. Such feelings can result in some carers who visit patients in hospital or care homes appearing to be 'demanding'. In such situations it is essential that the nurse shows empathy towards the carer and listens carefully to the concerns in an attempt to work with the carer, rather than dismissing the person as 'awkward'. Just as patients need to be involved in their own care, so carers can be a valuable resource for nurses.

ETHICAL CONSIDERATIONS

Ethics is said to be about the 'rights and wrongs' of a situation, the value judgements and decisions made relating to how people should and should not act. The promoting of individual responsibility for health is central to rehabilitation, but as Caplan (1997) suggests, such an approach may give rise to dilemmas, which grow out of differing political ideologies. On one side the responsibility of individuals for their own health is seen as paramount. Therefore if individuals do not reduce identified risk factors in their lifestyles they are viewed as responsible for their own ill health. The opposing argument suggests that there are extraneous factors that make it difficult for individuals to adopt healthy lifestyles, such as poverty and media pressure. Added to this is the suggestion that although the association between healthy lifestyles and good health outcomes is strong, it is not conclusive. Social factors, for instance, may have a large part to play in health. From this perspective the emphasis on individual responsibility is seen as making a scapegoat of the sick and blaming them for their own misfortune. Such a debate has implications for the allocation of resources.

Box 19.2 Areas of influence for rehabilitation nurses (Royal College of Nursing 2007b)

Essential skills – enabling the nurse to provide care that considers the physical, psychological and emotional needs of individuals in their care

Therapeutic practice – the combination of specialist knowledge and essential skills in such a way as to ensure that the patient receives the care most suited to their individual needs

Coordination – enabling all stakeholders to have a voice in the process, ensuring that the individual aspects of a process are delivered in a coherent and appropriate way, fostering a team approach to care

Empowerment and advocacy – enabling the patient to voice their own views and concerns and be part of decision making process. If the individual is unable to participate, nurses have a role in advocating for, or giving a voice to the patient's needs

Clinical governance – ensuring care is of high quality, delivered in a safe and effective way

Advice/counselling – in relation to both the emotional and practical needs of patients

Political awareness – to influence rehabilitation services, there is a need to be aware of developments and trends at local, national and international levels

Education – for all those involved in the rehabilitation process – patients, carers and other staff

---

Decision–making exercise

- Should people with cardiac problems be admitted to a rehabilitation programme if they continue to smoke?
- Should scarce resources be allocated only to those who show a willingness to adapt their behaviour or does everyone have a right to treatment regardless of their lifestyle?
- Is it possible to deliver a rehabilitation programme when care is based on availability of resources rather than the needs of patients?
- What should be the nurse's response in such circumstances?

Box 19.3 Factors for exploring clinical ethics (Sliwa et al (2002)

1. Patient competency – relates to patient understanding of issues, capacity for decision making and giving of informed consent
2. Patient autonomy – concerns the right of competent patients to be fully informed and involved in treatment decisions
3. Alternative decision makers – relates to patients with impaired capacity, the making of treatment decisions and the standing of advance directives
4. Decision making – relates to interdisciplinary team working, patient involvement and conflict resolution
5. Institutional issues – concerns resource availability and impact on treatment regimens

6. Community ethics – relates to value placed on different types of intervention, e.g. acute care versus rehabilitation and the allocation of resources by central and local government in relation to such values
7. Personal belief system – concerns the effect components such as culture, gender, spirituality may have on individual beliefs of patients, families and health professionals in relation to care/treatment
8. Medical futility – relates to inter-relationship between patient autonomy, resource availability and perceived need to continue treatment where the possibility of improvement is negligible

Associated with the dilemma relating to the allocation of resources is a suggestion that changes in social policy relating to resourcing of services and the prioritizing of need have a profound impact on those requiring rehabilitation programmes. Caplan (1997) talks of the stresses experienced by health carers in the conflict between the identification of those in greatest need when allocating resources and the belief in the right to equal access to care and treatment and provision of resources to all in need.

Within the general sphere of health care the individual's right to choose how his or her care is managed and the possible lack of clarity as to the right or wrong of a situation (for example, whether or not to provide care for someone with heart disease who continues to smoke) may leave the practitioner unsure about how to act and moral dilemmas arise. The same is true in the arena of rehabilitation, particularly in relation to goal setting. There may be times when the goals of the health professional and those of the client are diametrically opposed. Kuczewski & Fiedler (2001) identify the individual's right to self-determination and thus the right to refuse treatment or to participate in rehabilitation programmes. Thus informed consent is central to the process of rehabilitation, all information being made available to the individual allowing them to weigh the pros and cons and make informed decisions.

Sliwa et al (2002) offer eight factors which they suggest provide a framework through which clinical ethics in rehabilitation medicine can be explored and understood (see Box 19.3). Although generated in relation to medical practice in the USA, these have resonance for nursing practice in the UK.

Decision–making exercise

Gordon Hill is a 29-year-old sales representative. Recently, following a road traffic accident, he has become severely disabled. He sees life as worthless and a rehabilitation programme to maximize his abilities and independence as useless. The nurse, believing that disability does not devalue the individual, views the development of skills to promote independence as vital.

- Why do you think that Gordon feels this way?
- Gordon and the nurse have differing views on rehabilitation. What are the consequences of accepting each view?
- How might the nurse acknowledge Gordon's feelings, but also encourage him to take a more positive outlook?
- Devise a plan to reinforce Gordon's self-esteem by using appropriate goals.

PERSONAL AND REFLECTIVE KNOWLEDGE

REHABILITATION IN PROFESSIONAL PRACTICE

Recovery is a complex concept and rehabilitation a complex activity. They require an understanding of the psychological and social impact that illness has on an individual and how these can influence a client's progress to optimum functioning. The nurse must also consider policy issues in relation to the provision of care and address ethical dilemmas. The role of the nurse within the rehabilitation process is therefore multifaceted and requires a dynamic approach. The nurse must draw on wide ranging knowledge to promote the well-being of clients, facilitate multidisciplinary teamwork and deliver individualized care in partnership with service users and carers.

CASE STUDIES IN REHABILITATION

Four case studies now follow, one from each branch of nursing. Use the knowledge you have gained from this chapter to answer the questions set in each.

Case study: Mental health

Kevin is 20 years old and has been diagnosed with schizophrenia. He is an only child, has very few friends and normally lives with his parents. Kevin was attending university, but had to leave because of his illness. He has had a number of admissions to his local acute psychiatric unit, usually when his parents feel they can no longer cope with his 'odd' behaviour. Following his most recent admission he has been referred to the rehabilitation team with a view to placing him in a rehabilitation hostel. It is hoped to eventually enable Kevin to live independently in the community.

- What are the immediate problems that confront Kevin and the rehabilitation team?
- How would you involve Kevin and his parents in the planning of care?
- Consider the examples of motivation theories and suggest how these could be used to motivate Kevin to participate in his rehabilitation programme.
- Select one of the problems you have identified and construct a rehabilitation programme encompassing short-term and long-term goals.

Case study: Adult

Edna is 64 years old and lives with her 72-year-old husband, Sidney. They have three daughters, June aged 44 years, Mary aged 42 years and Joan aged 40 years, all of whom are married and live some distance away. Edna is the main carer for her husband who has dementia. She suffers a severe stroke and is admitted to hospital with a left-sided hemiplegia. Initially she is very reliant on the nursing staff for many of the basic requirements to sustain life. Gradually her condition improves.

- Identify the changes in body image Edna may experience following her stroke.
- What sort of labels may be applied to Edna and what impact could these have on her self-concept?

- What implications may the disability inclusion model have for Edna?
- Identify and prioritize the services that Edna may require to enable her to live in her own home following her recovery.

Case study: Learning disabilities

John is 45 years old, has a moderate learning disability and lives in a staffed group home with three other residents. Before this he lived in the local large institution, which closed 7 years ago. He is a popular member of the home, and takes part in many social activities. John is overweight, having a 'sweet tooth' and taking very little exercise. While attending the social education centre John has a heart attack and is admitted to hospital.

- What personal characteristics may be attributed to John and how might these affect his care?
- How might nurses address labelling and stigma issues related to John?
- What changes might John need to make because of his myocardial infarction?
- John is to undertake a fitness regimen. Identify a possible long-term goal and the sequential short-terms goals to meet such a requirement.

Case study: Child

Susan is 8 years old and is the middle child of three. Her family live in a three-bedroom semi-detached house on the outskirts of the city. Both her parents work: her father Paul is a police officer, her mother Sarah works part time as a nurse. While on her way home from school Susan is knocked down by a car. As she has suffered severe head injuries she is transferred from the local hospital to the nearest neurosurgical ward some 40 miles away.

- What impact might Susan's injuries have on her family members?
- Susan is referred to a rehabilitation team. What data would be needed to develop her rehabilitation programme and how could these be collected?
- Identify a selection of assessment tools that will aid this process.

SUMMARY

The main points covered in this chapter were as follows:

1. Rehabilitation is a process aimed at enabling an individual to gain his or her optimum level of functioning through interprofessional working. Involving service users and carers in the rehabilitation/recovery process is essential.

2. Recovery is an associated concept which is relevant to the individual's lived experience.

3. The nurse's role is multifaceted and requires a breadth and depth of knowledge relating to clients' physical, social and psychological needs and care management and delivery issues.

4. Good communication is essential to effective rehabilitation and recovery.

5. Integral parts of the nurse's role are those of health educator (this includes the identification of risk factors associated with various disorders) and facilitator of change.

6. Rigorous assessment is essential in providing a baseline from which to work, in identifying what is achievable and in monitoring progress.

7. Appropriate goal setting is a prerequisite to the identification of desired outcomes of care, ensuring effective communication, teamwork and the maintenance of client and carer motivation.

8. Social and psychological issues have a profound influence on the individual's experience of illness, provision of services and delivery of care.

See Evolve 19.3 for further resources.

19.3 – REHABILITATION AND RECOVERY: USEFUL WEBSITES

- Essential Internet resources on aspects of rehabilitation and recovery.

Annotated further reading and websites

Allvin R, Berg K, Idvall E, Nilsson U 2007 Postoperative recovery: a concept analysis. Journal of Advanced Nursing 57(5): 552–558

This paper presents a theoretical definition of postoperative recovery, using Walker & Avant's (2005) concept analysis approach.

Brennan J 1994 A vital component of care: the nurse's role in recognizing altered body image. Professional Nurse February:298

This paper offers the reader insight into the nurse's role in caring for clients with altered body image.

Long A, Kneafsey R, Ryan J et al 2002 The role of the nurse within the multiprofessional rehabilitation team. Journal of Advanced Nursing 37(1):70–78

This article describes a qualitative investigation into the role of the nurse in the rehabilitation setting.

Vahakangas, P, Noro, A. and Bjorkgren, M. 2006. Provision of rehabilitation nursing in long-term care facilities. Journal of Advanced Nursing. 55(1):29–35

A quantitative research study into rehabilitation nursing in Finland is reported. The authors conclude that the provision of rehabilitation nursing is determined by patient characteristics and nurses' views of rehabilitation potential.

Worden J W 1991 Grief counselling and grief therapy, 2nd edn. Routledge, London

Every change involves a loss and many people grieve or mourn, because of change. This is an area where people may be helped through the process of change. Worden identifies four tasks of mourning that must be completed for successful resolution. Although this was written with the bereaved in mind the principles may be applied to most loss.

By identifying that a person may be grieving we may assist them through the grieving process and consequently facilitate their successful adaptation to change.

References

Albery IP, Munafo M 2008 Key concepts in health psychology. Sage, London

Allvin R, Berg K, Idvall E, Nilsson U 2007 Postoperative recovery, a concept analysis. Journal of Advanced Nursing 57(5):552–558

Anthony P, Crawford P 2000 Service user involvement in care planning: the mental health nurses perspective. Journal of Psychiatric and Mental Health Nursing 7:425–434

Bandura A 1977 Self-efficacy: towards a unifying theory of behavioural change. Psychology Review 84(2):191–215

Barnes M, Carpenter J, Bailey D 2000 Partnerships with service users in interprofessional education for community mental health: a case study. Journal of Interprofessional Care 14(2):189–200

Beresford P, Croft S 1993 Citizen involvement: a practical guide for change. Macmillan, London

Blanche-Spelich M, Oluwole O, Ferrrio L 2004 The journey back to life. Chart, Journal of Illinois Nursing 101(2):15

Bloom L, Lapierre NM, Wilson KG, Curran D, Deforge DA, Blackmer J 2006 Concordance in goal setting between patients with multiple sclerosis and their rehabilitation team. American Journal of Physical Medicine and Rehabilitation 85(10):807–813

Brennan J 1994 A vital component of care: the nurse's role in recognizing altered body image. Professional Nurse 9(5):298

Caplan A 1997 The ethics of gatekeeping in rehabilitation medicine. Journal of Head Trauma Rehabilitation 12(1):29–36

Carers UK 2007 Our health, our care, our say for our caring future. Available online: www.carersuk.org (accessed 27 March 2007)

Costello J 1995 Helping relatives cope with the grieving process. Professional Nurse 11(2):89–92

Croghan E 2005 Assessing motivation and readiness to alter lifestyle behaviour. Nursing Standard 19(13):50–52

Deegan P 1988 Recovery: the lived experience of rehabilitation. Psychosocial Rehabilitation Journal 11:11–19

Department of Health and Social Security 1979 Patients first: consultative paper on the structure and management of the National Health Service in England and Wales. HMSO London

Department of Health 1989 Working for patients. HMSO, London

Department of Health 1990 NHS and Community Care Act. HMSO, London

Department of Health 1991a The health of the nation. HMSO, London

Department of Health 1991b The patient's charter. HMSO, London

Department of Health 1992 Local voices: the views of local people in purchasing for health. NHS Management Executive, London

Department of Health 1997 The new NHS: modern, dependable. HMSO, London

Department of Health 2000 The NHS plan. HMSO, London

Department of Health 2001a National service framework for older people. HMSO, London

Department of Health 2001b Intermediate care: HSC2001/01/LAC(2001) 1. HMSO, London

Department of Health 2001c The expert patient: a new approach to chronic disease management for the 21st century. HMSO, London

Department of Health 2005 National service framework for long-term (neurological) conditions. HMSO, London

Department of Health 2006 From values to action: the chief nursing officer's review of mental health nursing. Stationery Office, London

Dougherty L, Lister SE (eds) 2004 The Royal Marsden Hospital manual of clinical nursing procedures, 6th edn. Blackwell, Oxford

Dunne K 2005 Grief and its manifestations. Nursing Standard 18(45):45–53

Farrell C 2004 Patient and public involvement in health: the evidence of policy implementation. Department of Health, London

Faulkner A, Layzell S 2000 Strategies for living: a report of user-led research into people's strategies for living with mental distress. Mental Health Foundation, London

Finlay L 2005 Difficult encounters. Nursing Management 12(1):31–35

Frisby R 2001 User involvement in mental health branch education: client review presentations. Nurse Education Today 21:663–669

Gibbons B, Watkins C, Barer D et al 2002 Can staff attitudes to team working in stroke care be improved? Journal of Advanced Nursing 40(1):105–111

Gibson CH 1991 A concept analysis of empowerment. Journal of Advanced Nursing 16:354–361

Goffman E 1963 Stigma: notes on the management of a spoiled identity. Prentice-Hall, Englewood Cliff

Great Britain 2001 Health and Social Care Act 2001, Chapter 15. Available online: http://www.opsi.gov.uk/Acts/acts2001/ukpga_20010015_en_1 (accessed 22 August 2008)

Great Britain 2005 Disability Discrimination Act 2005, Chapter 50. Available online: http://www.opsi.gov.uk/acts/acts1995/1995050.htm (accessed 22 August 2008)

Gross R 2005 Psychology: the science of mind and behaviour, 5th edn. Hodder Arnold, London

Harrison R 2005 Psychological assessment during cardiac rehabilitation. Nursing Standard 19(27):33–36

Holliday RC, Ballinger C 2007 Goal setting in neurological rehabilitation: patients' perspectives. Disability and Rehabilitation 29(5):389–394

Hope R 2004 The ten essential shared capabilities: a framework for the whole of the mental health workforce. Department of Health, London

Huczynski A, Buchanan D 2001 Organizational behaviour: an introductory text, 4th edn. Prentice-Hall, London

Jinks A, Hope P 2000 What do nurses do? An observational survey of the activities of nurses on acute surgical and rehabilitation wards. Journal of Nursing Management 8:273–279

Karner A, Tingstorm P, Abrandt-Dahlgren M, Bergdahl B 2005 Incentives for lifestyle changes in patients with coronary heart disease. Journal of Advanced Nursing 51(3):261–275

Kubler Ross E 1975 Death: the final stage of growth. Prentice-Hall, London

Kuczewski M, Fiedler I 2001 Ethical issues in rehabilitation: conceptualizing the next generation of challenges. American Journal of Physical Medicine and Rehabilitation 80(11):848–851

Kvigne K, Kirkevoid M, Gjengedal E 2005 The nature of nursing care and rehabilitation of female stroke survivors: the perspective of hospital nurses. Journal of Clinical Nursing 14(7):897–905

Lemert E 1951 Social pathology. McGraw Hill, New York

Lewinter M, Mikkelsen S 1995 Patients' experience of rehabilitation after stroke. Disability and Rehabilitation 17(1):3–9

Lohne V, Severinsson E 2005 Patients' experiences of hope and suffering during the first year following acute spinal injury. Journal of Clinical Nursing 14(3):285–293

Long A, Kneafsey R, Ryan J 2002 The role of the nurse within the multiprofessional rehabilitation team. Journal of Advanced Nursing 37(1):70–78

Low G 2003 Developing the nurse's role in rehabilitation. Nursing Standard 17(45):33–38

McGrath J 2004 Beyond restoration to transformation: positive outcomes in the rehabilitation of acquired brain injury. Clinical Rehabilitation 18:767–775

Masterson M, Owen S 2006 Mental health service users' social and individual empowerment: using theories of power to elucidate far-reaching strategies. Journal of Mental Health 15(1):19–34

National Health Service and Community Care Act 1990 HMSO, London

Nazarko L 2001 Rehabilitation. Part 1: The evidence base for practice. Nursing Management 8(8):14–18

Newell R 2002 The fear-avoidance model: helping patients cope with disfigurement. Nursing Times 98(16):38–39

Ostir G, Goodwin JS, Markides K 2002 Differential effects of premorbid physical and emotional health on recovery from acute events. Journal of the American Geriatrics Society 50(4):713–718

Paquet M, Bolduc N, Xhignesse M, Vanasse A 2005 Re-engineering cardiac rehabilitation programmes: considering the patient's point of view. Journal of Advanced Nursing 51(6):567–576

Parsons T 1951 The social system. Routledge & Kegan Paul, London

Price B 1990 Body image: nursing concepts and care. Prentice-Hall, London

Prochaska JO, DiClemente CC 1983 Stages and processes of self-change of smoking: towards an integrative model of change. Journal of Consulting and Clinical Psychology 51:390–395

Pryor J, Smith C 2002 A framework for the role of registered nurses in the specialty practice of rehabilitation in Australia. Journal of Advanced Nursing 39(3):249–257

Resnick B 2002 The impact of self-efficacy and outcome expectation on the functional status in older adults. Topics for Geriatric Rehabilitation 17(4):1–10

Repper J, Perkins R 2003 Social inclusion and recovery: a model for mental health practice. Baillière Tindall, London

Royal College of Nursing 2007a Maximising independence: the role of the nurse in supporting the rehabilitation of older people. Royal College of Nursing, London

Royal College of Nursing 2007b Role of the rehabilitation nurse: RCN guidance. Royal College of Nursing, London

Ryles SM. 1999 A concept analysis of empowerment: its relationship to mental health nursing. Journal of Advanced Nursing 29(3):600–607

Sayce L 2000 From psychiatric patient to citizen: overcoming discrimination and social exclusion. Palgrave, Basingstoke

Scott C 2001 Nursing in the public sphere: health policy research in a changing world. Journal of Advanced Nursing 33(3):387–395

Shields P 1985 The consumer's view of psychiatry. Hospital and Health Services Review 81(3):117–119

Sherwood NE, Jeffery RW 2000 The behavioural determinants of exercise: implications for physical activity. Annual Review of Nutrition 20:21–44

Sliwa JA, McPeak L, Gitter M, Bodenheimer C, King J, Bowen J 2002 Clinical ethics in rehabilitation medicine: core objectives and algorithm for resident education. American Journal of Physical Medicine and Rehabilitation 81(9):708–717

Social Exclusion Unit 2001 Preventing social exclusion. Social Exclusion Unit, London

Vähäkangas P, Noro A, Björkgren M 2006. Provision of rehabilitation nursing in long-term care facilities. Journal of Advanced Nursing 55(1):29–35

Vaughan B, Pillmoor M 1989 Managing nursing work. Scutari, London

Wade DT 2005 Describing rehabilitation interventions. Clinical Rehabilitation 19:811–818

Walker LO, Avant KC 2005 Strategies for theory construction in nursing, 4th edn. Pearson Prentice Hall, Upper Saddle River

Walker J, Payne S, Smitth P, Jarrett N 2006 Psychology for nurses and the caring professions, 2nd edn. Open University Press, England

White A, Johnson, M 2005 Men making sense of their chestpain: niggles, doubts, denial. Journal of Clinical Nursing 9(4):534–541

Williams S 1987 Goffman, interactionism, and the management of stigma in everyday life. In: Scambler G (ed) Sociology theory and medical sociology. Tavistock, London

Wing J 1983 Schizophrenia. In: Watts FN, Bennet DH (eds) Theory and practice of psychiatric rehabilitation. John Wiley, Chichester, pp 45–67

Xyrichis A, Lowton K 2008 What fosters or prevents interprofessional teamworking in the primary and community care? A literature review. International Journal of Nursing Studies 45(1):140–153

Glossary

Ablution The act of washing or cleansing, especially the washing of hands.

Abrasion A superficial wound in the skin, where damage has been caused by some kind of scraping.

'Adverse event' In health care, any act or omission that leads to unintended or unexpected harm, loss or damage. Compare **Near miss**.

Advocacy Active support or representation. Advocacy is the expression of support for or opposition to a cause, argument or proposal. Advocacy may include influencing laws, legislation or attitudes. A nurse may act as the client's advocate, representing their interests and interpreting wishes to others involved in their care.

Aetiology The cause(s) or origin(s) of a disease. (Note that the US spelling is etiology.)

Ageism Prejudice and discrimination against elderly people solely on the grounds of their age.

Aggression A hostile or destructive attitude to other persons or objects, and which can include verbal attacks or physical violence.

Allograft A graft of tissue between individuals of the same species; in the medical context, between two humans. The tissue donor might be a cadaver or a living person, related or unrelated. Compare **Autograft, Xenograft**.

Amino acid An organic compound containing an amino ($-NH_2$) and a carboxyl ($-COOH$) group. Amino acids are combined into proteins and are thus an important element of the diet. See also **Essential amino acid**.

Analgesia The relief of pain without loss of consciousness.

Androgen Any of several steroid hormones produced in the testes (or synthetically), and promoting male secondary sexual characteristics.

Angiogenesis The development of blood vessels. This can be in the embryo and foetus during development, or during the growth of a tumour. It also occurs during a stage of wound healing.

Antibiotic A chemical substance produced by a microorganism or made synthetically that inhibits or destroys other microorganisms.

Antidepressant Any drug that stimulates the mood of a depressed patient, e.g. amitriptyline or fluoxetine.

Antipsychotic A drug used to treat psychotic disorders such as schizophrenia.

Anxiolytic Any drug that reduces anxiety; the most usual ones are in the benzodiazepine group, e.g. diazepam.

Arousal The state of responsiveness to sensory stimuli.

Asepsis The absence of microorganisms.

Assertiveness Confidently but sensitively claiming one's position or stating one's point of view.

Autograft A graft of tissue between one part of a patient's body to another. Compare **Allograft, Xenograft**.

Biofeedback A technique for controlling one's own body state, e.g. anxiety, by the aid of electronic devices that monitor and report functions, increasing self-awareness of the body's response to stress, such as pulse rate, respiration rate or blood pressure.

Burnout A condition that occurs following prolonged exposure to high levels of stress, characterized by emotional numbing and changes to personality that result in the individual becoming isolated and acquiring an overwhelmingly cynical attitude that belittles the achievement of self and others.

Carbohydrate Any of a large group of organic compounds having the general formula $C_m(H_2O)_n$. It includes the sugars (e.g. glucose) and polysaccharides (e.g. starch), which are important energy producing foods.

Catheter A tube that is inserted into the body to introduce or remove fluid.

Charting The technique of recording at regular time intervals aspects of a patient's state, e.g. fluid intake/urinary output.

Chemoreceptor A sensory receptor in a cell membrane which receives molecules from the external environment and gives rise to the sensation of smell or taste.

Chemotherapy The treatment of a disease with a chemical substance.

Circadian rhythm The pattern of biological processes that occur regularly at 25-hour intervals. These patterns persist even in the absence of environmental cues, e.g. in crews of spacecraft.

Circumcision Male – removal of foreskin; female – removal of clitoris (and sometimes also the labia majora and labia minora).

Clinical audit Examination or measurement of clinical practice quality standards and associated outcomes.

Clinical governance An initiative of the UK Department of Health begun in 1997 and defined by them as 'a system through which NHS organizations are accountable for continuously improving the quality of their services and safeguarding high standards of care by creating an environment in which excellence will flourish'.

Commensal Two different species of organisms that live together without one of them being dependent on the other or one being parasitic on the other.

Complementary medicines Treatments taken by patients that are not prescribed through conventional medical sources, but may complement such treatments; they are not alternative, as they do not replace medical treatments.

Compliance The act of obeying. In health care, compliance refers to the patient's/client's conduct in carrying out the agreed treatment or regimen, e.g. by taking the medications prescribed or by adhering to diet.

Compression Depression of the chest by a rescuer to 'squeeze' the heart between the sternum and spine as a means of emptying the heart of blood to pump the blood around the circulation.

Confidentiality The understanding that no information relating to a patient, such as personal or clinical details, may be divulged to unauthorized individuals or data sites without their consent.

Confusion Disturbance of a person's orientation as to place or time or their own personhood.

Consciousness The state of being aware of oneself, one's environment and one's physical and mental condition. Immediate knowledge or perception of the presence of any object, state or sensation.

Consent Agreement with a client/patient for a procedure to be undertaken or withheld. For the consent to be valid it is important that the client/patient has been fully informed of all relevant factors, is not under some form of coercion and is mentally fit to grant consent. In the UK the age at which a client/patient may give consent is 16.

Coroner In England and Wales, the public official responsible for the investigation of unexplained deaths, be they sudden, violent or otherwise suspicious. The coroner is usually, but need not be, medically qualified.

Counselling Support offered to a person who is trying to overcome a psychosocial problem. Broadly defined, it includes both 'therapy' and 'psychotherapy'. Counselling is a developmental process, in which one individual (the counsellor) provides to another individual or group (the client) guidance and encouragement, challenge and inspiration in creatively managing and resolving practical, personal and relationship issues, in achieving goals, and in self-realization. Counsellors are nowadays usually professionals specializing in particular problem areas, e.g. bereavement.

Cytoplasm The protoplasm of a cell, i.e. everything within the cell membrane except the nucleus. It consists of a fluid (the cytosol) in which are suspended the various cell organelles.

Deciduous Of teeth, the non-permanent of the infant and child, colloquially known as 'milk teeth'.

Decontamination Removal of a contaminant or pollutant.

Defibrillation A method of sending a controlled electrical shock through the chest wall to terminate a chaotic cardiac rhythm, allowing, when possible, the heart's own electrical conduction system to regain control. It does not 'restart' the heart.

Dehydration The condition resulting from excessive loss of body water.

Delirium A transitory state of disturbed consciousness, which can be caused by various factors including fever, brain injury or drug intoxication.

Dementia A clinical state characterized by progressive deterioration or impairment of brain function. Dementia is the mental deterioration (loss of intellectual ability) that is associated with old age. Two major types of senile dementia are identified: those due to generalized atrophy (Alzheimer type) and those due to vascular problems (mainly strokes).

Dependency Over-reliance by a person on some external form of support, most commonly some other person, or something that is psychologically or physically habit-forming (especially alcohol or narcotic drugs).

Deviation Behaviour that does not conform to what is considered acceptable, especially sexual behaviour.

Disinfection A process which reduces the number of microorganisms to a level at which they are no longer harmful.

Diuretic An agent that promotes the excretion of urine.

Dizygotic twins Non-identical twins, resulting from the separate fertilization of two ova by two spermatozoa; in effect brothers/sisters born at the same time. Compare **Monozygotic twins**.

Double voiding A technique which helps to empty the bladder completely. To do this the client voids, stands up and then sits down again to urinate a second time.

Duty of care The legal or moral obligations that a person has to perform actions for another's welfare.

Electrolyte A chemical compound that when in solution dissociates into ions.

Elimination The act of clearing waste from the body, including both urination and defaecation.

Emollient Any substance, especially an ointment, that has a softening effect when applied to the skin.

Emulsion A mixture in which both constituents are liquids.

Endemic The usual level or presence of an agent or disease in a defined population during a given period.

Endorphins Various polypeptides that occur naturally in the brain and can bind to pain receptors (**nociceptors**) thus blocking off the sensation of pain.

Energy The capacity to do work: in the body, it takes two forms, heat and chemical energy. It is measured in joules or calories.

Epidemic An unusual higher than expected level of infection or disease in a defined population in a given period.

Ergonomics The science that tries to adapt the task, the equipment and the working environment to suit the worker(s).

Essential amino acid One of the nine amino acids that cannot be synthesized in the human body so must be taken in the diet.

Ethics Moral standards and criteria for conduct. The socially agreed rules and principles that should be applied in decisions about actions towards others. Ethics is the field of study that is concerned with questions of value, that is, judgements about what human behaviour is 'good' or 'bad'.

Ethnicity The sense of belonging to a particular cultural or racial group, with its own customs, practices and beliefs.

Ethology The study of the behaviour of non-human animals in their natural habitats.

Euthanasia The practice of 'mercy killing', i.e. painlessly ending the life of a person with an incurable illness. It is not legal in the UK.

Exudate Matter that oozes from a blood vessel into surrounding tissues, usually as a result of inflammation.

Fat A non-technical term for the component in the diet more properly called lipids. In the diet these are mostly triglycerides, which consist of three fatty acids and a glycerol molecule.

Feedback loop A closed pathway in which the input signal directly controls the output. In positive feedback higher input leads to higher output. In negative feedback increased input results in a reduction of output, which is a common mechanism of **homeostasis**.

Fulcrum Of a lever, the point about which a lever turns.

Goal setting A technique in rehabilitation in which the patient and nurse agree step by step projects within a timeframe, to recover as much as possible of normal function.

Hazard An event or situation that has the potential to cause harm.

Heimlich manoeuvre Action taken by a rescuer when the victim has a partial or complete obstruction of the upper airway. The rescuer stands behind the victim, forming one hand into a fist, covering it with the other hand and applying pressure to the upper abdomen. The action should push upwards against the diaphragm so increasing the pressure in the chest cavity under the obstruction, helping to move it upwards.

Holistic A system of treatment that takes into account the whole person, i.e. their physical, psychological and social aspects.

Homeostasis A tendency to stability in the body's metabolism; the maintenance of a constant internal environment. It is achieved by a system in which the negative **feedback loop** is the basic mechanism.

Homeothermy The maintenance of a constant internal body temperature.

Homophobia Fearing or disliking of homosexual people or homosexuality. There are four basic levels of homophobia: (1) the fear and hatred of gays and lesbians, (2) the fear of being perceived as gay or lesbian, (3) the fear of one's own sexual or physical attraction for same-sex individuals, and (4) the fear of being gay or lesbian.

Hospice A nursing home that specializes in the care of the dying, either full-time as a place for the patient to die or part-time to give respite to the caring family.

Hydrotherapy The application of water in the treatment of disease, especially the use of swimming as therapeutic exercise to strengthen weak joints and wasted muscles.

Hygiene Strictly, the science of health, and its maintenance, but more generally used to mean the practices of bodily cleanliness that promote health.

Hypoallergenic Made of substances known to be unlikely to provoke an allergic reaction.

Immunity The ability of an organism to resist infection by means of circulating antibodies.

Immunocompromised Having impaired immune response that renders the host particularly susceptible to an infection.

Indemnity insurance Insurance that covers a professional person for damages resulting from being sued by a patient, colleague or member of the public.

Infection An invasion of the body by pathogenic microorganisms, or the disease resulting therefrom.

Infestation An invasion of the body by parasites, usually insects. Compare **Infection**.

Inflammation The self-protective reaction of tissue to infection or injury, the signs of which are swelling, redness, heat and pain.

Learning disabilities The arrested or incomplete development of mind or significant impairment to intellectual, adaptive or social functioning. The dimensions of this term are defined by the World Health Organization as: (1) a state of arrested or incomplete development of mind; (2) significant impairment of intellectual functioning; (3) significant impairment of adaptive/social functioning. One of the four branches of nursing concerns the care of clients with learning disabilities.

Lesion Any injury or ailment involving direct damage to tissue or loss of a body part.

Libido The urge towards sexual activity.

Living will A form of advance directive which can be verbal or something more formal, as found in the USA, in which the patient/client expresses what should happen within certain situations, e.g. refusal of resuscitation or life-prolonging treatment in the case of serious incapacity. The validity of a living will is recognized under UK common law.

Malnutrition Any disorder of nutrition. Although used most commonly referring to an insufficient quantity of nutrition, it can also mean oversupply of nutrition, or dietary imbalance.

Marginalization The act of relegating a person or group to the fringes of society, owing to some perceived short-coming, e.g. disability or age.

Menopause The ending of menstruation in a woman's life cycle, either naturally at the age of about 50, or as the result of surgical intervention (e.g. hysterectomy).

Menstruation The cyclic discharge of blood through the vagina in a non-pregnant woman of childbearing age.

Metabolism The chemical processes that drive the machinery of the body, giving rise to growth, movement and elimination of waste.

Microorganism Any organism of microscopic size, e.g. a virus, bacterium or protozoon. It may or may not be a **pathogen**, i.e. capable of causing a disease.

Mobilism Prejudice and discrimination against people with impaired mobility.

Monozygotic twins Identical twins, resulting from the fertilization of a single ovum by a single spermatozoon, with subsequent division of the early zygote into two independent embryos. Compare **Dizygotic twins**.

'Near miss' In health care any act or omission that could have led to unintended or unexpected harm, loss or damage but did not actually do so. (If it had done so it would have been an **adverse event**.)

Necrosis Death of a group of cells or part of a structure or organ, often resulting from failure of blood supply.

Negligence A civil wrong in which the defendant has breached a duty of care which has caused some injury, loss or damage to the claimant of a type that the law acknowledges.

Neurotransmitter A chemical by means of which a neurone passes on a message to another neurone or a muscle.

Nociceptor A receptor for pain. The stimulus may be either physical (e.g. heat, a blow or electric shock) or chemical (presence of a toxin).

Nomogram Graphical representation of relationship between two or more variables.

Non-verbal communication Communication by means other than speech, i.e. facial expressions, gestures, posture, non-word sounds, or non-verbal aspects of speech such as tone of voice, accent, pace of speaking. It may be both intentional and unintentional.

Norm An established standard of behaviour applicable to and upheld by a social group.

Nosocomial An infection that is acquired or occurring in hospital.

Oedema Swelling caused by accumulation of fluid in the inter-cellular spaces of tissue. (Note that US spelling is edema.)

Off-label The unlicensed use of a medication with a client group who are not included in the licensing criteria, or (off-licence) are given in a manner not included in the licensing criteria, e.g. an alternative route is used.

Oscillation A regular fluctuation above or below a mean value.

Palliation Any system of care that aims to provide relief from pain rather than cure.

Pathogen A microorganism that is capable of causing a disease.

Pathway In metabolism, a series of reactions that converts one biological substance to another.

Phagocytosis The process by which a white blood cell ingests objects such as microorganisms or foreign bodies.

Pharmacodynamics A study of the mechanism of a drug in relation to cellular physiology and biochemistry.

Pharmacokinetics A process of drug movement through the body; this includes phases of absorption, distribution, metabolism and excretion where drug action may take place.

Photoageing The process of premature ageing of the skin due to the action of sunlight.

Physiotherapy The use of physical means such as exercise, massage or manipulation in the treatment of musculo-skeletal problems.

Pigmentation Coloration in the skin or other tissue caused by the presence of pigments such as melanin in the cells.

Polypharmacy The practice of treatment with more than one prescribed medicine simultaneously.

Postmortem The examination (including dissection and possibly also tissue culture) of a dead body to ascertain the cause of an otherwise unexplained death.

Prognosis The prediction of the likely outcome of a disease, injury or inborn disorder.

Protein A chain of amino acids joined by peptide bonds and folded into a three-dimensional shape typical for each protein. Proteins are found in all cells of the body; some form the basic components of tissue, some function as enzymes, hormones or antibodies.

Psychoanalysis A method, pioneered by Sigmund Freud, of treating patients with psychological disorders based on investigating and bringing to light the unconscious and repressed processes of the mind.

Puberty The phase of maturation at which the sex glands become functional and the secondary sexual characteristics develop. In boys, spermatogenesis begins and the voice 'breaks'; in girls, menstruation commences.

Queen's Square stimulator A hand-held vibrating device which if put on the abdomen over the bladder may trigger a bladder contraction and initiate voiding.

Recumbency The state of being unable to maintain any body posture other than lying down.

Rehydration The restoration of normal body fluid content. This may be done orally, by feeding tube or intravenously.

Respiration Breathing, i.e. the process of exchange of air between the lungs and the external environment; it includes inspiration (breathing in) and expiration (breathing out). Breathing is known as external respiration, while internal respiration refers to the exchange of oxygen and carbon dioxide at cellular level.

Resuscitation Action taken to restore breathing and normal heart rhythm in a person in whom these have ceased.

Risk The possibility that a **hazard** will cause harm.

Risk assessment The science of assessing (1) the probability of a harmful outcome in any situation, and (2) the extent of the harm resulting.

Risk management The control of hazards in any situation so as to minimize the possibility of a harmful outcome and limit its extent.

Sociobiology The study of social behaviour in animals and humans, especially with a view to interpreting the evolutionary advantage of particular behaviours.

Stereotype A way of judging a person by simplistic (usually derogatory) generalizations about the group of which they are, or are supposed to be, a member.

Sterilization A process that completely removes or destroys all microorganisms.

Stigmatization The act or practice of marking out a person or group as being inferior due to some perceived failing, either mental, physical or social.

Stressor Any stimulus to which an individual responds either physically or psychologically.

Surveillance The systematic collection, collation, interpretation and dissemination of information essential to identifying outbreaks and trends of infectious disease.

Suture Anything used to secure the edges of a wound together to promote healing. Formerly always done with silk thread; now metal clips are often used, or absorbable threads that are dissolved by enzymes and do not need removal.

Telemedicine The use of medical information exchanged by electronic means.

Thermogenesis The production of heat by body processes. Shivering, producing heat by activity in the muscles, is a form of thermogenesis.

Thermoregulation The control of body heat. Warm-blooded animals (including humans) maintain a constant internal body heat despite fluctuations of external environmental temperature.

Trauma In psychology, an event causing a powerful shock that has long-lasting effects on the personality. In pathology, any injury or wound.

Ulceration The formation of an ulcer, i.e. a hole in the surface of a tissue or an organ due to **necrosis**.

Ultrasound Sound waves above the audible range (above 20 kHz) used for viewing internal structures of the body, or the fetus *in utero*.

Unlicensed Drugs that have no product licence and no data sheet/product specification.

Urinalysis Chemical analysis of the urine to test for signs of disease or malfunction.

Vaccination The process of inducing immunity by the giving of a vaccine which is an inactivated microbial toxin or microbial antigen.

Ventilation Movement of air in and out of the lungs either by the individual (self-ventilating) or by another person, e.g. a first-aider (mouth to mouth), or by artificial means using a machine.

Vitamin A general term for a number of unrelated organic substances that are essential in small quantities for the normal functioning of the body. Some can be synthesized in the human body, but others must be taken in the diet. Vitamins may be either water-soluble or fat-soluble.

Vocabulary The stock of words that a person has at their disposal; also the system of techniques or symbols serving as a means of expression. The number of words understood is always greater than the number that a person will themselves use in speech or writing.

Xenograft A graft of tissue between different species. Compare **Allograft**, **Autograft**.

Zeitgeber A stimulus that affects an organism's biological clock, e.g. a change in the level of light.

Zero tolerance The policy of applying penalties to even minor offences in order to enforce the overall principles of a code of behaviour.

Index